Emergency Radiology

Emergency Radiology

....

HELEN C. REDMAN, M.D.
Professor of Radiology
Department of Radiology
University of Texas
Health Sciences Center
Dallas, Texas

PHILLIP D. PURDY, M.D.
Director of Neuroradiology
Division of Neuroradiology
Department of Radiology
University of Texas
Health Sciences Center
Dallas, Texas

GEORGE L. MILLER, M.D.
Department of Radiology
University of Texas
Health Sciences Center
Dallas, Texas

NANCY K. ROLLINS, M.D.
Medical Director of Radiology
Department of Radiology
Dallas Children's Hospital
Dallas, Texas

W. B. SAUNDERS COMPANY
Harcourt Brace Jovanovich, Inc.
Philadelphia   London   Toronto   Montreal   Sydney   Tokyo

W. B. SAUNDERS COMPANY
Harcourt Brace Jovanovich, Inc.

The Curtis Center
Independence Square West
Philadelphia, Pennsylvania 19106

Library of Congress Cataloging-in-Publication Data

Emergency radiology/Helen C. Redman . . . [et al.].

    p. cm.

ISBN 0–7216–7491–7

1. Diagnosis, Radiologic.   2. Radiology, Medical.
   3. Medical emergencies.   I. Redman, Helen C.
   [DNLM: 1. Emergencies. 2. Radiography. WN 200 E531]

RC78.E58 1993

616.07′57—dc20

DNLM/DLC   92–7578

EMERGENCY RADIOLOGY   ISBN 0–7216–7491–7

Printed in the United States of America

Last digit is the print number: 9   8   7   6   5   4   3   2   1

CONTRIBUTORS

C. WILLIAM DEATON, JR., M.D.
Staff, Radiology Associates, P.A.;
Staff, St. Vincent Infirmary
Medical Center, Little Rock,
Arkansas
The Calvarium and the Extra-axial Spaces

STEVEN A. DUNNAGAN, M.D.
Staff, San Angelo Radiologists,
P.A.; Staff Radiologist, Shannon
Memorial Hospital, San Angelo,
Texas
Skull Base Trauma

DONALD A. ECKARD, M.D.
Assistant Professor of Diagnostic
Radiology and Chief,
Interventional Neuroradiology
Section, University of Kansas
Medical Center, Kansas City,
Kansas
Traumatic Brain Injury

GEORGIANA GIBSON, M.D.
Clinical Assistant Professor of
Radiology, University of Texas
Southwestern Medical Center at
Dallas, Dallas, Texas; Staff
Radiologist, HCA Plano Medical
Center, Plano, Texas
The Thoracic and the Lumbar Spine, and the Spinal Cord

**MARK S. GIRSON, M.B.B.CH.
(RAND)**
Clinical Assistant Professor of
Radiology, University of Texas
Southwestern Medical Center at
Dallas, Dallas, Texas; Staff
Neuroradiologist, Irving
Radiological Associates, P.A.,
Irving, Texas
Orbits and Eyes

MARGARET E. HANSEN, M.D.
Assistant Professor of Radiology,
University of Texas
Southwestern Medical Center at
Dallas; Staff, Parkland Memorial
Hospital, Zale Lipshy University
Hospital, and Department of
Veterans Affairs Medical Center,
Dallas, Texas
Emergency Evaluation of Vascular Injuries

LINDA O'CONNELL JUDGE, M.D.
Clinical Assistant Professor of
Radiology, University of Texas
Southwestern Medical Center at
Dallas; Staff Radiologist, Midway
Park Medical Center, Lancaster,
Texas
Soft Tissues of the Neck; The Esophagus

W. B. LOWRY, M.D., M.A.C.R.
Staff, Radiology Associates of
Tarrant County, P.A., Fort
Worth, Texas; Staff Radiologist,
Arlington Memorial Hospital,
Arlington, Texas; Staff, Cook–
Fort Worth Children's Medical
Center, St. Joseph Hospital,
Harris Methodist Fort Worth
Hospital, Harris Methodist
Southwest Hospital, HCA North
Hills Medical Center, and HCA
Medical Plaza Hospital, Fort
Worth, Texas
Facial Trauma

DIANNE B. MENDELSOHN, M.D.
Associate Professor of Radiology,
University of Texas
Southwestern Medical Center at

Dallas; Director of
Neuroimaging, Mary Nell and
Ralph Rogers Magnetic
Resonance Center, Dallas, Texas
*The Thoracic and the Lumbar Spine,
and the Spinal Cord*

GEORGE L. MILLER, M.D.
Assistant Professor of Radiology,
University of Texas
Southwestern Medical Center at
Dallas; Attending Faculty
Member, Parkland Memorial
Hospital, Zale Lipshy University
Hospital, and Department of
Veterans Affairs Medical Center,
Dallas, Texas
*Cardiac Trauma; Emergency
Evaluation of Vascular Injuries*

ANN R. MOOTZ, M.D.
Assistant Professor of Radiology,
University of Texas
Southwestern Medical Center at
Dallas; Staff, Zale Lipshy
University Hospital and Parkland
Memorial Hospital, Dallas, Texas
*Injuries of the Chest: The Lungs, the
Pleura, the Tracheobronchial Tree,
the Diaphragm, and the Chest Wall*

PHILLIP D. PURDY, M.D.
Associate Professor of Radiology,
Neurosurgery, and Neurology
and Director of Neuroradiology,
University of Texas
Southwestern Medical Center at
Dallas; Director of
Neuroradiology, Parkland
Memorial Hospital, Zale Lipshy
University Hospital, and
Department of Veterans Affairs

Medical Center, Dallas, Texas
*Traumatic Brain Injury; Skull Base
Trauma*

HELEN C. REDMAN, M.D.
Chief of Special Procedures and
Body Imaging and Professor of
Radiology, University of Texas
Southwestern Medical Center at
Dallas; Attending Faculty,
Parkland Memorial Hospital,
Zale Lipshy University Hospital,
and Department of Veterans
Affairs Medical Center, Dallas,
Texas
*The Gastrointestinal System; The
Genitourinary System*

NANCY K. ROLLINS, M.D.
Associate Professor of Radiology,
University of Texas
Southwestern Medical Center at
Dallas; Medical Director,
Department of Radiology,
Children's Medical Center;
Division Head, Pediatric
Radiology, Parkland Memorial
Hospital, Dallas, Texas
Imaging of the Injured Child

RICHARD A. SUSS, M.D.
Clinical Associate Professor of
Radiology, University of Texas
Southwestern Medical Center at
Dallas; Consulting Radiologist,
Parkland Memorial Hospital,
Zale Lipshy University Hospital,
and Children's Medical Center,
Dallas, Texas; Radiologist, North
Texas Health Imaging Center,
Grand Prairie, Texas
*Overview of the Spine; Cervical
Spine*

PREFACE

· ·

The rapid, efficient evaluation of a trauma victim is the most effective way of obtaining the best possible outcome for that patient. Clinical examination of trauma patients is frequently supplemented by both radiologic and laboratory procedures. The emergency department physicians and nurses must know which procedures are most likely to provide the required information as well as what these procedures require of the patient. Similarly, any radiologist who sees injured patients must be familiar with the problems these patients present and know how to most effectively use radiographic procedures to answer clinical questions. This book has been written to provide guidance in making these decisions, primarily in regard to injury to soft tissues. Discussions of the skull, facial bones, and spine are included because fractures of these bones occur in association with soft tissue injury to the brain, eyes, or spinal cord. There are several excellent books on bone radiology that thoroughly discuss the radiology of fractures. Therefore, we have decided to concentrate on the soft tissues.

The book consists of six sections. The first section addresses trauma to the brain and the bones of the head. The second section covers injury to the cervical, thoracic, and lumbar spine and the spinal cord. In the third section, the neck, heart, lungs, and esophagus are discussed. Section Four addresses trauma to the abdomen, including the gastrointestinal tract and genitourinary system. In the fifth section, injury to the blood vessels is covered. The final section addresses problems specific to the pediatric trauma patient.

Most chapters begin with an outline of procedures appropriate to that organ system and an abbreviated description of the nature of each procedure as well as its pros and cons. The chapters then provide a more detailed discussion of the various procedures and their demands on patients and, finally, cover the radiographic findings of injury using various techniques. There is no attempt to cover every minute detail of each radiographic procedure or the myriad subtle variations in the manifestations of injury. Rather, the book is intended to be a practical guide to initial patient evaluation. Experienced trauma surgeons or trauma radiologists may find some of the discussion simplistic, but we hope that they will agree with the overall approach. We believe that physicians who encounter trauma with a lesser frequency will find this volume useful and will consult the references for more in-depth information.

The illustrations are the heart of most radiology textbooks. We have included as many examples of various injuries as seemed useful, emphasizing observations on the most appropriate and commonly used examinations in this country. International readers may be disturbed by the paucity of ultrasound illustrations and their discussion. As is mentioned repeatedly throughout the book, ultrasound is rarely used in the United States during the initial evaluation of trauma because computed tomography is quite readily available, whereas skilled ultrasonographers are not as plentiful. Ultrasound is a very useful modality in the evaluation of injury to liver, spleen, and kidneys and has other applications in acute injury, and we are not implying otherwise by our limited discussion of the subject.

Most of the chapters are not extensively annotated so as to make reading more comfortable. However, bibliographies are provided at the end of each chapter to provide supplemental reading for those who desire it.

The approach to trauma presented in this book is derived in large part from our extensive experience at Parkland Memorial Hospital in Dallas, Texas. The authors of all of the chapters have worked at Parkland at some point in their careers. Although the experience at other major trauma centers may be different from ours, we believe we have presented a logical, straightforward approach to the radiology of trauma that we hope will be useful to our readers.

HELEN C. REDMAN, M.D.
GEORGE L. MILLER, M.D.
PHILLIP D. PURDY, M.D.
NANCY K. ROLLINS, M.D.

ACKNOWLEDGMENTS

The completion of a manuscript requires assistance from a number of individuals. In the case of a book, virtually the entire department of radiology is affected. We wish to thank all those who located radiographs of specific injuries, provided secretarial, editorial, and photographic skills, and were generally supportive of the project. In particular, Dianna Otterstad and Leslie Mihal were invaluable for their editorial assistance in the typing of draft after draft of these chapters. Irene Delgado kept track of galley and page proofs. Alison Russell, with some assistance from Jerry Cheek, willingly and efficiently photographed the numerous illustrations for the chapters. Drs. Jack Reynolds and Thomas S. Curry III provided important case material, and many other faculty members and residents found good examples of specific injuries for us. Dr. Robert Parkey provided departmental backing for this multiyear undertaking.

Most important, I want to thank my three coeditors for their efforts and, in particular, mention the individual chapter authors who responded with excellent chapters while fulfilling their clinical assignments. These include Drs. William Deaton, Donald Eckard, Bruce Lowry, Mark Girson, Dianne Mendelsohn, Georgiana Gibson, Linda Judge, Margaret Hansen, Richard Suss, Ann Mootz, and Steven Dunnagan, without whom this book would never have been completed.

Finally, this book would not have been undertaken if all the authors had not trained or worked at Parkland Memorial Hospital. The experience in trauma and radiology of trauma gained at Parkland is invaluable and provides the backbone of this book.

HELEN C. REDMAN, M.D.

CONTENTS

SECTION ONE
Head and Brain

CHAPTER 1
Traumatic Brain Injury 3
PHILLIP D. PURDY, M.D. • DONALD A. ECKARD, M.D.

CHAPTER 2
The Calvarium and the Extra-axial Spaces 41
C. WILLIAM DEATON, JR., M.D.

CHAPTER 3
Skull Base Trauma 77
STEVEN A. DUNNAGAN, M.D.

CHAPTER 4
Facial Trauma 95
W. B. LOWRY, M.D.

CHAPTER 5
Orbits and Eyes 123
MARK S. GIRSON, M.D.

SECTION TWO
Spine

OVERVIEW OF THE SPINE
RICHARD A. SUSS, M.D.

CHAPTER 6
Cervical Spine 179
RICHARD A. SUSS, M.D.

CHAPTER 7
The Thoracic and the Lumbar Spine, and the Spinal Cord 265
DIANNE B. MENDELSOHN, M.D. • GEORGIANA GIBSON, M.D.

SECTION THREE
Neck and Thorax

CHAPTER 8
Soft Tissues of the Neck 285
LINDA O'CONNELL JUDGE, M.D.

CHAPTER 9
*Injuries of the Chest: The Lungs, the Pleura, the Tracheobronchial
Tree, the Diaphragm, and the Chest Wall* 315
ANN R. MOOTZ, M.D.

CHAPTER 10
The Esophagus 355
LINDA O'CONNELL JUDGE, M.D.

CHAPTER 11
Cardiac Trauma 371
GEORGE L. MILLER, M.D.

SECTION FOUR
Abdomen

CHAPTER 12
The Gastrointestinal System 377
HELEN C. REDMAN, M.D.

CHAPTER 13
The Genitourinary System 407
HELEN C. REDMAN, M.D.

SECTION FIVE
Vascular Injuries

CHAPTER 14
Emergency Evaluation of Vascular Injuries 451
GEORGE L. MILLER, M.D. • MARGARET E. HANSEN, M.D.

SECTION SIX
Pediatric Trauma

CHAPTER 15
Imaging of the Injured Child 517
NANCY K. ROLLINS, M.D.

INDEX 533

SECTION ONE

Head and Brain

CHAPTER 1

• •

Traumatic Brain Injury

• • • • • • •

PHILLIP D. PURDY, M.D.
DONALD A. ECKARD, M.D.

Brain trauma is a broad-based subject that encompasses penetrating and nonpenetrating injury, diffuse injury, which is often difficult to image, and injuries caused by the mass effect of primary cerebral extra-axial trauma leading to herniation. Although the focus of this text is the radiologic appearance of acute trauma, understanding the clinical manifestations of brain injury requires some knowledge of functional neuroanatomy. More important, interpretation of the various diagnostic examinations as they relate to a specific patient demands a sophisticated correlation between the clinical presentation and the radiographic examinations. For instance, a right-handed patient with right frontal trauma and computed tomography (CT) evidence of a right frontal contusion should have his or her CT scan re-evaluated or repeated if the clinical presentation is one of a right hemiparesis and aphasia. These are symptoms of injury of the left side of the brain, and the probability is that a contrecoup injury is to be found. The importance of clinical correlation with radiographic image interpretation mandates that an overview of functional cerebral anatomy precede any discussion of specific injuries.

• • • •

CEREBRAL ANATOMY

This section serves as an overview of a very complex subject. The reader is referred to textbooks of neuroanatomy and neurology for more precise or detailed information.

The brain can be functionally subdivided into five components: the brain stem, the cerebellum, the diencephalon, the basal ganglia, and the cerebral cortex. The role of the hypothalamus in brain trauma and its extremely complex metabolic functions are only briefly discussed. Figures 1–1 and 1–2 show radiographic anatomy on CT and magnetic resonance (MR) scans.

The Brain Stem and the Cerebellum

The brain stem includes the medulla, the pons, and the midbrain. Although each of these structures has specific functions, in general the brain stem relays information from the cortex to the cerebellum

3

• • • • • APPROPRIATE RADIOGRAPHIC STUDIES

I. **Plain Films—Skull Series**

Comment: Rarely indicated because computed tomography (CT) and magnetic resonance (MR) imaging are both superior for visualizing the brain, and CT will demonstrate most fractures.

Exceptions: Recommended for children under 24 months in age or when child abuse is suspected. The severely injured adult may also benefit from portable views on the way to surgery if CT is not readily available.

II. **Computed Tomography**

A. In *noncontrast* study 10-mm sections at 10-mm intervals are used. Contrast-enhanced examinations are rarely indicated acutely. All other examinations that require contrast media should follow the head CT scan.

B. Sections for the orbits and the face can be added when clinically indicated.

Comment: At present, CT is the survey procedure of choice for acute head trauma. It is accessible, rapid, and requires that the patient hold still for only 2–3 seconds. The patient is not isolated, and ferromagnetic objects are not of concern. As MR technology develops it may supplant CT, even though it does not display bone well.

III. **Magnetic Resonance Imaging**

A. An axial projection is standard. Coronal and sagittal projections are performed as required.

Comment: At present, MR imaging has more uses later in the course of therapy as a prognosticator. However, the patient is isolated, study is lengthy, and equipment is not readily available 24 hours a day. All these factors may change as MR technology advances.

and the spinal cord, from the spinal cord to the cerebellum and the cortex, and from the cerebellum to the cerebral cortex. The brain stem also contains the group of nuclei responsible for the final output of signals to and from the cranial nerves. Since the 10th cranial nerve (the vagus) has important parasympathetic visceral functions, including cardiac innervation, cardiac modulation is also an important function of the brain stem, particularly of the medulla.

Another important function of the brain stem, which is located primarily in the upper pons and the lower midbrain, is the maintenance of consciousness. Coma can be produced by either diffuse bilateral cortical injury or by a very specific injury to the reticular formation located centrally in the lower midbrain and the upper pons. This is critical in the interpretation of the clinical presentation of patients following head trauma.

The medulla contains the nuclei for the 9th, the 10th, the 11th, and the 12th cranial nerves. These nerves control motor function of the pharynx, the larynx, and the tongue. They control both taste and tactile sensation in the pharynx and the larynx. The 11th cranial nerve (the spinal accessory nerve) receives some contribution from the upper cervical spinal cord. It controls motor function of the trapezius muscle. The 9th, the 10th, and the 11th cranial nerves exit the skull through the jugular foramen. The 12th cranial nerve (the hypoglossal) exits the skull through the hypoglossal foramen.

The eighth cranial nerve (the vestibulocochlear nerve) is associated with nuclei in the lateral medulla and traverses the pontomedullary junction. The vestibular and the cochlear functions of the vestibulocochlear nerve are controlled separately. The nerve exits at the pontomedullary junction along with the seventh (facial) cranial nerve, and both enter the internal auditory canal. The pons contains nuclei for the sixth and the seventh cranial nerves. The nuclear anatomy of the fifth cranial nerve is complex, extending from the midbrain to the upper cervical spinal cord, and involves several components. The third and fourth cranial nerves (the oculomotor nerve

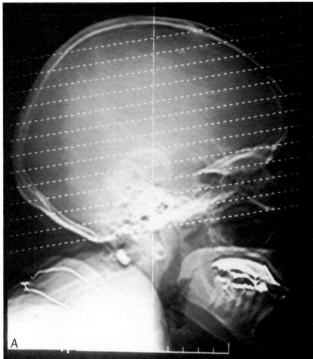

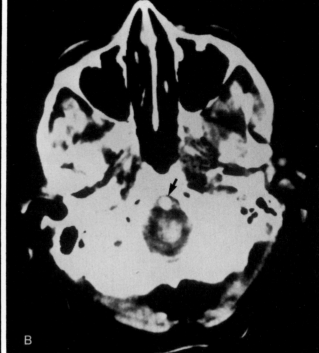

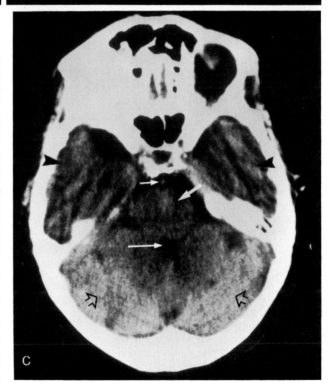

FIGURE 1–1. Normal Computed Tomography Anatomy Also Illustrating Some Commonly Encountered Artifacts

• • • •

A, A lateral "scout" film illustrating the levels at which the scans are taken. Note the dentures in this patient's mouth; dentures can create significant artifacts if the level of the scan includes them. The lateral scout film can serve the same function as a lateral skull film in patients with trauma. *B,* An image obtained through the level of the foramen magnum. Note the rounded density anterior to the spinal cord at the cervicomedullary junction. This is the tip of the odontoid process of C2 *(arrow). C,* This scan obtained through the posterior fossa illustrates the fourth ventricle *(long white arrow),* the basilar artery *(small white arrow),* the pons *(medium white arrow),* the cerebellum *(open black arrows),* and the temporal lobes *(arrowheads).* Note the streak artifact through the temporal lobes. This is caused by complex bone structures that surround brain tissue; multiple abrupt interfaces can be seen between high-density and low-density structures. As the x-rays strike these complex bones, differential absorptions of x-ray photons occur. The higher-energy photons pass through, and the lower-energy photons are absorbed. This causes so-called "beam hardening," which can appear homogeneous if the bone is simple but dense. If the bone is complex, it can appear as multiple streaks through the tissue, as in this case. This type of artifact can also be produced by small amounts of motion. Note the rounded appearance anterior to the basis pontis (pons).

Illustration continued on following page

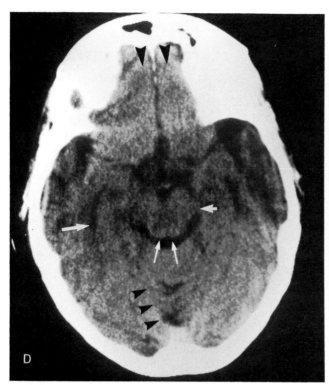

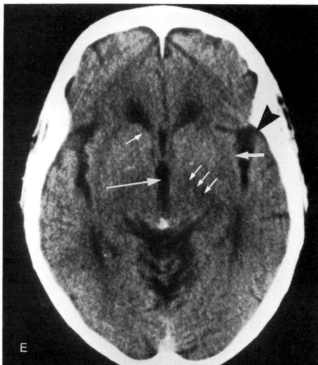

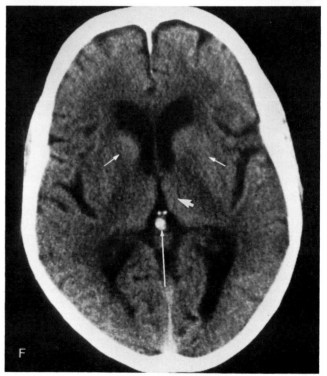

FIGURE 1–1 *Continued* **Normal Computed Tomography Anatomy Also Illustrating Some Commonly Encountered Artifacts**

• • • •

D, A slightly higher scan than that in *C* shows the midbrain. The quadrigeminal plate (colliculi) are indicated by the *small white arrows.* The *medium white arrow* points to the cerebral peduncle of the midbrain. The basilar artery lies anterior between the two peduncles. The *larger white arrow* points to the temporal horn of the lateral ventricle. The *small arrowheads* outline the edge of the tentorium, which is shown as a subtle interface between horizontally oriented sulci of the cerebellum and nonhorizontal sulci of the adjacent occipital lobe. If a contrast medium is administered intravenously, the tentorium becomes enhanced and is more conspicuous. The *large arrowheads* anteriorly point to the inferior frontal lobes. *E,* This scan is obtained at the level of the apex of the midbrain. The *three small arrows* aligned side-by-side point to the lower density of the posterior limb of the internal capsule. This normally appears with this density owing to the large content of myelinated fibers, which contain fat and are thus of lower density than the more proteinaceous gray matter of the nuclei or of the outer cortex. The *long white arrow* points to the third ventricle. The *large black arrowhead* is pointing toward the sylvian fissure, in the floor of which is the insula *(medium white arrow).* The *smallest white arrow* points to the head of the caudate nucleus, which lies in the lateral wall of the frontal horn of the lateral ventricle. *F,* This scan is obtained at the level of the pineal gland *(longest white arrow).* The *small white arrow* on the left of the image points to the head of the caudate nucleus, which is in the lateral wall of the frontal horn of the lateral ventricle. In this patient, some cerebral atrophy is present, and the ventricles are larger than they normally appear in younger patients. However, in elderly patients, this finding can be a normal variant. The widened cortical sulci located peripherally indicate that the ventricular enlargement is not caused by obstructive hydrocephalus. The *short large white arrow* points to the thalamus. The *small white arrow* on the right of the image points to the putamen.

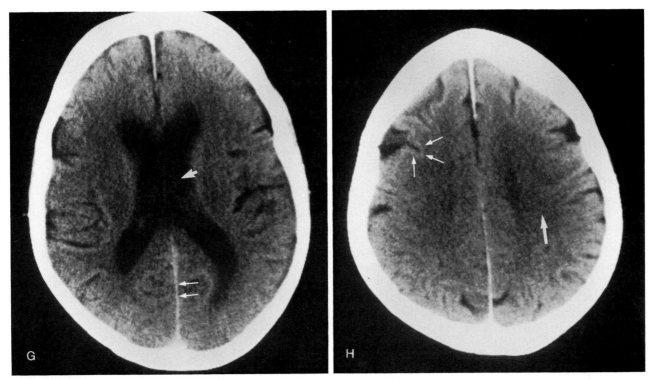

FIGURE 1–1 *Continued* **Normal Computed Tomography Anatomy Also Illustrating Some Commonly Encountered Artifacts**

• • • •

G, This scan was obtained through the body of the lateral venticles, which is indicated by the *short white arrow.* The slightly *longer small white arrows* that are aligned in a pair posteriorly point to the falx. *H,* This slice was obtained above the level of the lateral ventricles. It primarily contains the white matter of the centrum semiovale, which is shown as the large, slightly lower-density area *(large white arrow).* The *three small arrows* outline the junction between gray matter and white matter along the depths of a cortical sulcus.

and the trochlear nerve, respectively) arise from the midbrain.

The third, the fourth, and the sixth cranial nerves control eye movements. Conjugate lateral eye movement is achieved by simultaneous input to the nucleus of the sixth nerve on one side and to the nucleus of the third nerve on the other. Simultaneous communication to these contralateral nuclei is achieved by a fiber bundle called the *medial longitudinal fasciculus,* which lies immediately anterior to the fourth ventricle or the aqueduct of Sylvius. A lesion in the medial longitudinal fasciculus causes a gaze palsy called an *internuclear ophthalmoplegia.*

In addition to function of the cranial nerves, the brain stem transmits ascending sensory signals from the spinal cord and descending motor signals from the cerebral cortex. The motor signals are carried by a fiber bundle to the cerebral peduncles of the midbrain via the posterior limb of the internal capsule. From there, they descend ventrally along the length of the brain stem to the basis pontis and then to the medullary pyramids. It is the medullary pyramids that give these bundles the name *pyramidal tracts.* At

the cervicomedullary junction they decussate to the opposite side of the spinal cord, where they continue to descend.

The brain stem also transmits signals to the cerebellum via the inferior and the middle cerebellar peduncles. Basically, the inferior cerebellar peduncle carries afferent, predominantly proprioceptive sensory input from the spinal cord. The middle cerebellar peduncle carries afferent nerves from the pontine nuclei, which are interspersed in the basis pontis and receive their input from the cerebral cortex. The superior cerebellar peduncle transmits into the midbrain, where the nerves decussate and continue to the red nucleus in the midbrain and to the thalamus. From there they are transmitted to the cortex contralateral to the cerebellar hemisphere in which they arose. In the cortex, the cerebellar input modifies motor output. Since the motor output supplies body parts contralateral to the cerebral hemisphere in which they arise, the motor output is ipsilateral to the cerebellar hemisphere that modifies it. Thus, the cerebellum is "uncrossed," and a right cerebellar lesion results in a right hemiataxia.

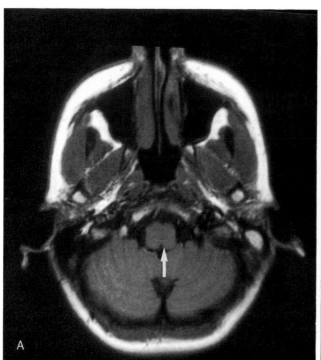

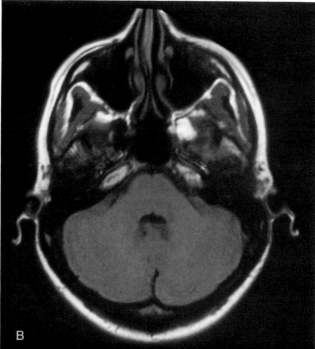

**FIGURE 1–2. Gross Anatomy on T₁-weighted Axial
Images**

• • • •

A, This image, acquired immediately above the foramen
magnum through the posterior fossa, shows the medulla
(white arrow). It is surrounded by cerebrospinal fluid, which
appears black on T₁-weighted images. Posterior to the
medulla are the cerebellar tonsils. *B,* An image acquired at
the level of the pons. Note the absence of any artifacts in
the posterior fossa on magnetic resonance images as compared with those seen with computed tomography in
Figure 1–1C. The ovoid black structure surrounded by
brain in the center of the posterior fossa is the fourth
ventricle. It separates the pons anteriorly from the cerebellum posteriorly. The structures on either side of the
fourth ventricle that connect the pons to the cerebellum
are the middle cerebellar peduncles. *C,* This image acquired
at the level of the lower midbrain shows the transition
from the basis pontis to the cerebral peduncles. Note the
black dot *(small arrow)* surrounded by dark gray cerebrospinal fluid anterior to the brain stem. This is the basilar
artery. Note how poorly it is seen on the T₁-weighted
images compared with how it appears on T₂-weighted
images (see Fig. 1–3A). Anterior to the basilar artery, the
pituitary gland can be seen within the sella turcica *(large
arrow).* Note also the appearance of the globes within the
orbits. The high-signal intensity fat provides good contrast
for the lower-signal intensity of the globes. The optic
nerves are seen passing posteriorly from the globe to the
optic foramen and are, again, well outlined by the orbital
fat. Note that some motion of the eyes that occurred during
imaging has caused a blurring effect.

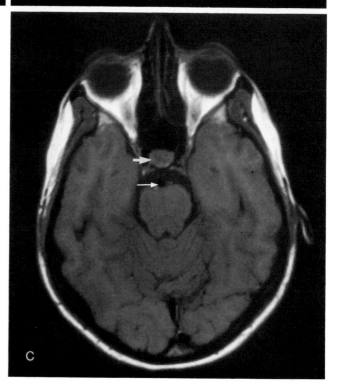

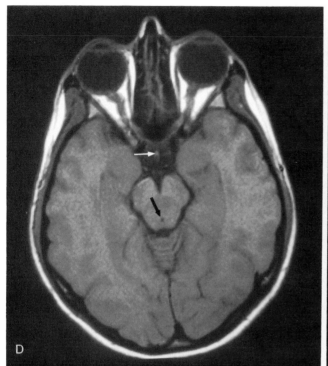

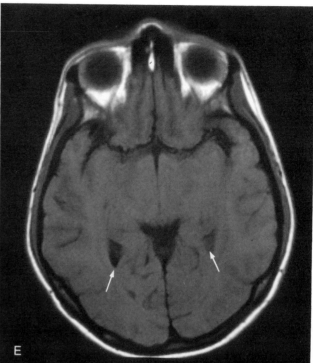

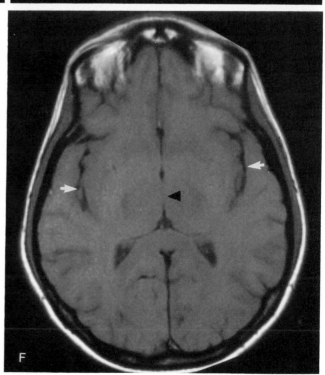

FIGURE 1–2 *Continued* **Gross Anatomy on T₁-weighted Axial Images**

• • • •

D, This image taken at the level of the midbrain shows good detail of the orbital anatomy. The small circular dot of soft tissue intensity anterior to the midbrain *(white arrow)* is the pituitary stalk. At this level, the cerebral peduncles are well defined. Posteriorly within the midbrain *(black arrow),* the small circular area of low signal intensity is the aqueduct of Sylvius. The temporal lobes are lateral to the midbrain on either side. The occipital lobes are separated only by the linear low-signal intensity of the falx posteriorly. *E,* A level slightly above that shown in *D* shows the lower part of the third ventricle centrally. The ventricular trigone (transition from the body of the lateral ventricles to the temporal horns) is shown on either side by the *white arrows.* Anteriorly, the linear signal void of the anterior and the middle cerebral arteries can be seen. *F,* An image acquired at the level of the thalami shows the slit-like third ventricle in the midline *(arrowhead).* The thalami form the lateral walls of the third ventricle. The sylvian fissures are well seen *(white arrows).* The undulating brain structure that forms the medial wall of the sylvian fissure in these images is the insula.

Illustration continued on following page

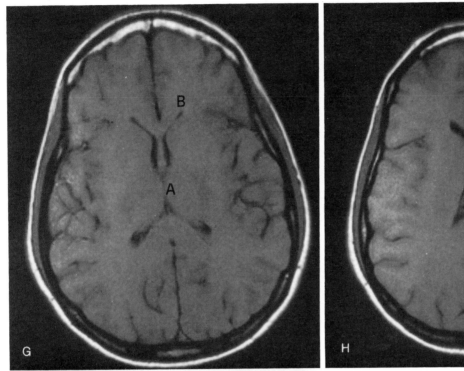

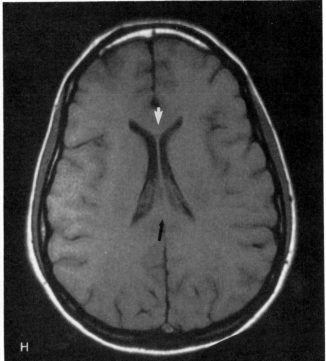

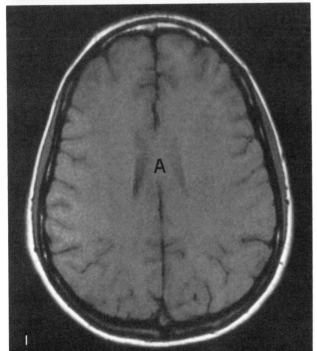

FIGURE 1–2 *Continued* **Gross Anatomy on T₁-weighted Axial Images**

• • • •

G, An image taken at the level of the frontal horns of the lateral ventricles. Note the similarity in the signal intensities of the gray matter and of the white matter on T₁-weighted images. Compare this similarity with the appearance of these signal intensities on T₂-weighted images in Figure 1–3C. In these images, the thalamus *(A)* is predominantly composed of gray matter. White matter in the periventricular region adjacent to the frontal horn of the left lateral ventricle is indicated by *B. H,* A level slightly above that seen in *G.* This image was acquired at the level of the bodies of the lateral ventricles. Note the genu *(white arrow)* and splenium *(black arrow)* of the corpus callosum. *I,* An image acquired superior to that in *H* shows the body of the corpus callosum *(A).* The white matter of the centrum semiovale is shown lateral to the upper body of the lateral ventricle.

The Diencephalon

The diencephalon includes the pineal gland, the thalamus, the subthalamus, and the claustrum. Of these, the most important nuclear complex is the thalamus, which performs vital relay tasks for both sensory and motor function. It is important for image interpretation to know that the thalamus lies immediately above the midbrain and forms the lateral walls of the third ventricle. When seen on CT and MR scans, the thalamus is the mass of gray matter that lies medial to the posterior limb of the internal capsule.

In addition to its somatic sensory function, the thalamus has special functions in both hearing and vision. The medial geniculate body is an intermediate synaptic structure for primary auditory signals; it receives input from the cochlear nucleus and projects this input to the auditory cortex. The lateral geniculate body is a primary visual relay station, receiving input from the optic tracts, which arise from the optic nerves, and projecting the information to the visual cortex in the occipital lobes and to the superior colliculi, which function in the visual motor system.

The pineal gland is a special endocrine organ that produces biogenic amines such as serotonin, norepinephrine, and melatonin. It also contains hypothalamic hormones and is known to function in the production of circadian rhythms. Both its midline location and its frequent calcification are important in imaging. At angiography, the pineal gland is outlined by the inferior and the superior sweep of the internal cerebral vein and the vein of Galen. It lies immediately anterior to the junction of the vein of Galen and the straight sinus.

The claustrum is a small nucleus immediately deep to a thin band of white matter underlying the insular cortex. Its function is poorly understood, and it is not significant to image interpretation in trauma.

Injury to the hypothalamus is important to the long-term outcome of head trauma as the hypothalamus has both endocrinologic and behavioral functions. The hypothalamus is a paired midline nuclear structure that produces hormones modulating pituitary function and communicates with the pituitary gland by way of the pituitary stalk. It lies immediately above the sella turcica and forms a portion of the anterior floor of the third ventricle. It is best imaged coronally with MR imaging, though it can be seen on coronal CT scans. When axial imaging is attempted, the hypothalamus is often obscured by other structures in the suprasellar cistern that are included in the section.

The Basal Ganglia

The basal ganglia include the caudate nucleus, the putamen, and the globus pallidus. The caudate nucleus and the putamen are separated by the anterior limb of the internal capsule to which they lend a striated appearance on axial sections. This complex is referred to as the *corpus striatum.* The caudate nucleus forms the lateral wall of the frontal horn of the lateral ventricle. It normally indents the ventricle when seen axially and gives a normal frontal horn the concavity on its lateral margin. The putamen is posterolateral to the caudate nucleus and medial to the claustrum. Immediately medial to the putamen is the globus pallidus. Together, the caudate nucleus, the putamen, and the globus pallidus function in the "extrapyramidal" motor system, which maintains muscle tone and smooth, coordinated muscle movements. They communicate broadly with the cerebellum, the thalamus, the subthalamus, and the cortex. Perhaps their best known communication is between the substantia nigra and the caudate nucleus. The substantia nigra is a bundle of pigmented nuclei underlying the pyramidal tracts in the cerebral peduncles of the midbrain. It is the nigrostriatal pathway that is most affected in Parkinson's disease.

Disorders of the basal ganglia and their connections result in behavioral manifestations such as tremor, rigidity, athetosis, and chorea. Their location deep within the brain and the severity of trauma that is required to injure the basal ganglia perhaps accounts for the infrequency of clinical manifestations of trauma to the basal ganglia. Patients with trauma severe enough to damage the basal ganglia usually have global injuries and paralysis, which obscure the injury (Fig. 1–3).

The Cerebral Lobes

Any discussion of the cerebrum in the context of trauma must acknowledge that information derived from elegant studies is being applied to gross and extremely inelegant pathology. This discussion is therefore broad, but interpretation of images in the light of neurologic abnormalities must be founded in a knowledge of functional neuroanatomy. The major cerebral lobes are the frontal, the parietal, the occipital, and the temporal lobes (Fig. 1–4). Although its behavioral significance is uncertain, the importance of the insula in brain imaging is undeniable and is therefore discussed as well.

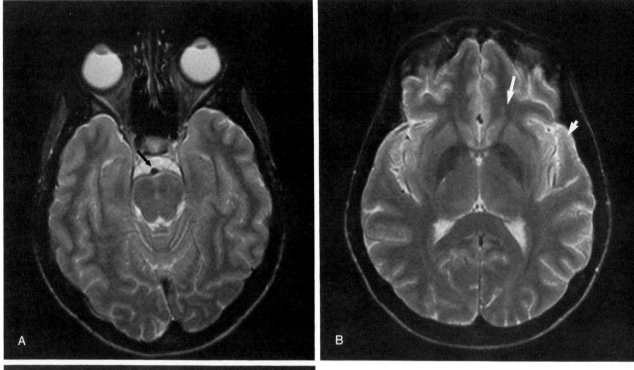

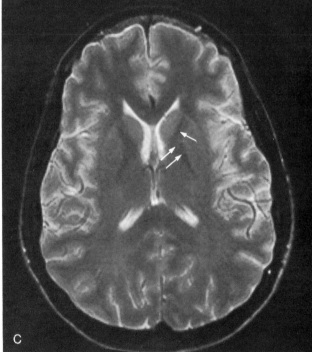

Figure 1–3. Demonstration of Signal Characteristics of T₂-weighted Images at 1.5 Tesla

• • • •

A, This image, acquired through the lower midbrain, shows the brain stem to be surrounded by high-signal-intensity cerebrospinal fluid. Note also the high-signal intensity of the globes. The small circular area of the signal void *(arrow)* anterior to the brain stem is the basilar artery. Note its better demonstration with this sequence than with the T₁-weighted image in Figure 1–2C. *B,* This image acquired at the level of the thalami shows the high-signal intensity of the cerebrospinal fluid within the ventricular system. Note also the better distinction between gray matter and white matter. In this image, the gray matter of the cortex is indicated by the *small arrow,* and the white matter of the frontal lobe is identified by the *large arrow.* *C,* At the level of the frontal horns of the lateral ventricle, the white matter of the anterior *(small arrow)* and the posterior *(double arrow)* limbs of the internal capsule are well outlined by the gray-matter nuclei surrounding them. The internal cerebral veins are the paired linear areas of signal void in the midline; they travel in the roof of the third ventricle.

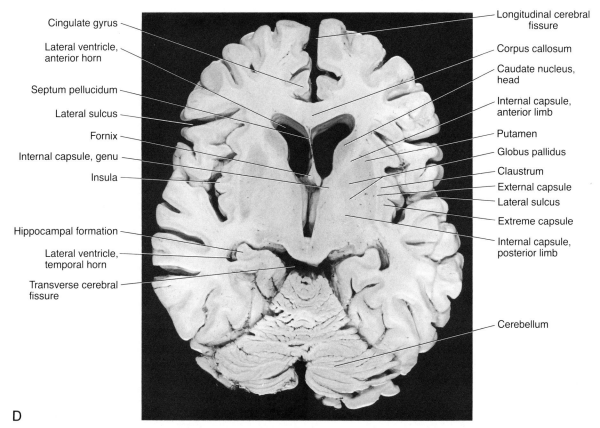

D

FIGURE 1–3 *Continued* **Demonstration of Signal Characteristics of T₂-weighted Images at 1.5 Tesla**

• • • •

D, This transaxial anatomic slice of the brain taken through the level of the frontal horns of the lateral ventricles and through the tentorium shows associated cerebral structures as they appear on a brain slice. (From Burt AM. Textbook of Neuroanatomy. Philadelphia: W. B. Saunders Co., 1993, p 158 [in press].)

The Frontal Lobe

The frontal lobes are the largest lobes in the brain. They extend from the rostral tip of the telencephalon posteriorly to the central sulcus. The frontal lobes are separated from the temporal lobes by the sylvian fissure and from each other by the interhemispheric fissure. They are connected by the anterior portion of the corpus callosum, a large bundle of white matter traversing the interhemispheric fissure at the level of the roof of the third ventricle and forming the medial margin of the bodies of the lateral ventricles.

The frontal lobes contain the associative cortex and function in higher-order problem solving. They are actually largely redundant, and patients generally function well after a unilateral resection of a frontal lobe tip. However, if bilateral frontal lobe lesions are found, some decline in function is common. In trauma, bilateral injury is frequent. In addition to the associative cortex, specific regions in the frontal lobes are responsible for rapid eye movements. The frontal lobe tends to drive the eyes contralaterally. Therefore, an irritative right frontal lobe lesion often results in deviation of the eyes to the left, whereas a destructive lesion results in deviation to the right.

Another frontal lobe function is the maintenance of the sphincters of the bowel and bladder. This function is bilateral; thus, unilateral lesions usually do not cause incontinence. These areas reside on the mesial surface of the frontal lobes. Incontinence is one symptom of a midline lesion compressing both medial frontal lobes.

The primary motor strip lies in the precentral gyrus in the posterior frontal lobes. It is organized as an inverted homunculus, so that the lateral surface adjacent to the sylvian fissure subserves the face and the hand. The inverted arm and trunk lie in the middle and the superior portion of the gyrus, respectively. The portion of the gyrus serving the movement of the leg and the foot is on the medial surface of the hemisphere. Rostral to the precentral gyrus on both the medial and the lateral surfaces of the hemisphere is a segment that also subserves motor function; this segment is referred to as the *precentral motor* and the *supplementary motor area*. It has associative functions for the motor system.

From the motor cortex, signals project through the corona radiata (the group of white matter projections lying deep to the cortex over the hemispheres) to the posterior limb of the internal capsule. From there

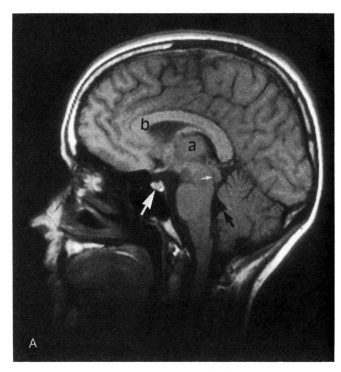

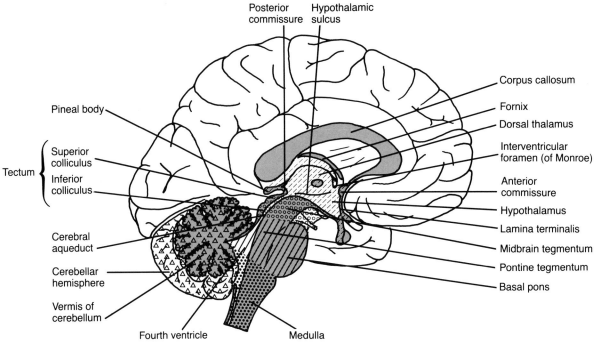

Posterior commissure   Hypothalamic sulcus

Corpus callosum

Fornix

Dorsal thalamus

Interventricular foramen (of Monroe)

Anterior commissure

Hypothalamus

Lamina terminalis

Midbrain tegmentum

Pontine tegmentum

Basal pons

Pineal body

Superior colliculus

Inferior colliculus

Tectum

Cerebral aqueduct

Cerebellar hemisphere

Vermis of cerebellum

Fourth ventricle

Medulla

B

Midsagittal View

FIGURE 1–4. Midline and Lateral Sagittal Magnetic Resonance Imaging Anatomy

• • • •

A, A midline sagittal image acquired with T_1 weighting shows many brain structures well. The fourth ventricle *(black arrow)* is shown as a dark area of low-signal intensity immediately posterior to the pons. Its triangular shape is characteristic. Cerebrospinal fluid traverses the aqueduct of Sylvius to enter the fourth ventricle from the third ventricle. The aqueduct is shown as a thin black streak *(white arrow)* extending through the midbrain. The posterior aspect of the aqueduct is formed by the quadrigeminal plate, which contains the superior and the inferior colliculi. The vermis of the cerebellum lies posterior to the fourth ventricle on this image. The round structure in the third ventricle *(a)* is the thalamus. The corpus callosum *(b)* forms the roof of the third ventricle. Midline gyral anatomy is well shown on this image. The pituitary gland is a small structure in the sella turcica *(larger white arrow). B,* This drawing of a mirror-image midline sagittal section of *A* shows other anatomic structures. (From Burt AM. Textbook of Neuroanatomy. Philadelphia: W. B. Saunders Co., 1993, p 133 [in press].)

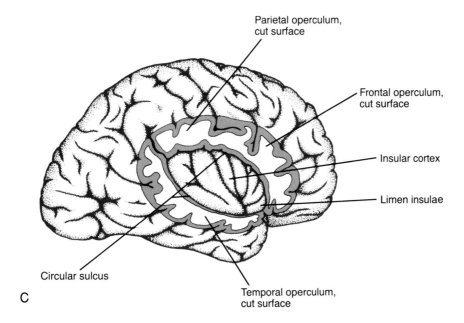

C

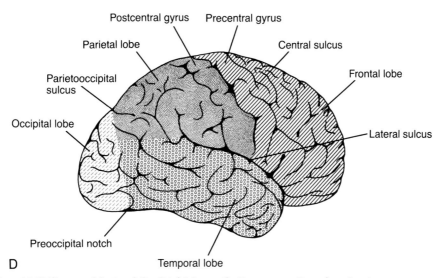

D

FIGURE 1–4 *Continued* **Midline and Lateral Sagittal Magnetic Resonance Imaging Anatomy**
• • • •
C, An image of the lateral brain surface showing the insula in the depths of the sylvian fissure. *D*, This lateral view of the brain shows the division between the major cerebral lobes. (From Burt AM. Textbook of Neuroanatomy. Philadelphia: W. B. Saunders Co., 1993, pp 157, 159 [in press].)

they continue to the cerebral peduncles and traverse the brain stem to the spinal cord as the pyramidal tracts. Lesions in any location along this pathway can result in a spastic hemiparesis contralateral to the lesion if it occurs in the brain. In the spinal cord, inferior to the decussation of the pyramids at the cervicomedullary junction, the motor deficit becomes ipsilateral to the lesion.

The Parietal Lobe

The parietal lobe begins at the central sulcus and continues posteriorly to its junction with the occipital lobe. On the mesial surface of the brain this junction occurs at the parieto-occipital sulcus. On the lateral surface, the border extends along a line drawn from the superior extent of the parieto-occipital sulcus to the preoccipital notch on the inferior surface. The inferior surface of the parietal lobe is not crisply defined at its junction with the temporal lobe. The temporal lobe includes the superior, middle, and inferior temporal gyri on its lateral surface. The junction of the parietal lobe with the temporal lobe must be extrapolated from the supramarginal and the angular gyri and their junction with the temporal gyri. The function of the posterior temporal lobe merges into the function of the parietal lobe in these locations, where many associative tasks are performed.

The anterior margin of the parietal lobe is formed by the postcentral gyrus. Just as the precentral gyrus is the primary motor strip, the postcentral gyrus is the primary sensory strip for tactile and kinesthetic senses. Its organization is also that of an inverted homunculus, closely resembling that of the motor strip. In addition to associative and supplementary sensory function, the remainder of the parietal lobe functions in higher order processes, such as spatial orientation, calculation, naming, the orientation of body parts and their identification, and dressing. There are significant interhemispheric differences between the parietal lobes in these higher intellectual functions, but the right side of the body is recognized from the left hemisphere, and the left side of the body is recognized from the right hemisphere. Therefore, patients with large right parietal lesions may deny the left side of their body.

Another center responsible for eye movements lies in the posterior parietal lobe or the anterior occipital lobe. The parieto-occipital center controls slow, smooth movements following an object through the visual field to the ipsilateral side, whereas the frontal lobe controls rapid eye movements to the contralateral side. Therefore, for instance, the right hemisphere causes rapid eye movements to the left and slow, smooth movements to the right. These visual centers are connected so that they operate in concert, following one object through the visual field and then jumping to another object to follow it through the visual field. Disorders in the frontal eye fields, parieto-occipital eye fields, or their connections can produce abnormalities of optokinetic nystagmus.

The Temporal Lobe

The temporal lobe is demarcated superiorly by the sylvian fissure and posteriorly by the same line extending from the parieto-occipital sulcus to the pre-occipital notch. On the lateral surface of the temporal lobe there are three gyri called the superior, the middle, and the inferior temporal gyri. The medial surface of the temporal lobe is more complex. Here lie the parahippocampal gyrus, the uncus, the occipitotemporal gyrus, and the lingula. The superior temporal gyrus contains the primary auditory cortex, which receives input from the eighth cranial nerve. Surrounding the primary auditory cortical area is a region of the secondary associative auditory cortex. The posterior superior temporal lobe of the dominant hemisphere contains Wernicke's area, where signals from the auditory cortex and the visual cortex converge to lend comprehension to words. A white matter bundle called the *arcuate fasciculus* carries these signals around the posterior aspect of the sylvian fissure and then anteriorly to Broca's area in the

frontal lobe, near the portion of the motor strip concerned with the face. Broca's area is responsible for the primary motor output of speech. There are supplementary comprehension areas in the inferior temporal lobe and motor areas for speech in the superior frontal lobe. Not coincidentally, "watershed" infarcts involving the supplementary areas can create aphasia. Aphasias resulting from lesions in the central language areas include Broca's aphasia, Wernicke's aphasia, conduction aphasia, and global aphasia. The type of aphasia corresponds to the specific area of the brain involved. These syndromes are classified according to their effect on fluency, repetition, comprehension, and the naming of objects.

While propositional language arises from the dominant hemisphere, affective or emotional language is theorized to arise from the nondominant hemisphere. This occurs in an anatomic organization that is perhaps analogous to that in the dominant hemisphere for propositional language.

The medial temporal lobe functions extensively in the domain of recent memory. In some patients this is a predominantly unilateral function, whereas in others it is almost equal bilaterally. In fact, closed head trauma is a leading cause of recent memory loss, especially when the injury has caused loss of consciousness for a short time. Partial or even complete recovery of memory may occur over the weeks or months following the injury.

In addition to recent memory function, the medial temporal lobe contains important portions of the "limbic lobe." Although not a true lobe, the limbus is linked functionally to olfactory sensory and emotional regulation. Limbic emotional regulation should be separated from affective language function, which arises from the nondominant hemisphere. In the case of affective language function, the perception and the expression of emotion is involved, not the visceral emotional state itself. Patients can have pathologic depression, as witnessed by the vegetative signs of depression, yet not have extremely flat affective output. The structures in the medial temporal lobe include the amygdala and the hippocampal formation. The parahippocampal gyrus communicates with the cingulate gyrus, which is the most inferior gyrus in the mesial frontal lobe, lying immediately above the corpus callosum. This communication occurs through the isthmus of the cingulate gyrus. The amygdala is one of the primary sensory receptive areas for smell.

The Occipital Lobe

The margins of the occipital lobe on the lateral cortical surface have been described in the discussion of the parietal lobe. On the medial surface, the occipital lobe is demarcated anteriorly by the parieto-occipital sulcus and the calcarine sulcus. The occipital lobes control vision and contain both the primary and the supplementary visual areas. The primary visual cortex in each hemisphere subserves the contralateral visual hemifield. Images are inverted so that the more inferior cortex represents the superior visual field. Macular vision (finely detailed visual perception) is represented at the occipital tips. There is a poorly demarcated oculomotor functional area subserving smooth pursuit eye movements located near the occipitoparietal junction. In the process of reading, visual signals are carried to the posterior parietal lobe and then to Wernicke's area. If the patient is left hemisphere dominant, signals from the right visual cortex traverse the splenium of the corpus callosum in order to reach the language areas. Lesions in the splenium, the surrounding white matter fiber tracts, and the left occipital lobe produce alexia (i.e., the inability to read) and visual agnosia (i.e., the inability to recognize objects in the visual field unaccompanied by a loss of primary visual perception).

The Insula

The insula, a triangular cortical region in the floor of the sylvian fissure, is an important boundary in neuroimaging. Lateral to the insula is the sylvian fissure. Medial to the insula are the basal ganglia. The insula contains a group of shallow folds, the short gyri of insula and the long gyri of insula, which are oriented slightly oblique to the sylvian fissure. These are readily apparent on transaxial CT and MR images and demarcate the medial extent of the sylvian fissure. This is important in deciding whether blood is intraparenchymal or subarachnoid. The middle cerebral artery branches, which course superiorly along the surface of the insula and then loop inferiorly to exit the sylvian fissure, are deviated upward or medially by temporal lobe masses, anteriorly by parietal or occipital masses, and inferiorly by frontal masses. They can also be deviated laterally by frontal lobe masses. These "insular" loops form the *sylvian triangle*, a major landmark in the interpretation of cerebral angiograms.

The Ventricular System

The ventricular system is shown quite elegantly by both CT and MR imaging. In each hemisphere there is a lateral ventricle that begins in the frontal lobes as the *frontal horns*, extends posteriorly as the *body of the lateral ventricle*, and finally angles inferiorly and anteriorly at the *trigone* to enter the *temporal horn* in the temporal lobe. There is also an *occipital horn*, which extends posteriorly from the trigone into the anterior occipital lobe. The lateral ventricles contain choroid plexus and drain medially into the single third ventricle by way of the foramen of Monro. These foramina are located medial and posterior to the head of the caudate nucleus. From the third ventricle, cerebrospinal fluid passes into the fourth ventricle in the posterior fossa through the cerebral aqueduct (i.e., the aqueduct of Sylvius). The fourth ventricle begins in the inferior midbrain and traverses the pons to the upper medulla. Posteriorly, the roof of the fourth ventricle is formed by the cerebellum (Fig. 1–5). Cerebrospinal fluid exits into the subarachnoid space via two lateral foramina (the foramina of Luschka) and one medial foramen (the foramen of Magendie) at the level of the medulla.

• • • •

IMAGING OF HEAD TRAUMA

Imaging Strategies in Head Trauma

The modalities of concern in evaluating suspected brain trauma include plain film radiography, CT, MR imaging, and angiography. Prior to the decision as to what modality to employ, clinical evaluation must be performed and an assessment regarding the need for any imaging made (see "Appropriate Radiographic Studies" for Chapter 1).

Patients examined in the emergency room for minor head injuries who have not lost consciousness have a low probability of significant intracranial injury. Scalp lacerations and even linear skull fractures may be present, but little radiographic evaluation is warranted if the patients are observed to be stable over time. Patients who have had either a short-lived loss of consciousness or transient neurologic symptoms are at increased or moderate risk for brain injury. These patients may or may not have a skull fracture, but brain injury may be seen in as many as 20% of patients seen for head injury. Although a skull series does demonstrate a fracture when present, CT is the appropriate procedure for the evaluation of intracranial injury in these patients. Patients who have had prolonged or ongoing loss of consciousness and persistent neurologic abnormalities are at high risk for brain injury.

Children less than 2 years of age with potential intracranial injury are at somewhat higher risk because the more flexible cranial vault provides less protection to the brain. Child abuse with its attendant medicolegal aspects often warrants skull films for documentation and follow-up, even when brain injury is not a clinical concern.

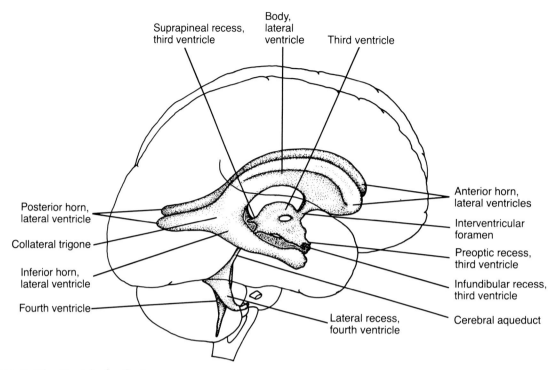

FIGURE 1–5. The Ventricular System

• • • •

This lateral view (with brain tissue shown as transparent) demonstrates the orientation of the ventricular system within the brain. The anterior horn of the lateral ventricles is the same structure as the frontal horn. (From Burt AM. Textbook of Neuroanatomy. Philadelphia: W. B. Saunders Co., 1993, p 173 [in press].)

The decision to use CT or MR imaging in the evaluation of intracranial injury is not yet straightforward. Pragmatically, CT is much more available on an emergency basis, and the patient is less isolated than in most MR scanners. No attention needs to be directed toward the avoidance of ferromagnetic equipment or the presence of ferromagnetic foreign bodies with CT. These are a serious concern with MR imaging.

Comparative data about the clinical efficacy of CT and MR imaging in acute injury is preliminary and uncontrolled at present. In general, CT has been used as the first diagnostic procedure, and MR imaging has been performed days or weeks later. Acute hemorrhage is usually better demonstrated by CT, whereas subacute and chronic hemorrhage is seen better on MR images. MR imaging is more sensitive in the recognition of brain swelling or contusion, but these abnormalities can be identified at CT. MR imaging is more accurate in finding all areas of abnormality, especially at a time removed from the acute trauma, and therefore may be a better prognostic test (Fig. 1–6). On the other hand, MR imaging does not evaluate bone well at all, whereas CT is excellent in this regard. Knowledge of fractures that can lead to infections or cerebrospinal fluid leaks can

be quite important; such fractures are discussed to some degree in subsequent chapters.

Therefore, CT currently remains the procedure of choice in acute intracranial injury. MR imaging has a significant role in the delineation of brain injury both to evaluate the complete extent of injury and to predict the potential for recovery. It must be recognized that CT can miss significant brain injury acutely, especially when no bleeding is involved. This is especially seen in anoxic injuries such as near-drowning.

In the past, angiography played a major role in the evaluation of epidural and subdural hematomas. CT and MR imaging have completely obviated the need for angiography to make these diagnoses. Angiography continues to have a role in the evaluation of the extracranial carotid and the vertebral arteries in both penetrating and blunt trauma to the neck or at the skull base. It also has a role in intracranial penetrating injury when the projectile has a course near the major intracranial arteries or when subarachnoid or parenchymal blood is found in an unexpected location at CT. In addition, angiography may be of use when CT or MR imaging has raised the question of a pre-existing lesion. In blunt trauma to the head, angiography is sometimes indicated to determine the

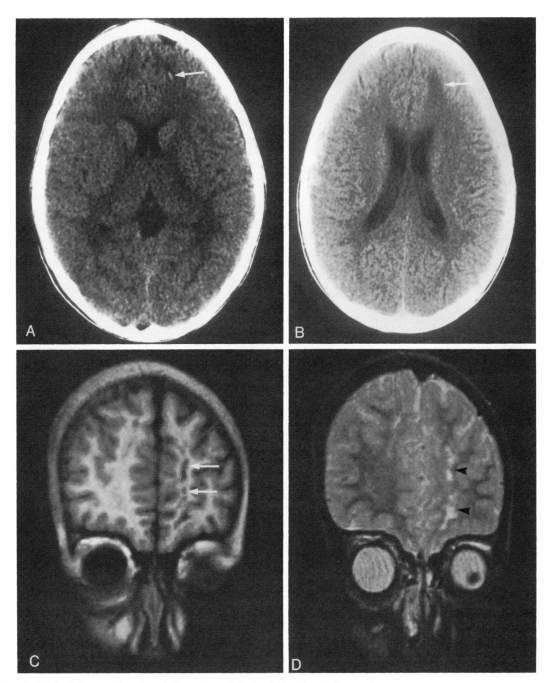

FIGURE 1–6. White Matter Shearing Injury Associated with a Small Contusion
• • • •
A, A patient with a closed head injury who was scanned acutely shows only a small area of increased density in the left frontal lobe *(arrow)*. *B,* This delayed computed tomography scan shows the white matter's low density *(arrow)*. *C,* This magnetic-resonance scan better demonstrates the area of white matter injury. Coronal T_1-weighted images show low signal intensity in the frontal white matter *(arrows)*. *D,* This injury is demonstrated in a more conspicuous fashion on T_2-weighted images as areas of increased signal intensity *(arrowheads)*. (Case courtesy of Dianne Mendelsohn, M.D.)

etiology of a sylvian fissure hematoma that could have resulted from a ruptured aneurysm or trauma. We perform angiography several times a year in motor vehicle accident patients with subarachnoid hemorrhage because it can be difficult to distinguish traumatic subarachnoid hemorrhage from primary aneurysmal hemorrhage, the latter of which resulted in the initial loss of consciousness and subsequently caused the original motor vehicle accident.

Another indication for angiography is unexplained neurologic deficit. The introduction of foreign bodies in the chest or the neck may result in cerebral embolization (Fig. 1–7). Stretch injuries to carotid arteries (Fig. 1–8) may result in anoxia or, if associ-

ated with intimal disruption (Fig. 1–9) may cause thromboembolic events. Penetrating trauma in the neck may also be seen with associated injury of nearby structures, such as the esophagus (Fig. 1–10).

Brain Response to Trauma

Types of Trauma

The traditional and convenient classification of the mechanism of head injury is a division between blunt and penetrating trauma. There is some overlap of

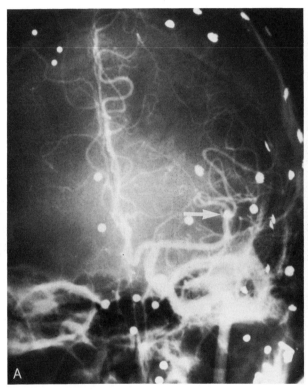

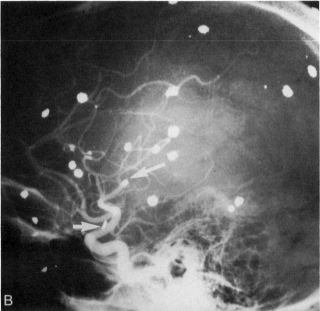

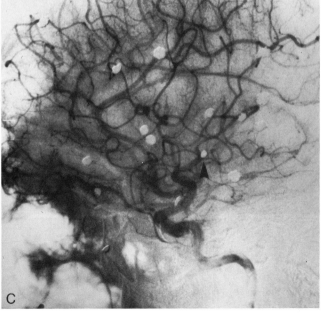

FIGURE 1–7. Unusual Embolic Complication of a Gunshot Wound

• • • •

A, This anteroposterior (AP) view shows no pellets overlying the distal carotid or the proximal anterior or middle cerebral arteries. However, a pellet is seen in the sylvian fissure in the region of the middle cerebral artery branches *(arrow). B,* On the lateral view, a pellet overlying the distal carotid *(short arrow)* was suspicious but had been cleared on the AP view. However, the angular branch of the middle cerebral artery is occluded by a pellet *(long arrow)* that had embolized to that location by way of an entry wound in the neck. *C,* The embolus is shown to greater advantage by use of subtraction techniques on the lateral view *(arrowhead).*

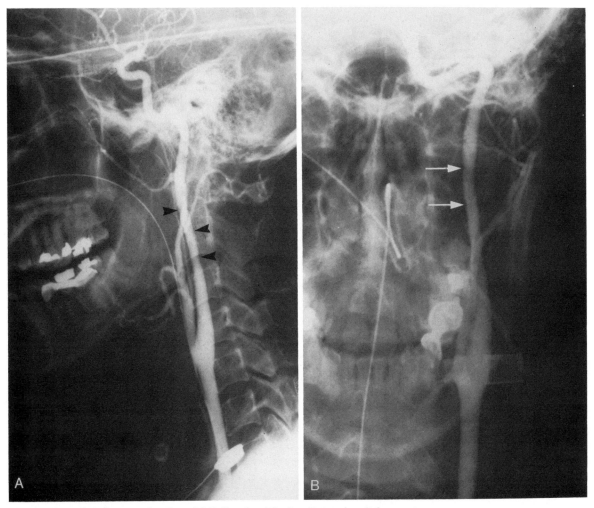

FIGURE 1–8. Stretch Injury to the Carotid Following Flexion Extension Injury
• • • •
A, Subtle irregularities along the wall of the internal carotid *(arrowheads)* indicate stretch injury. *B,* On the anteroposterior view, subtle irregularities are again seen. Note the segmental decrease in caliber of the internal carotid proximal to the skull base *(arrows).*

these two mechanisms of brain injury when depressed fractures with brain penetration by bone fragments is present in blunt injury.

Blunt injuries can be further divided into acceleration and deceleration injuries. This subdivision is of some utility in understanding the forces that have been applied to the brain but is of limited utility in guiding patient management. With acceleration injury, such as that which occurs in assault, a focal hematoma or a contusion can occur in the part of the brain underlying the point of impact. However, since assault often involves multiple blows, a simplistic view of the injury is not possible. Deceleration injuries are seen with falls or motor vehicle accidents. Both deceleration and acceleration injuries are capable of causing coma. However, if the injury involves a rotatory force in addition to either acceleration or deceleration, the potential for neurologic injury is

enhanced. Rotation adds a shearing force to the linear translation so that white matter injury occurs.

The extent of damage produced by penetrating injuries is a function of both the size and the velocity of the penetrating agent. The most frequent source of penetrating injury is a gunshot wound, although nail guns, knives (often transorbital), pencils, ice picks, or other more exotic materials can produce penetration (Fig. 1–11). Penetration can also result from a fall onto an object or from impact with a moving object. Angiographic exclusion of vascular injury can be difficult in a setting with multiple foreign bodies (see Fig. 1–7).

Injury from blunt or penetrating injury can be at the site of trauma or may be remote from it. Due to the movement of the brain with respect to the skull, contusion is often seen in the brain opposite the point of impact. Such injury is referred to as a

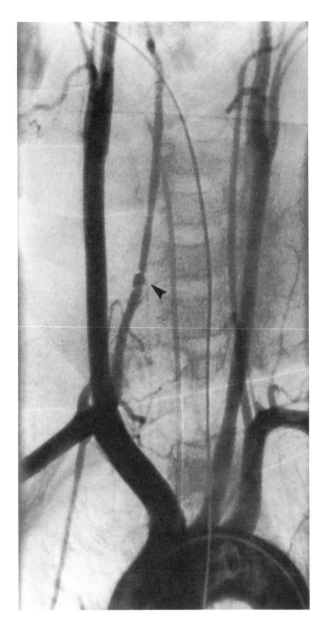

FIGURE 1–9. Intimal Disruption Associated with Penetrating Injury

• • • •

This patient suffered a penetrating injury to the neck and underwent angiography for possible proximal injury. The arch aortogram reveals an intimal defect of the right vertebral artery *(arrowhead).* This can be seen with penetrating injury (blast effect) or with soft tissue injury, particularly when lines of force create fractures involving the vertebral foramina. Such an arterial defect can serve as a nidus for embolic strokes.

contrecoup injury. Additionally, the gelatinous consistency of the brain results in the transmission of the energy of impact through much of the brain in severe trauma. Such transmission can result in *axonal shearing,* causing diffuse or focal brain injury. Such injury, though clinically evident, may be obvious, subtle, or absent on CT and MR examinations. Either blunt or high-velocity penetrating injury can cause axonal shearing (Fig. 1–12).

Imaging Appearance of Specific Entities

It is arguable that skull films are useful for screening in the emergency room for skull fractures. It is even more important to recognize that the historic importance of fracture detection was as a clue to the

severity of the underlying intracranial injury. Such observation could lead to the decision to observe the patient closely to rule out either severe brain injury or an incipient subdural or epidural hematoma. In the era of readily available CT scanning, the ability to directly image the underlying brain injury, subdural hematoma, or epidural hematoma has made the use of plain films obsolete as a screening tool. This discussion will therefore center on CT and MR imaging.

Although CT is clearly preferable for the demonstration of bone injury, CT and MR imaging are often complementary with respect to the information they provide, and the performance of both is sometimes necessary. Patients with acute brain injury present a particular problem in MR imaging because of the physical constraints of the magnet and because of

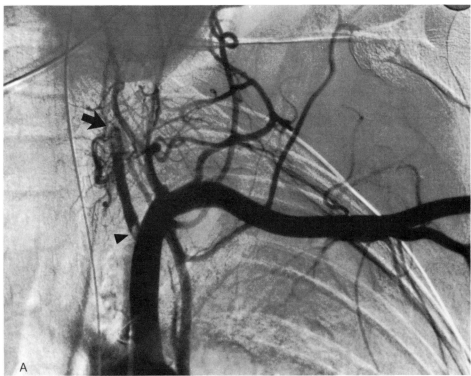

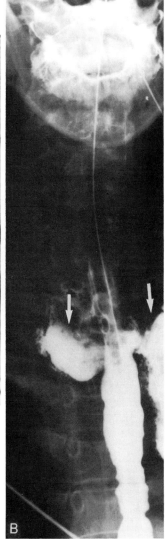

FIGURE 1–10. Vertebral Artery Injury Associated with Esophageal Injury

• • • •

A, This patient suffered a gunshot wound to the neck and was found to have an occluded left vertebral artery on angiography *(arrow)*. Note also the intraluminal clot at the origin of that vertebral artery *(arrowhead)*. The occlusion protects the patient from potential embolization of the intraluminal thrombus. *B,* There was an associated esophageal tear, as shown by extravasation of the contrast material into the periesoph-ageal space *(arrows)* on a contrast swallow examination.

the confused and often unstable state of the patient. The time required to acquire an MR study, during which the patient must remain motionless, presents a particular difficulty. The use of imaging protocols that shorten the acquisitions while retaining image quality improves the applicability of MR imaging in trauma. Devices using more open and permanent magnets are now on the market. Although patient availability is increased, the signal-to-noise ratio in the images is sometimes decreased by lower field strength, and acquisition times are lengthened.

The ability to acquire a single CT slice in 1–2 seconds and to repeat that individual slice if the patient moves is very important in obtaining a diagnostic study in a short period of time. Although MR imaging demonstrates subtle edema and contusion better than CT, the clinical utility of observations of these abnormalities in the acute setting is unclear. An MR image may demonstrate a subdural hema-toma in some patients with an unexplained mass

effect at CT. In general, MR imaging is more effec-tively utilized when the patient has stabilized as a secondary modality to demonstrate the extent of brain injury, either for medicolegal reasons or for examining unexplained deficits. In general, CT re-mains the primary modality in an acute traumatic brain injury. MR technology is particularly superior in imaging brain injury in the posterior fossa.

Brain injury can be primary or secondary. Primary injuries include contusion, laceration, and swelling. Secondary injuries include compression, hydroceph-alus, and ischemic injury. Subarachnoid hemorrhage, with or without other injury, is also frequent. Venous sinus thrombosis should also be considered if there is disproportionate brain edema or evidence of in-creased intracranial pressure. This diagnosis is es-pecially pertinent now that direct interventional ther-apies are available (Fig. 1–13).

When secondary ischemic injury occurs, the changes can be focal or diffuse. Diffuse ischemic

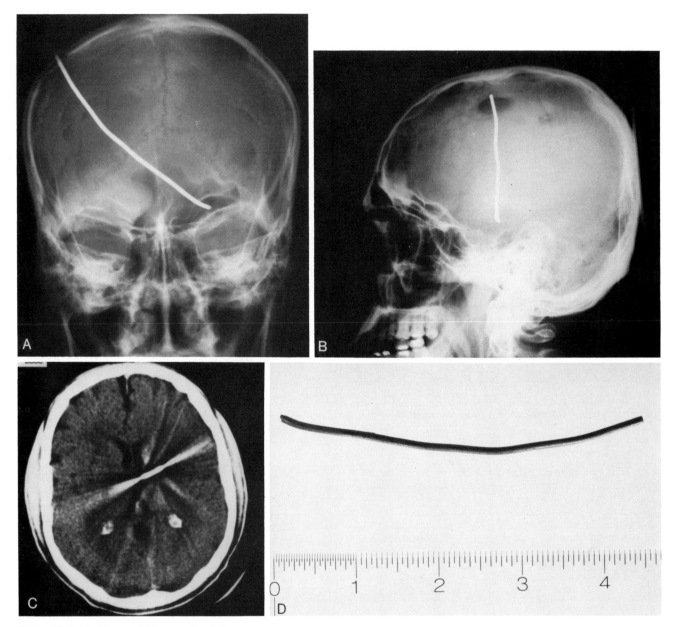

FIGURE 1–11. Unusual Penetrating Injury

• • • •

This deranged patient had a history of prior burr-hole placement in the right frontal region. He sought to remove demons from his brain by inserting a coat hanger through the burr hole. *A* and *B,* These anteroposterior and lateral radiographs show the course of the coat hanger fragment. *C,* A computed tomography scan reveals no evidence of intracerebral hemorrhage. The patient was treated by withdrawal of the coat hanger, followed by a short course of antibiotic therapy. He suffered no neurologic sequelae. *D,* The surgical specimen is shown.

injury can result from systemic effects such as anoxia or hypotension. This is seen in drowning or in severe hemorrhage from injuries remote from the brain. Initially, brain imaging studies in these patients are most frequently normal. Delayed imaging reveals diffuse cerebral swelling if the insult is diffuse. The area of the cortex most vulnerable to anoxic or ischemic insult is that most peripheral in the vasculature. This is in the so-called *watershed area* in the

superolateral frontoparietal region. If carotid occlusion has been produced, the lesion may involve only the middle cerebral artery distribution or both the anterior and the middle cerebral distributions. Ischemic injury results in a low-density appearance with a loss of the distinction between gray matter and white matter. This is seen as a wedge of low density on the CT images or as a wedge of high signal

Text continued on page 30

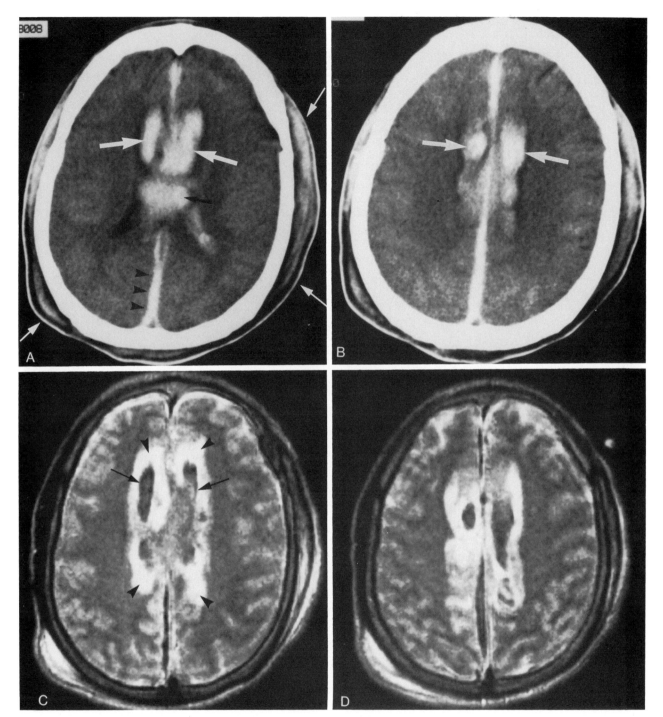

FIGURE 1–12. Multiple Computed Tomography, Magnetic-Resonance, and Angiographic Findings in Severe Closed Head Injury

• • • •

A, Following a severe injury in a motor vehicle accident, a computed-tomography scan shows diffuse swelling of the soft tissues of the scalp *(small white arrows).* Also, note the intraventricular blood *(large white arrows)* and the hematoma on the corpus callosum *(black arrow).* Additionally, there is an interhemispheric fissure subdural hematoma *(arrowheads). B,* A higher cut better demonstrates the interhemispheric subdural hematoma. In this slice note also the size and the extent of the intraventricular hematoma *(arrows). C,* T$_2$-weighted magnetic resonance (MR) scan at the level of that in *A* shows the acute blood to be dark *(small black arrows)* in both the ventricles and in the interhemispheric subdural hematoma. Note the bright area in the periventricular white matter *(arrowheads).* This represents an axonal shearing injury in the periventricular white matter. *D,* The T$_2$-weighted MR slice at the level of that in *B* shows a greater prominence of the interhemispheric subdural hematoma and also illustrates the shearing injury.

Illustration continued on following page

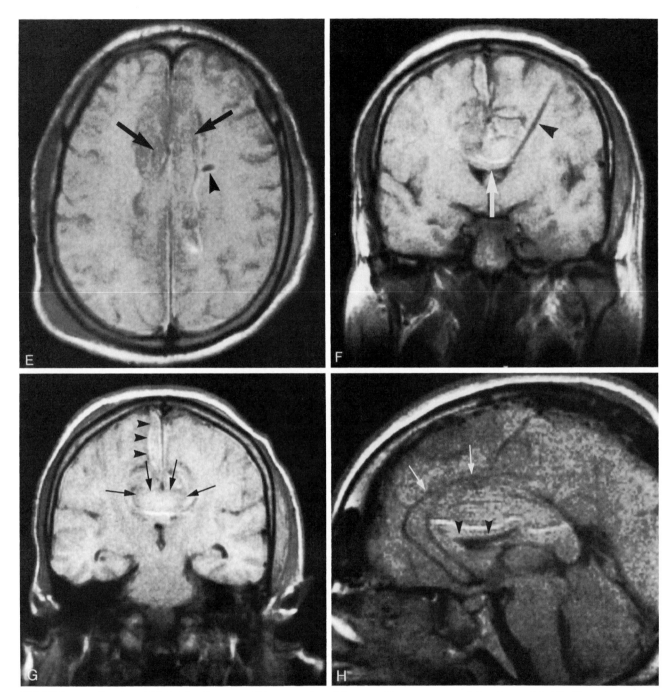

FIGURE 1–12 *Continued* **Multiple Computed Tomography, Magnetic-Resonance, and Angiographic Findings in Severe Closed Head Injury**

• • • •

E, This T$_1$-weighted transaxial MR scan at approximately the level of that used in *A* demonstrates the acute blood to be isointense with brain *(arrows).* Note the ventriculostomy catheter *(arrowhead).* The interhemispheric subdural hematoma is poorly seen on this study. *F,* A coronal image demonstrates the ventriculostomy catheter *(arrowhead).* Also, note the depression of the corpus callosum *(white arrow)* by the clot above it. Note the mixed signal intensity in the blood. *G,* A slice further posterior to that shown in *F* better demonstrates the hematoma above the corpus callosum *(arrows).* As this is a T$_1$-weighted image, it is relatively isointense with brain. Also, note the interhemispheric subdural hematoma *(arrowheads). H,* This T$_1$-weighted sagittal image clearly demonstrates the depression of the corpus callosum *(arrowheads)* by the clot. Note elevation of the pericallosal artery by the clot *(arrows).*

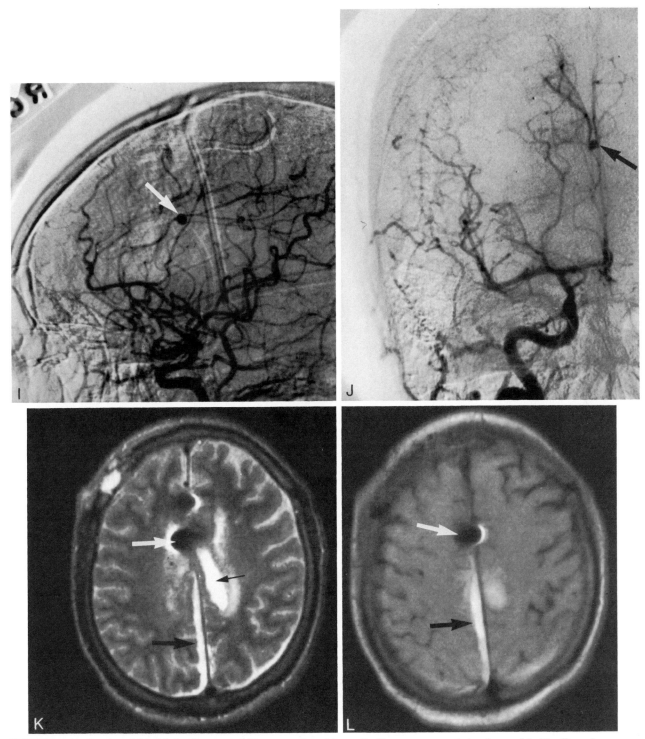

FIGURE 1–12 *Continued* **Multiple Computed Tomography, Magnetic-Resonance, and Angiographic Findings in Severe Closed Head Injury**

• • • •

I, Lateral view of the patient's arteriogram shows a pericallosal artery in an approximately normal location (the clot and depression of the corpus callosum are counterbalanced angiographically). There is an aneurysm on the pericallosal artery *(arrow)*. *J*, An anteroposterior view of the arteriogram shows the aneurysm *(arrow)*. Note the splaying of the anterior cerebral arteries by the subdural hematoma (seen in this view immediately above the aneurysm). At surgery, this was a traumatic pseudoaneurysm produced by arterial shearing under the falx. *K*, MR scan obtained approximately 2 weeks later shows an artifact from the metallic clip that was placed on the aneurysm *(white arrow)*. Note that the intraventricular blood *(small black arrow)* and subdural hematoma *(large black arrow)* have now become bright on this T$_2$-weighted image. *L*, A T$_1$-weighted image obtained at the same time as *K* also shows the artifact from the clip *(white arrow)* and the increased signal intensity in the interhemispheric fissure subdural hematoma *(black arrow)*. This case illustrates the change in signal intensity observed over time with the MR scan of blood. These images were obtained at 0.35 Tesla.

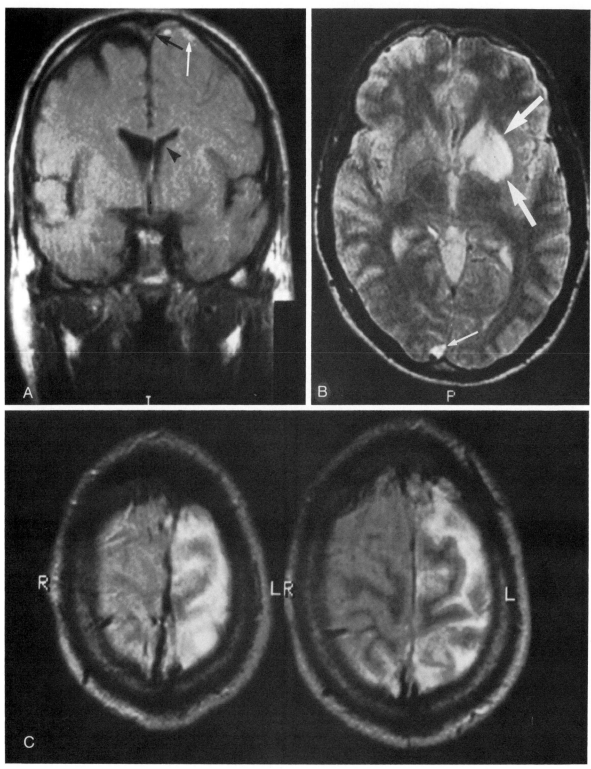

FIGURE 1–13. Sagittal Sinus Thrombosis Treated with Thrombolytic Infusion

• • • •

Sagittal sinus thrombosis, a rare complication of trauma, is more frequently seen idiopathically or in association with tumors. In this patient, progressive hemiparesis was seen following a weekend of heavy physical activity and presumed dehydration. *A*, A coronal magnetic resonance (MR) scan demonstrates absence of signal void in the superior sagittal sinus *(arrow)*. Note also the effacement of sulci in the left hemisphere and the compression of the lateral ventricle *(arrowhead)*. A small amount of increased signal in the vertex region *(small white arrow)* indicates some hemorrhagic diathesis. *B*, This transaxial MR scan shows increased signal intensity in the basal ganglia on the left *(large arrows)*. Note also the increased signal in the sagittal sinus posteriorly *(small arrow)*. *C*, A proton density-weighted image of the upper part of the brain (in the region where the sulcal effacement was seen on the coronal image) shows increased signal in the left hemisphere.

28

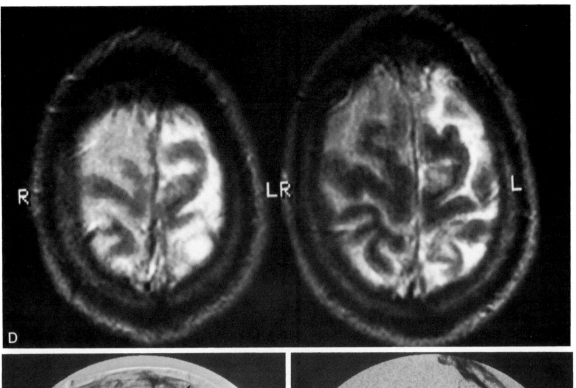

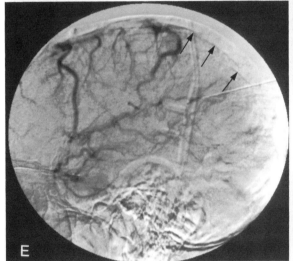

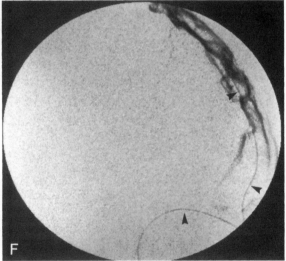

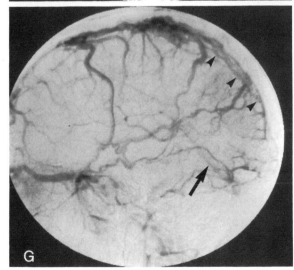

FIGURE 1–13 *Continued* **Sagittal Sinus Thrombosis Treated with Thrombolytic Infusion**

• • • •

D, The increased signal is also shown on the T₂-weighted image. This is consistent with cerebral edema resulting from venous congestion. *E,* Angiography shows the absence of the filling of the superior sagittal sinus *(arrows).* *F,* The absence of filling was treated by retrograde catheterization of the sagittal sinus through the thrombus and the infusion of 1.8 million units of urokinase for 8 hours. In this figure, the catheter is shown traversing the transverse sinus into the superior sagittal sinus *(arrowheads).* Note the filling defects within the sagittal sinus; they are consistent with intraluminal thrombus. *G,* The patient was returned to the intensive care unit and received another infusion of 500,000 units of urokinase over the ensuing 5 hours. Following catheter withdrawal, this arteriogram shows improved canalization of the superior sagittal sinus *(arrowheads).* The straight sinus is now seen as filling on the arteriogram *(arrow),* whereas it was previously nonfilling. The patient subsequently made a complete neurologic recovery.

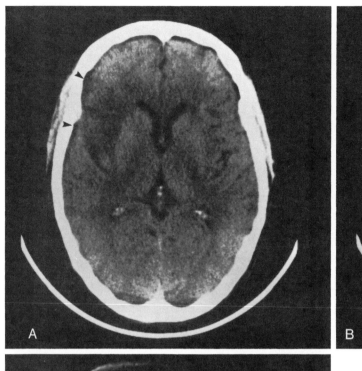

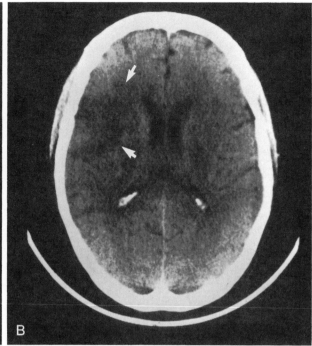

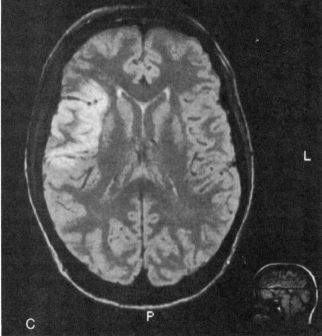

FIGURE 1–14. Magnetic Resonance and Computed Tomography Appearance of an Infarct in the Distribution of the Middle Cerebral Artery

• • • •

A, A computed tomography (CT) scan at the level of the lateral ventricles shows a wedge of low density in the right frontal lobe, near the frontal horn of the lateral ventricles *(arrowheads).* *B,* A slightly higher slice again shows the same wedge of low density *(arrows).* *C,* A magnetic resonance (MR) scan with either spin-density or T_2-weighting shows cerebral edema prominently. In this image, the area of infarction is shown as a wedge of high signal intensity in the same distribution as was seen on the CT scan. The MR appearance of the infarct is more conspicuous than its CT appearance.

intensity on T_2-weighted MR images in the distribution of the vascular territory involved (Fig. 1–14).

Both contusion and laceration of the brain present as blood on imaging studies. Acute blood appears dense on CT scans. On MR images extremely acute blood can appear isointense or hypointense, but in the subacute phase blood becomes intense on both T_1- and T_2-weighted images. One must be aware that these changes occur over time. The ability of MR techniques to image multiple properties of the tissue

(T_1, T_2, and proton density) can be used to advantage to separate normal from abnormal structures.

MR imaging detects subarachnoid blood poorly. The abnormal collection of blood can be diffuse in patients with contusion. This is largely a function of the severity of the injury. The blood can also be punctate and scattered. Small contusions may be subtle at CT but should be sought as an indicator of the extent of injury. Since blood induces swelling in the surrounding brain, MR is particularly useful in a delayed setting for verification of the extent of injury (see Fig. 1–12). In that setting, contusions appear bright on T$_2$-weighted images.

In laceration, the hemorrhage is seen along the track of the projectile (Fig. 1–15), and can be used to localize the path of the projectile (Fig. 1–16). This may be useful during a forensic analysis. Another consideration in a setting of laceration is the possibility of vascular injury, which can result in severe or even fatal intracranial hemorrhage. However, the development of clot around the injury can stop active bleeding, leading to survival. The possibility of vascular injury must be entertained when the path of a projectile crosses the potential course of major cerebral arteries. Angiography can be performed to exclude vascular injury (laceration, occlusion, or pseudoaneurysm formation) in that setting. Iatrogenic vascular injury may be seen following some surgical procedures (Fig. 1–17).

Brain swelling presents as low density on CT scans. On MR images it presents as low signal intensity on T$_1$-weighted images and high signal intensity on T$_2$-weighted images. Associated findings include effacement of the ventricular system, the cerebral sulci, and the junction between gray matter and white matter. When the edema is focal, the mass effect can produce significant shifts in the midline or in posterior fossa structures. In more extreme examples of midline shift, transtentorial herniation can result. The shift of the midline gradually pushes the midbrain against the contralateral tentorial incisura. Because the oculomotor (third) nerve exits the brain stem near that location, it is compressed, and the patient develops a palsy of both the pupillomotor ("blown pupil") and oculomotor components. Since the cerebral aqueduct (aqueduct of Sylvius) passes through the midbrain near that location, compression of the midbrain results in compression of the aqueduct.

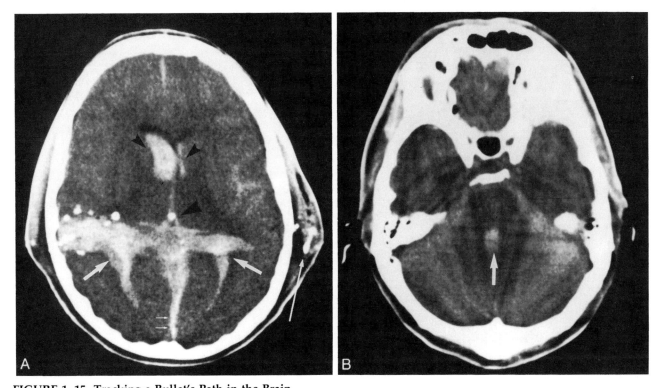

FIGURE 1–15. Tracking a Bullet's Path in the Brain

• • • •

A, The course of a projectile that has traversed brain tissue can often be traced by studying the hematoma left in its place or the fragments of the projectile. In this patient, a bullet entered the right parietal region and traversed the ventricular trigonal area bilaterally *(large arrows).* It also traversed the region of the vein of Galen and left a subdural hematoma in the interhemispheric fissure (seen on this cut posteriorly *[small arrows]).* Note also the presence of a bullet fragment and blood in the third ventricle *(large arrowhead),* blood in the frontal horns of the lateral ventricles bilaterally *(small arrowheads),* and some subarachnoid blood in the left sylvian fissure. There is soft tissue swelling on the scalp bilaterally that corresponds to the regions of entry and exit. A bone fragment is seen in the scalp swelling on the left *(long white arrow).* This suggests that this is the exit zone (bone fragments in the entry zone are pushed intracranially rather than extracranially as a rule). *B,* On a lower cut, blood is seen in the fourth ventricle *(arrow).* Additionally, lateral to the cut on either side, increased density peripheral to the cerebellum and brain stem indicates subarachnoid blood.

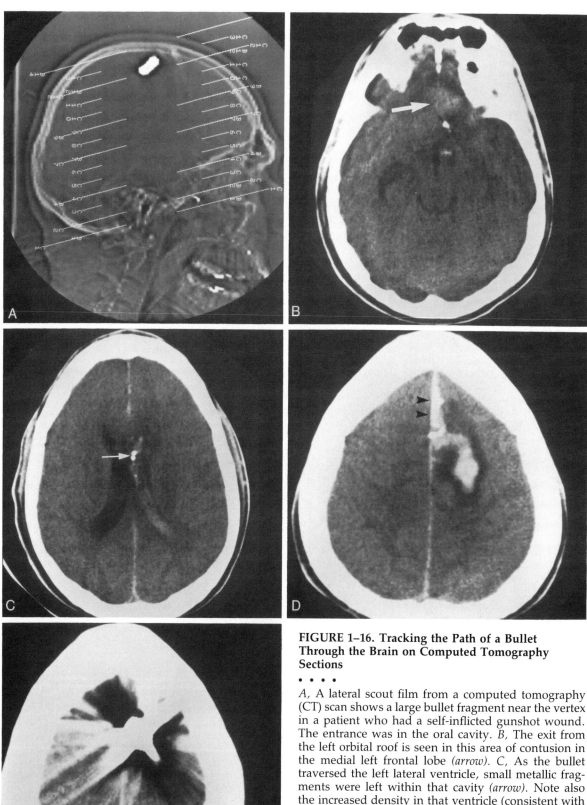

FIGURE 1–16. Tracking the Path of a Bullet Through the Brain on Computed Tomography Sections

• • • •

A, A lateral scout film from a computed tomography (CT) scan shows a large bullet fragment near the vertex in a patient who had a self-inflicted gunshot wound. The entrance was in the oral cavity. *B,* The exit from the left orbital roof is seen in this area of contusion in the medial left frontal lobe *(arrow). C,* As the bullet traversed the left lateral ventricle, small metallic fragments were left within that cavity *(arrow).* Note also the increased density in that ventricle (consistent with blood). *D,* A focal hematoma in the upper frontal lobe is seen on this cut where the bullet traversed the brain. The hemorrhage dissects toward the midline from the hematoma. Note also the subdural hematoma in the interhemispheric fissure on the left *(arrowheads). E,* The metallic artifact in this high cut obscures anatomic detail because the scan includes the bullet fragment.

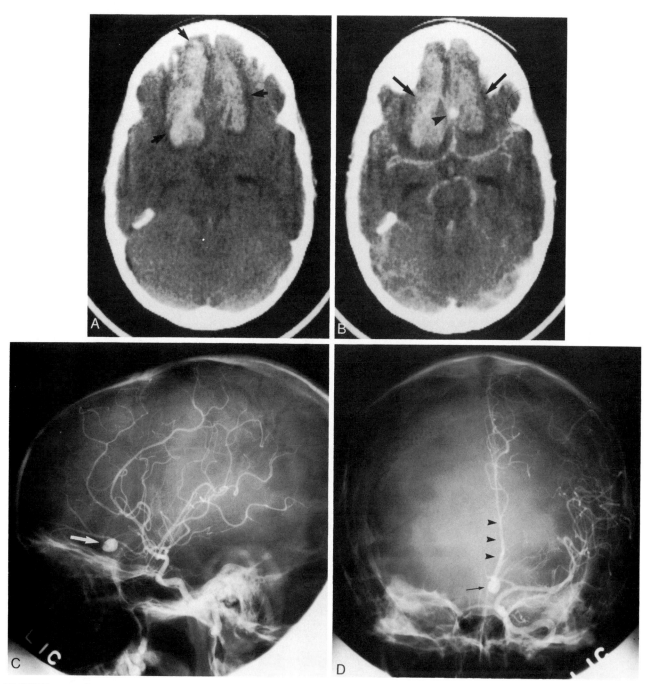

FIGURE 1–17. Iatrogenic Brain Injury

• • • •

A, An 11-year-old white male underwent sinus surgery at an outside hospital. He presented with declining mental status. This computed tomography (CT) scan showed bifrontal hematomas *(arrows). B,* A CT scan after contrast material administration shows the same bifrontal hematomas *(arrows)* and a rounded enhancing lesion *(arrowhead),* suspected to represent an aneurysm. *C,* A lateral view from a left internal carotid arteriogram showing a pseudoaneurysm of the frontopolar artery *(arrow). D,* An AP view showing an aneurysm *(arrow)* as well as right-to-left shift of the anterior cerebral artery *(arrowheads).* At surgery, a defect in the cribriform plate was found adjacent to the aneurysm, presumably where the biopsy instrument perforated the cribriform plate.

This impedes the drainage of cerebrospinal fluid from the lateral and the third ventricles, resulting in hydrocephalus. However, since the ventricle ipsilateral to the mass effect is compressed, the contralateral lateral ventricle is often the only one to dilate. Often, dilatation of the temporal horn of the lateral ventricle is the earliest sign of this phenomenon. Therefore, in a setting of midline shift, dilatation of the lateral ventricle opposite the mass effect is an indication of transtentorial herniation (Fig. 1–18).

The effects of compression can be difficult to separate from the effects of ischemia and the direct effects of trauma but should be considered. This can be especially important in the posterior fossa, where the brain is relatively unforgiving of any mass effect, and where important brain stem structures are compressed by hematomas of small volume. This is seen most commonly with subdural or epidural collections.

As mentioned earlier, hydrocephalus can result from the herniation and the compression of the cerebral aqueduct. However, it can also result from a defect of cerebrospinal fluid resorption following trauma. This can be a consequence of subarachnoid hemorrhage. In the elderly or in the chronic state following trauma, the separation of hydrocephalus occurring on a hydrodynamic basis from that occurring as a result of atrophy—known as *hydrocephalus ex vacuo*— can be difficult. Generally, atrophic processes produce relatively less dilatation of the temporal horns than the bodies of the lateral ventricles, whereas hydrodynamic hydrocephalus often causes early temporal horn enlargement. If the lateral and the third ventricles are significantly dilated, but the fourth ventricle is small, obstruction at the level of the cerebral aqueduct should be considered. Lumbar puncture may be performed to help ascertain cerebrospinal fluid pressures as well.

Ischemic injury can be a result of direct injury to vascular structures or be caused by compression. When compression is a consequence of local mass effect, infarction may occur in the territory of the compressed artery. The most common example of this is occipital infarction resulting from the compression of the posterior cerebral artery at the tentorial incisura at the time of transtentorial herniation.

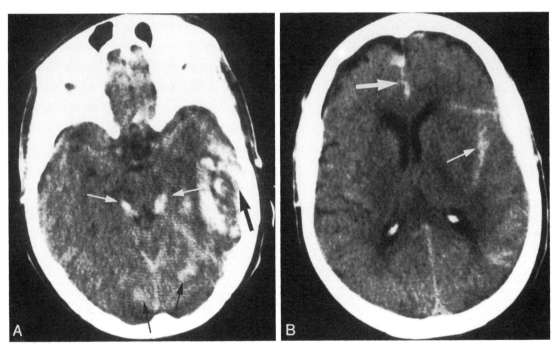

FIGURE 1–18. Progressive Edema, Infarction, and Transtentorial Herniation in a Closed Head Injury

• • • •

A, This patient was a pedestrian struck by a motor vehicle. In this lower cut, taken on the first day, focal hematoma in the ambient cisterns lateral to the midbrain can be seen bilaterally *(small white arrows).* Additionally, note the large contusion in the temporal lobe laterally on the left *(larger black arrow).* There are also scattered punctate contusions *(small black arrows)* posteriorly bilaterally, suggesting that the patient suffered diffuse brain injury. *B,* At the level of the frontal horns of the lateral ventricles, notice the subarachnoid blood in the sylvian fissure on the left *(small arrow)* and in the interhemispheric fissure *(large arrow).* There is perhaps an early appearance of asymmetry between the two hemispheres, with a slightly lower density appearance and a slightly less well defined junction between the gray matter and the white matter on the left as compared with that on the right. This finding is subtle but may be the earliest indication of diffuse edema.

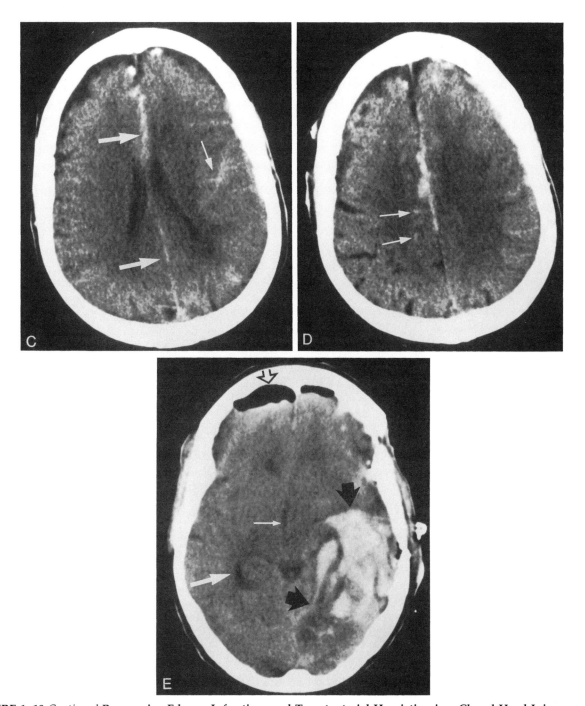

FIGURE 1–18 *Continued* **Progressive Edema, Infarction, and Transtentorial Herniation in a Closed Head Injury**
• • • •
C, At the level of the bodies of the lateral ventricles and the corpus callosum, note again the collection of blood in the interhemispheric fissure *(larger arrows)* and in the depths of a cerebral sulcus *(smaller arrow)*. Again, we see evidence of diffuse cerebral edema, indicated by effacement of sulci in the left hemisphere as compared with those in the right and by a less well defined junction between gray matter and white matter. D, Note the punctate contusions in the white matter *(arrows)* above the ventricles in the centrum semiovale. E, On the second day the patient's temporal lobe hematoma was evacuated (note the craniotomy over the left temporal lobe). However, the contusion has continued to evolve posteriorly and is now extending toward the occipital lobe *(closed black arrows)*. Note the pneumocephalus anteriorly from the patient's craniotomy *(open black arrow)*. Emerging signs of early transtentorial herniation include the left-to-right shift of the third ventricle *(small white arrow)* and the early dilatation of the temporal horn on the right *(large white arrow)*.

Illustration continued on following page

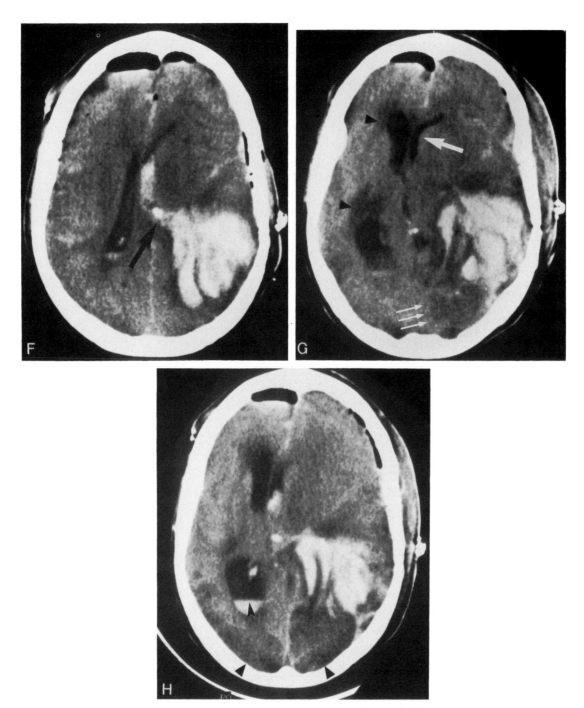

FIGURE 1–18 *Continued* **Progressive Edema, Infarction, and Transtentorial Herniation in a Closed Head Injury**
• • • •

F, In a higher cut also taken on the second day note the extension of the hematoma medially. It has now ruptured into the ventricular cavity *(arrow)* and in its medial extent forms a cast within the lateral ventricle. Note the midline shift in this ventricular cast from left to right. *G,* On the third day the patient has evidence of full-blown transtentorial herniation. The frontal horn of the left lateral ventricle is compressed and shifted to the right *(large white arrow)*. The right lateral ventricle is dilated. Anteriorly we see the frontal horn, and posteriorly we see the temporal horn in this slice *(arrowheads)*. Posteriorly, there is a margin between low density and normal density *(small white arrows)*; this is the margin between the infarcted occipital lobes and the more normal, uninfarcted cerebellum underlying the tentorium. *H,* In a higher cut we see the diffuse occipital lobe infarctions bilaterally *(large arrowheads)*. This is observed in transtentorial herniation when the posterior cerebral arteries become kinked between the swollen brain and the tentorium as they pass laterally around the midbrain. This results in the restriction of flow and in the infarction of the occipital lobes. On the left, note the diffuse low density in the brain with diffuse effacement of the junction between gray matter and white matter. In the medial frontal area this indicates anterior cerebral artery involvement. In the large wedge laterally this indicates middle cerebral artery involvement. In the occipital lobe it indicates posterior cerebral artery involvement. Thus, the entire left hemisphere is infarcted. The small arrowhead shows the fluid-fluid level within the ventricle. This signifies the layering of blood within the cerebrospinal fluid, with the higher density representing blood and the lower density representing cerebrospinal fluid. Subsequently the patient expired.

CT will demonstrate low density in the occipital lobe opposite the mass effect (see Fig. 1–18).

When diffuse brain swelling occurs, compression can result from diffuse mass effect. Both hydrocephalus and diffuse brain swelling can produce a sufficient increase in intracranial pressure to impede blood flow. The existence of gradations of injury from diffuse ischemia has not been thoroughly explored. The most extreme example of diffuse mass effect, however, is brain death. In this entity, diffuse swelling causes such a significant rise in intracranial pressure that circulatory arrest is produced. Thus, there is no flow to the brain on an angiogram performed to evaluate for that entity. The CT scan shows diffuse effacement of the junction between gray and white matter, effacement of the sulci, and a homogeneous low density in the brain. Multifocal injury from ischemia can also be seen as a consequence of severe subarachnoid hemorrhage resulting in vasospasm. Vasospasm is a much more frequent consequence of hemorrhage; however, it results from aneurysmal rupture due to the formation of a local clot around the artery. Intracranial angioplasty has been shown to be effective in a setting of severe vasospasm in association with subarachnoid hemorrhage and should be considered if the patient fails a brief trial of aggressive medical management.

Bibliography

Adams JH, Doyle D, Graham DI, Lawrence AMDR. Diffuse axonal injury in head injuries caused by a fall. Lancet 1984; 2:1420–1421.

Adams JH, Graham DI, Scott G, et al. Brain damage in fatal non-missile head injury. J Clin Pathol 1980; 33:1132–1145.

Adams JH, Mitchell DE, Graham DI, Doyle D. Diffuse brain damage of immediate impact type. Brain 1977; 100:489–502.

Al-Mefty O, Holoubi A, Fox JL. Value of angiography in cerebral nail-gun injuries. AJNR 1986; 7:164–165.

Anderson DW, Kalsbeek WD. The national head and spinal cord injury survey: Assessment of some uncertainties affecting the findings. J Neurosurg 1980; 53:532–534.

Bakay L. The value of CT scan in gunshot injuries of the brain. Acta Neurochir (Wien) 1984; 71:189–204.

Bingas B, Vogt U. The traumatic aneurysm of intracranial vessels. Neurosurg Rev 1980; 3:197–199.

Braakman R. Depressed skull fracture: Data, treatment, and follow-up in 225 consecutive cases. J Neurol Neurosurg Psychiatry 1972; 35:395–402.

Brown FD, Mullan S, Duda EE. Delayed traumatic intracerebral hematomas: Report of three cases. J Neurosurg 1978; 48:1019–1022.

Bruce DA, Alavi A, Bilaniuk L, et al. Diffuse cerebral swelling following head injuries in children: The syndrome of "malignant brain edema." J Neurosurg 1981; 54:170–178.

Bruce DA, Schut L, Sutton L. Brain and cervical spine injuries occurring during organized sports activities in children and adolescents. Prim Care 1984; 11:175–194.

Brunetti J, Zingesser L, Dunn J, Rovit RL. Delayed intracerebral hemorrhage as demonstrated by CT scanning. Neuroradiology 1979; 18:43–46.

Bullock R, Smith R, Favier J, et al. Brain specific gravity and CT scan density measurements after human head injury. J Neurosurg 1985; 63:64–68.

Cao M, Lisheng H, Shouzheng S. Resolution of brain edema in severe brain injury at controlled high and low intracranial pressures. J Neurosurg 1984; 61:707–712.

Carey ME, Tutton RH, Strub RL, et al. The correlation between surgical and CT estimates of brain damage following missile wounds. J Neurosurg 1984; 60:947–954.

Carey ME, Young HF, Mathis JL. The neurosurgical treatment of craniocerebral missile wounds in Vietnam. Surg Gynecol Obstet 1972; 135:386–390.

Casson IR, Sham R, Campbell EA, et al. Neurological and CT evaluation of knocked-out boxer. J Neurol Neurosurg Psychiatry 1982; 45:170–174.

Clifton GL, Grossman RG, Makela ME, et al. Neurological course and correlated computerized tomography findings after severe closed head injury. J Neurosurg 1980; 52:611–624.

Clifton GL, McCormick WF, Grossman RG. Neuropathology of early and late deaths after head injury. Neurosurgery 1981; 8:309–314.

Cohen WA, Kricheff II. Craniocerebral trauma. In McCort JJ (ed): Trauma Radiology. New York: Churchill Livingstone, Inc., 1990, pp 1–29.

Cooper PR, Maravilla K, Kirkpatrick J, et al. Traumatically induced brain stem hemorrhage and the computerized tomographic scan: Clinical, pathological, and experimental observations. Neurosurgery 1979; 4:115–124.

Cooper PR, Maravilla K, Moody S, Clark WK. Serial computerized tomographic scanning and the prognosis of severe head injury. Neurosurgery 1979; 5:566–569.

Cordobes F, Lobato RD, Rivas JJ, et al. Post-traumatic diffuse axonal brain injury. Analysis of 78 patients studied with computed tomography. Acta Neurochir 1986; 81:27–35.

Dacey RG, Alves WM, Rimel RW, et al. Neurosurgical complications after apparently minor head injury. J Neurosurg 1986; 65:203–210.

Davidoff G, Morris J, Roth E, Bleiberg J. Closed head injury in spinal cord injured patients. Retrospective study of loss of consciousness and post-traumatic amnesia. Arch Phys Med Rehabil 1985; 66:41–43.

Davis RA, Cunningham PS. Prognostic factors in severe head injury. Surg Gynecol Obstet 1984; 159:597–604.

Diaz FG, Yock DH, Larson D, Rocksworld GL. Early diagnosis of delayed post-traumatic intracerebral hematomas. J Neurosurg 1979; 50:217–223.

Doron Y, Gruszkiewica J, Peyser E. Penetrating craniocerebral injuries due to unusual foreign bodies. Neurosurg Rev 1982; 5:35–40.

Dublin AB, French BN, Rennick JM. Computed tomography in head trauma. Radiology 1977; 122:365–369.

Echizenya K, Satoh M, Nakagawa T, et al. Bitemporal compression injury caused by static loading mechanism. J Neurosurg 1985; 62:438–441.

Esparza J, M-Portillo J, Sarabia M, et al. Outcome in children with severe head injuries. Childs Nerv Syst 1985; 1:109–114.

Espersen JO, Petersen OF. Computerized tomography (CT) in patients with head injuries: Relation between CT scans and clinical findings in 96 patients. Acta Neurochir 1981; 56:201–217.

Fleischer AS, Huhn SL, Meislin H. Post-traumatic acute obstructive hydrocephalus. Ann Emerg Med 1988; 17:165–167.

Freytag E. Autopsy findings in head injuries from firearms. Arch Pathol 1963; 76:111–121.

Gandy SE, Snow RB, Zimmerman RD, Deck MD. Cranial nuclear magnetic resonance imaging in head trauma. Ann Neurol 1984; 16:254–257.

Gennarelli TA, Spielman GM, Langfitt TW, et al. Influence of the type of intracranial lesion on outcome from severe head injury. J Neurosurg 1982; 56:26–32.

Gentry LR, Godersky JC, Thompson B. MR imaging of head trauma: Review of the distribution and radiopathologic features of traumatic lesions. AJR 1988; 150:663–672.

Gentry LR, Godersky JC, Thompson B. MR imaging of head trauma: Review of the distribution and radiopathologic features of traumatic lesions. AJNR 1988; 9:101–110.

Gentry LR, Godersky JC, Thompson B, Dunn VD. Prospective comparative study of intermediate-field MR and CT in the evaluation of closed head trauma. AJR 1988; 150:673–682.

Gentry LR, Godersky JC, Thompson B, Dunn VD. Prospective comparative study of intermediate-field MR and CT in the evaluation of closed head trauma. AJNR 1988; 9:91–100.

Gomori JM, Grossman RI, Hackney DB, et al. Variable appearances of subacute intracranial hematomas on high-field spin-echo MR. AJNR 1987; 8:1019–1026.

Graham DI, Adams JH, Doyle D. Ischaemic brain damage in fatal non-missile head injuries. J Neurol Sci 1978; 39:213–234.

Greenberg JO. Neuroimaging in brain swelling. Neurol Clin 1984; 2:677–694.

Groswasser Z, Reider-Groswasser I, Soroker N, Machtey Y. Magnetic resonance imaging in head injured patients with normal late computed tomography scans. Surg Neurol 1987; 27:331–337.

Gutierrez A, Gil L, Sahuquillo J, Rubio E. Unusual penetrating craniocerebral injury. Surg Neurol 1983; 19:541–543.

Haas DC, Lourie H. Trauma-triggered migraine: An explanation for common neurological attacks after mild head injury. J Neurosurg 1988; 68:181–188.

Hadley DM, Teasdale GM, Jenkins A, et al. Magnetic resonance imaging in acute head injury. Clin Radiol 1988; 39:131–139.

Hagan RE. Early complications following penetrating wounds of the brain. J Neurosurg 1971; 34:132–141.

Han JS, Kaufman B, Alfidi RJ, et al. Head trauma evaluated by magnetic resonance and computed tomography: A comparison. Radiology 1984; 150:71–77.

Hansen JE, Gudeman SK, Holgate RC, Saunders RA. Penetrating intracranial wood wounds: Clinical limitations of computerized tomography. J Neurosurg 1988; 68:752–756.

Healy JF, Crudale AS. Computed tomographic evaluation of depressed skull fractures and associated intracranial injury. Comput Radiol 1982; 6:323–330.

Helmke K, Kuhne D. Balloon embolisation of intracranial arteriovenous fistulas in children and juveniles. Pediatr Radiol 1985; 15:85–91.

Hesselbrock R, Sawaya R, Tomsick T, Wadhwa S. Superior sagittal sinus thrombosis after closed head injury. Neurosurgery 1985; 16:825–828.

Hesselink JR, Dowd CF, Healy ME, et al. MR imaging of brain contusions: A comparative study with CT. AJR 1988; 150:1133–1142.

Holland BA, Brant-Zawadzki M, Pitts LH. The role of CT in evaluation of head trauma. In Federle MP, Brant-Zawadzki M (eds): Computed Tomography in the Evaluation of Trauma. 2nd ed. Baltimore: Williams & Wilkins, 1986, pp 1–63.

Hume JH, Graham DI, Murray LS, Scott G. Diffuse axonal injury due to nonmissile head injury in humans: An analysis of 45 cases. Ann Neurol 1982; 12:557–563.

Hyman RA, Gorey MT. Imaging strategies for MR of the brain. Radiol Clin North Am 1988; 26:471–503.

Hyrshko FG, Deeb ZL. Computed tomography in acute head injuries. J Comput Tomogr 1983; 7:331–344.

Jacobs LM, Berrizbeitia LD, Ordia J. Crowbar impalement of the brain. J Trauma 1985; 25:359–361.

Jenkins A, Teasdale G, Hadley MDM, et al. Brain lesions detected by magnetic resonance imaging in mild and severe head injuries. Lancet 1986; 445–446.

Jennett B, Bond M. Assessment of outcome after severe brain damage. Lancet 1975; 480–484.

Jinkins JR. Post-traumatic ethmoidal pseudomeningoencephalocele. AJNR 1987; 8:649–651.

Jooma R, Bradshaw JR, Coakham HB. Computed tomography in penetrating cranial injury by a wooden foreign body. Surg Neurol 1984; 21:236–238.

Kaiser MC, Rodesch G, Capesius P. CT in a case of intracranial penetration of a pencil. Neuroradiology 1983; 24:229–231.

Katayama Y, Yoshida K, Ogawa H, Tsubokawa T. Traumatic homonymous hemianopsia associated with a juxtasellar hematoma after acute closed head injury. Surg Neurol 1985; 24:289–292.

Kaye EM, Herskowitz J. Transient post-traumatic cortical blindness: Brief vs. prolonged syndromes in childhood. J Child Neurol 1986; 1:206–210.

Keane JR. Traumatic internuclear ophthalmoplegia. J Clin Neuro Ophthalmol 1987; 7:165–166.

Kelly AB, Zimmerman RD, Snow RB, et al. Head trauma: Comparison of MR and CT: experience in 100 patients. AJNR 1988; 9:699–708.

Kim CH, Tanaka R, Kawakami K, Ito J. Traumatic primary intraventricular hemorrhage. Surg Neurol 1981; 16:415–417.

Kishore PRS, Lipper MH, Becker DP, et al. Significance of CT in head injury: Correlation with intracranial pressure. AJR 1981; 137:829–833.

Klauber MR, Barrett-Connor E, Marshall LF, Bowers SA. The epidemiology of head injury. Am J Epidemiol 1981; 113:500–509.

Klauber MR, Toutant SM, Marshall LF. A model for predicting delayed intracranial hypertension following severe head injury. J Neurosurg 1984; 61:659–699.

Kline LB, Morawetz RB, Swaid SN. Indirect injury of the optic nerve. Neurosurgery 1984; 14:756–764.

Kobayashi S, Nakazawa S, Otsuka T. Acute traumatic intraventricular hemorrhage in children. Childs Nerv Syst 1985; 1:18–23.

Kraus JF. A comparison of recent studies on the extent of the head and spinal cord injury problem in the United States. J Neurosurg 1980; 53:535–543.

Kraus JF, Black MA, Hessol N, et al. The incidence of acute brain injury and serious impairment in a defined population. Am J Epidemiol 1984; 119:186–201.

Kraus JF, Fife D, Conroy C. Pediatric brain injuries: The nature, clinical course, and early outcomes in a defined United States' population. Pediatrics 1987; 79:501–507.

Kraus JF, Fife D, Cox P, et al. Incidence, severity, and external causes of pediatric brain injury. Am J Dis Child 1986; 140:687–693.

Kriel RL, Sheehan M, Krach LE, et al. Pediatric head injury resulting from all-terrain vehicle accidents. Pediatrics 1986; 78:933–935.

Langfitt TW, Obrist WD, Alavi A, et al. Computerized tomography, magnetic resonance imaging, and positron emission tomography in the study of brain trauma. J Neurosurg 1986; 64:760–767.

Lesoin F, Viaud C, Pruvo J, et al. Traumatic and alternating delayed intracranial hematomas. Neuroradiology 1984; 26:515–516.

Levin HS, Amparo E, Eisenberg HM, et al. Magnetic resonance imaging and computerized tomography in relation to the neurobehavioral sequelae of mild and moderate head injuries. J Neurosurg 1987; 66:706–713.

Lindenberg R, Freytag E. The mechanism of cerebral contusions. Arch Pathol 1960; 69:440–469.

Lobato RD, Cordobes F, Rivas JJ, et al. Outcome from severe head injury related to the type of intracranial lesion. J Neurosurg 1983; 59:762–774.

MacEwan DW, Bristow GK, Gordon WL. Managed reduction of unnecessary skull radiography. J Can Assoc Radiol 1984; 35:287–290.

Macpherson P, Graham DI. Correlation between angiographic findings and the ischaemia of head injury. J Neurol Neurosurg Psychiatry 1978; 41:122–127.

Macpherson P, Teasdale E, Dhaker S, et al. The significance of traumatic haematoma in the region of the basal ganglia. J Neurol Neurosurg Psychiatry 1986; 49:29–34.

Manfredini M, Marliani AF. CT and plain X-ray examination of the skull in pure traumatic laceration of the brain. Neuroradiology 1983; 24:249–252.

Masters SJ, McClean PM, Arcarese JS, et al. Skull X-ray examinations after head trauma: Recommendations by a multidisciplinary panel and validation study. N Engl J Med 1987; 316:84–91.

Mauser HW, van Nieuwenhuizen O, Veiga-Pires JA. Is contrast-enhanced CT indicated in acute head injury?. Neuroradiology 1984; 26:31–32.

McMicken DB. Emergency CT head scans in traumatic and atraumatic conditions. Ann Emerg Med 1986; 15:274–279.

Meyers CA, Levin HS, Eisenberg HM, Guinto FC. Early versus

late lateral ventricular enlargement following closed head injury. J Neurol Neurosurg Psychiatry 1983; 46:1092–1097.

Mills ML, Russo LS, Vines FS, Ross BA. High-yield criteria for urgent cranial computed tomography scans. Ann Emerg Med 1986; 15:1167–1172.

Misra JC, Chakravarty S. A study on rotational brain injury. J Biomech 1984; 17:459–466.

Narayan RK, Greenberg RP, Miller JD, et al. Improved confidence of outcome prediction in severe head injury. J Neurosurg 1981; 54:751–762.

Okamoto H, Harada K, Yoshimoto H, Uozumi T. Acute epidural hematoma caused by contrecoup injury. Surg Neurol 1983; 20:461–463.

Papo I, Caruselli G, Luongo A, et al. Traumatic cerebral mass lesions: Correlations between clinical, intracranial pressure, and computed tomographic data. Neurosurgery 1980; 7:337–346.

Parkinson D, West M. Traumatic intracranial aneurysms. J Neurosurg 1980; 52:11–20.

Pasqualin A, Vivenza C, Rosta L, et al. Cerebral vasospasm after head injury. Neurosurgery 1984; 15:855–858.

Perini S, Beltramello A, Pasut ML, et al. CNS trauma: Head injuries. Neurol Clin 1984; 2:719–743.

Plum F, Posner JB (eds). The Diagnosis of Stupor and Coma. 3rd ed. Philadelphia: F.A.Davis Co., 1980.

Rahimizadeh A, Shakeri M, Amirdjamshidi A. Unusual craniocerebral injuries by glass fragments. Neurosurgery 1987; 21:427–428.

Rao N, Jellinek HM, Harvey RF, Flynn M. Computerized tomography head scans as predictors of rehabilitation outcome. Arch Phys Med Rehabil 1984; 65:18–20.

Rivara F, Tanaguchi D, Parish RA, et al. Poor prediction of positive computed tomographic scans by clinical criteria in symptomatic pediatric head trauma. Pediatrics 1987; 80:579–584.

Rosenberg RN, Grossman RG, Schochet SS Jr, et al. (eds). The Clinical Neurosciences. Vol 2. New York: Churchill Livingstone, Inc., 1983, pp 786–787, 1282.

Sahuquillo-Barris J, Lamarca-Ciuro J, Vilalta-Castan J, et al. Acute subdural hematoma and diffuse axonal injury after severe head trauma. J Neurosurg 1988; 68:894–900.

Seelig JM, Marshall LF, Toutant SM, et al. Traumatic acute epidural hematoma: Unrecognized high lethality in comatose patients. Neurosurgery 1984; 15:617–620.

Servadel F, Ciucci G, Pagano F, et al. Skull fracture as a risk factor of intracranial complications in minor head injuries: A prospective CT study in a series of 98 adult patients. J Neurol Neurosurg Psychiatry 1988; 51:526–528.

Smith MS, Buchsbaum HW, Masland WS. One and a half syndrome: Occurrence after trauma with computerized tomographic correlation. Arch Neurol 1980; 37:251.

Snoek J, Jennett B, Adams JH, et al. Computerized tomography after recent severe head injury in patients without acute intracranial haematoma. J Neurol Neurosurg Psychiatry 1979; 42:215–225.

Soloniuk D, Pitts LH, Lovely M, Bartkowski H. Traumatic intracerebral hematomas: Timing of appearance and indications for operative removal. J Trauma 1986; 26:787–794.

Stanley LD, Suss RA. Intracerebral hematoma secondary to lightning stroke: Case report and review of the literature. Neurosurgery 1985; 16:686–688.

Sweet RC, Miller JD, Lipper M, et al. Significance of bilateral abnormalities on the CT scan in patients with severe head injury. Neurosurgery 1978; 3:16–21.

Taylor SB, Quencer RM, Holzman BH, Naidich TP. Central nervous system anoxic-ischemic insult in children due to near-drowning. Radiology 1985; 156:641–646.

Thornbury JR, Campbell JA, Masters SJ, Fryback DG. Skull fracture and the low risk of intracranial sequelae in minor head trauma. AJR 1984; 143:661–664.

Toutant SM, Klauber MR, Marshall LF, et al. Absent or compressed basal cisterns on first CT scan: Ominous predictors of outcome in severe head injury. J Neurosurg 1984; 61:691–694.

Tsai FY, Teal JS, Itabashi HH, et al. Computed tomography of posterior fossa trauma. J Comput Assist Tomogr 1980; 4:291–305.

Tsai FY, Teal JS, Quinn MF, et al. CT of brain stem injury. AJR 1980; 134:717–723.

Tsementzis SS, Hitchcock ER. Head injury from firework explosion. Neurosurgery 1984; 15:719–723.

van Dongen KJ, Braakman R. Late computed tomography in survivors of severe head injury. Neurosurgery 1980; 7:14–22.

van Dongen KJ, Braakman R, Gelpke GJ. The prognostic value of computerized tomography in comatose head-injured patients. J Neurosurg 1983; 59:951–957.

Wilberger JE, Deeb Z, Rothfus W. Magnetic resonance imaging in cases of severe head injury. Neurosurgery 1987; 20:571–576.

Wilson JTL, Wiedmann KD, Hadley DM, et al. Early and late magnetic resonance imaging and neuropsychological outcome after head injury. J Neurol Neurosurg Psychiatry 1988; 51:391–396.

Yamamoto I, Yamada S, Sato O. Unusual craniocerebral penetrating injury by a chopstick. Surg Neurol 1985; 23:396–398.

Yano M, Ikeda Y, Kobayashi S, Otsuka T. Intracranial pressure in head-injured patients with various intracranial lesions is identical throughout the supratentorial intracranial compartment. Neurosurgery 1987; 21:688–692.

Yonas H, Snyder JV, Gur D, et al. Local cerebral blood flow alterations (Xe-CT method) in an accident victim. J Comput Assist Tomogr 1984; 8:990–991.

Young HA, Gleave JRW, Schmidek HH, Gregory S. Delayed traumatic intracerebral hematoma: Report of 15 cases operatively treated. Neurosurgery 1984; 14:22–25.

Young HA, Schmidek HH. Complications accompanying occipital skull fracture. J Trauma 1982; 22:914–920.

Zimmerman RA, Bilaniuk LT, Genneralli T. Computed tomography of shearing injuries of the cerebral white matter. Radiology 1978; 127:393–396.

Zimmerman RA, Bilaniuk LT, Hackney DB, et al. Head injury: Early results of comparing CT and high-field MR. AJNR 1986; 7:757–764.

Zimmerman RD, Heier LA, Snow RB, et al. Acute intracranial hemorrhage: Intensity changes on sequential MR scans at 0.5 T. AJR 1988; 9:47–57.

CHAPTER 2

The Calvarium and the Extra-axial Spaces

WILLIAM DEATON, JR., M.D.

THE CALVARIUM

Skull Fractures

Fractures of the calvarium occur frequently with trauma to the head. In the past, a calvarial fracture associated with neurologic deficits was an indication to perform emergency angiography to look for a subdural or an epidural hematoma or brain contusion and swelling. Since the development of computed tomography (CT) and magnetic resonance (MR) imaging, however, angiography is no longer a screening technique for intracranial injury. At the same time, the importance of the plain film diagnosis of a skull fracture has markedly diminished. Radiographs of the skull are no longer a routine part of the evaluation of head trauma. Patients who have had a minor injury that causes a scalp laceration or a minor headache should not have skull films and usually can be discharged after a brief period of observation. Patients with more serious trauma and more impressive symptoms, such as amnesia, vomiting, or palpable depressed skull fractures, need CT evaluation of the intracranial contents; their skulls can be eval-

uated by CT using bone windows. Skull series rarely add any useful information to the CT study, which must be performed to evaluate the brain and extra-axial spaces. The patient who has a rapidly deteriorating mental status generally needs emergency CT and emergency surgery. If CT is not readily available, a portable anteroposterior (AP) and lateral skull series on the way to the operating room may occasionally aid the neurosurgeon in his or her approach to the treatment of a patient.

Skull films, therefore, are rarely needed in the evaluation of head trauma. Although injury to the box may affect the contents, it is the injury to the contents of the box that is important. Skull films should be reserved for use only when they may provide an answer to a specific question. In the pediatric population where the possibility of child abuse may exist, skull films may be helpful for medicolegal documentation even though they are not important in the medical management of the patient.

Linear Skull Fractures

Calvarial fractures fall into two categories, linear fractures and depressed fractures. A linear fracture

---

• • • • • *APPROPRIATE RADIOGRAPHIC STUDIES*

    I. **Skull Series**
       A. Includes lateral view, anteroposterior (AP) view, and Towne's view.
       B. Portable examination usually includes one lateral view and an AP view.
      Comment: No longer indicated routinely but may have use in patients who are too seriously injured to undergo computed tomography (CT).

    II. **Computed Tomography**
       A. A noncontrast enhanced study is performed using contiguous 10-mm sections from the foramen magnum to the top of the brain.
       B. Contrast enhancement may aid in the evaluation of acute problems superimposed on chronic disease.
      Comment: Although high-resolution scans are desirable, short scanning time studies may be performed in agitated patients. CT is the current scanning procedure of choice. Thinner (5-mm) sections through the posterior fossa may be advantageous.

    III. **Magnetic Resonance Imaging**
       A. Both T_1- and T_2-weighted sequences are generally needed.
       B. In addition to the axial plane, coronal or sagittal sequences may be of use.
      Comment: Not readily available everywhere for emergency studies. Acute blood is often isointense with brain. Magnetic resonance (MR) imaging is not as useful for studying bone injury as CT. The technique isolates a seriously injured patient who may be unstable. It is, however, excellent for identifying subacute hemorrhage.

    IV. **Angiography**
      Comment: No longer indicated to study subdural and epidural hematomas, but may be needed in selected patients for associated injuries.

---

has virtually no clinical significance unless it crosses the path of a meningeal artery, potentially injuring that vessel. The exception occurs in the pediatric age group, since leptomeningeal cysts may develop at the site of linear fracture. Tears of the middle meningeal arteries can cause epidural hematomas. Linear skull fractures are seen on skull radiographs as sharply defined dark lines that are often angular in course (Fig. 2–1). They may branch. Vascular grooves are generally less sharply defined and have a gently curving, smooth, rounded course (Fig. 2–2). Vascular grooves also branch. Sutures in general have serrated edges and are symmetric and bilateral. As fractures heal their margins become less distinct. A healing fracture may resemble a vascular groove, but generally fractures do not follow the usual course of the meningeal arteries and can be easily distinguished. Linear fractures are seen as cortical discontinuity on CT scans. Bone windows are necessary (Fig. 2–3).

Depressed Skull Fractures

Depressed skull fractures are usually caused by a direct, highly localized blow to the calvarium. Multiple fragments are present. These often radiate from a central point, but any pattern of fragments is possible. The important consequence of depressed fractures is the pushing of bone fragments into the cranial cavity; these fragments may press upon or actually penetrate the brain. The depth of depression is very easily determined by CT (Fig. 2–4). Tangential skull films of the fracture were needed to determine the depth of depression before CT was developed. Many depressed fragments need surgical elevation of the fragments and repair of the dural rents.

The skull film findings of a depressed fracture include more than one fracture line, overlapping bone fragments causing areas of added bone density,

Text continued on page 48

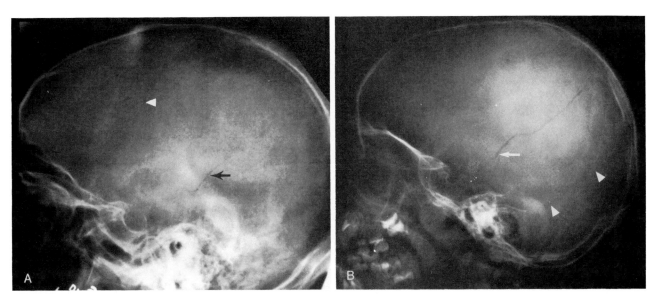

FIGURE 2–1. Linear Skull Fracture

• • • •

A, A short, sharply defined linear skull fracture *(arrow)* is seen in the posterior temporoparietal region. It is much more sharply defined than are the vascular grooves *(arrowhead). B,* A longer linear skull fracture is sharply defined. It crosses a vascular groove *(arrow).* A serrated occipital suture *(arrowheads)* is easily seen and is quite different from the sharply defined fracture line.

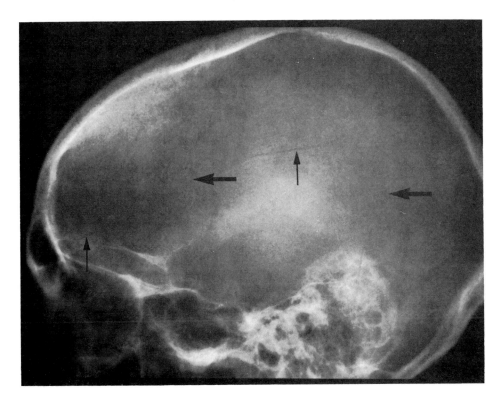

FIGURE 2–2. Vascular Grooves Contrasted with Linear Fractures

• • • •

This patient was the victim of an aggravated assault and was found unconscious under a bridge. Two sharply defined linear skull fractures *(small arrows)* contrast with the less distinct vascular grooves *(large arrows).*

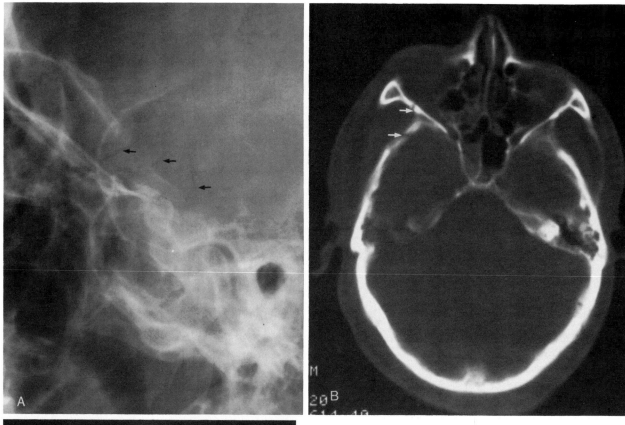

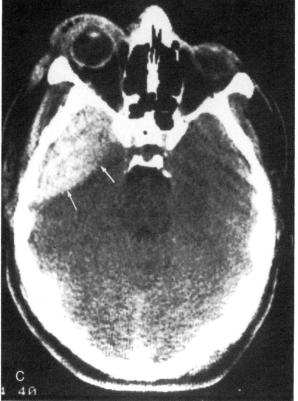

FIGURE 2–3. Computed Tomography (CT) Demonstration of Linear Skull Fracture

• • • •

A, This skull film demonstrates several linear skull fractures *(arrows).* *B,* A CT section of the same patient displayed appropriately for bone demonstrates the linear fractures *(arrows).* In addition, there are air-fluid levels in both halves of the sphenoid sinus and opacification of the dorsal right ethmoid air cells. Soft tissue swelling is noted over the fractures and the right orbit. *C,* The same CT section displayed for soft tissue detail demonstrates a large, right-middle-fossa epidural hematoma *(arrows)* and air in the soft tissues over the right globe.

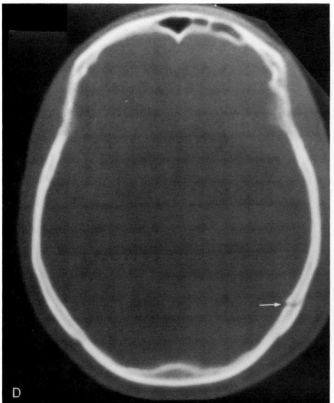

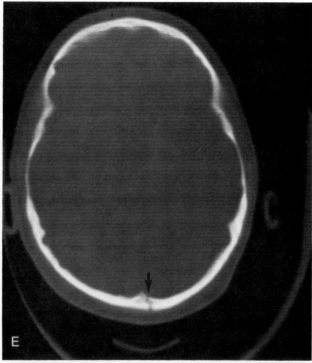

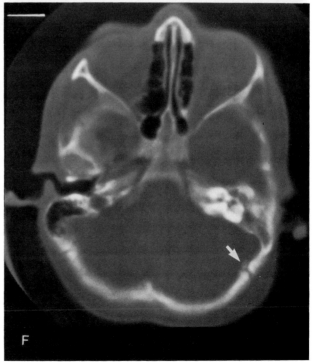

FIGURE 2–3 *Continued* **Computed Tomography (CT) Demonstration of Linear Skull Fracture**

• • • •

D, A CT bone window display on a second patient demonstrates another linear skull fracture *(arrow).* There is some associated soft tissue swelling. *E,* A linear fracture *(arrow)* near the confluens sinuum. A fracture in this location should raise concern for venous injury and possible venous epidural hematoma. *F,* Sutures *(arrow)* must not be confused with fractures at CT. In this patient the head is not quite straight and therefore the sutures are not symmetric. An accessory bone could confuse the issue further unless the reader is careful.

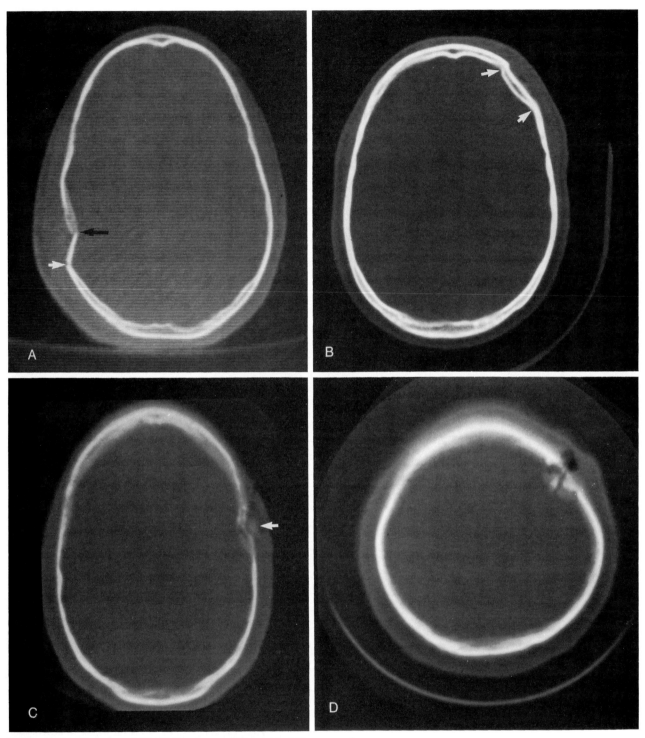

FIGURE 2–4. Depressed Skull Fractures at Computed Tomography
• • • •
A, A depressed fracture is demonstrated in the posterior parietal bone. Such fractures are always comminuted. The point of greatest depression *(black arrow)* and another fracture line *(white arrow)* can be seen. *B,* A frontal-bone depressed fracture *(arrows)* has associated air in the soft tissues and demonstrates some swelling. *C,* The skull is more fragmented in this depressed fracture. In addition, packing *(arrow)* is seen in the scalp laceration. *D,* The depressed fragments are easily seen and their depth can be measured. Air is seen in the scalp. This display used a window of 4000 Hounsfield units (H) and a level of 400 H.

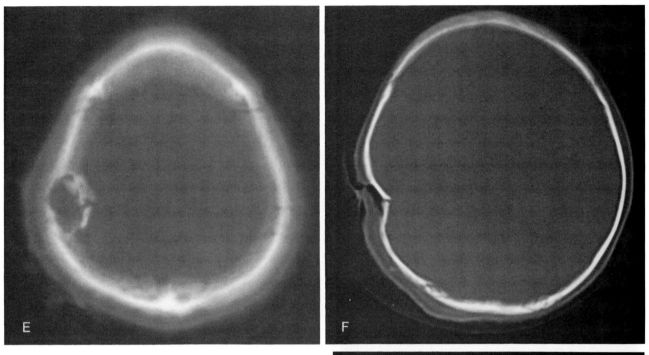

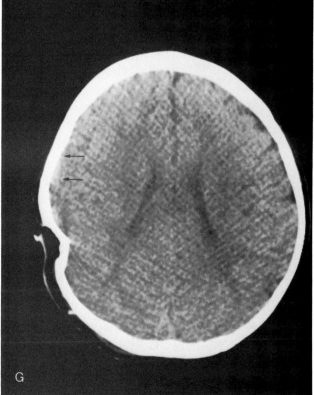

FIGURE 2–4 *Continued* **Depressed Skull Fractures at Computed Tomography**

• • • •

E, In this patient, the fracture fragments are displaced well into the brain. *F,* Bone window display of another depressed fracture. *G,* The same section displayed for soft tissue provides much less information about the skull but does demonstrate effacement of the sulci on the right and also a small subdural hematoma *(arrows).*

actual deformity of the skull contour, and fracture lines of varying widths (Fig. 2–5). The fracture lines are often very jagged. The depth of depression is an important observation and should be assessed by CT in all but critically emergent situations.

• • • •
TRAUMATIC EXTRA-AXIAL HEMORRHAGE

Subdural and epidural hematomas can occur with even minor head trauma. Both can become rapidly symptomatic and require prompt reliable diagnosis in order to minimize patient morbidity and mortality. At the present time, the screening procedure of choice is CT, which is both generally available and highly sensitive in the detection of both subdural and epidural hematomas. In the future, MR imaging may replace CT because MR imaging has even greater sensitivity, no bone artifact, and multiplanar capabilities. Scan times and degradation by motion artifacts limit its current utility in such often uncooperative or unstable patients.

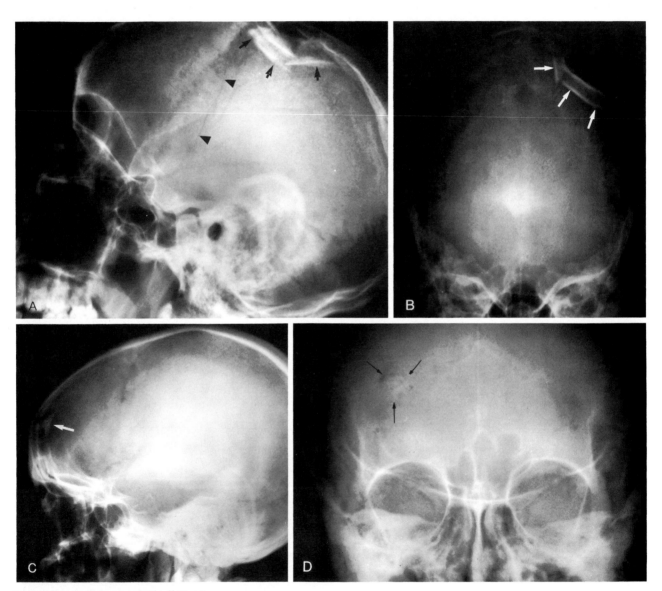

FIGURE 2–5. Depressed Skull Fracture
• • • •
A, This lateral view of the skull demonstrates a comminuted, depressed skull fracture *(arrows)*. Areas of increased density are caused by bone fragments that are seen on edge or overlapping bone. Linear fracture is also present *(arrowheads)*. *B*, Towne's view of the same patient demonstrates the fracture *(arrows)*. Note that the depth of depression cannot be precisely evaluated from either view. *C*, This lateral view of the skull of another patient demonstrates a more subtle depressed fracture *(arrow)* identified by increased bone density only on this projection. *D*, This anteroposterior view demonstrates both increased and decreased bone density in this depressed fracture *(arrows)*.

Radiographic Studies

As stated earlier, the skull series has no current place as a screening technique. In the past it was used to look for skull fractures, especially those crossing the middle meningeal artery (Fig. 2–6), which may lead to an epidural hematoma, and for depressed skull fractures, which often require surgical intervention (see Fig. 2–5). The skull series was also used to look for shifts from the midline of a calcified pineal gland. All these findings can be evaluated by CT and, more important, the extra-axial space and the brain itself can be seen using this modality. There is now virtually no indication for a skull series in the evaluation of extra-axial fluid collections.

Radionuclide imaging can also demonstrate extra-axial fluid collections, but this procedure has relatively low sensitivity and detects only about 50% of all small subdural collections on a flow study. Because of the lack of specificity or sensitivity, radionuclide scanning is a poor technique and should not be considered in the care of patients with suspected traumatic extra-axial fluid collections.

For years, angiography was the procedure of choice in the evaluation of both subdural (Fig. 2–7) and epidural (Fig. 2–8) hematomas. It is very accurate in the detection of most of these lesions, though small collections and those at the base of the brain can be difficult to define. Tangential views were often needed. Angiography is invasive and more time-consuming than CT and, therefore, should no longer be a primary screening technique for extra-axial fluid. However, when angiography is performed for penetrating trauma or any other reason, extra-axial fluid should not be overlooked.

Midline ultrasound is another technique that was devised to look for shifts of midline structures when a calcified pineal gland was not present. This procedure was difficult to perform accurately and at best indicated only that one half of the contents of the skull was different in size than the other. This procedure is no longer needed and has been forgotten by most radiologists and technologists who had mastered it. As transcranial imaging techniques improve, however, it may undergo resurgence in a new form.

CT is therefore the current survey procedure of choice. MR imaging lurks in the wings as rapid imaging techniques evolve. In hospitals where it is readily available for emergency procedures, MR imaging is a very reasonable technique for the detection of small subacute subdural hematomas and for those hematomas in nonconvexity locations. Therefore, both CT and MR imaging are discussed in this chapter.

FIGURE 2–6. Middle-Meningeal-Artery Injury Caused by Temporoparietal Fracture

• • • •

An early arterial film demonstrates prominent fracture lines *(arrows)*. The anterior extent of the fracture crosses the middle meningeal artery. Extravasation is seen at the site of the injury *(arrowhead)*. The patient had a rapid loss of consciousness. An epidural hematoma was evacuated at surgery.

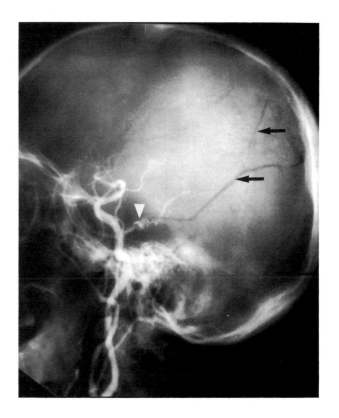

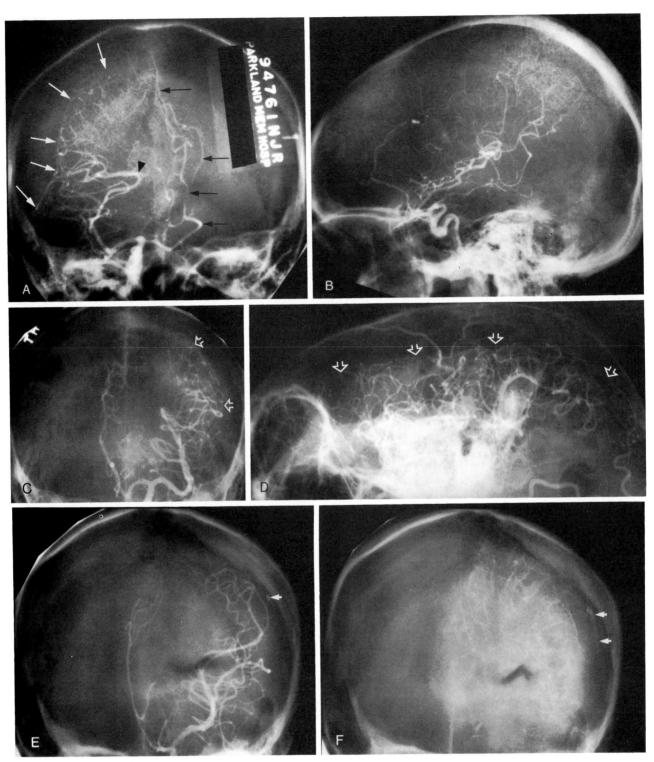

FIGURE 2–7. Angiography of Subdural Hematoma

• • • •

A, An anteroposterior (AP) arterial film of a right carotid angiogram demonstrates marked shift of the anterior cerebral circulation *(black arrows)* across the midline. The sylvian point *(arrowhead)* is displaced nearly to the midline and is depressed. The middle cerebral arteries are displaced from the calvarium by a large subdural hematoma *(white arrows). B,* A lateral film from the same injection is less obviously abnormal, except that the arteries of the sylvian triangle are compressed (there is a metallic artifact superimposed on the pericallosal artery). *C,* An AP left carotid angiogram in a second patient demonstrates a similar left-sided subdural hematoma *(arrows). D,* A view tangential to the subdural hematoma was performed in order to determine the full extent of this subdural hematoma *(arrows). E,* An AP arterial phase film on a third patient demonstrates shift of the anterior cerebral circulation to the right and the displacement of the middle cerebral circulation. In addition, extravasation of contrast material *(arrow)* is seen, indicating that this subdural hematoma arises from a parenchymal injury. *F,* This later film from the same series demonstrates further extravasation *(arrows).*

50

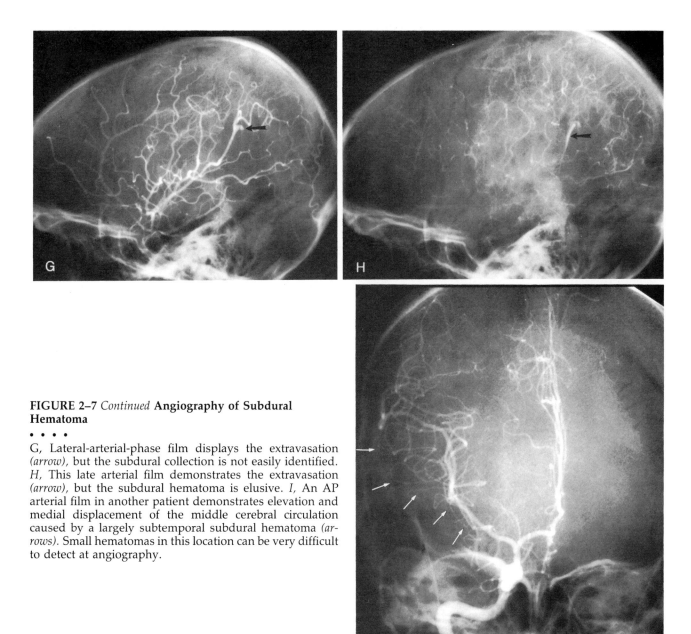

FIGURE 2–7 *Continued* **Angiography of Subdural Hematoma**

• • • •

G, Lateral-arterial-phase film displays the extravasation *(arrow)*, but the subdural collection is not easily identified. H, This late arterial film demonstrates the extravasation *(arrow)*, but the subdural hematoma is elusive. I, An AP arterial film in another patient demonstrates elevation and medial displacement of the middle cerebral circulation caused by a largely subtemporal subdural hematoma *(arrows)*. Small hematomas in this location can be very difficult to detect at angiography.

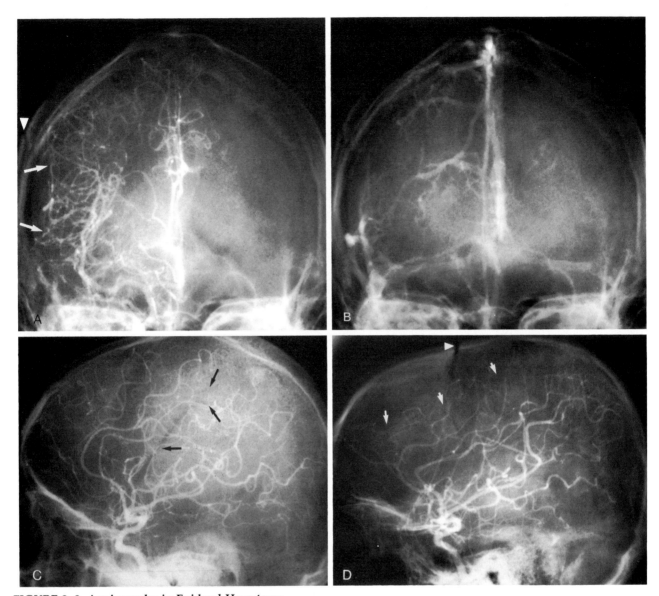

FIGURE 2–8. Angiography in Epidural Hematoma

• • • •

A, This anteroposterior (AP) arterial film of a right carotid angiogram demonstrates a typical lenticular extra-axial collection *(arrows).* The temporoparietal fracture *(arrowhead)* is also seen. *B,* In this film the extra-axial collection is again seen. *C,* The temporoparietal fracture *(arrows)* crosses the distribution of the middle meningeal artery. Notice that it branches dorsally. However, the epidural hematoma could easily be overlooked in this projection. *D,* A second patient with diastasis of the coronal suture *(arrowhead)* and bilateral parietal fractures has a large frontoparietal lenticular extra-axial epidural hematoma *(arrows).*

Epidural Hematoma

Clinicopathology

Epidural hematomas occur in fewer than 10% of patients with head trauma. However, since many epidural hematomas accumulate blood rapidly under high pressure and can quickly cause severe brain damage, they can be serious medical emergencies. Most patients with an epidural hematoma recover completely if the problem is recognized early and is treated appropriately. Failure to consider the diagnosis may lead to permanent brain damage or to death.

Epidural hemorrhage is caused by bleeding between the inner table of the skull and the dura. There is no normal epidural space because the dura is firmly attached to the inner table of the skull and can be stripped from the inner table of the skull only by direct force. The meningeal vessels lying between the inner table and the dura are vulnerable to injury, especially when the skull is fractured. Although any

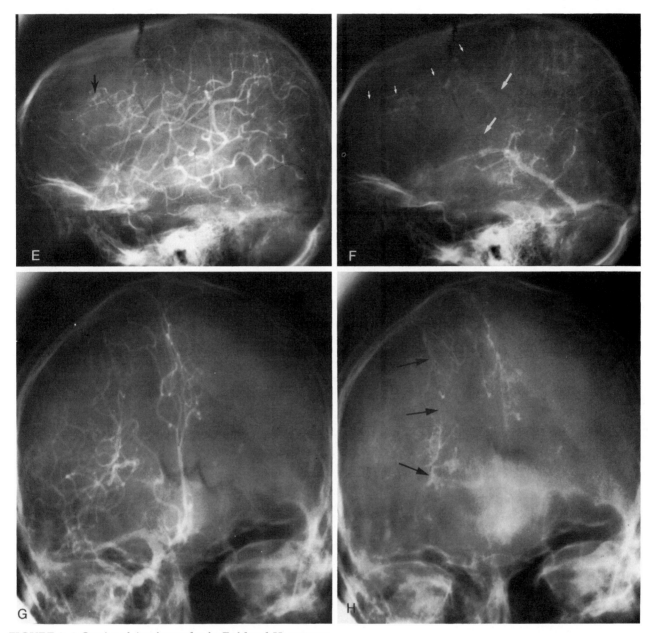

FIGURE 2–8 *Continued* **Angiography in Epidural Hematoma**

• • • •

E, A later arterial-phase film demonstrates some extravasation *(arrow) F,* In the venous phase, the epidural hematoma is well defined *(small arrows).* The extravasation was from bridging veins that had been torn from the sagittal sinus. The parietal fractures are easily seen *(large arrows). G,* The AP arterial phase film from a third patient demonstrates compression and displacement of middle cerebral arteries. *H,* This venous phase film demonstrates the typical lenticular configuration of a large epidural hematoma *(arrows).*

meningeal artery injury can cause an epidural hematoma, it develops most commonly from an injury to the anterior or the posterior branches of the middle meningeal artery resulting from a fracture of the thin squamous portion of the temporal bone (see Fig. 2–6). When one of these arteries is torn, the arterial pressure is sufficient to strip the dura away from the skull, forming the epidural hematoma. Because the dura is more firmly attached to the skull at the

sutures, epidural hematomas rarely cross the suture lines. Therefore, most epidural hematomas are localized and assume a lenticular or biconvex shape defined by the sutures (Fig. 2–9). When a fracture crosses a suture, an epidural hematoma may occasionally assume a bilobate appearance because the dural attachment is often disrupted (Fig. 2–10).

Occasionally, a venous epidural hematoma develops. Such hematomas are also usually caused by

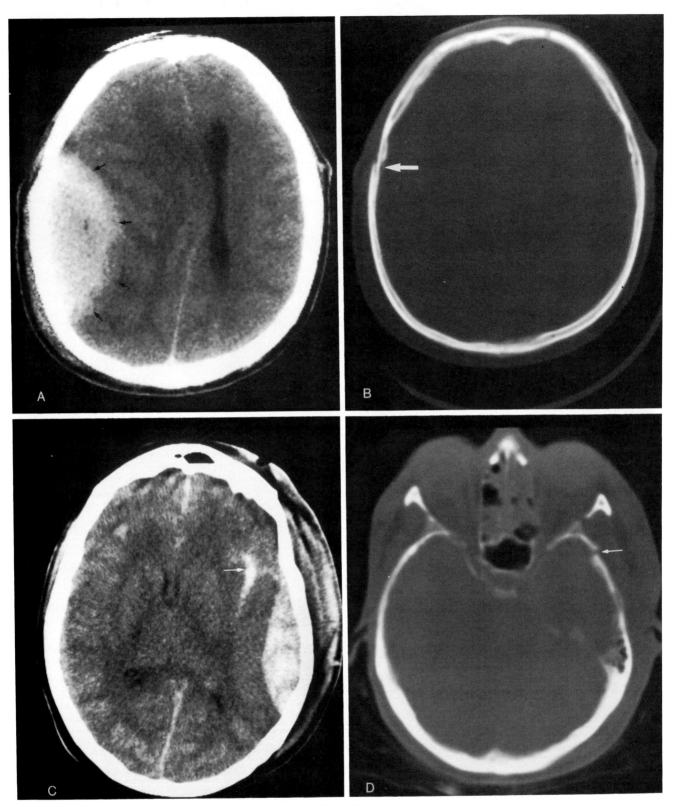

FIGURE 2–9. Typical Lenticular Shape of an Acute Epidural Hematoma

• • • •

A, The large epidural hematoma *(arrows)* has a typical lenticular or biconvex shape. The inhomogeneous density is probably caused by different ages of thrombus, implying sequential thrombus formation. The right lateral ventricle is completely effaced, and there is a shift of midline structures. The dark area within the hematoma may represent unclotted blood. When seen acutely this indicates active bleeding. *B,* A bone window display at the same level demonstrates a slightly depressed fracture *(arrow). C,* A second patient has a right parietal epidural hematoma. In addition, hemorrhage is present in the sylvian fissure *(arrow).* Small parenchymal hemorrhages are also found. *D,* Bone window display of a lower section demonstrates the temporal bone fracture *(arrow).*

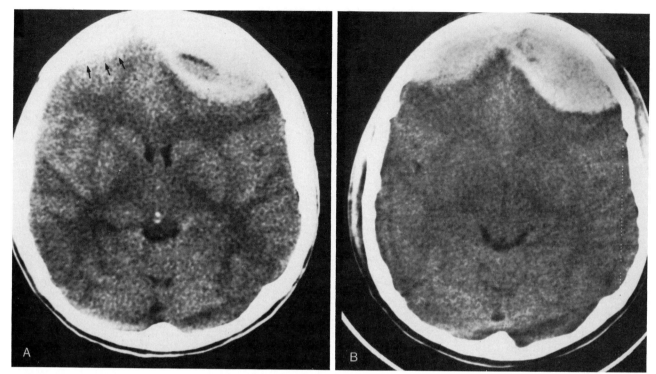

FIGURE 2–10. Bilobate Epidural Hematoma Crossing the Falx

• • • •

A, This computed tomography section is from an examination performed at about 9:00 AM. There is a large epidural hematoma with a swirling pattern seen in the left frontal region. A smaller abnormality in a similar location on the right *(arrows)* may also be questioned. *B,* A similar section taken at 1:00 PM after transfer of the patient demonstrates a bilobate epidural hematoma that has crossed the suture line through a dural tear.

skull fractures. Most venous epidural hematomas are small and expand slowly, primarily owing to the low pressure in the venous system. Blood may accumulate within a space created by dura stripped at the time of the trauma. Large hematomas occur when the major dural sinuses are ruptured; these hematomas may produce symptoms. Venous hematomas may also develop just external to the attachment of the falx or the tentorium, or both. A tear of the superior sagittal sinus can produce a bilateral lentiform venous hematoma extending over both cerebral hemispheres. A tear of the transverse sinus or the torcula may cause an epidural hematoma that has both infratentorial and supratentorial components.

A skull fracture is present in 85% of patients with an epidural hematoma. If the calvarium is somewhat flexible or resilient, as it is in a child, the dura is occasionally torn without an accompanying fracture. Epidural hematomas are less likely to be associated with parenchymal injuries, such as cerebral contusion, than are subdural hematomas. However, parenchymal injury may be present (Fig. 2–11). The parenchymal damage that occurs is usually secondary to the compression produced by the rapidly expanding hematoma, which causes ischemia or infarction.

The symptoms caused by an epidural hematoma are produced by the rapid accumulation of blood under arterial pressure. This quickly growing mass can compress or displace vital structures and produce herniation with its accompanying respiratory compromise and brain infarction (Fig. 2–12). Most patients with enlarging epidural hematomas present with rapid loss of consciousness, and emergent surgical evacuation is necessary. The efficient diagnosis of an epidural hematoma by CT or MR imaging has contributed to a decrease in mortality from approximately 30% to about 7% in one series.

Computed Tomography Imaging

The CT technique used for detecting a suspected epidural hematoma is the same as for brain trauma in general. The CT scan should be performed before the administration of any intravenous contrast material. Although clinically important epidural hematomas are rarely subtle lesions, contrast material administered for urography or angiography may obscure some small lesions. The scan can be performed using contiguous 10-mm sections from the brain stem through to the vertex. Bone windows will help to define any skull fractures. The soft tissue images •

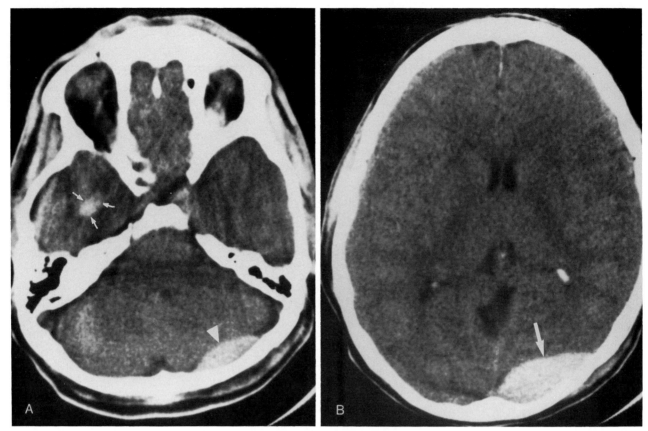

FIGURE 2–11. Parenchymal Hemorrhage in a Patient with Infratentorial and Supratentorial Epidural Hematomas
• • • •

A, The lower computed tomography section demonstrates a typical epidural hematoma *(arrowhead)* located in the left posterior fossa. There is a right temporal parenchymal hemorrhage *(arrows)*, which is the result of a contrecoup injury. *B,* A section located several centimeters cephalad demonstrates a supratentorial component of the epidural hematoma *(arrow).* The force of the blow to the left parieto-occipital region caused the right temporal lobe to impact the skull, resulting in the contrecoup hemorrhage.

must also be displayed appropriately. Contrast material is rarely needed in the evaluation of an acute epidural hematoma, though subacute and chronic epidural hematomas may be better seen with intravenous contrast material because their membranes are enhanced and because hematomas do pass through an isodense stage as they age. Thin (5-mm) sections through the posterior fossa help in the definition of anatomy and in the limitation of artifact.

The typical appearance of an epidural hematoma at CT is a focal, smoothly marginated, biconvex, or lenticularly shaped high-density (40–90 H) mass intimately related to the inner table of the skull. The content of many epidural hematomas is nonhomogeneous. This has been called a swirling pattern but is probably caused by the varying ages of the blood within the hematoma (Fig. 2–13; see also Figs. 2–9 and 2–10). Less specific findings caused by any mass

include midline shift, ventricular compression, and the effacement of sulci. Cerebral herniation may be demonstrated. Bilateral epidural hematomas are uncommon but must not be forgotten as they can occur. Occasionally, a small epidural hematoma does not produce clinical symptoms that require immediate surgery (Fig. 2–14). These hematomas may be treated conservatively and followed to resolution. Delayed epidural hematomas do develop and can be identified on CT scans several days after injury. They are usually caused by slow venous oozing or by an arterial injury that had severe spasm delaying the development of the epidural hematoma. Late rupture of a pseudoaneurysm at the site of injury may also cause an epidural hematoma to form remotely from the time of injury. Subacute and chronic epidural hematomas may be isodense or hypodense in relation to the brain. The membrane that forms around a

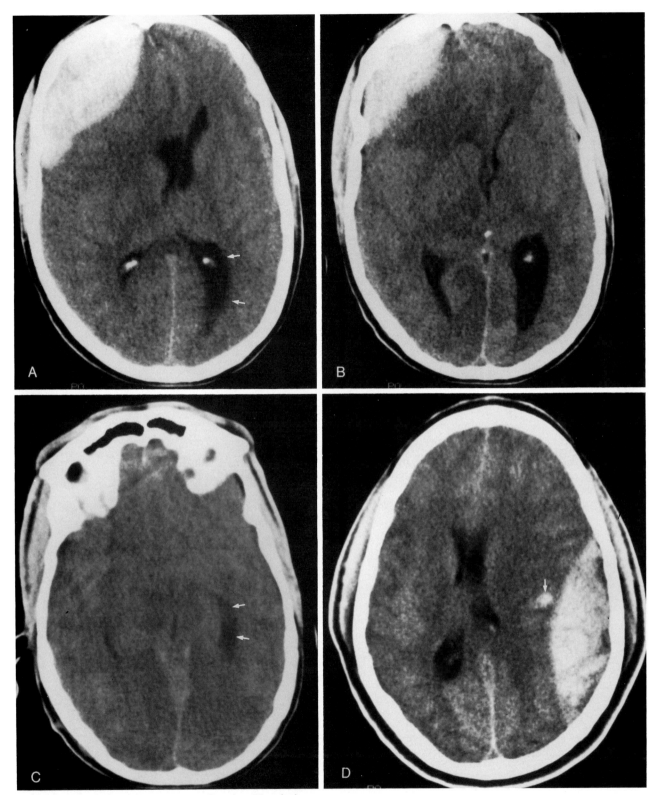

FIGURE 2–12. Epidural Hematoma Causing Herniation

• • • •

A, A very large acute epidural hematoma is situated in the right frontoparietal area. The lateral ventricles are shifted to the left, and the posterior horn on the left *(arrows)* is much larger than that on the right. *B*, A computed tomography section taken 10 mm caudal to the first still demonstrates the epidural hematoma as well as the dilated left posterior horn and the shift of anterior structures. *C*, A third section located 2 cm caudal to that shown in *B* displays the trapped contralateral temporal horn *(arrows)* and the effaced third ventricle. Other findings not demonstrated in this patient include effacement of the ipsilateral suprasellar cistern and the contralateral perimesencephalic cistern. *D*, A posterior parietal epidural hematoma in a 16-year-old has displaced the lateral ventricles to the right and effaced much of the left posterior horn. A small parenchymal hemorrhage *(arrow)* is present.

Illustration continued on following page

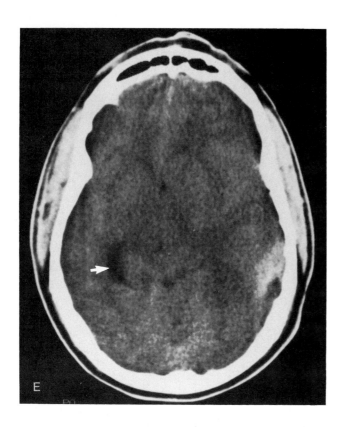

FIGURE 2–12 *Continued* **Epidural Hematoma Causing Herniation**

• • • •

E, A caudal section demonstrates the trapped right temporal horn *(arrow).* Again, the mass effect makes evaluation of the various cisterns around the brain stem difficult.

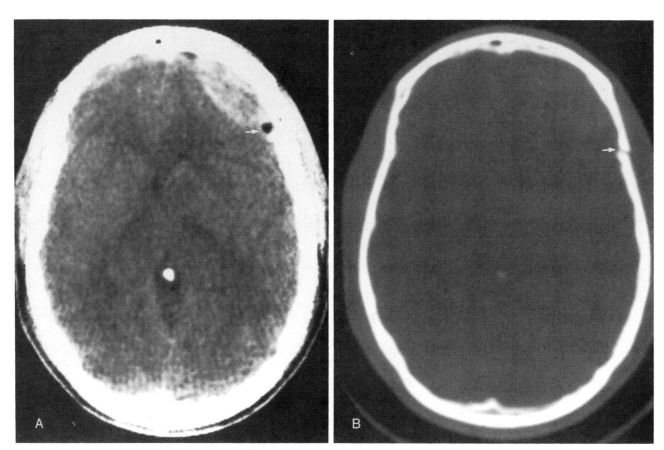

FIGURE 2–13. Swirl-like Pattern in Epidural Hematoma

• • • •

A, An epidural hematoma in the left frontal region demonstrates the swirl-like pattern that is seen in over half of all acute epidural hematomas. A small air collection *(arrow)* is also seen. *B,* This bone window display of the same section demonstrates a slightly diastatic coronal suture fracture *(arrow).*

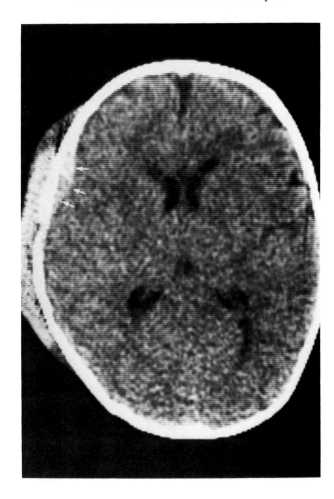

FIGURE 2–14. Small Epidural Hematoma

• • • •

This newborn had a large cephalohematoma that prompted a computed tomography scan. A small epidural hematoma *(arrows)* is seen at the coronal suture. As no neurologic abnormalities could be detected, this hematoma was treated conservatively.

chronic epidural collection is often enhanced with contrast material.

Subdural Hematoma

Clinicopathology

The subdural space is a pre-existing potential space between the dura and the arachnoid membrane. If blood gains access to this potential space, it can spread throughout the subdural space and extend over the entire hemisphere (Fig. 2–15), limited medially by the falx or the tentorium. Blood may also extend around the occipital or the frontal lobes along the falx into the interhemispheric fissure (Fig. 2–16). Hemorrhage into the subdural space may be caused by cortical contusion, laceration of meningeal membranes, or a tear of a vein bridging the subdural space. Hemorrhagic collections in the subdural space are classified as either acute or chronic. Acute and chronic subdural hematomas differ in history, have different associated rates of mortality and morbidity, and differ in the pattern of resolution. They can usually be distinguished by CT scanning.

Acute subdural hematoma is the most common traumatic lesion that requires neurosurgical intervention, occurring in about 5% of all patients with head trauma and in over 50% of those with severe head injury. The mortality rate in patients with acute subdural hematomas accompanying severe head injury ranges from 50 to 88%. Advancing patient age, the increasing size of the hematoma, and the delay in the evacuation of the hematoma are all factors associated with a poor prognosis. Most chronic subdural hematomas, in contrast, occur in elderly or alcoholic patients with cortical atrophy and are often found in the absence of a history of trauma. The enlarged extra-axial space allows a large accumulation of blood in the subdural space before the collection becomes clinically apparent in these patients. The mortality rate from chronic subdural hematoma is less than that seen with acute subdural hematoma and ranges from 0 to 23%. Confusion in terminology has been caused by cerebrospinal fluid-like collections of various origins in the subdural space that are often called *hygromas*. Inflammatory conditions, especially in children, produce low-density proteinaceous transudates in the subdural space and are more properly referred to as *subdural effusions*. The hallmark of a true subdural hygroma is its cerebro-

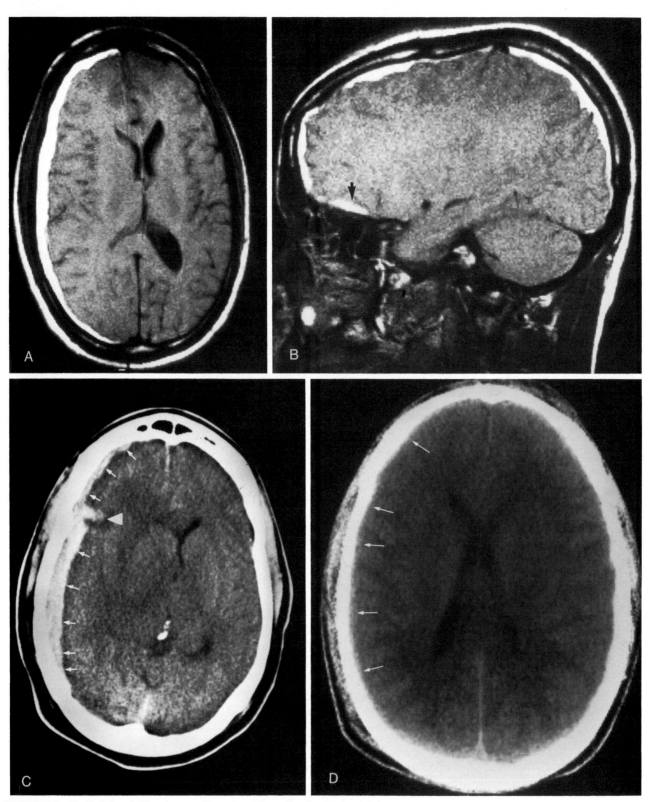

FIGURE 2–15. Subdural Hematoma Covering Virtually the Entire Right Hemisphere

• • • •

A, An axial MR section (T₁-weighted) demonstrates that this subdural hematoma surrounds the right hemisphere. The sulci are slightly effaced, and there is compression of the right lateral ventricle. *B,* A sagittal section (T₁-weighted) to the right of the midline in the same patient demonstrates that the subdural hematoma extends under the frontal lobe *(arrow)* but does not involve the tentorium. *C,* An axial computed tomography (CT) section of another patient demonstrates another subdural hematoma that nearly covers the hemisphere *(arrows).* There is also a small parenchymal hemorrhage *(arrowhead).* The lateral ventricles are displaced to the left as is the calcified pineal gland. No sulci are seen. *D,* A CT scan on another patient demonstrates a very thin subdural hematoma covering most of the hemisphere. It is easier to detect this lesion by looking at the slight displacement of the brain from the calvarium than by defining the subdural hematoma itself *(arrows).*

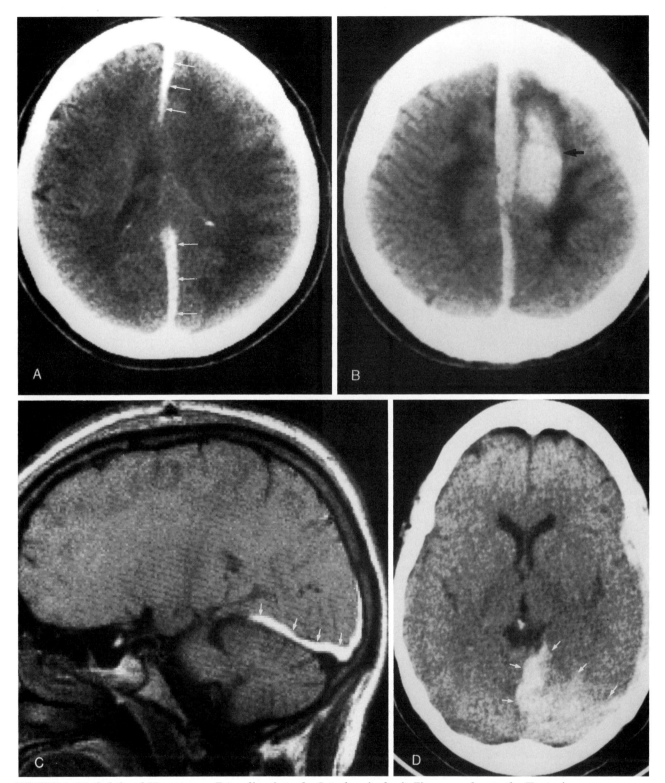

FIGURE 2–16. Subdural Hematomas Extending into the Interhemispheric Fissure and onto the Tentorium

• • • •

A, This computed tomography (CT) section at the level of the lateral ventricles demonstrates apparent thickening of the falx both anteriorly and posteriorly. The sharp edge of the falx is to the right, and the subdural hematoma is to the left *(arrows).* The hematoma is somewhat less sharply defined than the falx. *B,* A higher section demonstrates subdural hematoma along the entire falx. There is also a large intraparenchymal hemorrhage *(arrow). C,* A sagittal MR scan (TR = 500 msec, TE = 40 msec) in another patient demonstrates a subdural hematoma *(arrows)* extending onto the tentorium. *D,* An axial CT section in another patient demonstrates a small subdural hematoma along the left parieto-occipital area. The subdural hematoma is layered on the tentorium *(arrows).* The indistinctness of this part of the subdural hematoma is caused by the angle of the tentorium and the angle of the section. This finding must not be confused with parenchymal hemorrhage.

Illustration continued on following page

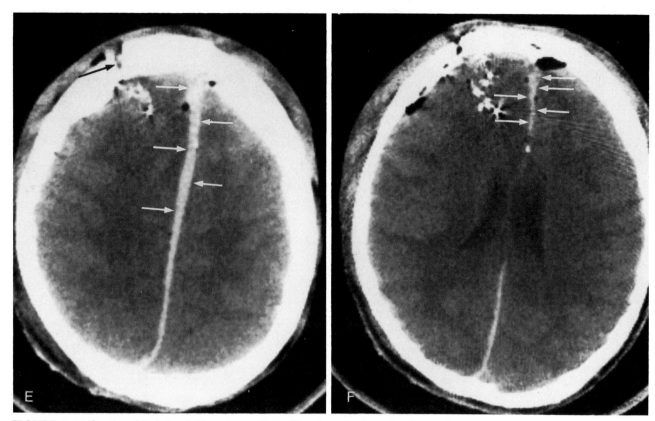

FIGURE 2–16 *Continued* **Subdural Hematomas Extending into the Interhemispheric Fissure and onto the Tentorium**
• • • •
E, This CT section after a gunshot wound to the head demonstrates the bony defect *(black arrow)*, metallic fragments, and pneumocephalus. In addition, there is an interhemispheric subdural hematoma *(white arrows)* on both sides of the falx that has been disrupted by the gunshot wound. *F,* A lower CT section demonstrates the irregular thickening of the falx *(arrows)* caused by the hematoma.

spinal fluid-like appearance and the lack of blood products and membranes. The distinction between subdural hygroma and chronic subdural hematoma is more easily made using MR imaging than CT because signal intensity with a hygroma is that of cerebrospinal fluid.

Acute Subdural Hematoma

Acute subdural hematomas typically originate from cortical contusions or lacerations associated with tears of the leptomeningeal membranes. Patients who have such hematomas probably suffered severe head trauma, which produced both the subdural bleeding and the concomitant parenchymal injury (Fig. 2–17; see also Figs. 2–11 and 2–12). Most of these patients are immediately symptomatic and are frequently unconscious when they reach the emergency room. Because of the high incidence of underlying serious brain injury, the prognosis in acute subdural hematoma is poor. In patients who are comatose at the time of initial examination, the mortality rate approaches 100% without surgery. Even

with surgical intervention, the mortality rate remains at 60–80%. This high mortality rate has been attributed to the irreversible parenchymal damage. Mortality incidence does decrease to below 50% if surgical intervention occurs within 3–4 hours of the injury. These patients are therefore surgical emergencies, so that immediate CT and appropriate surgical intervention are needed. In patients who survive, the residual disability is greater than in patients with epidural hematomas or chronic subdural hematomas because these entities generally have a lesser degree of associated cerebral damage. With moderate head injury, the acute subdural hematoma may be small and the underlying brain injury minimal or absent. These patients may have no neurologic dysfunction, and the attending physician may even choose to treat them conservatively by following the subdural collection with serial CT examinations (Fig. 2–18). These small and moderately sized acute subdural hematomas do not develop into chronic subdural hematomas. As an acute subdural collection resolves, it not only becomes more lucent and smaller, but it also has a decreasing mass effect. It can resemble a typical

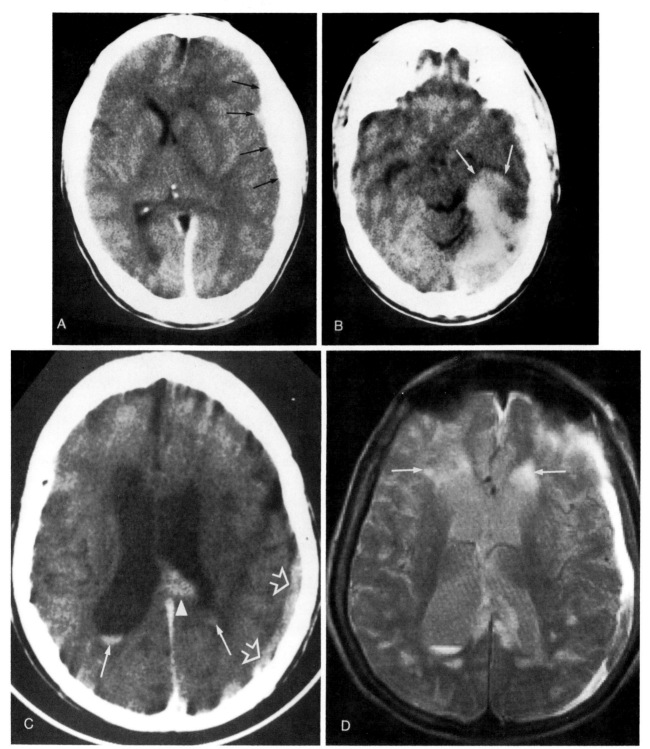

FIGURE 2–17. Subdural Hematoma with Concomitant Parenchymal Injury

• • • •

A, A computed tomography (CT) section at the level of the anterior horns demonstrates a modest acute left subdural hematoma *(arrows)* as well as marked shift of the midline structures and near complete effacement of the left lateral ventricular system. The subdural hematoma extends along the falx posteriorly. *B,* A more caudal section demonstrates that the subdural hematoma covers the tentorium on the left but also that there is parenchymal hemorrhage *(arrows). C,* A CT section in another patient who has hydrocephalus. There is an acute left parietal subdural hematoma *(open arrows).* A more chronic subdural hematoma is seen in the left frontal region. In addition, there is blood in both occipital horns *(arrows)* and parenchymal hemorrhage *(arrowhead). D,* An MR section (TR = 2000 msec, TE = 90 msec) in the same patient demonstrates additional parenchymal abnormalities *(arrows)* that are caused by transependymal edema. The intraventricular blood and acute subdural hematoma are easily seen.

Illustration continued on following page

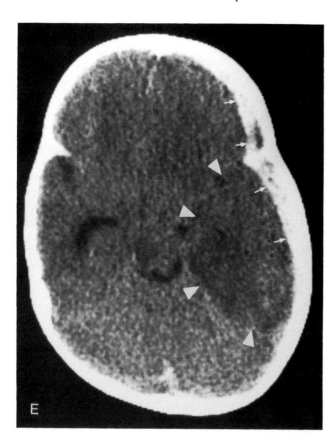

FIGURE 2–17 *Continued* **Subdural Hematoma with Concomitant Parenchymal Injury**

• • • •

E, This single CT section in a young child demonstrates a small left subdural hematoma *(arrows)*. There is also a large low-density area, which is a contusional infarct *(arrowheads)*.

chronic subdural hematoma during resolution. Acute subdural hematomas that do not require surgery usually resolve spontaneously and do not have as great a tendency to rebleed as do chronic subdural hematomas.

Subdural hematomas usually occur over one parietal or frontal convexity but may extend over an entire hemisphere. In 25% of the patients, subdural hematomas are bilateral (Fig. 2–19). Bilateral collections are often asymmetric, and one of the subdural hematomas may not be identified on the initial examination. After drainage of the larger subdural collection, the smaller contralateral collection may enlarge due to a decrease in the tamponade effect of the larger lesion. It may then become both more clinically and radiographically apparent.

On CT scans, an acute subdural hematoma usually is a homogeneous, high-density (40–90 H) crescent that conforms to the calvarium laterally and to the cerebral cortex medially. Acute subdural hematomas may also be isodense or hypodense when first seen. This variation in density is caused by a low blood hemoglobin level or is a result of the mixing of cerebrospinal fluid with blood due to a tear in the arachnoid. An acute subdural hematoma in a patient with a hemoglobin level of 8–10 mg/dl can have the same density as normal brain tissue and therefore be difficult to visualize as a distinct collection. A medial

"beak" may be seen at the pterion when the subdural hematoma extends into the lateral portion of the sylvian fissure.

When isodense subdural hematoma is suspected, MR imaging is helpful in verifying that diagnosis. MR imaging is superior in detecting subtle lesions owing to its increased sensitivity, but a lack of patient cooperation is often a technical problem in obtaining diagnostic studies. A characteristic of acute subdural hematomas is that the mass effect is frequently out of proportion to the actual size of the collection. When the collection extends around the entire hemisphere, it produces a circumferential compressing force on the underlying cortex. The mass effect is also due in part to underlying cerebral contusion and edema.

Subdural hematomas may also be located in the interhemispheric fissure. The collection of blood in these cases is generally thicker than that observed with subarachnoid hemorrhage (see Fig. 2–16). Interhemispheric fissure subdural hematomas are usually caused by damage to the small bridging veins between the medial cortex and the venous sinuses. Many of these interhemispheric collections are found in adults who experience a whiplash-type injury, which produces stress on the bridging veins. They have also been described in battered children who have been shaken violently. The subdural space

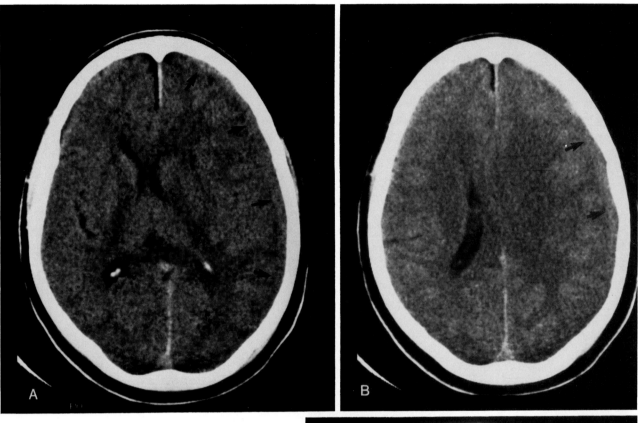

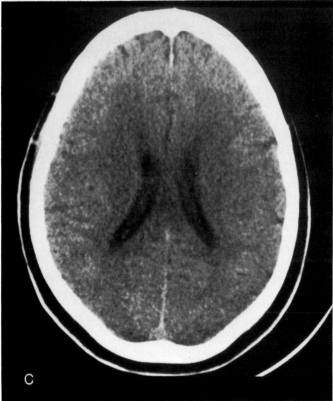

FIGURE 2–18. Conservatively Treated Subdural Hematoma

• • • •

A, This computed tomography (CT) section demonstrates an acute subdural hematoma that is nearly isodense *(arrows)*. The patient had suffered a traumatic amputation at the time of injury, with massive hemorrhage probably accounting for the diminished density of the hematoma. B, A higher section demonstrates effacement of the left lateral ventricle in addition to the subdural hematoma *(arrows)*. Sulci are also effaced. C, The patient was neurologically intact but had serious problems caused by blood loss. The subdural hematoma was treated conservatively. This CT section performed 3 months after the injury is normal.

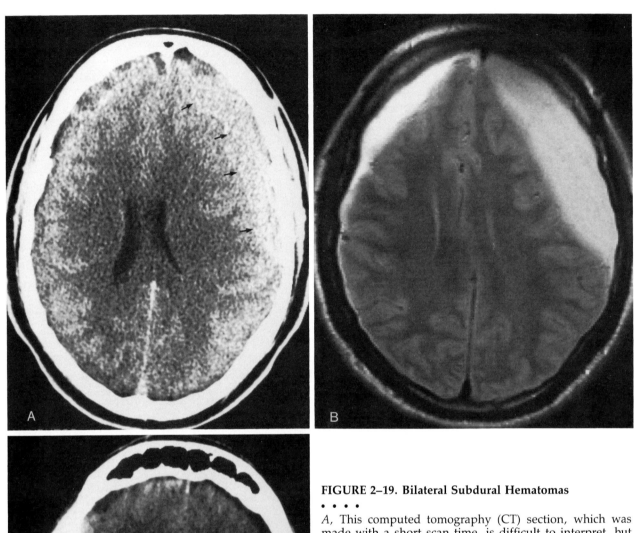

FIGURE 2–19. Bilateral Subdural Hematomas

• • • •

A, This computed tomography (CT) section, which was made with a short scan time, is difficult to interpret, but there clearly is a shift to the right with effacement of the left lateral ventricle and a peripheral semilunar increase in density *(arrows)* that is suggestive of a subdural hematoma. At the same time, it is difficult to assert that the sulci on the right reach the calvarium. *B,* An MR section (TR = 2000 msec, TE = 30 msec) at a similar level performed on the same patient under sedation demonstrates bilateral frontoparietal subdural hematomas of different ages. The left hematoma had high signal intensity on T_2- and decreased intensity on T_1-weighted images, whereas the right hematoma had high signal intensity on both T_1- and T_2-weighted images. *C,* This single CT section on another patient demonstrates an acute right subdural hematoma with effacement of the right frontal horn. On the left there is a chronic subdural hematoma that has rebled because there is a fluid-blood level *(arrow)* in the dependent portion of the subdural collection.

extends into the interhemispheric fissure along both sides of the falx, but because of the firm attachments of the inferior sagittal sinus, the two portions of the interhemispheric fissure are not in communication. Interhemispheric subdural hematomas are therefore generally unilateral. They usually have a flat medial border formed by the falx and a convex or straight lateral border caused by the subdural hematoma pressing into the ipsilateral hemisphere (see Fig. 2–16). Bilateral interhemispheric subdural hematomas are uncommon and are usually caused by penetrating trauma with rupture of the falx. Most interhemispheric subdural hematomas lie in the posterior superior portion of the interhemispheric fissure above and behind the splenium of the corpus callosum. Interhemispheric subdural hematomas often extend inferiorly over the ipsilateral tentorial surface, but in less than 50% of patients do they extend anteriorly into the precallosal portion of the fissure. This differs from subarachnoid hemorrhage, which produces an interhemispheric hematoma that is usually confined to the anterior portion of the fissure. Subarachnoid hemorrhage also usually conforms to the shape of the fissure rather than that of the falx.

In the pediatric population, the interhemispheric fissure is the most common site of subdural hemorrhage. The hemorrhagic collections are often small and difficult to recognize. Most young patients also have a parenchymal abnormality, such as a contusion or an infarction, adjacent to the collection. In both pediatric and adult patients the normal posterior falx is visualized on unenhanced scans as a thin midline hyperdense line. Eccentric thickening of the falx and inferior extension over the tentorial surface are important observations differentiating blood from a normal falx. Subfrontal, subtemporal, high-convexity, and occipital acute subdural hematomas also occur occasionally. These are difficult to visualize on axial CT scans. If mass effect causing sulcal effacement or ventricular displacement is identified without an obvious cause on the axial CT scan, direct coronal scanning, coronal reformation, or MR imaging with its multiplanar capabilities may be helpful for further evaluation.

Most subdural hematomas remain hyperdense on CT scans relative to adjacent brain tissue for 5–10 days after trauma. The collection passes through an isodense phase between the 7th and the 21st days (Fig. 2–20). After this time the hematoma is hypodense (Fig. 2–21). However, the sequence of density change is quite variable, making accurate aging of subdural hematomas difficult. This is especially true in patients with a low hematocrit or when there has been an admixture of blood and cerebrospinal fluid. Subacute subdural hematomas may also appear hyperdense or isodense if there has been a recent rehemorrhage. The density within a subdural hematoma of any age may be inhomogeneous. Layering occurs with a hyperdense dependent portion and a hypodense nondependent portion (Fig. 2–22; see also Fig. 2–19C). This phenomenon has been called the *hematocrit effect* and occurs after liquefaction of the clotted blood, most often in the subacute or the chronic phase. Layering may produce any combination of hypodensity, isodensity, and hyperdensity. Occasionally, the layering phenomenon is seen within an acute subdural hematoma. It is indicative of a failure of extravasated blood to clot, usually secondary to a bleeding diathesis or anticoagulation. Acute bleeding into a chronic subdural hematoma can also produce a layering phenomenon.

Detection of an isodense subdural hematoma can be difficult with CT and has been the subject of many studies. Additional techniques may be required to confirm a suspected isodense subdural hematoma. These include contrast-enhanced scanning, delayed scanning, and high-dose contrast scanning. With modern CT scanners, however, almost all subdural hematomas can be diagnosed using routine CT techniques. On unenhanced CT scans there are several diagnostic features that generally permit detection of an isodense subdural hematoma. The most specific finding is the diffuse mass effect, displacing the entire cerebral hemisphere away from the calvarium (Fig. 2–23). The position of the brain surface is determined by identifying the cortical sulci and also the corticomedullary junction as it extends into each gyrus. Sulci that extend to the calvarial edge exclude the possibility of an isodense subdural hematoma. This may be confusing when atrophic changes are confined to one hemisphere, such as in hemiatrophy and following a large healed infarction. In these cases, an isodense subdural hematoma may be incorrectly suggested on the side that is actually normal unless other indirect signs of an isodense subdural hematoma are recognized. One of the more reliable indirect signs of an isodense subdural hematoma is *buckling of the white matter*. Normally, the centrum semiovale has a convex lateral border, but with an extra-axial mass this white matter is displaced medially and has a flat or concave border; this is called buckling (Fig. 2–24). The finger-like projections of white matter that extend into each gyrus are also displaced medially. Because the corticomedullary junction is visible on unenhanced scans on most modern CT scanners, this white matter displacement can be recognized. The administration of contrast material produces cortical enhancement and improved delineation of the corticomedullary junction or the separation between cortex and subdural hematoma, or both. Contrast material may also opacify

Text continued on page 72

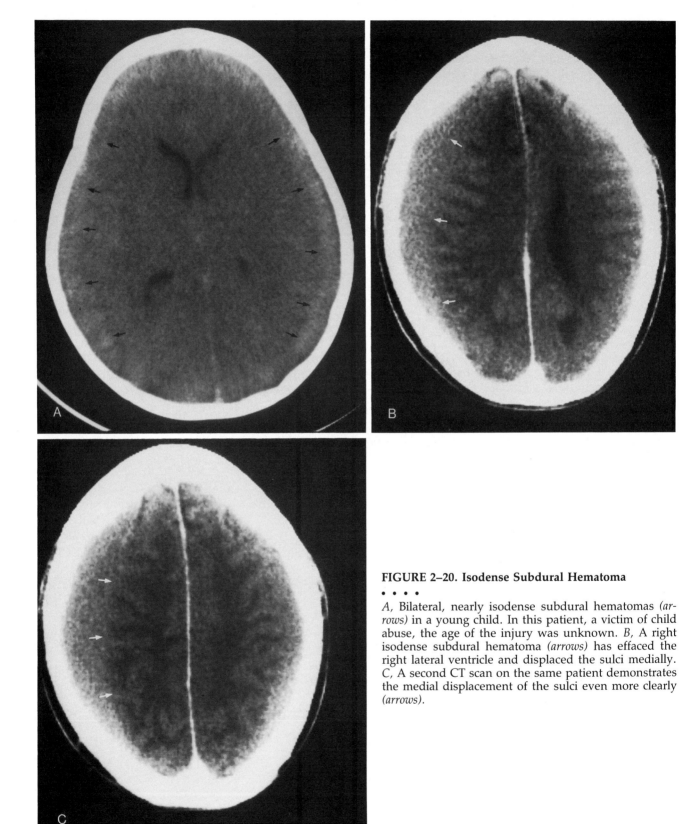

FIGURE 2–20. Isodense Subdural Hematoma

• • • •

A, Bilateral, nearly isodense subdural hematomas *(arrows)* in a young child. In this patient, a victim of child abuse, the age of the injury was unknown. *B*, A right isodense subdural hematoma *(arrows)* has effaced the right lateral ventricle and displaced the sulci medially. *C*, A second CT scan on the same patient demonstrates the medial displacement of the sulci even more clearly *(arrows)*.

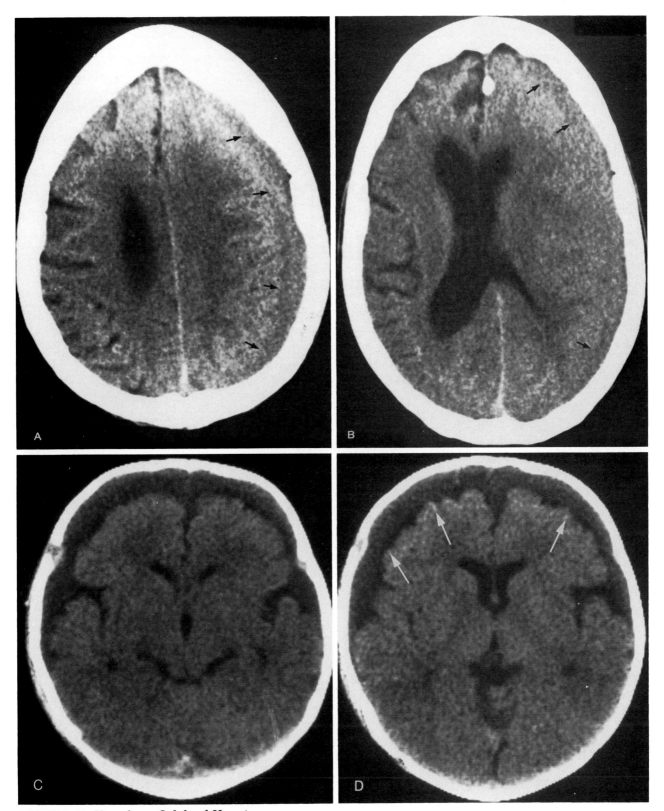

FIGURE 2–21. Hypodense Subdural Hematoma

• • • •

A, This computed tomography (CT) section demonstrates effacement of the left lateral ventricle and left-sided sulci near a large hypodense subdural hematoma *(arrows)*. *B*, A more caudal section still demonstrates compression of the left lateral ventricle and effacement of the left-sided sulci, but the subdural hematoma *(arrows)* is less easily seen. *C*, Hypodense bilateral chronic subdural hematoma in another patient who has atrophy. No mass effect is seen. *D*, A second section on this patient demonstrates some of the vessels *(arrows)* on the surface of the brain that are visible on this noncontrast scan because of the hypodense subdural hematoma.

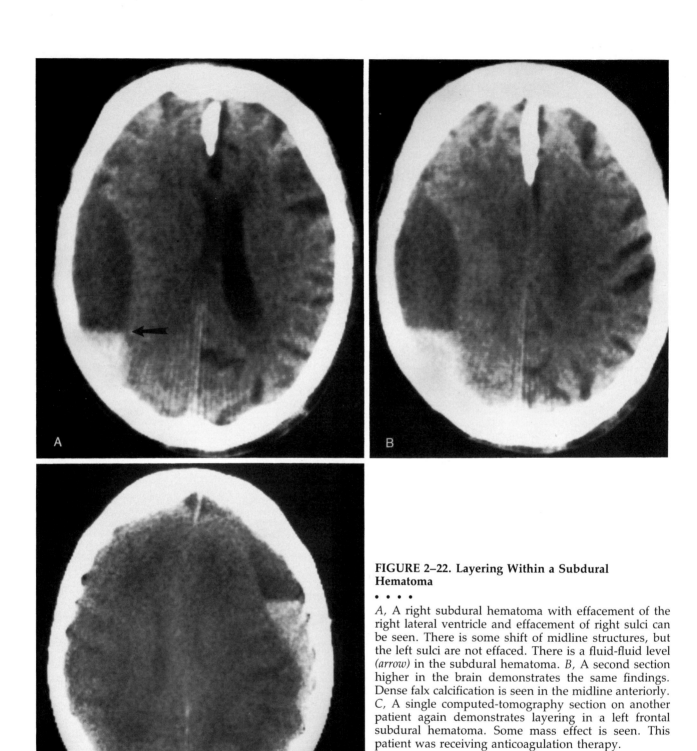

FIGURE 2–22. Layering Within a Subdural Hematoma

• • • •

A, A right subdural hematoma with effacement of the right lateral ventricle and effacement of right sulci can be seen. There is some shift of midline structures, but the left sulci are not effaced. There is a fluid-fluid level *(arrow)* in the subdural hematoma. *B,* A second section higher in the brain demonstrates the same findings. Dense falx calcification is seen in the midline anteriorly. *C,* A single computed-tomography section on another patient again demonstrates layering in a left frontal subdural hematoma. Some mass effect is seen. This patient was receiving anticoagulation therapy.

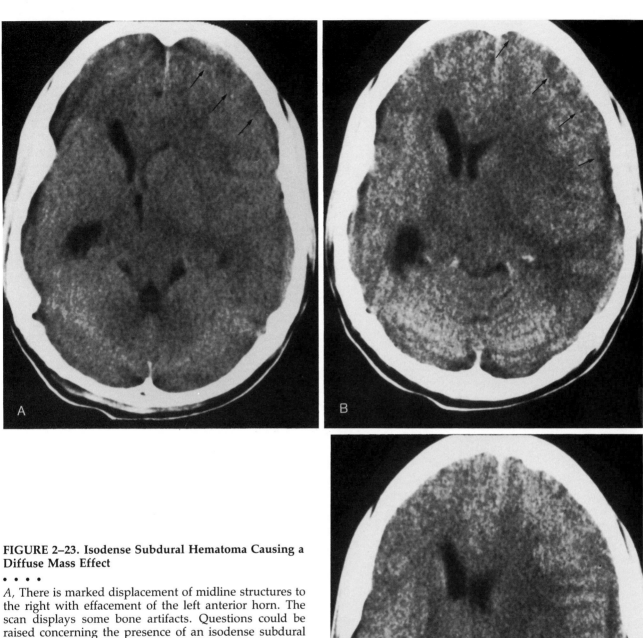

FIGURE 2–23. Isodense Subdural Hematoma Causing a Diffuse Mass Effect

• • • •

A, There is marked displacement of midline structures to the right with effacement of the left anterior horn. The scan displays some bone artifacts. Questions could be raised concerning the presence of an isodense subdural hematoma in the left frontoparietal region *(arrows). B,* The section located 10 mm cephalad presents similar findings but diminished artifacts. The left frontoparietal region again looks medially displaced *(arrows). C,* A third section does not clearly demonstrate a subdural hematoma; however, the cortex appears too thick, again supporting the diagnosis of isodense subdural hematoma.

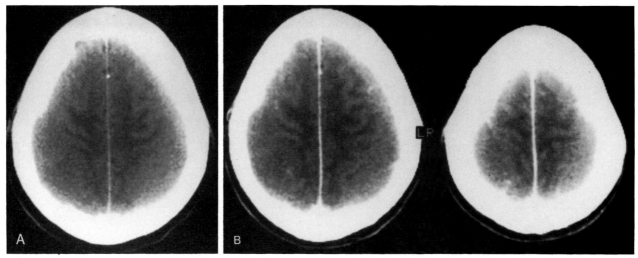

FIGURE 2–24. Buckling of the White Matter with Isodense Subdural Hematoma

• • • •

A, The white matter is displaced medially and bilaterally by the isodense subdural hematomas, resulting in a flattened and even concave border. *B,* Two cephalad sections scanned on the same patient following administration of a contrast material again demonstrate buckling of the white matter.

medially displaced cortical veins and enhances the vascular membrane that forms around subdural hematomas 1–4 weeks after injury (Fig. 2–25). Rarely, contrast material may seep into the hematoma and produce a fluid-fluid level.

Other features on unenhanced CT scans that suggest an isodense subdural hematoma include characteristic ventricular distortion and displacement patterns. There is usually symmetric compression of the ipsilateral ventricle (see Figs. 2–17 to 2–19, and 2–22). When transfalcine herniation has occurred, the ventricles are displaced toward each other. With bilateral subdural hematomas, ventricular shift is prevented, and there is bilateral compression of the lateral ventricles (see Fig. 2–20). The frontal horns become parallel and point anteriorly rather than anterolaterally. The atria and the occipital horns also do not normally diverge. This compression produces narrow, elongated ventricles that are nearly parallel. In reality, very few subdural collections are completely isodense. The density is usually slightly greater or less than that of the adjacent brain tissue. Careful imaging using modern CT scanners is usually able to demonstrate these small differences in density using subtle manipulation of both window width and level settings by an experienced radiologist. If doubt persists, MR imaging should be performed.

Identification of the isodense or the subacute subdural hematoma with MR imaging is straightforward because the MR technique relies on different factors for imaging. Whereas acute subdural hematomas may rarely be isointense with brain tissue on either

T_1- or T_2-weighted images, subacute subdural hematomas are hyperintense to brain tissue on T_1-weighted images (Fig. 2–26). Chronic subdural hematomas are usually hyperintense on T_2-weighted images and more variably hyperintense on T_1-weighted images.

Chronic Subdural Hematoma

Chronic subdural hematomas typically occur when a bridging vein is torn and a slow effusion of venous blood into the subdural space occurs. These bridging veins are most vulnerable to tearing when the subdural space is enlarged, as occurs with atrophy in elderly and alcoholic patients. Chronic subdural hematomas are usually the product of rather trivial head injury, and often no history of head trauma can be elicited. Symptoms occur solely because of the mass effect of the chronic subdural hematoma itself. Associated brain injury is rare. Patients with chronic subdural hematomas may complain of headaches, display minor changes in mental status, or have a gait disturbance. Chronic subdural hematomas are very susceptible to rebleeding caused by repeated minor injury owing to the thin-walled, fragile vessels that develop in the membrane on the dural side of the hematoma. Such a sudden increase in mass effect may produce more dramatic changes, including unconsciousness and herniation. Patients with these symptoms are encountered in the emergency room often after seemingly minor trauma. Patients do well after the drainage of chronic sub-

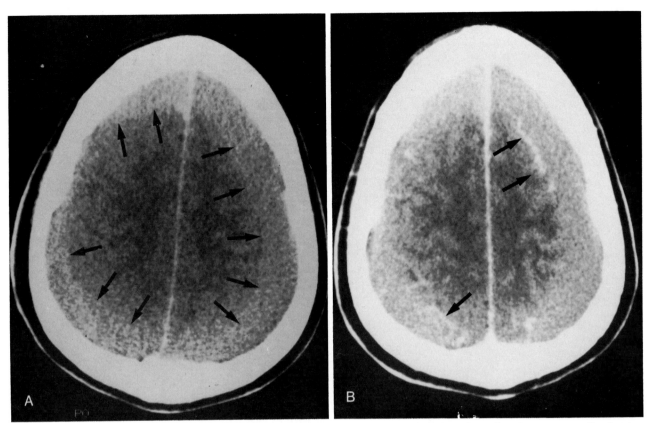

FIGURE 2–25. Bilateral Isodense Subdural Hematomas Before and After Administration of an Intravenous Contrast Material

• • • •

A, A section prior to administration of the contrast material demonstrates the slightly hyperdense subdural hematomas *(arrows).* *B,* After contrast material has been given, cortical veins are seen *(arrows),* demonstrating the cortical surface margin.

dural hematomas because there is usually no associated cerebral parenchymal injury. The subdural space frequently remains enlarged after evacuation of a chronic subdural hematoma. This is owing to the length of time that the chronic subdural hematoma has been present and also to cerebral atrophy.

The classic CT appearance of a chronic subdural hematoma is a peripheral crescent-shaped hypodense collection (see Fig. 2–21C), but because of the propensity for rebleeding, a chronic subdural hematoma can be hypodense, isodense, or even hyperdense. Chronic subdural hematomas may also be composed of layers of differing density (see Fig. 2–22). Membranes may form within the chronic subdural hematoma, causing compartmentalization; episodes of rebleeding may occur in only one portion of the collection. These same fibrous membranes also occasionally result in a biconvex configuration of a chronic subdural hematoma. Chronic subdural hematomas are most frequently located at the convexities. In 25% of patients chronic subdural hematomas are bilateral.

• • • •

POSTERIOR FOSSA EXTRA-AXIAL HEMATOMAS

Extra-axial hematomas in the posterior fossa comprise less than 5% of all extracerebral hematomas. However, the posterior fossa is a confined compartment, and even a small volume mass can seriously compromise vital brain stem function. Prompt diagnosis and treatment are essential for survival.

Epidural hematomas of the posterior fossa may occur as a result of either arterial or venous bleeding. Arterial hemorrhage is usually from the anterior or the posterior meningeal branches of the vertebral artery. These epidural hematomas are frequently located centrally because of the midline location of the arteries, but they may also occur elsewhere (Fig. 2–27). Venous epidural hematomas usually occur following a rupture of the torcula or the transverse sinus and are typically biconvex. Epidural hematomas in the posterior fossa occasionally cross the

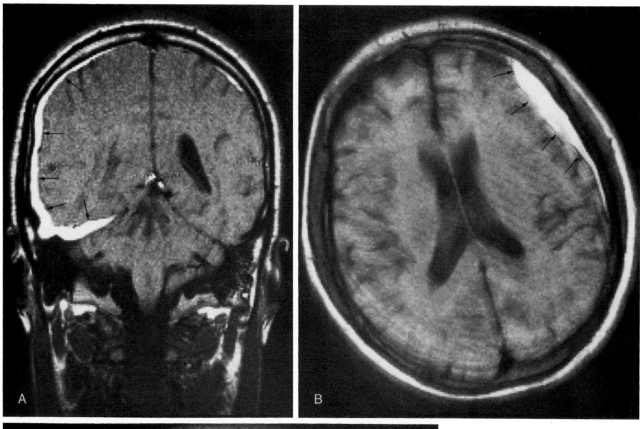

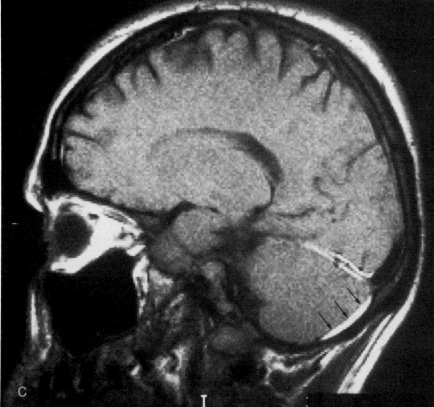

FIGURE 2–26. Subacute Subdural Hematoma at Magnetic Resonance Imaging

• • • •

A, A coronal section (TR = 500 msec, TE = 40 msec) demonstrates a right subdural hematoma *(arrows)* effacing the lateral ventricle. There is also a small left vertex contusion. B, A second patient has a left frontoparietal subdural hematoma *(arrows)*, which is easily seen on this T_1-weighted scan. C, A third patient has a subacute subdural hematoma in the posterior fossa *(arrows)* and along the tentorium; it is easily seen on a T_1-weighted image (TR = 500 msec, TE = 40 msec).

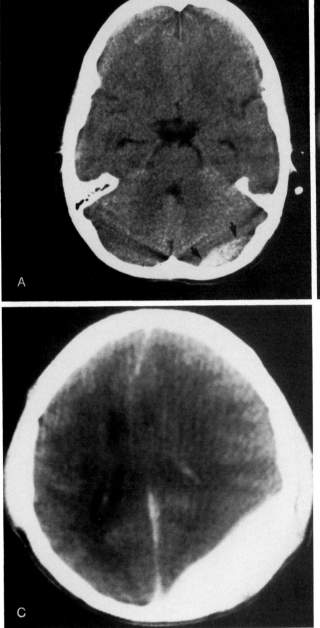

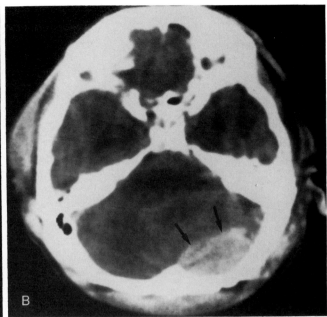

FIGURE 2–27. Posterior Fossa Epidural Hematoma

• • • •

A, Computed tomography (CT) demonstrates a typical bi-convex epidural hematoma *(arrows)* in the posterior fossa. *B,* A CT scan in a second patient demonstrates a posterior fossa hematoma *(arrows)*. *C,* A higher section demonstrates a large supratentorial component to the epidural hematoma. The left lateral ventricle has been effaced by the mass.

tentorium, whereas subdural hematomas do not (see Fig. 2–11). Posterior fossa extra-axial collections may produce hydrocephalus by compressing the cerebral aqueduct. The clinical implications are serious, and rapid surgical decompression is needed for the vast majority of patients. CT is the screening procedure of choice, but bone artifacts may degrade the CT image sufficiently in some patients to necessitate MR imaging to identify the hematoma. Precise localization may be difficult with either modality and should not be allowed to delay surgery if the situation is adequately defined for surgical planning in a setting of rapid neurologic deterioration.

Subdural hematomas in the posterior fossa may be produced by the rupture of a dural sinus, the rupture of bridging veins, or by trauma to cerebellar tissue. This lesion is occasionally seen in newborn infants after difficult deliveries and is secondary to a tear in the tentorium produced by severe pressure during birth. A posterior fossa subdural hematoma is usually crescentic, but occasionally a biconvex collection that is indistinguishable from an epidural hematoma is seen. When a posterior fossa subdural hematoma extends superiorly, it has a sharp lateral margin where it abuts the tentorium.

Bibliography

Amendola MA, Ostrum BJ. Diagnosis of isodense subdural hematomas by computed tomography. AJR 1977; 129:693–697.

Cohen WA, Kricheff II. Craniocerebral trauma. In McCort JJ (ed). Trauma Radiology. New York: Churchill Livingstone, Inc., 1990, pp 1–29.

Dublin AB, French BN, Rennick JM. Computed tomography in head trauma. Radiology 1977; 122:365–369.

Gandy SE, Snow RB, Zimmerman RD, Deck MDF. Cranial nuclear magnetic resonance imaging in head trauma. Ann Neurol 1984; 16:254–257.

Gentry LR, Godersky JC, Thompson B, Dunn VD. Prospective comparative study of intermediate-field MR and CT in the evaluation of closed head trauma. AJNR 1988; 9:91–100.

George AE, Russell EJ, Kricheff II. White matter buckling: CT sign of extraaxial intracranial mass. AJR 1980; 135:1031–1036.

Gomori JM, Grossman RI, Hackney DB, et al. Variable appearances of subacute intracranial hematomas on high-field spin-echo MR. AJNR 1987; 8:1019–1026.

Han JS, Kaufman B, Alfidi RJ, et al. Head trauma evaluated by magnetic resonance and computed tomography: A comparison. Radiology 1984; 150:71–77.

Hayman LA, Evans RA, Hinck VC. Rapid-high-dose contrast computed tomography of isodense subdural hematoma and cerebral swelling. Radiology 1979; 131:381–383.

Holland BA, Brant-Zawadzki M, Pitts LH. The role of CT in evaluation of head trauma. In Federle MP, Brant-Zawadzki M (eds). Computed Tomography in the Evaluation of Trauma. 2nd ed. Baltimore: Williams & Wilkins, 1986, pp 1–63.

Hryshko FG, Deeb ZL. Computed tomography in acute head injuries. J Comput Tomogr 1983; 7:331–344.

Kelly AB, Zimmerman RD, Snow RB, et al. Head trauma: Comparison of MR and CT-experience in 100 patients. AJNR 1988; 9:699–708.

Kim KS, Hemmati M, Weinberg PE. Computed tomography in isodense subdural hematoma. Radiology 1978; 128:71–74.

Masters SJ, McClean PM, Arcarese JS, et al. Skull x-ray examinations after head trauma. N Engl J Med 1987; 316:84–91.

New PFJ, Aronow S. Attenuation measurements of whole blood and blood fractions in computed tomography. Radiology 1976; 121:635–640.

Patronas NJ, Duda EE, Mirfakhraee M, Wollmann RL. Superior sagittal sinus thrombosis diagnosed by computed tomography. Surg Neurol 1981; 15:11–14.

Royal College of Radiologists. A study of the utilisation of skull radiography in 9 accident and emergency units in the U.K. Lancet 1980; 1234–1237.

Scotti G, Terbrugge K, Melancon D, Belanger G. Evaluation of the age of subdural hematomas by computerized tomography. J Neurosurg 1977; 47:311–315.

Sipponen JT, Sepponen RE, Sivula A. Chronic subdural hematoma: Demonstration by magnetic resonance. Radiology 1984; 150:79–85.

Smith WP Jr, Batnitzky S, Rengachary SS. Acute isodense subdural hematomas: A problem in anemic patients. AJR 1981; 136:543–546.

Thornbury JR, Masters SJ, Campbell JA. Imaging recommendations for head trauma: A new comprehensive strategy. AJR 1987; 149:781–783.

Tsai FY, Teal JS, Itabashi HH, et al. Computed tomography of posterior fossa trauma. J Comput Assist Tomogr 1980; 4:291–305.

Weinstein MA, Alfidi RJ, Duchesneau PM. Computed tomography versus skull radiography. AJR 1977; 128:873.

Zimmerman RA, Bilaniuk LT. Computed tomographic staging of traumatic epidural bleeding. Radiology 1982; 144:809–812.

Zimmerman RA, Bilaniuk LT, Gennarelli T, et al. Cranial computed tomography in diagnosis and management of acute head trauma. AJR 1978; 131:27–34.

CHAPTER 3

•••••••••••••••••••••••••••••••

Skull Base Trauma

•••••••

STEVEN A. DUNNAGAN, M.D.
PHILLIP D. PURDY, M.D.

The base of the skull is formed by the floors of the anterior, the middle, and the posterior cranial fossae. Recognized skull base fracture usually occurs in association with other injuries, especially those of the face, the cranial vault, and the cervical spine. In fact, fracture of the skull base is probably more common than is recognized because uncomplicated skull base fractures require no special attention and therefore are not subjected to the extensive evaluation that is required to confirm their presence. It is injury to the brain itself, to the paranasal sinuses, or to the arteries, the veins, and the cranial nerves that pass through the base of the skull that requires a full and often immediate radiographic evaluation.

•••
ANATOMY

Anterior Cranial Fossa

The skull base of the anterior cranial fossa is formed by the orbital plates of the frontal bones, the cribriform plate, the crista galli, and the upper surface of the lesser sphenoid wing. This part of the skull

base supports the underlying surface of the frontal lobes and separates the anterior fossa from the upper nasal passages, the ethmoid sinuses, and the orbits. Portions of the frontal sinuses and the ethmoid air cells may extend into the orbital roof. This pneumatization is quite extensive in some individuals. The cribriform plate of the ethmoid bone transmits branches of the olfactory nerve and is in intimate apposition to the upper nasal cavity. No other major nerves or blood vessels pass through the skull base of the anterior fossa (Figs. 3–1 and 3–2).

Middle Cranial Fossa

The base of the middle cranial fossa cradles the temporal lobes. The greater wing of the sphenoid bone forms the anterior and the medial walls of the middle cranial fossa as well as the medial portion of its floor. The lateral portion of the middle cranial fossa is formed by the squamous portion of the temporal bone. The sella turcica occupies the midline of the middle cranial fossa.

The sella and the medial aspects of the middle cranial fossa form the superior and the lateral walls of the sphenoid sinus. This is an important associa-

---

• • • • *APPROPRIATE RADIOGRAPHIC STUDIES*

I. **Plain Films**
   A. A routine series includes posteroanterior, lateral, Water's, Towne's, and submentovertex views.
   Comment: A submentovertex view must *not* be attempted if any cervical spine injury is suspected.
   B. Stenver's view, Law's view, and Schüller's view should be used when indicated.
   C. Plain films have been replaced by computed tomography (CT) for evaluation of the skull base.
   Comment: Although skull base fractures can often be identified on plain films, CT demonstrates not only the fractures but also the associated and more important soft tissue injury. Because CT is mandatory in patients requiring evaluation, there is no longer any indication for plain films.

II. **Computed Tomography**
   A. The procedure of choice in skull base fracture.
   B. A survey CT scan can use 5-mm sections in an axial plane to examine for fracture.
   C. Thin sections, preferably 1–2 mm in thickness, must be used to evaluate the ossicles of the middle ear and subtle fractures of the skull base.
   D. Direct coronal sections may further define skull base fractures.
   Comment: Must not be performed if cervical spine injury is suspected.
   E. Care must be taken to display images well and to use appropriate reconstruction algorithms.
   F. CT cisternography may demonstrate a cerebrospinal fluid leak.
   Comment: Remember that the diagnosis and the treatment of most skull base injury is less urgent than the therapy for other brain and facial injuries that often occur with skull base trauma.

III. **Magnetic Resonance Imaging**
   Comment: Not recommended at the present time.

IV. **Angiography**
   A. May be required to define arterial injury for surgical or neurointerventional therapy
   Comment: Angiography is occasionally needed in the immediate post-trauma workup but is more commonly used later in the patient's course. The neurointerventionist should be consulted early during patient evaluation when vascular injury is of concern. Rarely is surgical therapy now needed for traumatic vascular injury in the face or neck in centers where endovascular therapy is available. Surgical exploration is sometimes needed if injury cannot be confirmed radiographically.

---

tion since the sphenoid sinus is frequently involved in skull base trauma. Progressing laterally, the greater wing of the sphenoid bone borders the posterior orbit, the pterygopalatine fossa, and the infratemporal space.

Many important neural and vascular structures are adjacent to or pass through the skull base of the middle cranial fossa. The optic chiasm lies just anterior to the sella turcica; anterolaterally from the chiasm, the optic nerves exit and pass under the anterior clinoids to enter the orbits through the optic foramina. Cranial nerves III, IV, and VI and the ophthalmic (frontal) division of cranial nerve V are intimately associated with the cavernous sinus before they pass through the superior orbital fissure into the orbit. The superior orbital fissure is bounded by the greater and lesser wings of the sphenoid bone. Just inferior to the superior orbital fissure is the

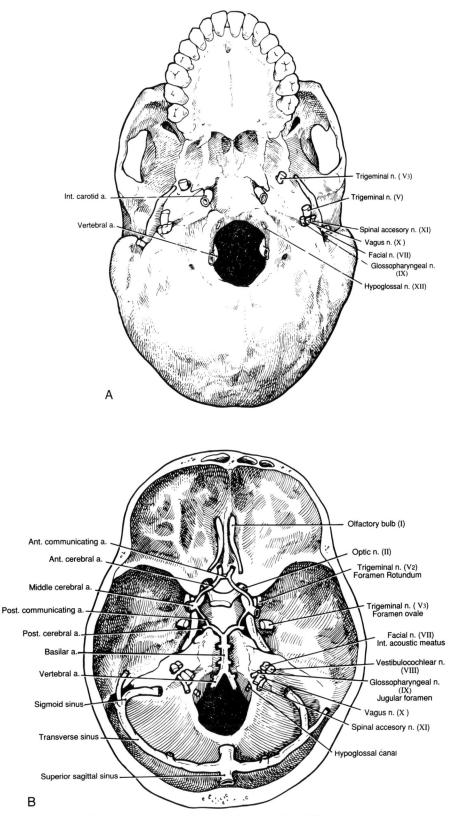

FIGURE 3–1. Cranial Nerves and Vascular Structures Involved in the Skull Base

• • • •

A, This view from below shows the entry of the carotid arteries and the vertebral arteries as well as the exits of the various cranial nerves. *B,* The view from above shows the same, as well as the arterial circle of Willis, the optic nerves, the olfactory nerves, and the transverse and sigmoid sinuses. Fractures or penetrating injuries in the region of the structures in the intracranial or extracranial space can cause neural or vascular injuries. (Drawing by Mary Ann Zapalac, Medical Illustration, University of Texas Southwestern Medical Center at Dallas.)

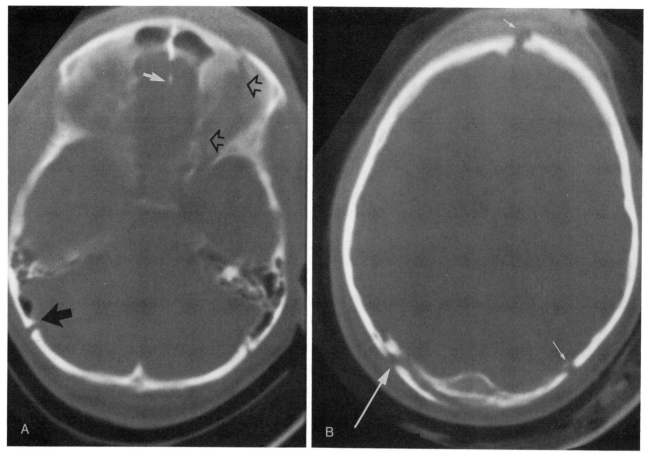

FIGURE 3–2. Fracture Through the Orbital Roof with a Fracture Line Extending to the Occipital Bone

• • • •

A, A computed tomography slice at the level of the orbital roof reveals a linear fracture along the axis of the left orbit *(open arrows)*. The apex of the ethmoid spine *(white arrow)* marks the cribriform plate region. The fracture line is seen also on the occiput; the small amount of air adjacent to it may represent a small area of pneumocephalus but more likely is a pocket of mastoid air cells *(black arrow)*. *B*, A higher cut reveals a midline frontal fracture and bilateral occipital fractures. The frontal and left occipital fractures are shown *(small arrows)*. Note the depression and the comminution of the right occipital fracture *(large arrow)*.

foramen rotundum through which the maxillary branch of the fifth cranial nerve enters the pterygopalatine fossa. The mandibular branch of the fifth cranial nerve exits through the foramen ovale, which is lateral and posterior to the foramen rotundum. The foramen spinosum lies just lateral to the foramen ovale and carries the middle meningeal artery.

The internal carotid artery enters the skull base through the carotid foramen, traverses the petrous bone in an anteromedial direction, and enters the middle cranial fossa posteromedially. It then travels through the cavernous sinus along with cranial nerves III, IV, and VI and the ophthalmic and the maxillary branches of cranial nerve V (Fig. 3–3). The internal carotid artery does not actually become intradural until it turns superiorly and leaves the cavernous sinus just medial to the anterior clinoids.

The cavernous sinus is a venous confluence lateral to the sella and the sphenoid sinus. The third, the fourth, and the sixth cranial nerves, the ophthalmic and the maxillary branches of the fifth cranial nerve, and a portion of the internal carotid artery pass through the cavernous sinus. The veins communicating with the cavernous sinus include the superior ophthalmic vein, the superficial middle cerebral vein, and the sphenoparietal sinus. The sella turcica and the clivus support an extensive venous plexus. The cavernous sinuses communicate with each other via this plexus and the petrosal sinuses, which also communicate with the transverse sinuses and the internal jugular veins. The large number of important neurologic functions of the cavernous sinuses as well as the extensive venous connections assist in the localization of trauma to this area.

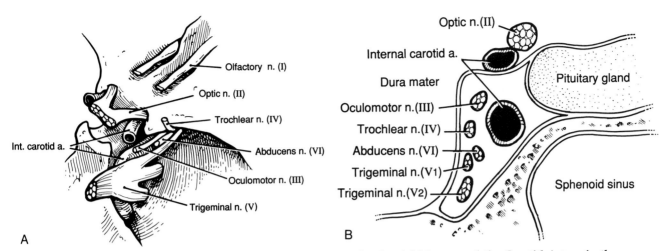

FIGURE 3–3. Diagrams Illustrating the Relationships between the Cranial Nerves and the Carotid Artery in the Cavernous Sinus

• • • •

A, This lateral view shows the third, fourth, and sixth cranial nerves as well as the first two divisions of the fifth nerve lateral to the carotid artery in the cavernous sinus. The carotid enters the subarachnoid space at the level of the anterior clinoid process (in close proximity to the optic nerve). *B,* A cross section of the cavernous sinus again shows the relationships between the carotid artery in both the cavernous sinus and in the subarachnoid space near the anterior clinoid process; related nerves, the pituitary gland, and the sphenoid sinus are also shown. (Drawing by Mary Ann Zapalac, Medical Illustration, University of Texas Southwestern Medical Center at Dallas.)

Posterior Cranial Fossa

The posterior cranial fossa contains the cerebellum and the brain stem. The petrous ridges form the anterolateral boundaries that converge medially on the clivus. The remainder of the posterior fossa skull base is formed by the occipital bone.

Cranial nerves VII and VIII enter the posterior aspect of the petrous bone through the internal auditory canal. The seventh cranial nerve has a complicated path that brings it in close proximity to the semicircular canals, the vestibule, the middle ear, and the external auditory canal before exiting inferiorly at the stylomastoid foramen. The eighth cranial nerve has its end organs (the cochlea, the vestibule, and the semicircular canals) within the petrous bone. Even with this short course it may be injured by a fracture traversing the internal auditory canal.

The roof of the jugular foramen is formed by the petrous bone, and the floor is formed by the occipital bone. The foramen is divided into two components, the superomedial pars nervosa and the inferolateral pars vasculosa. Cranial nerve IX travels in the pars nervosa. Cranial nerves X and XI and the jugular vein travel in the pars vasculosa. Inferior and medial to the jugular foramen on the anterolateral rim of the foramen magnum is the hypoglossal canal, which transmits cranial nerve XII. The spinal cord leaves the posterior cranial fossa through the foramen magnum at its articulation with the cervical spine.

• • • •

RADIOLOGIC MANAGEMENT OF SKULL BASE INJURIES

Fractures of the skull base are rarely themselves important. They become important owing to their associated clinical manifestations. Problems often encountered with skull base fracture include orbital and periorbital fractures, swelling and hematoma, hematotympanum, leakage of cerebrospinal fluid, cranial nerve palsy, major vascular injury, and cerebrovascular accident associated with trauma. Skull base fracture should be a consideration in any obtunded trauma patient and in patients with significant facial or cervical spine injuries.

It is important to keep in mind that most skull base fractures are not life-threatening and in and of themselves do not require emergency evaluation. Cranial nerve palsies and cerebrospinal fluid leaks often resolve spontaneously. Delay in their evaluation is not only acceptable but also appropriate when there are other more pressing clinical problems. Proper positioning for radiographic skull base examinations is impossible in the acutely injured uncooperative patient and dangerous in the presence

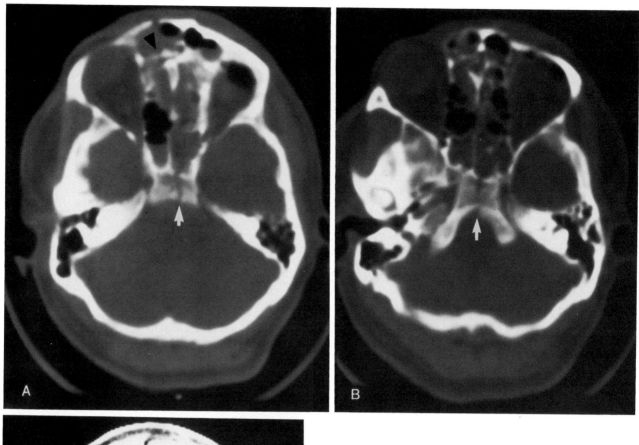

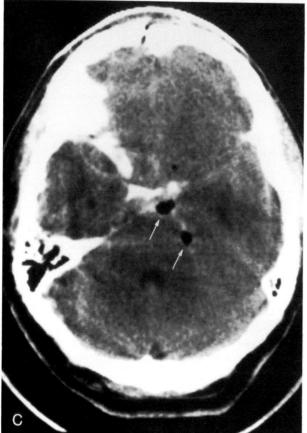

FIGURE 3–4. Fracture of the Skull Base Involving the Clivus

• • • •

A, A patient with severe head trauma had a complex basilar skull fracture that split the clivus *(arrow).* Note also the fracture through the anterior wall of the frontal sinus at the front of the skull and the comminuted fracture in the region of the cribriform plate *(arrowhead). B,* Note the step-off of the fracture in the clivus *(arrow). C,* Pneumocephalus *(arrows)* indicates communication between the pneumatized sinuses and the intracranial space.

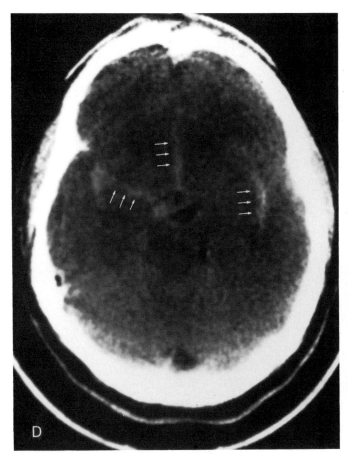

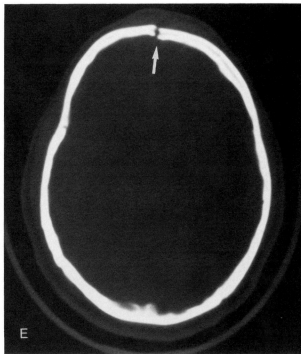

FIGURE 3–4 *Continued* **Fracture of the Skull Base Involving the Clivus**

• • • •

D, Density indicating subarachnoid hemorrhage *(arrows).* Trauma is a frequent cause of subarachnoid hemorrhage. *E,* This higher computed tomography slice indicates the separated fracture in the midline in the frontal bone *(arrow).* Note the soft tissue swelling superficial to the fracture.

of cervical spine injury. As a rule, evaluation of the skull base should be of secondary concern to the physician involved in the initial management of the trauma patient *except* in the setting of expanding hematoma or other significant vascular injury, progressive neurologic deficit, or obvious disruption of skull base integrity (Fig. 3–4).

Plain Film Examination

Skull base fractures are frequently not seen at plain film evaluation. They should be suspected when the paranasal sinuses or the mastoid air cells are opacified or when there is intracranial air. Visualization of an air-fluid level in the sphenoid sinus (Fig. 3–5) or opacification of the sphenoid sinus in the setting of trauma is strongly indicative of skull base fracture. Fracture lines are sometimes seen on submentovertex views, but their full extent is rarely apparent. Evaluation of skull base fractures requires a computed

tomography (CT) scan, and plain film evaluation is largely of historic interest only.

The condition of the patient will determine which if any plain films can be obtained. Ideally, the patient should have films taken using a dedicated head unit; they should include posteroanterior, lateral, Water's, Towne's, and submentovertex views, with the addition of Stenver's, Law's, or Schüller's views as indicated. Often, portable films with suboptimal positioning, collimation, and filming technique are all that is possible in these severely injured patients. The management of more important injuries must not be delayed by the effort to obtain a complete plain film evaluation of the skull base.

Opacification of paranasal sinuses is associated with skull base fracture. Although this finding is nonspecific, in the presence of other clinical or radiographic evidence of skull base fracture the opacification of a paranasal sinus or mastoid air cell is presumptive evidence of the site of injury in planning further evaluation. Unfortunately, facial bone

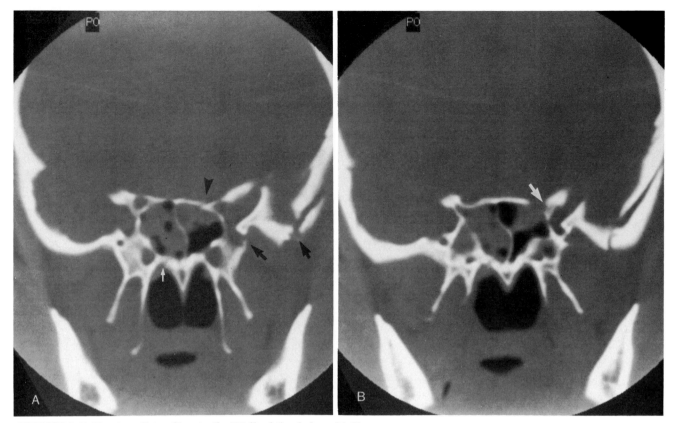

FIGURE 3–5. Fracture Extending to the Wall of the Sphenoid Sinus

• • • •

A, This patient had a comminuted fracture of the left temporal bone *(black arrows)* with a bony fragment impacting into the middle cranial fossa. Note the proximity of the depressed fragment to the superior orbital fissure. This type of fracture can present with ophthalmoparesis. Note also the extension of the fracture line to involve the wall of the sphenoid sinus both superiorly *(arrowhead)* and inferiorly *(white arrow). B,* This view further demonstrates the depressed bony fragment and the fracture line extending across the level of the anterior clinoid process to the planum sphenoidale *(arrow).*

trauma, any nasopharyngeal bleeding, or sinusitis also causes paranasal sinus opacification. This is especially true of the frontal, the ethmoidal, and the maxillary sinuses; opacification of the sphenoid sinus and the mastoid air spaces is a more specific indicator of skull base fracture.

Just as cerebrospinal fluid or blood may enter the paranasal sinuses through a basal skull fracture, air may also enter the cranial vault from the paranasal sinuses. In the absence of penetrating injury, pneumocephalus (see Fig. 3–4) is a highly significant finding. Pneumocephalus is strongly suggestive of basal skull fracture when it is accompanied by sinus opacification. The finding of sinus opacification or pneumocephalus on a plain film or CT scan should initiate a review for other signs of skull base fracture.

The visualization of fractures of the surrounding bones should also trigger a search for a basal skull fracture. Fracture of the anterior wall of the frontal sinus is frequently associated with a fracture of the posterior wall. A fracture of the squamous portion

of the temporal bone may be associated with a fracture of the petrous ridge. To a lesser degree, fractures of the face, the cervical spine, and the cranial vault are associated with the fracture of the skull base.

Computed Tomography

CT is the modality of choice for definitive evaluation of skull base fractures. Thin section and magnification techniques along with an inherently better depiction of bone anatomy make it superior to planar tomography, plain films, and magnetic resonance (MR) imaging. Images may be obtained in the coronal or the axial plane directly, though coronal images require a cooperative patient; in addition, positioning necessitates neck extension, so caution must be exercised in patient selection. Direct CT examination of the skull base in the coronal plane should not be

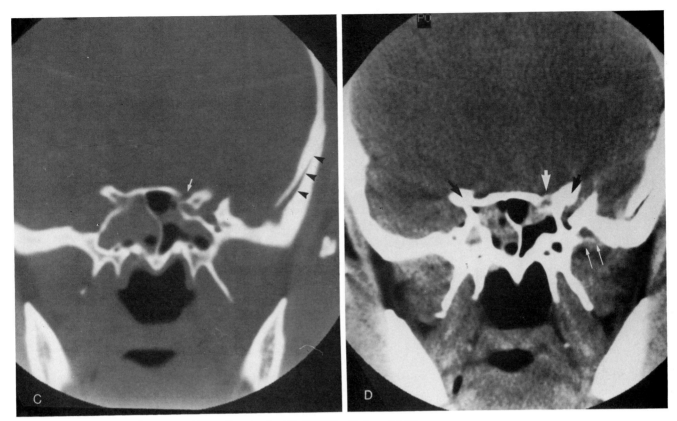

FIGURE 3–5 *Continued* **Fracture Extending to the Wall of the Sphenoid Sinus**

• • • •

C, A fracture in the planum sphenoidale *(arrow)* associated with the depression of the wall of the sphenoid sinus is seen. Note the fracture line in the diploic space in the temporal bone laterally *(arrowheads). D,* These soft tissue windows show density underlying the depressed fragment *(small arrows),* indicating a small area of hematoma. Also, note the density associated with the fracture of the planum sphenoidale *(large white arrow),* indicating the leakage of fluid into the sphenoid sinus (the two anterior clinoid processes are marked with black arrows).

performed in a patient with an unstable or an uncharacterized cervical spine injury.

Computer-generated images that have been reformatted from transaxial images may show three-dimensional relationships in other planes when direct imaging in those planes is not possible. Coronal or sagittal reconstructions may be especially valuable in individual cases as they eliminate dental artifacts that are seen on direct coronal cuts. Although three-dimensional reconstructions can be performed, the lack of significant displacement in most skull base fractures impedes fracture visualization on these reconstructed images.

Large fractures and the opacification of the paranasal sinuses and mastoid air cells may be demonstrated on routine head CT scans with sections as thick as 1 cm. Full characterization of fractures, however, requires thin cuts of 3 mm or less in thickness. Examination of the ossicles of the middle ear or of the facial canal should be done with cuts of 1–1.5 mm in thickness with targeting of the scan on

the region in question. If reconstruction of the images is planned, contiguity of cuts enhances quality, and overlap should be employed if thicker slices (5 mm) are used. Image viewing must be performed at suitable bone and soft tissue windows and levels.

The usual approach in a CT examination for head trauma is to evaluate the brain and the surrounding structures with contiguous axial 10-mm cuts from the foramen magnum to the top of the head. If special attention to the posterior fossa is desired, 5-mm cuts from the foramen magnum to the petrous ridges are obtained. Routine 5-mm cuts of the posterior fossa are employed in some centers. This screening examination includes portions of the ethmoid, the frontal, and the sphenoid sinuses as well as the mastoid air cells, the external auditory canal, and the middle ear. Opacification of these normally air-filled structures or the finding of pneumocephalus must raise suspicion of fracture of the skull base. Further evaluation of many skull base fractures can safely be deferred if there is a more life-threatening injury present. Isolated cerebrospinal fluid leak, hearing loss, and hematotympanum can sometimes continue for weeks before there is irreversible damage. Some delay in the evaluation of facial nerve injury is also acceptable, but generally treatment is initiated within 72 hours of the development of a traumatic facial nerve palsy. On the contrary, open fractures, progressive neurologic deficit, expanding hematoma, and active bleeding are indications for immediate work-up of a skull base fracture. Extreme cases occur in which the radiologic evaluation must be deferred for immediate surgical treatment of an acutely life-threatening problem related to a basal skull fracture. In the case of carotid-cavernous fistula, the onset of visual decline adds urgency to evaluation and treatment.

A proper reconstruction algorithm is necessary for diagnostic CT of the skull base. Algorithms designed for the sella turcica are excellent for the remainder of the skull base. There are other suitable algorithms designed to provide optimal resolution of bone structures. Prospective magnification, or *targeting*, of the areas of interest is important and can be tailored to the specific patient. Two-millimeter cuts are usually satisfactory for the evaluation of fractures; 1–1.5-mm contiguous cuts are necessary for the evaluation of ossicles of the middle ear.

Bone detail can also generally be appreciated using lower radiation doses during slice acquisition than that which is required to eliminate graininess and give soft tissue detail, especially on thinner sections. Therefore, we often use thicker sections (5 mm) to examine soft tissues and localize for bone imaging and then use thinner sections (1–2 mm) to rescan and reconstruct using a *bone algorithm* for fracture anatomy. The scout view acts as a lateral skull film and can sometimes indicate fracture extent (Fig. 3–6).

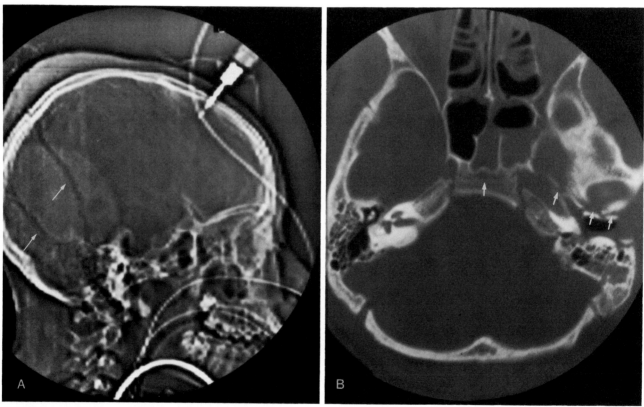

FIGURE 3–6. Horizontal Fracture Through the Clivus

• • • •

A, This scout view from a computed tomography (CT) scan shows a large occipital fracture bilaterally *(arrows)* and a large scalp hematoma superiorly. *B,* A thin CT cut through the skull base shows linear fracture extending from the external auditory canal longitudinally along the anterior aspect of the petrous apex, through the carotid canal, and across the clivus horizontally *(arrows).* Note also the fluid in the sphenoid sinus. Thinner cuts using bone algorithms result in improved definition of fracture detail.

CT cisternography can confirm the presence of a cerebrospinal fluid leak and often identifies the site of the leak. Skull base fractures are often multiple; thus, demonstration of a fracture does not necessarily locate the leak site. CT cisternography is performed by instilling 8–10 ml of a nonionic water-soluble myelographic contrast agent (200 mg/ml of organically bound iodine) into the intrathecal space using a lumbar injection site. The patient is placed in a lateral decubitus head-down position (Trendelenburg's position) for 10 minutes. Thin-section CT is performed immediately, with the area of suspected leak placed in a dependent position.

Some patients with a cerebrospinal fluid leak do not have sufficient clinical evidence to direct the CT examination. In these patients, nuclear cisternography can be performed. Pledgets are packed at strategic points in the nasal cavities just before the instillation of a solution of indium diethylenetriaminepentaacetic acid (DTPA) into the thecal sac via a lumbar puncture. The nasal pledgets are left in place for 12–24 hours. When they are removed, they are individually assessed for uptake of the radioactive tracer and compared with one another and to a background radiation reading from a plasma sample. A pledget (or pledgets) showing an elevation in activity three times greater than that of the background sample is a fairly accurate localizer for further CT investigation.

Every effort to obtain localizing information for CT evaluation fails in some patients. CT evaluation should then be performed in the areas statistically most likely to have a cerebrospinal fluid leak. The frontal and the ethmoid sinuses and the cribriform plate are the most frequent sites. The sphenoid sinus and the petrous bone are less often involved. The floor of the sella turcica, the clivus, and the sphenoid wings may also be sites of a post-traumatic cerebrospinal fluid rhinorrhea.

Magnetic Resonance Imaging

MR imaging is not recommended for the evaluation of skull base fractures. The imaging of the cranial nerves with MR techniques may augment bone imaging with CT but is generally not required to triage the patient in the emergency room. MR angiography may eventually replace angiography for the screening of the petrous and the cavernous internal carotid artery, though if an arteriovenous fistula or an aneurysm is suspected, angiography remains the procedure of choice. If intravascular intervention is being considered, angiography is mandatory and should be performed by or in consultation with the neurointerventionist.

Angiography

Angiography is sometimes required to evaluate new neurologic deficits in a patient with a skull base fracture, especially if there is active hemorrhage or an expanding hematoma. Injury to the intracranial carotid artery may not be obvious when the patient is first seen, though injury to the internal carotid artery may occur where the artery passes through the skull base, even in the absence of a fracture. Symptoms include cranial nerve palsy (especially of those nerves associated with the cavernous sinus), a bruit audible to the patient, a carotid-cavernous fistula, a cerebrovascular accident, or a frank intracranial hemorrhage. Epistaxis from the internal carotid artery usually occurs in patients undergoing treatment for tumors of the head and the neck, but may occur in the post-traumatic period. Angiography is the modality of choice in demonstrating injury to the artery itself and may be used in conjunction with CT or MR imaging to assess surrounding structures.

Angiographic evidence of arterial injury includes significant displacement of the artery, the presence of an intimal flap, an occlusion, a pseudoaneurysm, a carotid-cavernous fistula, and active hemorrhage. In addition to determination of the actual arterial injury, angiography can assess the adequacy of collateral arterial blood supply in the event that the sacrifice of the damaged artery becomes necessary.

In the past, injury to the internal carotid artery at the skull base has been treated either surgically or expectantly. Interventional neuroradiologic techniques can now either decrease the surgical risks or actually provide a definitive cure for the arterial injury. These techniques require advanced training but are becoming more widely available. Arterial occlusion is easily accomplished by the placement of detachable balloons when arterial sacrifice is planned (Fig. 3–7). Carotid-cavernous sinus fistulas can also be occluded with detachable balloons (Fig. 3–8), and some pseudoaneurysms can be obliterated with balloons or metallic coils. Planning for an occlusive procedure involves detailed knowledge of intracranial collateral blood supply and testing for the tolerance of arterial sacrifice using temporary occlusion techniques coupled with cerebral blood flow assessment during balloon inflation. Therefore, the interventional neuroradiologist should be involved early on in the evaluation and the treatment of these injuries. If no interventional neuroradiologist is available, patient referral should be considered.

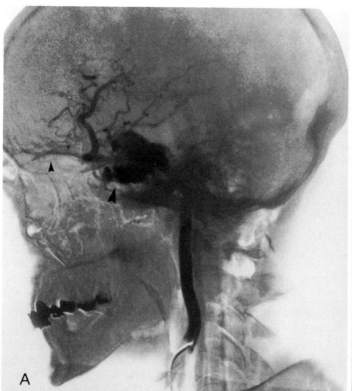

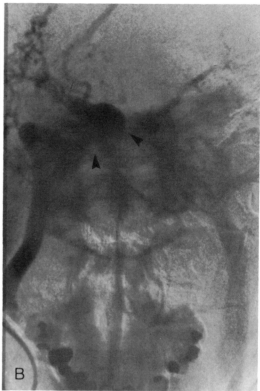

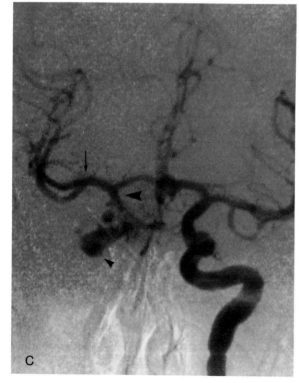

FIGURE 3–7. Carotid Cavernous Fistula Following Penetrating Trauma to the Orbit

• • • •

A, This lateral view from a right carotid arteriogram demonstrates gross extravasation of contrast in the cavernous sinus *(large arrowhead).* The superior orbital vein is seen to be filling *(small arrowhead).* All vascular structures that are visualized distal to the fistula are venous. No intracranial arterial filling is seen. *B,* An anteroposterior view shows a cloud of extravasated contrast in the cavernous sinus *(arrowheads).* Additionally, several smaller venous structures are seen. *C,* Injection of a contrast material into the contralateral carotid artery reveals filling across the anterior communicating artery to the right hemisphere. There is retrograde filling in the distal right internal carotid artery *(large arrowhead).* The contrast material flows into the fistula, and filling of the orbital vein on the right is seen *(small arrowhead).* Additionally, the right middle cerebral artery fills well via the left carotid injection *(arrow).*

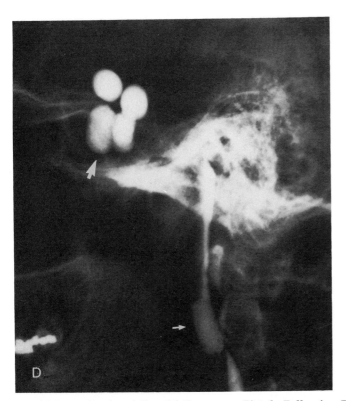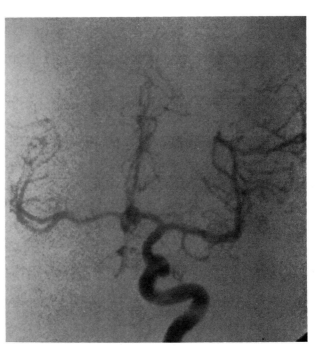

FIGURE 3–7 *Continued* **Carotid Cavernous Fistula Following Penetrating Trauma to the Orbit**
• • • •
D, Balloon embolization of the fistula was undertaken. Four balloons were placed in the cavernous sinus without occluding the carotid artery *(large arrow).* However, with the fourth balloon the fistula remained patent until the balloon was inflated to a point at which the carotid artery was occluded. We decided that the carotid must have been transected and, following a period of observation during which the patient tolerated carotid occlusion, the balloon was detached inflated to the point that the carotid remained permanently occluded. A fifth balloon was placed in the cervical carotid to ensure occlusion *(small arrow).* Note the static dye column proximal and distal to that balloon. E, Injection of a contrast material into the left internal carotid reveals continued filling of the right anterior and the middle cerebral arteries but no retrograde flow into the distal right carotid.

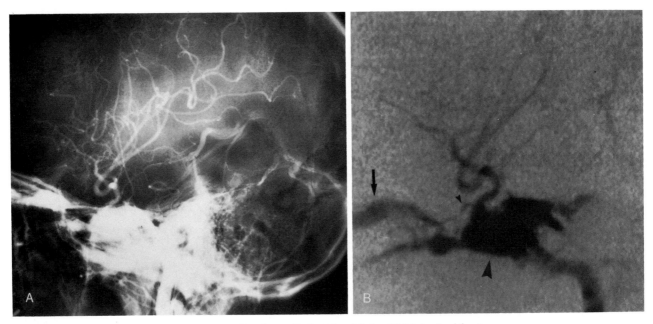

FIGURE 3–8. Carotid Cavernous Fistula Following a Pedestrian Motor Vehicle Accident

• • • •

This 15-year-old male was struck by a motor vehicle and suffered a basilar skull fracture. The development of a sixth nerve palsy and chemosis on the left was discovered. *A,* This lateral view arteriogram shows increased density in the region of the cavernous carotid; visualization of this segment of the carotid is poor. However, bone structures obscure some visualization of the precise anatomy. *B,* Using subtraction techniques, the bones can be eliminated. The study demonstrates the presence of extravasation of contrast from the cavernous carotid artery *(large arrowhead).* The ophthalmic artery is seen to be filling *(small arrowhead).* However, an additional, large venous structure (the superior orbital vein) is filling abnormally *(arrow).*

• • • •

PETROUS BONE FRACTURE

The petrous portion of the temporal bone has numerous important neurologic and vascular associations as well as external communications via the eustachian tube and the external auditory canal. Fracture of the petrous bone is relatively common, and clinical symptoms requiring evaluation and therapy are frequent. Fractures involving the petrous bone have been categorized as transverse, longitudinal, and mixed. Overlap in clinical symptoms among the fracture types does occur, but classification remains radiologically and clinically useful.

The majority of petrous bone fractures are longitudinal (70–90%), with the fracture line oriented along the long axis of the petrous ridge (see Fig. 3–6*B*). Longitudinal fractures are usually caused by a blow to the side of the head and are associated with fractures of the squamous portion of the temporal bone, which may be visible on plain films. The external auditory canal, the tympanic membrane, and the middle ear are traversed by the fracture line,

which then can extend anterolaterally to the carotid canal and as far medially as the foramen spinosum. The bony labyrinth, the facial nerve, and the internal auditory canal are usually spared by longitudinal fractures. Facial nerve palsy may appear late following this fracture and is often incomplete when it does develop (Fig. 3–9).

Hearing loss associated with longitudinal fracture is usually of the conductive type. Hemotympanum is a common cause of hearing loss and usually resolves spontaneously. Rupture of the tympanic membrane is also frequent and should be visible otoscopically. These causes of conductive hearing loss do not require radiologic investigation. Persistent conductive hearing loss with a normal tympanic membrane should prompt examination of the ossicular chain. Traumatic disruption of the ossicles should be evaluated by targeted CT using 1–1.5-mm contiguous cuts in both the axial and the coronal planes. Most ossicular disruptions involve the incudostapedial joint, the most common site of injury to the ossicles of the middle ear. Patients with longitudinal petrous bone fractures are also at increased risk of the late development of an acquired cholestea-

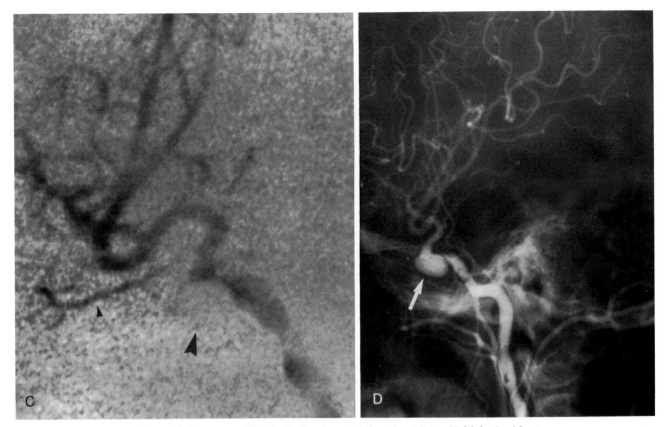

FIGURE 3–8 *Continued* **Carotid Cavernous Fistula Following a Pedestrian Motor Vehicle Accident**
• • • •
C, A single detachable balloon was introduced through the fistula, inflated, and then detached *(large arrowhead).* Note that when static structures are seen, the use of subtraction techniques obscures their presence. Therefore, the balloon is only a shadow on the subtracted arteriogram. The ophthalmic artery continues to fill *(small arrowhead).* However, the abnormally dilated and filling superior orbital vein is no longer seen. *D,* Without using the subtraction techniques, the contrast-material–filled balloon is more obvious *(arrow).*

toma. Cholesteatomas that occur following trauma are often more aggressive than those that develop as a sequel of inflammatory disease.

Transverse fractures of the petrous ridge are less common (20%) than longitudinal ones and usually result from a blow to the occiput. The fracture line extends from the jugular foramen or the foramen magnum through the petrous ridge and may involve the labyrinth and the seventh or the eighth cranial nerves. Ossicular disruption is not common with transverse fractures.

Labyrinthine involvement with fracture may cause sensorineural hearing loss or persistent, incapacitating vertigo. Evaluation of the bony labyrinth is also performed using thin-section CT (1- or 1.5-mm contiguous cuts). Sensorineural hearing loss and persistent vertigo may occur in the absence of any demonstrable CT abnormality.

Traumatic facial nerve palsy may also occur without a fracture. Contusion or compression of the facial nerve by a hematoma as it passes through its canal or in the middle ear causes this dysfunction in the affected portion. The complex course of the facial nerve makes examination by 1- or 1.5-mm CT cuts in both the axial and the coronal planes necessary. Although there are reports of the delayed recovery of facial nerve function over intervals as long as a year, therapy should be initiated within 72 hours to minimize the risk of wallerian degeneration of an otherwise normal distal facial nerve segment.

As in other skull base fractures, cerebrospinal fluid leakage, pneumocephalus, and meningitis may result. A cerebrospinal fluid leak resolves spontaneously in the majority of petrous bone fractures and may be observed over a period of several months or until meningitis supervenes. When evaluation is indicated, attempts to localize the site of the leak using clinical findings or nuclear cisternography, or both, should be made. CT cisternography may also be helpful in the petrous bone.

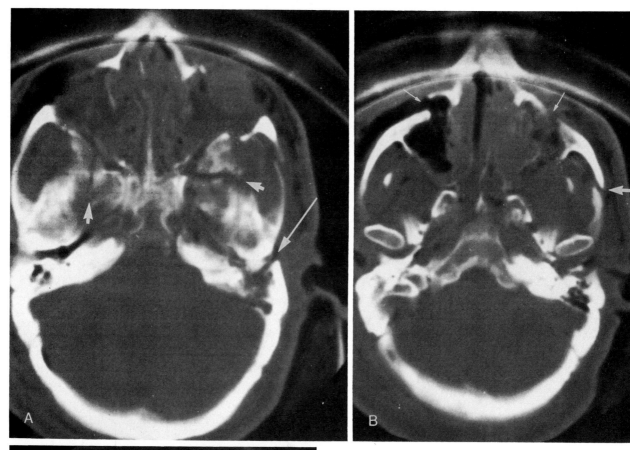

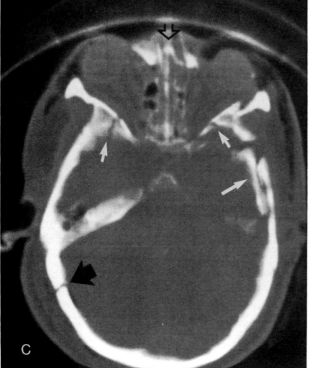

FIGURE 3–9. Complex Fracture of the Floor of the Middle Cranial Fossa

• • • •

A, A patient with severe head injury has fractures extending through the floor of the middle cranial fossa bilaterally *(short arrows).* There is also a fracture extending into the petrous apex through the inner ear on the left *(long arrow).* This fracture is perpendicular to the axis of the petrous apex. *B,* Fracture of zygomatic arch *(large arrow)* and of the anterior walls of both maxillary sinuses *(small arrows)* is evident. *C,* Fracture lines extend superiorly from the floor of the middle fossa to involve the lateral orbital walls bilaterally *(short white arrows).* Note also the depressed bony fragment from the squamous portion of the temporal bone *(long white arrow).* There is also a complex nasal fracture *(open arrow)* and an occipital fracture on the right *(large black arrow)* with underlying pneumocephalus.

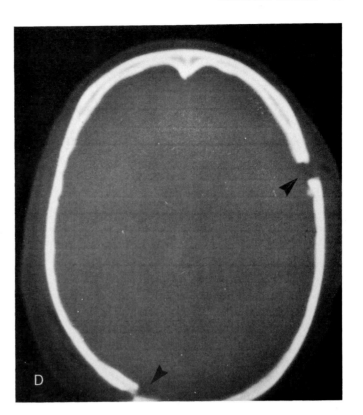

FIGURE 3–9 *Continued* **Complex Fracture of the Floor of the Middle Cranial Fossa**

• • • •

D, A higher cut indicates a large skull fracture extending into the frontal bone as well as the occipital bone *(arrowheads)*.

Bibliography

Azar-Kia B, Sarwar M, Batinitzky S, Schechter MM. Radiology of intracranial gas. AJR 1975; 124:315.

Cannon CR, Jahrsdoerfer RA. Temporal bone fractures. Review of 90 cases. Arch Otolaryngol 1983; 109:285.

Davis KR. Embolization of epistaxis and nasopharyngeal juvenile angiofibromas. AJNR 1986; 7:1953.

Freeman J. Temporal bone fractures and cholesteatoma. Ann Otol Rhinol Laryngol 1983; 92:558.

Goodwin WJ. Temporal bone fractures. Radiol Clin North Am 1983; 16:651.

Kleid MS, Miller HS. Internal carotid artery epistaxis. Otolaryngol Head Neck Surg 1986; 94:480.

Lantz EJ, Forbes GS, Brown ML, Laws ER Jr. Radiology of CSF rhinorrhea. AJR 1980; 135:1023.

Lindeman RC. Temporal bone trauma and facial paralysis. Otolaryngol Clin North Am 1979; 12:403.

McKusick KA, Malmud LS, Cardella PA. Radionuclide cisternography: Normal values for nasal secretions of intrathecally injected indium 111 DTPA. J Nucl Med 1973; 14:933.

Meschan I. An Atlas of Anatomy Basic to Radiology. Philadelphia: W.B. Saunders Company, 1975, pp 319–349.

Neely JG, Neblett CR, Rose JE. Diagnosis and treatment of spontaneous CSF otorrhea. Laryngoscope 1982; 92:609.

Potter GD. Trauma to the temporal bone. Semin Roentgenol 1969; 4:143.

Reynolds DF. Traumatic effusion of the sphenoid sinus. Clin Radiol 1961; 12:171–176.

Robinson A, Meares BM, Goree JA. Traumatic sphenoid sinus effusion. AJR 1967; 101:795.

Rogers LF (ed). Radiology of Skeletal Trauma. Vol 1. New York: Churchill Livingstone, Inc., 1982, pp 211–227.

Sandler MP, Price AC, Runge VM, et al. Cerebrospinal fluid cisternography. In Gottschalk A, Hoffer PB, Potchen EJ (eds). Diagnostic Nuclear Medicine. Vol 2. Baltimore: Williams & Wilkins, 1988, pp 888–898.

Swartz JD (ed). Imaging of the Temporal Bone. New York: Thieme Medical Publishers, Inc., 1986, pp 33–202.

Swartz JD, Swartz NG, Korsvik H, et al. Computerized tomographic evaluation of the middle ear and mastoid for post-traumatic hearing loss. Ann Otol Rhinol Laryngol 1985; 94:263.

Tamakawa Y, Hanafee W. CSF rhinorrhea: Significance of an air-fluid level in the sphenoid sinus. Radiology 1980; 135:101.

Tos M. Course of and sequelae to 248 petrosal fractures. Acta Otolaryngol 1973; 75:353.

CHAPTER 4

·····································

Facial Trauma

········

W. B. LOWRY, M.D.

RADIOGRAPHIC VIEWS, NORMAL ANATOMY, AND EVALUATION

Waters's view is the single best view for evaluating the facial bones (Fig. 4–1). The lateral and the inferior orbital rim, the orbital floor, the nasal arch and the septum, the maxillary and the frontal sinuses, and the zygoma are all well demonstrated on this view. There is a normal groove in the lateral wall of the maxillary sinus for passage of the posterior superior alveolar nerve. This groove is most easily seen in an opacified antrum and should not be mistaken for a fracture.

The Caldwell (Fig. 4–2) projection demonstrates the superior, the medial, and the lateral orbital rims, the frontal and the ethmoid sinuses, the oblique orbital line, and the nasal septum to good advantage. The fovea ethmoidalis (roof of the ethmoid sinus), the cribriform plate, the crista galli, the floor of the sella, and the superior orbital fissures are also seen.

Proper positioning is mandatory on the lateral view (Fig. 4–3). When positioning is truely lateral, the lack of superimposition of the normally superimposed structures suggests a fracture with displacement of the fracture fragments. The anterior and the posterior walls of the frontal and the maxillary sinuses are delineated on the lateral view. The oval densities outlining the maxillary recesses of the zygoma are normally well seen as are the pterygoid plates and the pterygopalatine fossa. The lateral rims of the orbits, the floor of the anterior cranial fossa, the sphenoid sinus, and the retropharyngeal soft tissues can also be evaluated.

A good submentovertex view is often hard to obtain in the injured patient and is contraindicated if there is an associated cervical spine injury. The structures well visualized on this view are the ethmoid and the sphenoid sinuses (Fig. 4–4), the anterior and the lateral walls of the maxillary sinuses, the lateral walls of the orbits, the greater wing of the sphenoid bone, the pterygoid plates, and the basal foramina. The anterior and the posterior walls of the frontal sinus may be demonstrated, though they are often obscured by the mandible. The nasopharynx is also seen superimposed on the sphenoid sinus. The zygomatic arches are not well delineated because the technique needed for a good base view is overpenetrated for these bones. An underpenetrated view should be obtained when the zygomatic arches need to be evaluated.

When reading films of the face, whether they are plain films, tomograms, or computed tomography (CT) scans, several direct and suggestive findings should raise the question of fracture. Soft tissue swelling and fluid in the paranasal sinuses are such signs. Swelling of the soft tissues in the clinical

• • • • APPROPRIATE RADIOGRAPHIC STUDIES

I. **Nasal Fractures, and Frontal Sinus and Ethmoid Air Cell Injury**
   A. Plain films
      1. Waters's view
   Comment: Best overall view for visualizing facial fractures in general. Demonstrates the nasal septum and the arch well. The frontal sinuses are also well seen.
      2. Caldwell view
   Comment: Excellent for visualization of the frontal sinus and the ethmoid air cells.
      3. Lateral view
   Comment: Demonstrates the anterior and the posterior walls of the frontal sinus. A lateral view using soft tissue technique is the best view for visualizing nasal bone fractures.
      4. Submentovertex view
   Comment: Demonstrates the ethmoid air cells to advantage. Must not be attempted when cervical spine injury is possible.
   B. Computed tomography
   Comment: Contiguous thin (2–3-mm) sections must be obtained. Axial and coronal scanning is preferable. When direct coronal sections are not possible, reconstructed images may be helpful. Computed tomography (CT) is useful in evaluation of the floor of the frontal sinus and the ethmoid air cells and when nasofrontal or nasolacrimal duct injury is of concern. Overall, CT is the technique of choice to assess facial fractures if they are seriously suspected.

II. **The Mandible**
   A. Plain films
      1. Anteroposterior view
      2. Bilateral oblique lateral views
   Comment: Best view for evaluation of the mandibular body, the ramus, and the angle.
      3. Towne's view
   Comment: Useful for studying the symphysis and the condyles in particular.
      4. Waters's view
      5. Panoramic view
   Comment: Equipment for performing panoramic views is uncommon in emergency facilities. However, these views can demonstrate the entire mandible well on a single film.
      6. Submentovertex view
   Comment: Useful in studying condylar displacement and in the evaluation of symphysis.

• • • • APPROPRIATE RADIOGRAPHIC STUDIES Continued

7. Polytomography

Comment: Can evaluate the temporomandibular joints well but has been virtually replaced by CT.

B. Computed tomography

Comment: Not routinely indicated. Excellent for the evaluation of the temporomandibular joints; can be used to study the entire mandible.

C. Magnetic resonance imaging

Comment: No acute application. Provides excellent demonstration of the temporomandibular joints and the post-traumatic problems of condyles.

III. **The Midface**

A. Plain films

1. Waters's view

Comment: Best overall projection for visualizing facial bones. Demonstrates the lateral and the inferior orbit rim, the floor of the orbit, the zygoma, the nasal arch and the septum, and the maxillary and the frontal sinuses.

2. Caldwell projection

Comment: Demonstrates the superior, the medial, and the lateral orbit rim, the frontal and the ethmoid sinuses, the nasal septum, and the floor of the sella.

3. Lateral view

Comment: Performing a true lateral projection is mandatory. Demonstrates the anterior and the posterior walls of the frontal and the maxillary sinuses, the sphenoid sinus, and the floor of the anterior cranial fossa.

4. Submentovertex view

Comment: The ethmoid and the sphenoid sinuses are well seen on this view, as are the greater wing of the sphenoid bone, the basal foramina, and the anterior and the lateral maxillary antral walls. An underpenetrated view demonstrates the zygomatic arches well.

B. Polytomography

Comment: Provides excellent evaluation of the midface but has been largely replaced by CT. Requires significant patient cooperation.

C. Computed tomography

Comment: Thin-section contiguous sections in the axial and the coronal planes are performed when feasible.

IV. **Zygomatic Fractures**

Comment: Same as for the midface. CT may be especially useful in planning reconstructive surgery.

V. **Le Fort Fractures and Facial Smashes**

Comment: Same as for the midface, but CT scans are often more easily interpreted than plain films. Three-dimensional CT is often important prior to reconstructive surgery.

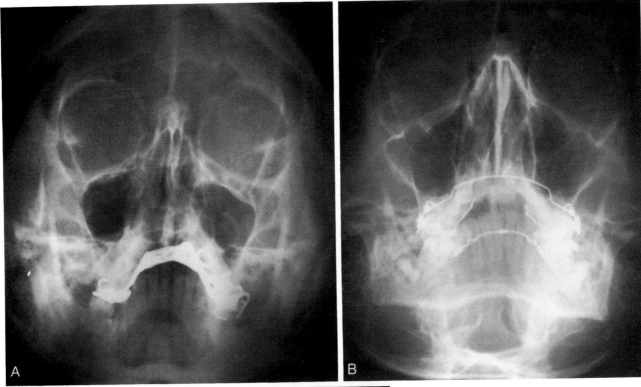

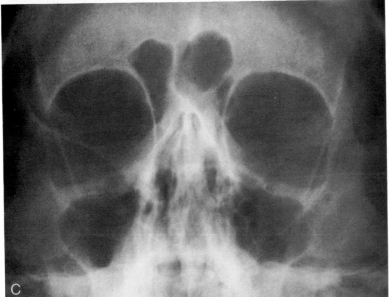

FIGURE 4–1. Waters's View

• • • •

This view is taken in the posteroanterior position with the canthomeatal line at approximately 37 degrees to the film surface. The actual angulation varies with neck extension. *A*, A Waters view with standard positioning. Note the interference of visualization caused by the patient's dentures. *B*, A Waters view showing increased neck extension placing petrous ridges well below the maxillary sinuses. *C*, A Waters view with decreased neck extension superimposes the petrous bone on the maxillary antra and could obscure a fluid level.

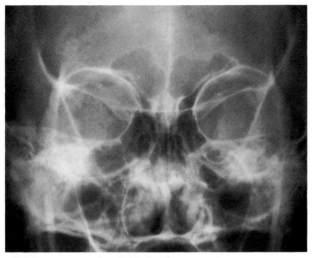

FIGURE 4–2. Caldwell Projection

• • • •

This view is obtained in the posteroanterior projection. The patient must place his or her forehead and nose against the film. The tube is then angled about 23 degrees caudad to the canthomeatal line. The petrous ridges are superimposed over the lower part of the orbit.

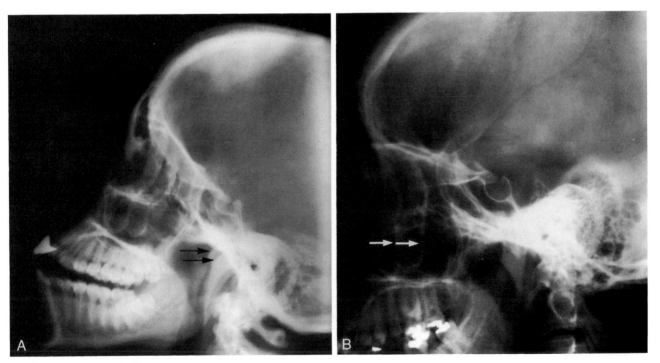

FIGURE 4–3. Lateral Film

• • • •

The goal is to obtain a true lateral projection without either tilt or rotation so that the paired structures are superimposed. In the trauma patient this goal is elusive, and lateral films must be interpreted with an understanding of the rotation and the tilt seen. *A,* This lateral film for the facial bones has rotation demonstrated by the lack of superimposition of the posterior maxillary sinus walls and the mandibular condyles *(arrows).* In addition, there is some tilt, which is most easily identified by the presence of two margins of the floor of the anterior cranial fossa. *B,* A second lateral film demonstrates more marked rotation, demonstrated by the zygomatic recesses of the maxillary sinuses *(arrows);* however, it shows very little tilt.

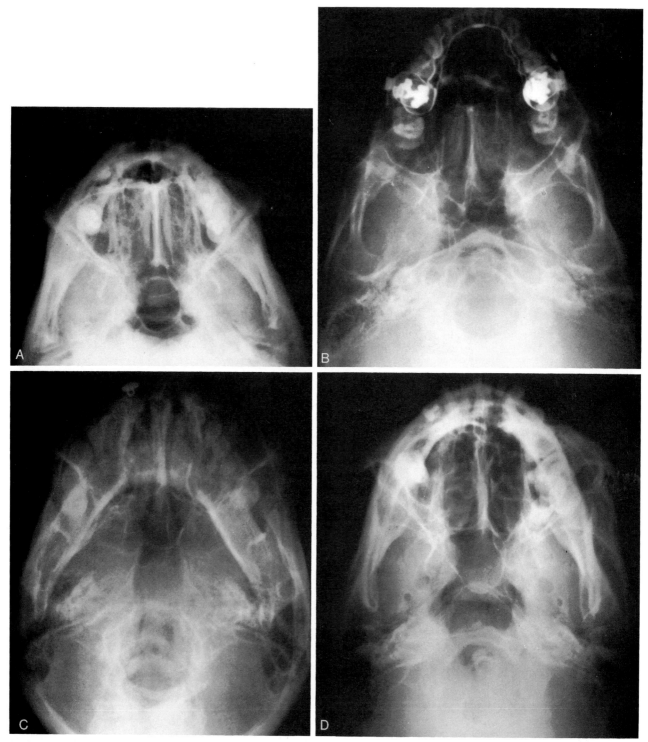

FIGURE 4–4. Submentovertex Projection

• • • •

This view requires extension of the neck and therefore must not be attempted if a cervical spine injury is possible. The vertex of the head is placed against the film, and the central x-ray beam is projected midline and perpendicular to the infraorbital line. *A,* In this case the extension is appropriate, and there is little rotation or tilt. *B,* Excessive extension superimposes the frontal sinuses on the hard palate, but the sphenoid sinus is well seen. *C,* Too little flexion superimposes the mandible over many of the facial bones. *D,* Rotation and decreased extension limit this example significantly.

setting of trauma indicates injury and helps to localize the area of primary concern. Fluid in the sinuses suggests bleeding from a fracture but could also be due to a nosebleed or pre-existing sinusitis. Direct signs are cortical defects, fragment displacement, and fragment rotation.

• • • •

NASAL FRACTURES AND INJURY TO THE FRONTAL SINUS AND ETHMOID AIR CELLS

The nasal bones are the most frequently fractured bones of the face. Injuries range from simple isolated fractures (Fig. 4–5) to components of complex fractures, such as the Le Fort II and the Le Fort III injuries (Fig. 4–6). The nasal bones are two predominantly flat bones that abut each other at a midline suture. They also adjoin the frontal bone and the frontal process of the maxilla. The ethmoid air cells lie posterior to the nasal bones. The nasal septum (Fig. 4–7) is composed of the perpendicular plate of the ethmoid bone posteriorly and superiorly, by the vomer posteriorly and inferiorly, and by a cartilaginous plate centrally and anteriorly. The center of growth for the cartilaginous septum is located at the septovomerine angle. The hard palate forms the floor of the nasal cavity, and the cribriform plate forms the roof. The anterior nasal spine is a triangular bony protuberance extending anteriorly from the maxilla at the inferior aspect of the nose.

Fractures of the nasal bones are usually transverse in orientation and best seen on a lateral view obtained using soft tissue technique. Longitudinal fractures also occur, but care must be taken not to mistake the normal sutures or the longitudinally oriented nasociliary grooves, which contain the nasociliary nerves, for longitudinal fractures. Fractures are generally more sharply delineated and have greater lucency than the normal sutures and grooves. Waters's view is used to evaluate the nasal arch for fracture, displacement, and soft tissue swelling (see Fig. 4–7). Isolated nasal fractures are often so obvious clinically that radiographic evaluation is unnecessary. However, soft tissue swelling can be great enough to obscure the extent of injury at clinical examination. Nasal septal fractures are also demonstrated on Waters's views by the displacement and the sharp angulation of the septum (Fig. 4–8). Septal hematomas can be identified by the presence of unilateral or bilateral swelling around the septum in the absence of any angulation or displacement. A septal injury can cause acute airway obstruction when swelling and displacement are sufficiently great.

When the growth center at the septovomerine angle is involved, physiologic as well as cosmetic deformity can cause obstruction, deformed growth, and the elevation of the hard palate in the young.[34]

More severe injuries to the nasofrontal region cause fractures of the walls of the frontal sinus, the ethmoid air cells, and the cribriform plate. The nasofrontal duct travels from the floor of the frontal sinus in a posterior caudal direction through the anterior ethmoid air cells to enter the nose at the anterior aspect of the middle meatus. Fractures of the floor of either the frontal sinus or the anterior ethmoid air cells, or both, involve the nasofrontal duct in more than two thirds of all patients. CT is the best way to evaluate this region radiographically. Contiguous thin sections (2–3 mm in thickness) in the axial and the coronal planes should be obtained. If associated injuries prevent direct coronal scanning, reconstructions of the CT scan in the coronal projection may be important. However, subtle disruptions of the cribriform plate may be missed without direct thin coronal CT scanning. Complications of fractures of the frontal sinus and the cribriform plate include pneumocephalus, cerebrospinal fluid rhinorrhea, and intracranial infection. Fortunately, most cerebrospinal fluid leaks stop spontaneously with conservative management.[41]

The lateral wall of the ethmoid air cells is the lamina papyracea, the paper-thin medial wall of the orbit. Fractures of this region are discussed in Chapter 5 on orbital trauma. Anterior to the lamina papyracea is the lacrimal bone. The frontal process of the maxilla lies anterior to the lacrimal bone. Fractures of this region often injure the medial canthal tendon, the lacrimal sac, and the nasolacrimal duct.[23] Epiphora or excessive tear formation associated with trauma to this region may make clinical assessment of the nasolacrimal duct difficult. Thin section axial CT scans can identify fractures of the nasolacrimal duct and by delineating the extent of injury can also suggest associated canthal injury. Dacrocystography is still the best radiographic method of demonstrating the integrity of the nasolacrimal duct itself but is virtually never indicated in the acutely injured patient. Waters's and Caldwell projections can sometimes demonstrate this injury, but detailed anatomic delineation is most successfully achieved with CT.

Fracture of the ethmoid air cells is rarely an isolated injury. There is usually also either orbital or nasofrontoethmoidal complex trauma. The plain film finding of ethmoid air cell opacification is suggestive of injury, but opacification also may be caused by mucosal edema, blood, or even pre-existing sinusitis. The Caldwell and base views are the best plain film projections for evaluation of the ethmoid air cells. The bony septa are too thin to be visualized on plain

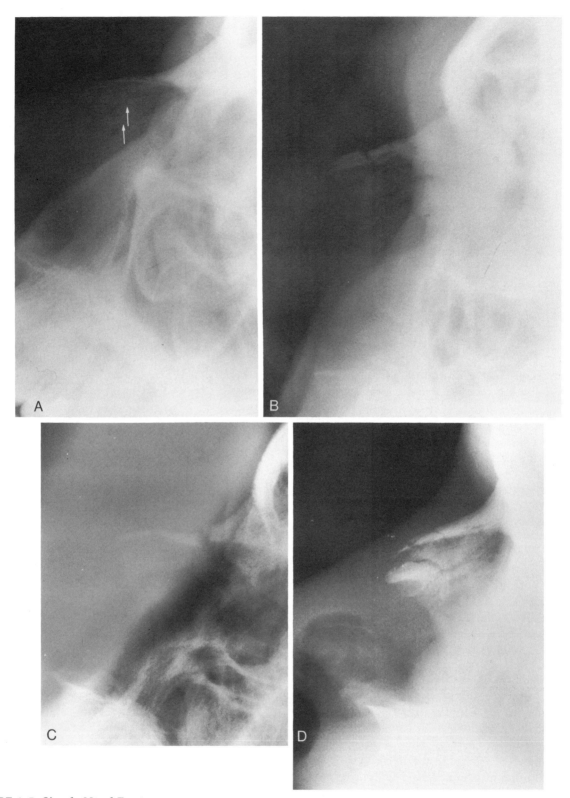

FIGURE 4–5. Simple Nasal Fracture

• • • •

A, This normal lateral view of the nasal bones reveals the normal sutures *(arrows),* which are longitudinally oriented. *B,* Transverse nasal bone fractures. *C,* A transverse nasal fracture with displacement of the distal fragment. *D,* This view of a more complex fracture of the nasal bones shows fracture lines that are somewhat longitudinal but which can be distinguished from the sutures owing to their sharpness and orientation.

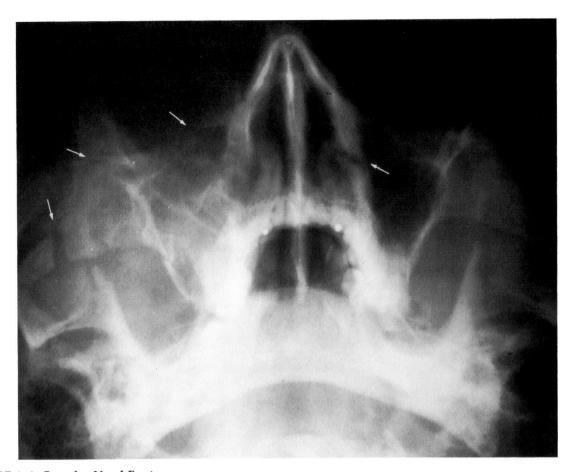

FIGURE 4–6. Complex Nasal Fracture

• • • •

A nasal fracture as part of a complex facial fracture is shown *(arrows)*.

FIGURE 4–7. Nasal Septum

• • • •

The nasal septum is best evaluated on a Waters view. In this patient the nasal arch is well seen as is a fracture of the right nasal bone *(arrow)*. Notice the associated soft tissue swelling.

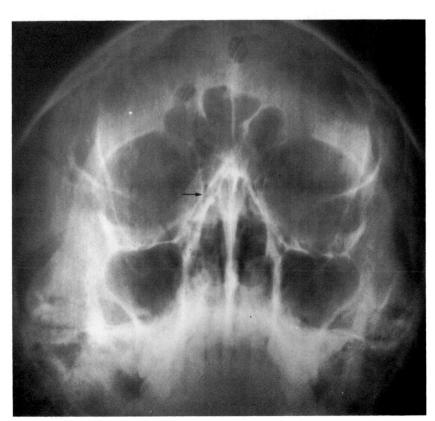

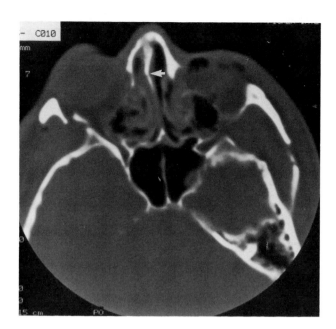

FIGURE 4–8. Nasal Septal Fracture and Hematoma in a Patient with a Facial Smash

• • • •

The nasal septum is fractured and deviated near its base *(arrow)*, and there is a bilateral septal hematoma. Many other abnormalities are also seen, including air in the soft tissues, opacification of ethmoid air cells, and fractures of the right lateral orbital wall.

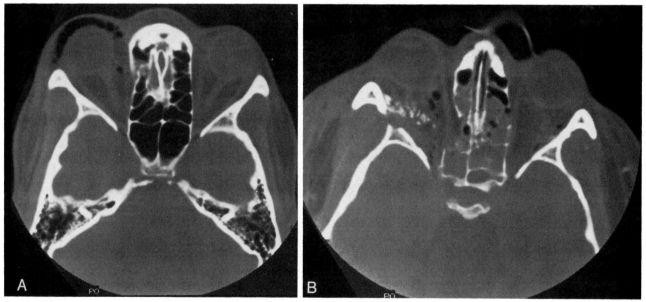

FIGURE 4–9. Opacification of Ethmoid Air Cells at Computed Tomography

• • • •

A, This computed tomography (CT) section in a patient with orbital emphysema and a medial orbital wall fracture demonstrates opacification of a few ethmoid air cells. The remainder of the air cells are normal, and the fine bony septa are well seen. B, This CT section in another patient taken following a gunshot wound demonstrates to advantage both the bony abnormalities and the degree of ethmoid air cell opacification. Bilateral intraorbital emphysema and hematoma are also seen. Note the entry wound in the lateral orbital wall on the patient's right, with bony fragments in the orbit traversing the expected course of the optic nerve. Note also the exit area from the medial right orbital wall, with medial displacement of the medial rectus muscle and cribriform plate. The medial rectus muscle does not appear entrapped in this case.

films, on which sinus opacification occurs; CT is required to visualize the septa (Fig. 4–9).

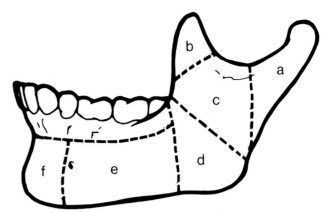

FIGURE 4–10. Diagram of the Mandible in Lateral Projection
• • • •
The condyle (a), the coronoid process (b), the ramus (c), the angle (d), the body (e), and the symphysis (f) are the six components of the hemimandible.

• • • •

THE MANDIBLE

The mandible is the horseshoe-shaped bone that forms the lower jaw. It is the largest of the facial bones and is second only to the nasal bones in frequency of injury.[40] The cause of mandibular injury varies.[5] In large urban hospitals aggravated assault with a blunt object is the most common cause of fracture. Motor vehicle accidents, falls, and gunshot wounds follow in frequency of incidence. However, in more suburban or private hospitals motor vehicle accidents are the common source of injury. The body and the angle of the mandible are most frequently injured during an aggravated assault. The condyles and the symphysis are more commonly injured in falls and in motor vehicle accidents; they are also the most commonly injured bones in children. Associated injuries are more common following motor vehicle accidents, but they are not at all unusual as the result of aggravated assaults. Additional facial fractures are the most frequently encountered associated injuries, but intracranial, cervical spine, thoracoabdominal, and appendicular skeletal injuries also occur. Airway obstruction is always a serious potential problem with significant facial trauma.

The mandible is a partial ring and therefore is injured in more than one location in more than 50% of fractures. The temporomandibular joints act as shock absorbers that may prevent some multiple fractures. The temporomandibular joints themselves can be injured by the blow but usually develop symptoms at a later time. Dislocation of the temporomandibular joints is a more immediate complication. Many systemic disorders predispose the patient to mandibular fracture and include, among others, hyperparathyroidism, Paget's disease, and osteoporosis. Focal abnormalities, such as impacted molar teeth, mandibular neoplasm, cysts, and tooth root abscesses, also predispose the patient to fracture.

The mandible is divided into six segments: the condyle, the coronoid process, the ramus, the angle, the body, and the symphysis (Fig. 4–10). The majority of mandibular growth emanates from the condyles, which are epiphyseal regions. Therefore, fractures of the condyles in the young can lead to asymmetric or abnormal growth, causing occlusal and cosmetic deformities.

The plain film evaluation includes an anteroposterior view, right and left oblique lateral views with 25-degree caudad angulation, a Towne view, and also a Waters projection as needed (Fig. 4–11). A single panoramic film (Fig. 4–12) of the mandible also suffices if the equipment is available and the patient is not too severely injured, is cooperative, and is able to sit up and hold still for a long exposure. The routine use of CT is not indicated except during evaluation of the condylar heads for fracture with displacement (Fig. 4–13), dislocation, and chip fractures.

Additional CT cuts through the temporomandibular joints can easily be obtained following a facial or head CT scan. Coronal and sagittal reconstructions can also be performed. Polytomography can also be used to study the temporomandibular joints, though this is seldom indicated during emergency evaluation. Magnetic resonance (MR) imaging can evaluate the soft tissues of the temporomandibular joints and also post-traumatic complications such as avascular necrosis and osteochondritis of the condyle.

Patients with mandibular fractures often have clinically obvious deformities of the mandible. Bruising, chin laceration, malocclusion, trismus, pain over the temporomandibular joints, and limited ability to open the mouth also occur. However, mandibular fractures may have little displacement, and more than half of such fractures are multiple. It is important to trace the cortical margins of the mandible and the mandibular canal, carefully searching for any irregularity or step-off to avoid missing fractures (Fig. 4–14). Mach lines from the air and soft tissues in the oropharyngeal space can be quite deceptive (Fig. 4–15). These are most problematic on the lateral oblique view, often the best projection for evaluating the mandibular body, the angle, and the ramus. The condyles are best seen on the Towne and the lateral

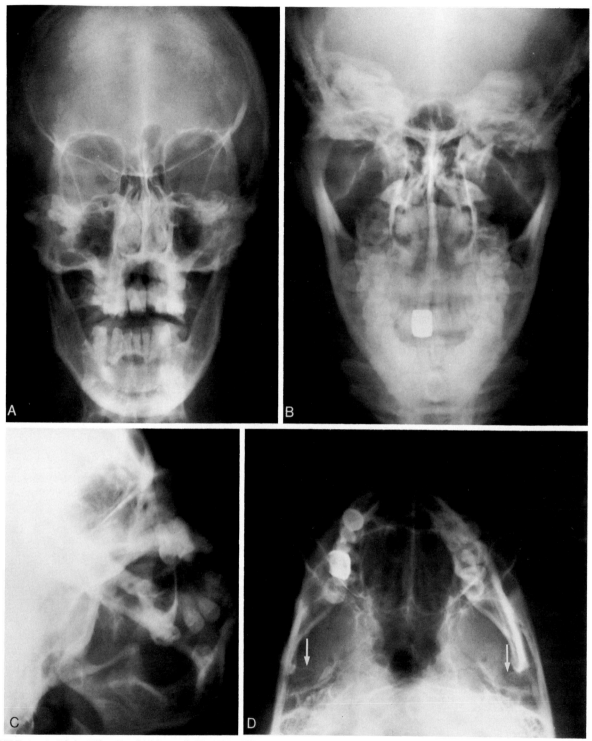

FIGURE 4–11. Plain Film Evaluation of the Mandible

• • • •

A, The anteroposterior (AP) view of the mandible demonstrates well this bone from ramus to ramus. The condyles and coronoid processes are obscured. *B,* The Towne view includes the condyles, but the coronoid processes are obscured. The elongation of the mandible may either obscure or improve the visualization of fractures seen on the AP view. *C,* The lateral oblique view is excellent for study of the body, the angle, the ramus, the coronoid process, and the condyle on the side being evaluated. *D,* A base view demonstrates the condylar head to advantage *(arrows).*

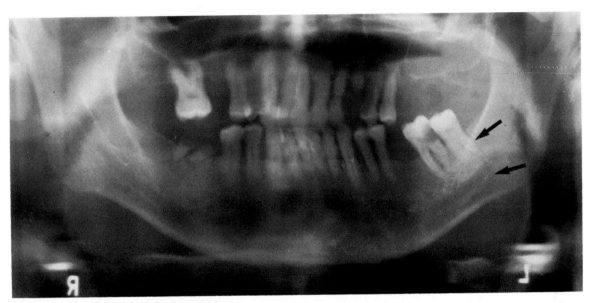

FIGURE 4–12. Panorex View of the Mandible

• • • •

The mandibular rami, angles, body, and symphysis are well displayed by this technique. In this patient a fracture of the left mandible at the junction of the body and the angle is demonstrated *(arrows)*. Panorex views require that the patient hold still for a longer time than for the usual radiograph and that he or she be able to assume an upright position. In this patient, the condyles are not demonstrated completely.

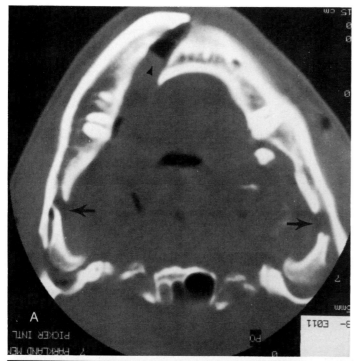

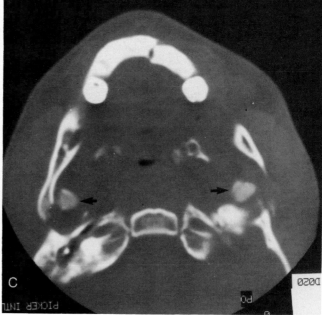

FIGURE 4–13. Computed Tomographic Demonstration of Condylar Fractures and the Dislocation of the Condylar Heads

• • • •

A, A fracture of the mandibular symphysis *(arrowhead)* is quite separated. In addition, bilateral condylar head fractures *(arrows)* are present. The condylar heads are displaced from the temporomandibular joint bilaterally. *B* and *C,* A second patient has a less displaced fracture of the symphysis. There are bilateral condylar fractures with more marked displacement of the condylar heads *(arrows)* from the temporomandibular joints.

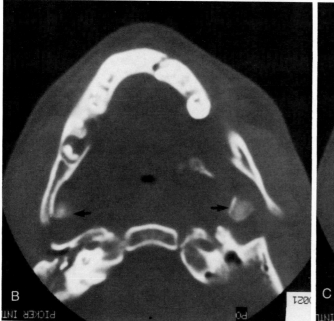

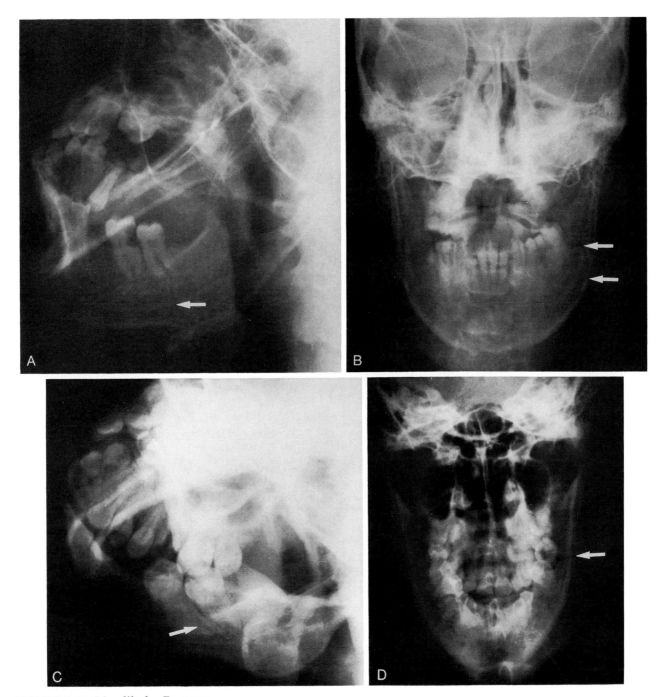

FIGURE 4–14. Mandibular Fractures

• • • •

A, A lateral oblique view demonstrates a subtle fracture of the body of the mandible near the angle *(arrow)* extending into a molar root. On this projection there is virtually no displacement. *B,* The fracture *(arrows)* is slightly more obvious on the anteroposterior view. *C,* A subtle mandibular fracture *(arrow)* in another patient is seen on a lateral oblique view. There is virtually no displacement. *D,* A minimally displaced left angle fracture *(arrow)* seen on a Towne view.

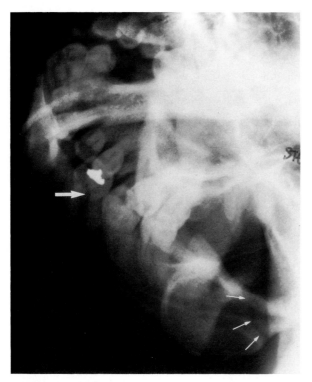

FIGURE 4–15. Mach Line From the Oropharyngeal Air Simulating a Fracture

• • • •

This patient has a mandibular fracture of the right body extending into a tooth root *(large arrow)*; this fracture was better demonstrated on other views. A second fracture is simulated by oropharyngeal air between the condyle and the coronoid process *(small arrows)*.

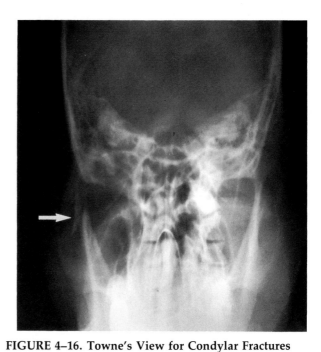

FIGURE 4–16. Towne's View for Condylar Fractures

• • • •

A fracture of the right condyle with inferior displacement of the condylar head is well demonstrated *(arrow)*.

oblique views (Fig. 4–16). The submentovertex view is useful for delineating condylar displacement and also to demonstrate the symphysis. Water's view also can evaluate the symphysis (Fig. 4–17). Whereas specific views are generally most suited to examine a specific aspect of the mandible, an entire series should always be obtained if fracture is suspected. More than one half of all mandibular fractures are multiple, but only one fracture may be clinically suspected (Fig. 4–18).

The condyles articulate with the temporal bone at the glenoid fossae. An empty glenoid fossa is indicative of either dislocation, which is usually anterior due to the pull of the lateral pterygoid muscle (Fig. 4–19), or of fracture with associated displacement/dislocation of the condylar head. A condyle can actually be driven up through the glenoid fossa into the middle cranial fossa, though this is rare.[11, 39]

The treatment of mandibular fractures depends on the nature of the fracture, the number of fractures, the displacement of the fragments, the state of dentition, and any associated facial injuries. The two most common methods are intermaxillary fixation (Fig. 4–20) and open reduction with internal fixation.

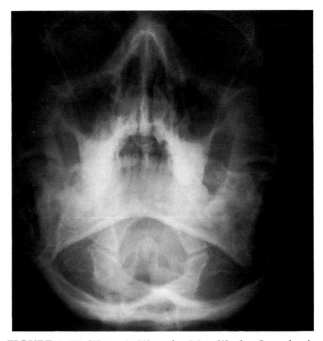

FIGURE 4–17. Waters's View for Mandibular Symphysis

• • • •

Water's view provides an excellent demonstration of the mandibular symphysis.

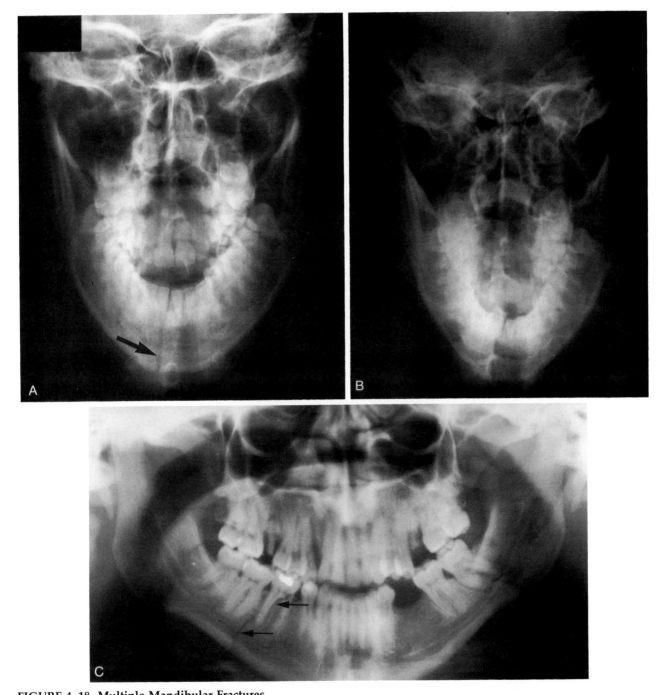

FIGURE 4–18. Multiple Mandibular Fractures

• • • •

A, An anteroposterior projection on a patient presenting with marked left facial swelling demonstrates an obvious fracture with displacement at the angle. A more subtle fracture at the symphysis is also seen *(arrow). B,* The Towne projection demonstrates both fractures, but the one at the symphysis is obscured by the laryngeal air column. *C,* A panoramic film on a second patient demonstrates two virtually nondisplaced fractures: the first of the right body traverses a molar root *(arrows);* the other is near the left angle and also extends to a molar root.

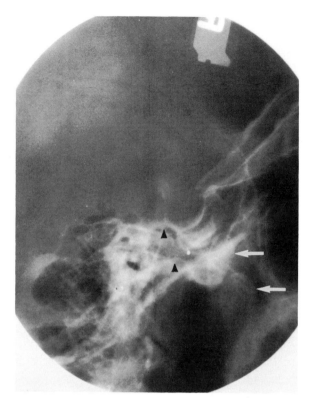

FIGURE 4–19. Bilateral Condylar Head Dislocation Without Fracture

• • • •

A lateral view reveals that both condylar heads *(arrows)* are located anterior and slightly inferior to their respective glenoid fossae *(arrowheads)*.

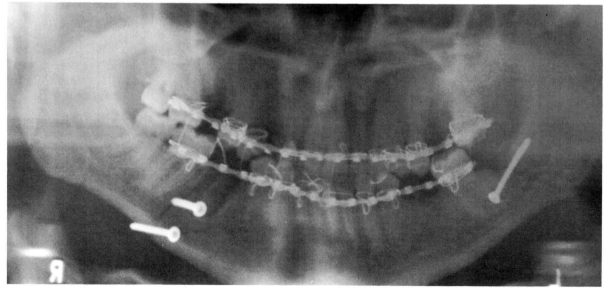

FIGURE 4–20. Intermaxillary Fixation

• • • •

The fractures demonstrated by a panoramic view in Figure 4–18C have been treated with intermaxillary fixation. Small threaded screws have been placed across the fractures, and the jaw has been wired shut.

On occasion, elaborate external stabilization is required.

THE MIDFACE

The nasal bones are the most commonly fractured bones of the midface and are discussed earlier in this chapter. The second most common isolated fracture of the midface, and the most common fracture involving the paranasal sinuses, is fracture of the zygoma. Approximately 40% of midface fractures not isolated to the nose are tripod fractures.[44] Isolated zygomatic arch fractures constitute another 10%. The third most common midface fracture is a blow-out fracture of the orbital floor, which may be associated with medial orbital wall blow-out fractures (see Chapter 5). The remainder of the fractures are complex in nature and include Le Fort II and Le Fort III fractures and facial smashes. Less than 10% of all facial fractures occur in children.[34, 44]

The cause of midface trauma usually varies with the type of hospital where a patient is treated. Motor vehicle accidents, aggravated assaults, falls, and sports injuries are the most common causes. Large urban medical centers treat more patients who have been assaulted, whereas private suburban centers treat a greater number of patients who have been in motor vehicle accidents. Motor vehicle accidents, falls (including bicycle accidents), and abuse are the most common causes of midface fractures in children. Associated craniocerebral injuries, such as contusion and subdural or epidural hematoma, occur in about one third of juvenile patients. Cervical spine injuries are seen in 1–2% of patients. Cervical spine injuries limit positioning for submentovertex films and also for coronal CT, and the cervical spine should be cleared prior to radiographic evaluation for facial fractures. The management and the evaluation of facial injuries is always secondary to airway, cardiovascular, and neurologic stabilization because midface injuries are rarely life-threatening.

Plain film radiographic evaluation of the face routinely includes four views. These are the Waters (see Fig. 4–1), the Caldwell (see Fig. 4–2), the lateral (see Fig. 4–3), and the submentovertex views (see Fig. 4–4). Coned-down views should primarily not be used, and when possible Waters's and Caldwell views should be obtained in a posteroanterior projection so as to provide the least geometric distortion of the facial bones. Stereo Waters's views are obtained routinely at some institutions and are helpful for the delineation of comminuted fractures and fragment displacement. Interpretation of plain films is quite difficult due both to the complex anatomy and to the many superimposed structures. This is particularly true of the lateral projection. However, careful analysis of good-quality plain films permits detection of most simple fractures and the majority of more complex ones. In the past, pluridirectional tomography was performed in the coronal and the sagittal planes to evaluate many of these complex fractures. This procedure has been replaced by thin section (2–5-mm) CT in the axial and the direct coronal planes. Often, direct coronal CT scans cannot be performed because of associated injuries, but reconstruction programs can be used. Three-dimensional CT has been advocated for routine use in the presurgical evaluation of facial trauma. If the facial injury is sufficiently severe to merit CT evaluation, then a screening head study should probably also be performed in order to rule out associated intracranial injury. Conversely, it is easy to add thin sections through the face at the end of a head examination if there is evidence of a severe facial injury. Our routine scan for multiplanar or three-dimensional reformatting utilizes a 3- or 5-mm section thickness and a 3-mm interslice separation, yielding a 2-mm overlap between contiguous slices when 5-mm slices are used. Contiguous thinner slices (2-mm) are better if fine bone detail on axial slices is desired. CT is superior to plain film examination. It may require significant sedation in patients who are uncooperative because of pain or confusion.

ZYGOMATIC FRACTURES

The zygoma is a complex bone that forms the malar eminence of the cheek. It articulates with the maxilla, the frontal bone, the sphenoid bone, and the temporal bones. It is part of the inferior and the lateral orbital rims, a portion of the floor and the lateral wall of the orbit, and a portion of the anterior and the lateral wall of the maxillary antrum. The zygoma is a commonly fractured facial bone. Isolated fractures involving the zygomatic arch occur frequently and are usually caused by a direct blow. Arch fractures are usually V-shaped with the apex toward the infratemporal fossa (Fig. 4–21). This inward displacement may impinge on the coronoid process of the mandible and limit the normal range of motion of the mandible. A localized comminuted fracture of the remainder of the zygoma can be caused by the impact from a high-velocity small object. However, the most common result of trauma to the zygoma is a tripod fracture (Fig. 4–22). This fracture has three main components: a fracture of the frontal process of the zygoma or separation of the frontozygomatic suture; a fracture of the zygomatic arch; and a fracture of the maxillary process of the zygoma, including inferior orbital rim, orbital floor,

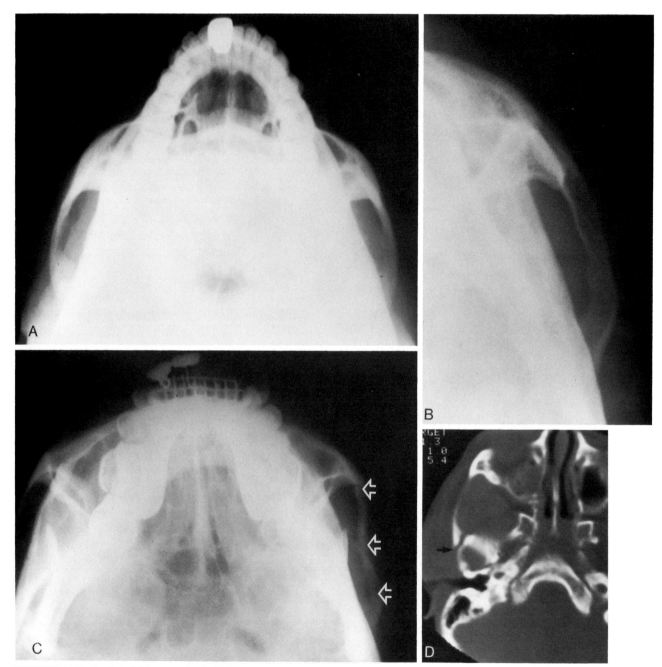

FIGURE 4–21. Isolated Zygomatic Arch Fractures

• • • •

A, These normal zygomatic arches are seen on a base view. Notice that the technique is underpenetrated for evaluation of the skull base. *B,* A tilted base view is sometimes required to see the entire zygomatic arch. *C,* A submentovertex view clearly demonstrates the depressed left zygomatic arch, which is fractured in three places *(arrows). D,* Computed tomography easily demonstrates a right zygomatic arch fracture *(arrow).*

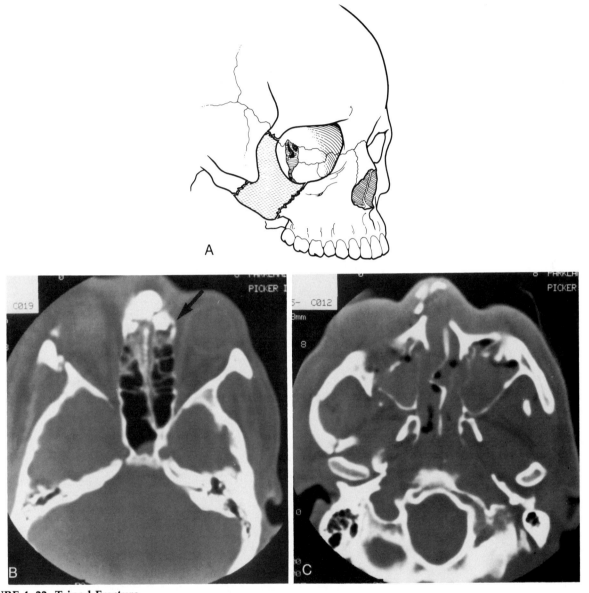

FIGURE 4–22. Tripod Fracture

• • • •

A, A diagram showing a tripod fracture. The stippled area indicates the segment of bone that has been separated from the facial strut. Note the zygomatic, the inferior orbital, and the lateral orbital components of the fracture. *B*, This transaxial image shows the lateral orbital component of a tripod fracture in a patient who suffered a complex facial injury. Notice also the fracture of the nasoethmoid complex *(arrow)*. *C*, An image taken slightly lower than that in *B* shows a compound fracture of the zygoma. Note again the nasoethmoid-complex fracture as well.

Illustration continued on following page

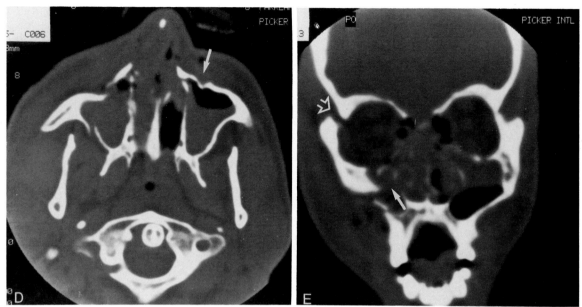

FIGURE 4–22 *Continued* **Tripod Fracture**

• • • •

D, This image in the maxillary region shows anterior and lateral maxillary wall fractures on the right in the same patient. Note also the left maxillary fracture *(arrow). E,* A direct coronal computed tomography scan shows a superolateral maxillary fracture extending into the inferior orbit *(arrow)* as well as a lateral orbital fracture *(open arrow).* Compare the appearance of the bony mass on the patient's right, which has been separated from the orbit and the maxilla, with the stippled area shown in *A.* Note also the nasoethmoid-complex injury. Involvement of the nasal process of the maxilla and the lacrimal bone regions raises the possibility of nasolacrimal duct injury as well.

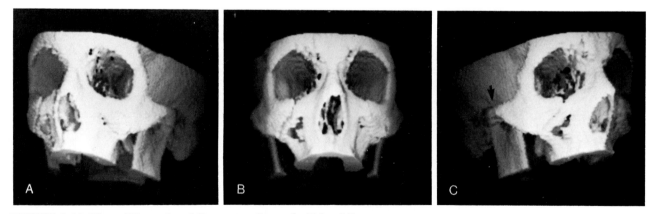

FIGURE 4–23. Three-Dimensional Reconstructions of a Tripod Fracture

• • • •

Three-dimensional reconstructions of the tripod fracture in the patient described in Figure 4–22 are shown. These reconstructions can sometimes be used to gain an improved appreciation of the bony displacements. Different hardware and software vendors supply packages with different capabilities. Images can be obtained in different obliquities and projections. *A,* The complexity of the anterior maxillary wall fracture is demonstrated, but not that of the zygomatic fracture. The left zygoma is well seen. *B,* Maxillary and orbital components are seen owing to the direct anteroposterior projection. *C,* The zygomatic component, though potentially better displayed using an inferior-to-superior projection, is demonstrated.

and anterior and lateral maxillary sinus wall fractures. Depending on the force and the direction of the blow, the tripod fracture may be nondisplaced, depressed, rotated about the x-, y-, or z-axis, be in various stages of comminution, or be associated with more complex facial fractures. Management ranges from no treatment to extensive open reduction and internal fixation with wires, screws, plates, and grafts. Three-dimensional reconstructions of CT scans may assist preoperative planning (Fig. 4–23).

LE FORT FRACTURES AND FACIAL SMASHES

In 1900 and 1901 French physician Rene Le Fort published a series of articles about fractures of the upper jaw. These studies included a literature review, an autopsy study, and also experimentally produced trauma to the face followed by careful dissection. In his work Le Fort determined reproducible planes of weakness in the facial skeleton, the fractures of which have come to bear his name (Fig. 4–24).

The Le Fort I fracture, described earlier by Guerin, is a transverse fracture through the lower face that results in the separation of the palate and the alveolar process of the maxilla from the maxillary antra. The fracture extends through the inferior aspects of both maxillary sinuses and posteriorly through the pterygoid plates. There is frequently a sagittal fracture through the hard palate. The fragment, which includes the alveolar processes and the palate, is clinically mobile.

The Le Fort II fracture, also known as the pyramidal fracture, is much more complex. The fracture extends from the nasion obliquely and inferolaterally through the medial orbital wall, through the floor of the orbit and the inferior orbital rim adjacent to the zygomaticomaxillary suture, obliquely through the maxillary sinuses, and posteriorly through the pterygoid plates. This results in the mobilization of a large pyramidal central facial fragment. The fracture may be asymmetric, and sagittal splitting of the palate may occur. The zygomas usually remain at-

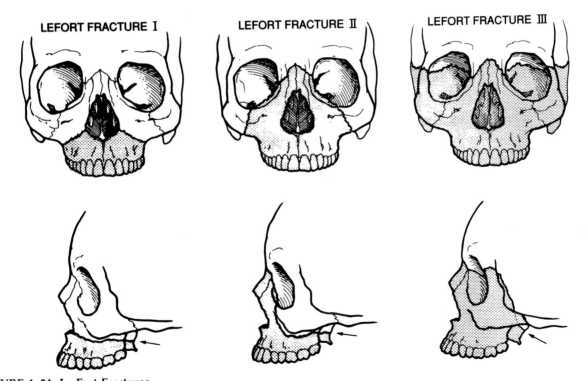

FIGURE 4–24. Le Fort Fractures

• • • •

This class of midface fractures has three subcategories, which are numbered I, II, and III. In the Le Fort I fracture, the alveolar ridge is separated from the maxilla, but the nasal and orbital areas are not involved. In the Le Fort II fracture, there is involvement of the medial orbital areas and the nasal bone, but the fracture does not extend through the lateral orbits and the zygoma. In the Le Fort III fracture, also known as a midface separation, the fracture extends through the medial and lateral orbital walls and the zygoma, and the midface is essentially freed from the skull in terms of its bony attachments. In this illustration these fractures are shown as stippled areas. Note the extension of the fracture through the pterygoid plate in all three types *(arrows)*.

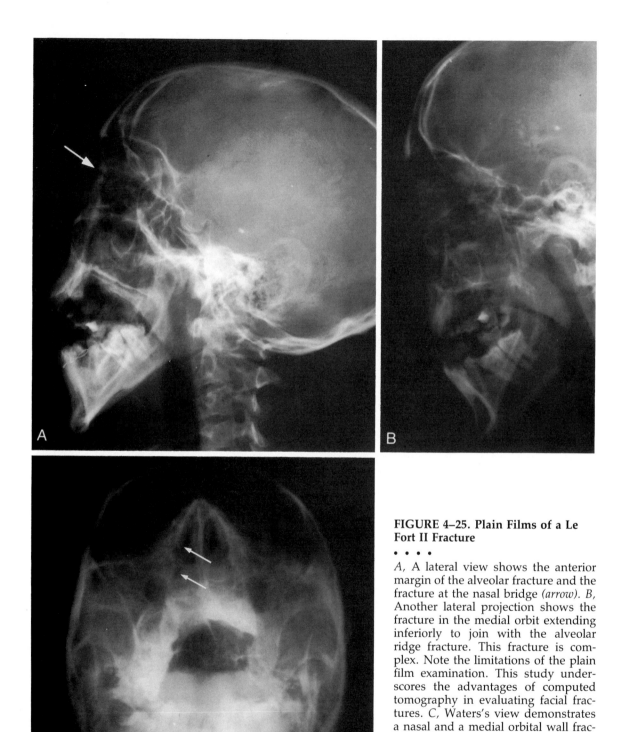

FIGURE 4–25. Plain Films of a Le Fort II Fracture

• • • •

A, A lateral view shows the anterior margin of the alveolar fracture and the fracture at the nasal bridge *(arrow). B,* Another lateral projection shows the fracture in the medial orbit extending inferiorly to join with the alveolar ridge fracture. This fracture is complex. Note the limitations of the plain film examination. This study underscores the advantages of computed tomography in evaluating facial fractures. *C,* Waters's view demonstrates a nasal and a medial orbital wall fracture *(arrows).*

tached to the skull by the zygomatic arches and the frontozygomatic processes.

The Le Fort III fracture, also known as craniofacial dissociation, is the most complex and severe of the Le Fort fractures. The fracture extends from the nasion posteriorly through the medial orbital walls, down through the inferior orbital fissures, and back through the pterygoid plates. It also extends through the lateral orbital wall and rim and travels obliquely and posteroinferiorly through the zygomatic arches and into the pterygoid plates. As in other Le Fort injuries, there can be asymmetry in the degree of injury, and multiple fragments are more common than single fragments.

The facial smash is the most severe of the complex facial fractures (Fig. 4–25). Its name is descriptive because there is severe comminution of virtually all of the facial skeleton such that the fractures fail to fit into any of the describable classifications. The best method for evaluation of these complex fractures is thin-section axial and coronal CT. In fact, since the development of CT it has become increasingly clear that many facial fractures do not fit neatly into a specific category and that combinations are quite common.

A three-dimensional CT scan (Fig. 4–26) is useful in preoperative planning for reconstructive surgery in these complex fractures and is often very illustrative, though fractures that were not previously seen at axial or coronal imaging are not frequently discovered (Fig. 4–27). Current software algorithms tend to use a surface-rendering approach based on a CT density interface between bone and soft tissues. Smoothing functions create a more visually pleasing surface contour. However, some anatomic detail is invariably lost during reconstruction. Reconstructions can create an appreciation for three-dimensional relationships between structures, which may be inapparent on transaxial images, and thus should be used liberally.

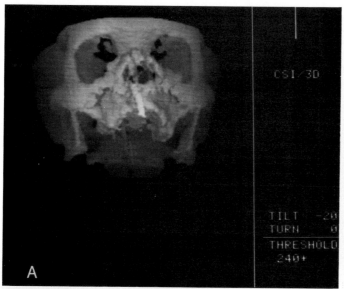

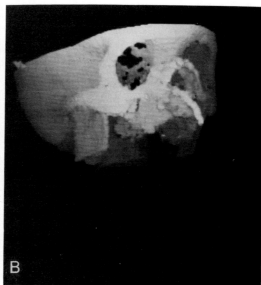

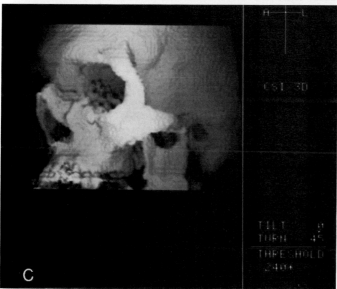

FIGURE 4–26. Three-Dimensional Reconstruction of a Le Fort II Fracture

• • • •

A three-dimensional reconstruction of the Le Fort II fracture in the patient described in Figure 4–25. Note the improved appreciation of the anatomy of the fracture. *A*, This anteroposterior projection shows the fracture across the nasal bridge angling inferiorly in the maxilla to join the fracture separating the alveolar ridge from the maxilla. *B* and *C*, Here the oblique projections better show the angle of the fracture line extending inferiorly from the nasal bridge to join with the alveolar fracture.

Illustration continued on following page

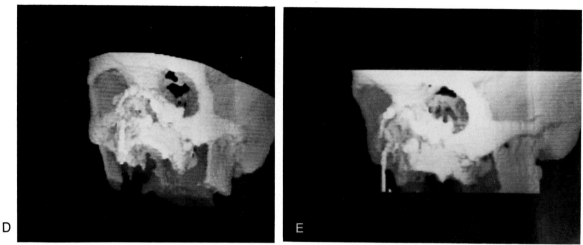

FIGURE 4–26 *Continued* **Three-Dimensional Reconstruction of a Le Fort II Fracture**

• • • •

D, The alveolar fracture is appreciated to extend into the pterygoid plate. *E,* The angle of the view is selected to illustrate the separation of the medial bony midface from its cranial support structures. Note also the complexity of this bony fracture. It is not a clean Le Fort II fracture, but rather a complex midface fracture, the planes of which follow the plane of a Le Fort II fracture.

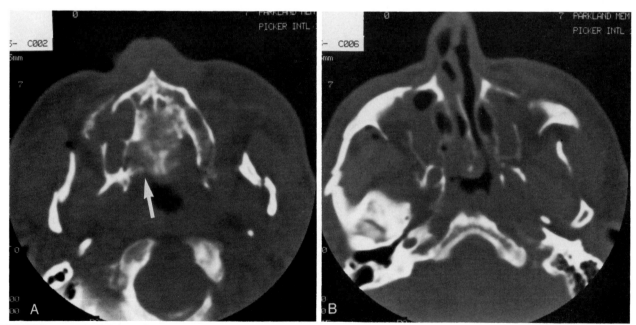

FIGURE 4–27. Facial Smash

• • • •

Bony fragments can be so complex that some fractures cannot be placed in any simple category. *A,* An axial section at the level of the hard palate shows a bilateral mandibular fracture. There is probable involvement of the hard palate as well *(arrow),* indicating a component of fracture that would place this into a Le Fort–type categorization. *B,* Bilateral maxillary components are seen, as well as a right zygomatic component. At times, direct coronal computed tomography provides the greatest information in these cases.

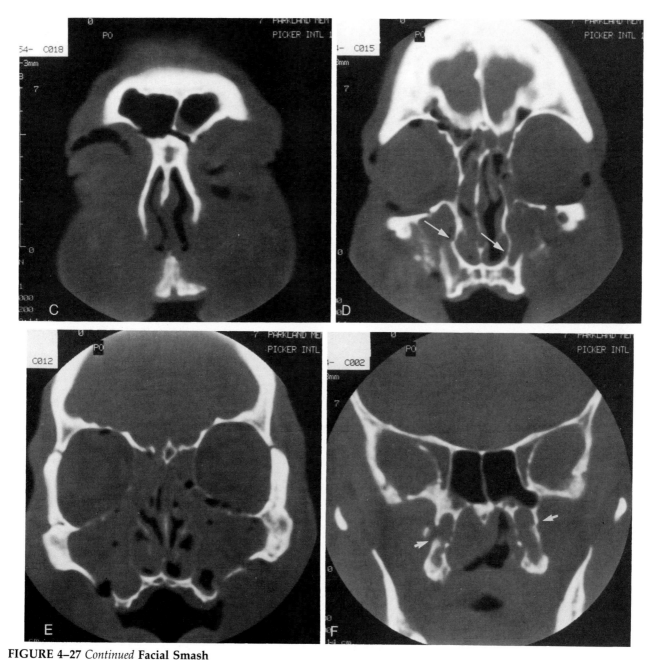

FIGURE 4–27 *Continued* **Facial Smash**
• • • •

C, The nasal fracture is seen to extend into the frontal sinuses. *D,* Inferior and lateral maxillary components are seen, as is a medial orbital fracture on the left. Note the intraorbital emphysema bilaterally. Note also the fracture lines along the medial maxillary area bilaterally *(arrows)*, completing the components of alveolar separation that would qualify part of this fracture as a variant of a Le Fort fracture. *E,* This scan through the orbits and the maxillary sinuses shows bilateral medial and lateral maxillary fractures and bilateral orbital fractures. *F,* A scan through the region of pterygoid plates shows them to be fractured bilaterally *(arrows)*.

References

1. Ahrendt D, Swischuk LE, Hayden CK Jr. Incomplete (bending?) fractures of the mandibular condyle in children. Pediatr Radiol 1984; 14:140–141.
2. Avrahami E, Horowitz I. Chip fractures of the mandibular condyle. Head Neck Surg 1984; 6:978–981.
3. Bailey BJ, Clark WD. Management of mandibular fractures. Ear Nose Throat J 1983; 62:371–378.
4. Bochlogyros PN. Non-union of fractures of the mandible. J Maxillofac Surg 1985; 13:189–193.
5. Busuito MJ, Smith DJ Jr, Robson MC. Mandibular fractures in an urban trauma center. J Trauma 1986; 26:826–829.
6. Chakeres DW. Computed tomography of the ethmoid sinuses. Otolaryngol Clin North Am 1985; 29–42.
7. Chan DM, Demuth RJ, Miller SH, Jastak JT. Management of mandibular fractures in unreliable patient populations. Ann Plast Surg 1984; 13:299–303.
8. Chayra GA, Meador LR, Laskin DM. Comparison of panoramic and standard radiographs for the diagnosis of mandibular fractures. J Oral Maxillofac Surg 1986; 44:677–679.
9. Ching M, Hase MP. Comparison of panoramic and standard radiographic radiation exposures in the diagnosis of mandibular fractures. Med J Aust 1987; 147:226–228.
10. Christiansen EL, Thompson JR, Hasso AN. CT evaluation of trauma to the temporomandibular joint. J Oral Maxillofac Surg 1987; 45:920–923.
11. Copenhaver RH, Dennis MJ, Kloppedal E, et al. Fracture of the glenoid fossa and dislocation of the mandibular condyle into the middle cranial fossa. J Oral Maxillofac Surg 1985; 43:974–977.
12. Daffner RH, Gehweiler JA Jr, Osborne DR, Roberts L Jr. Computed tomography in the evaluation of severe facial trauma. Comput Radiol 1983; 7:91–102.
13. Daffner RH, Apple JS, Gehweiler JA. Lateral view of facial fractures: New observations. AJR 1983; 141:587–591.
14. Dolan KD. The ethmoid sinus, plain film and tomographic anatomy. Otolaryngol Clin North Am 1985; 18:15–28.
15. Doyle T. Arthrography of the temporomandibular joint: A simple technique. Clin Radiol 1983; 34:147–151.
16. Ellis E, El-Attar A, Moos KF. An analysis of 2,067 cases of zygomatico-orbital fracture. J Oral Maxillofac Surg 1985; 43:417–428.
17. Fujii N, Yamashiro M. Classification of malar complex fractures using computed tomography. J Oral Maxillofac Surg 1983; 41:562–567.
18. Gentry LR, Manor WF, Turski PA, Strother CM. High-resolution CT analysis of facial struts in trauma: 1. Normal anatomy. AJR 1983; 140:523–532.
19. Gentry LR, Manor WF, Turski PA, Strother CM. High-resolution CT analysis of facial struts in trauma: 2. Osseous and soft-tissue complications. AJR 1983; 140:533–541.
20. Godoy J, Mathog RH. Malar fractures associated with exophthalmos. Arch Otolaryngol 1985; 111:174–177.
21. Harris L, Marano GD, McCorkle D. Nasofrontal duct: CT in frontal sinus trauma. Radiology 1987; 165:195–198.
22. Hohmann A, Wilson K, Nelms CR Jr. Surgical treatment in temporomandibular joint trauma. Otolaryngol Clin North Am 1983; 16:549–562.
23. Holt GR, Holt JE. Nasoethmoid complex injuries. Otolaryngol Clin North Am 1985; 18:87–98.
24. Horowitz I, Abrahami E, Mintz SS. Demonstration of condylar fractures of the mandible by computed tomography. Oral Surg 1982; 54:263–268.
25. Janecka IP. External stabilization of the mandible with the mini-H-fixator. Plast Reconstr Surg 1984; 73:840–842.
26. Kaplan PA, Tu HK, Koment MA, et al. Radiography after orthognathic surgery. Radiology 1988; 167:191–194.
27. Kaplan PA, Tu HK, Williams SM, Lydiatt DD. The normal temporomandibular joint: MR and arthrographic correlation. Radiology 1987; 165:177–178.
28. Kassel EE. Fractures of upper third of the face including the frontal sinuses. Otolaryngol Clin North Am 1988; 21:476–493.
29. Kinnunen J, Gothlin JH. Effect of alcohol intake on the radiographic quality in patients with midfacial trauma. Acta Radiol 1988; 29:217–221.
30. Kinnunen J, Gothlin JH, Totterman S. Effect of training and experience on radiologic diagnostic performance in midfacial trauma. Acta Radiol 1988; 29:83–87.
31. Kneeland JB, Ryan DE, Carrera GF, et al. Failed temporomandibular joint prostheses: MR imaging. Radiology 1987; 165:179–181.
32. Kreipke DL, Moss JJ, Franco JM, et al. Computed tomography and thin-section tomography in facial trauma. AJR 1984; 142:1041–1045.
33. Lello GE, Makek M. Stafne's mandibular lingual cortical defect. J Maxillofac Surg 1985; 13:172–176.
34. Maniglia AJ, Kline SN. Maxillofacial trauma in the pediatric age group. Otolaryngol Clin North Am 1983; 16:717–730.
35. Manzione JV, Katzberg RW, Brodsky GL, et al. Internal derangements of the temporomandibular joint: Diagnosis by direct sagittal computed tomography. Radiology 1984; 150:111–115.
36. Mathog RH. Non-union of the mandible. Otolaryngol Clin North Am 1983; 16:533–546.
37. Mattox DE, Delaney RG. Anatomy of the ethmoid sinus. Otolaryngol Clin North Am 1985; 18:3–14.
38. Mayer JS, Wainwright J, Yeakley JW, et al. The role of three-dimensional computed tomography in the management of maxillofacial trauma. J Trauma 1988; 28:1043–1053.
39. Musgrove BT. Dislocation of the mandibular condyle into the middle cranial fossa. Br J Oral Maxillofac Surg 1986; 24:22–27.
40. Myall RWT, Sandor GKB, Gregory CEB. Are you overlooking fractures of the mandibular condyle? Pediatrics 1987; 79:639–641.
41. Noyek AM, Kassel EE, Wortzman G, et al. Contemporary radiologic evaluation in maxillofacial trauma. Otolaryngol Clin North Am 1983; 16:473–508.
42. Prendergast ML, Wildes TO. Evaluation of the orbital floor in zygoma fractures. Arch Otolaryngol Head Neck Surg 1988; 114:446–450.
43. Robbins KT, Harris J Jr, Zaluzec D, Jahrsdoerfer R. Radiological evaluation of mid-third facial fractures. J Otolaryngol 1986; 15:366–372.
44. Rogers LF. Radiology of Skeletal Trauma. New York: Churchill Livingstone, Inc., 1982, pp 229–271.
45. Sataloff RT, Grossman CB, Gonzales C, Naheedy N. Computed tomography of the face and paranasal sinuses: Part II. Abnormal anatomy and pathologic conditions. Head Neck Surg 1985; 7:369–389.
46. Schwimmer AM, Greenberg AM. Management of mandibular trauma with rigid internal fixation. Oral Surg 1986; 62:630–637.
47. Schwimmer A, Stern R, Kritchman D. Impacted third molars: A contributing factor in mandibular fractures in contact sports. Am J Sports Med 1983; 11:262–266.
48. Thompson JR, Christiansen E, Hasso AN, Hinshaw DB Jr. Temporomandibular joints: High-resolution computed tomographic evaluation. Radiology 1984; 150:105–110.
49. Thompson R, Myer CM. Sagittal palate fracture. Ann Otol Rhinol Laryngol 1988; 97:432–433.
50. Tyndall DA, Matteson SR, Gregg JM. Computed tomography in diagnosis and treatment of mandibular fractures. Oral Surg 1983; 56:567–570.
51. Winstanley RP. The management of fractures of the mandible. Br J Oral Maxillofac Surg 1984; 22:170–177.
52. Zachariades N. Recurrent fractures of the mandible. Oral Surg 1985; 60:562–564.
53. Reitzik M, Lawnie JF, Cleaton-Jones P, et al. Experimental fractures of monkey mandibles. Int J Oral Surg 1978; 7:100–103.

CHAPTER 5

. . . .

Orbits and Eyes

. . . .

MARK S. GIRSON, M.D.

. . . .

ORBITAL FRACTURES

Blow-out Fractures of the Orbital Floor

In 1957 the orbital floor blow-out fracture was defined by Smith and Reagan as a fracture of the orbital floor without fracture of the orbital rim but with entrapment of the orbital contents. Two mechanisms have been proposed to account for orbital floor fracture in the absence of disruption of the orbital rim. The *hydraulic theory*, proposed by Converse and Smith, was developed after extensive experimentation with cadavers and exenterated eyes. They demonstrated that blow-out fractures are caused by a sudden increase in the intraorbital pressure, resulting from a traumatic force to the orbital soft tissues. This force is transmitted through the soft tissues, causing the blow-out fracture to occur through the weakest part of the orbit, most often the orbital floor. Less commonly, the lamina papyracea or medial orbital wall is fractured, usually in association with an orbital floor blow-out fracture but occasionally as an isolated injury. Orbital roof blow-out fractures are far less common than fractures involving the floor and the medial wall. The second

theory has been termed the *buckling force theory*, in which direct trauma to the orbital rim causes the rim's transient deformation. The force is then transmitted to the orbital floor. The orbital floor is far more delicate than the orbital rim and is less resistant to deformation. Therefore, fractures occur through the orbital floor without associated fracture of the orbital rim.

Blow-out fractures may result from either of these mechanisms or a combination of the two. Depending upon the force applied and the intrinsic resistance of the bone, the blow-out fracture may be as simple as a minor crack in the orbital floor or as complex as inferior displacement of the entire comminuted orbital floor and contents.

The typical history of a patient presenting with a blow-out fracture is that of a direct blow to the eye, such as that caused by a fist or a racquetball. Primary clinical signs of a blow-out injury include enophthalmos, paralysis of upward gaze secondary to entrapment of soft tissues by the fracture, orbital emphysema, and anesthesia in the distribution of the inferior orbital nerve. Nonspecific signs include periorbital swelling, subconjunctival hemorrhage, and exquisite tenderness over the lower orbit. Local swelling and tenderness may impede physical examination and forced duction testing, which is important in the assessment of the extent of orbital entrapment.

• • • • APPROPRIATE RADIOGRAPHIC STUDIES

Orbital Fractures

I. **Plain Films**
   A. Waters's view
   B. Caldwell view
   Comment: Plain film radiography is a survey technique for the cooperative patient.

II. **Polytomography**
   Comment: Requires patient cooperation and gives significant radiation to the lens; however, equipment for this modality is not universally available.

III. **Computed Tomography**
   A. Coronal plane
   B. Axial plane
   Comment: Not all patients can assume the position required for coronal scanning. Coronal reconstructions may be performed if the patient cannot cooperate for direct scanning. Direct coronal thin-section CT is the screening technique of choice.

IV. **Magnetic Resonance Imaging**
   A. Coronal plane
   B. Oblique sagittal plane
   Comment: Magnetic resonance (MR) imaging does not use ionizing radiation. It provides excellent soft tissue definition. However, it may not demonstrate the actual fracture.

Blow-out Fractures of the Orbital Floor

I. **Plain Films**
   A. Waters's view
   B. Caldwell view
   Comment: Waters's view and the Caldwell projection are the primary screening views that demonstrate most blow-out fractures in patients who are able to cooperate.
   C. Exaggerated Waters's views at 10 degrees, 20 degrees, and 30 degrees
   D. Lateral oblique views
   Comment: Exaggerated Waters's views and lateral oblique views increase sensitivity.

II. **Polytomography**
   A. Waters's view position
   Comment: Requires a high degree of patient cooperation and produces a high lens radiation dose.

III. **Computed Tomography**
   A. The coronal plane is preferred.
   B. Towne's computed tomography (CT) projection should be used if a coronal plane is not possible.
   Comment: An axial plane may provide added information, but it does not demonstrate the orbital floor well. High-resolution 2–3-mm cuts are preferable. CT is used to study enophthalmos and entrapment.

IV. **Magnetic Resonance Imaging**
   A. Oblique sagittal plane
   B. Coronal plane
   Comment: Provides excellent demonstration of soft tissues but does not demonstrate the actual fracture. Five-millimeter images should be used.

••••• *APPROPRIATE RADIOGRAPHIC STUDIES* Continued

Medial Wall Blow-out Fractures

I. Plain Films
   A. Waters's view
   B. Caldwell view
II. Polytomography
III. Computed Tomography
   A. Axial plane
   B. Coronal plane
   Comment: Provides excellent demonstration of both osseous and soft tissue abnormalities.
IV. Magnetic Resonance Imaging

Orbital Roof Fractures

I. Plain Films
   A. Facial films including Waters's view and the Caldwell view
   B. Skull series
II. Computed Tomography
   A. Coronal plane
   B. Axial plane
   Comment: Since orbital roof fractures are generally part of a complex craniofacial injury, both coronal and axial plane scans are generally required. The coronal plane is preferred to the axial plane because of the orientation of the orbital roof.

Tripod Fracture

I. Plain Films
   A. Facial bones
   B. Zygomatic arch views
   Comment: See Chapter 4.

Orbital Apex Fractures

I. Plain Films
   A. Angled anteroposterior (AP) view for the superior orbital fissure
   B. Oblique optic foramen view
   C. Caldwell view
   D. Reese's view
   E. Submentovertex view (when not contraindicated by other injuries)
II. Polytomography
   Comment: CT is preferred, but polytomography provides excellent visualization.
III. Computed Tomography
   A. Axial and coronal views

Other Fractures

Comment: This topic includes complex fractures, which are covered in Chapters 2–4.

• • • • *APPROPRIATE RADIOGRAPHIC STUDIES* Continued

Injuries to the Soft Tissues of the Orbit

Penetrating Injuries and Foreign Bodies

Comment: These injuries are always unique. The appropriate radiographic procedure depends on the injury and on the nature of the foreign material. Ophthalmoscopy and ultrasound scanning are the primary procedures in many patients.

 I. **Plain Films**
  A. Orthogonal views are required.
  B. AP and lateral views are usual.
  Comment: CT and MR imaging provide vastly superior localization.
 II. **Computed Tomography**
  A. Axial and coronal views using a thin-section high-resolution technique.
  Comment: Metal and glass are generally easily seen at CT. The visualization of plastic and wood requires narrow windows. CT also demonstrates the presence of any bone fragments.
  Caution: Because foreign bodies move, definitive localization should take place *immediately* before surgery.
 III. **Magnetic Resonance Imaging**
  A. Coronal and axial views
  Caution: No metallic foreign body should be evaluated by MR imaging unless it is known to be nonferromagnetic.

Rupture of the Globe

Comment: Generally a clinical diagnosis, but occult perforations may require study.

 I. **Computed Tomography**
  A. Axial projection
  Comment: Use a high-resolution thin-slice technique.

Optic Nerve Avulsion or Hematoma

 I. **Computed Tomography**
  A. Axial and coronal planes
  Comment: Use a high-resolution thin section.

• • • • **APPROPRIATE RADIOGRAPHIC STUDIES** Continued

Subperiosteal Hematomas of the Orbit

    I. Computed Tomography
       A. Coronal plane (the best view)
       B. Axial plane
    II. Magnetic Resonance Imaging
       A. Coronal plane (the best view)
       B. Axial plane

Vitreous Hemorrhage

    I. Computed Tomography

Subconjunctival Hemorrhage

    I. Computed Tomography

Proptosis/Enopthalmos

    I. Computed Tomography

Lens Injury

    I. Computed Tomography

Choroidal Detachment

    I. Computed Tomography
    II. Magnetic Resonance Imaging

Retinal Detachment

    I. Not a radiologic diagnosis.

Hyphema

    I. Not a radiologic diagnosis.

Radiographic examination of the orbit in the patient suspected of orbital fracture should include standard Waters's and Caldwell views. Direct radiographic signs of fracture include visualization of the fracture line itself (Fig. 5–1), the overlapping of bone structures, which produces a dense white line in the orbital floor, and abnormal linear opacities that are caused by displaced fragments. A fracture fragment may be well seen on one view but not identified on another view if the beam is tangential to the cortical line on only one of the views. Orbital emphysema may be seen radiographically. Prolapse of soft tissue into the maxillary sinus can be visualized as a polypoid-like soft tissue mass protruding from the roof of the maxillary sinus (Fig. 5–2). Indirect, nonspecific signs include opacification of the maxillary or the ethmoid sinuses and an air-fluid level within the maxillary sinus. Associated fractures of the orbital roof or the medial orbital wall may also be noted as may other facial fractures.

Blow-out fractures of the orbital floor can be diagnosed in nearly all cooperative patients using the standard Waters and Caldwell views. However, additional radiographic procedures are sometimes required. Exaggerated Waters's views using angulation of the beam at 10 degrees, 20 degrees, and 30 degrees in the caudad direction (while the patient's head is in the Waters position) and oblique lateral views of the orbital floor, which produce a tangential view of the orbital floor in the lateral projection, increase the sensitivity for the diagnosis of this injury.

Computed tomography (CT), magnetic resonance (MR) imaging, and polytomography all demonstrate blow-out fractures very well. Polytomography produces a relatively high level of radiation to the lens and has a significantly high proportion of false negatives to false positives. CT scans of the orbital floor should be performed in the coronal plane. High-resolution CT scans utilizing 2–3-mm cuts should be obtained, and images should be viewed with both

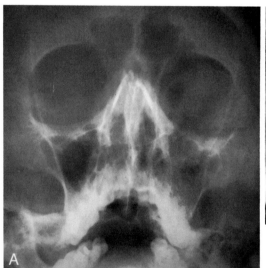

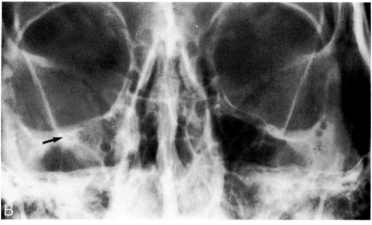

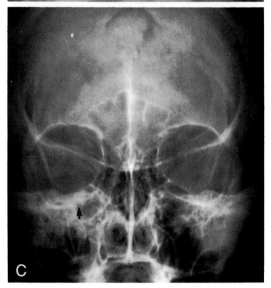

FIGURE 5–1. Blow-out Fractures on Waters's and Caldwell Views

• • • •

A, A Waters view of the face demonstrates a blow-out fracture of the left orbital floor. The discontinuity of the left orbital floor can be seen. In addition, there is opacification of the left maxillary sinus, and there is air within the orbit. *B,* A single Waters view in a second patient demonstrates a blow-out fracture of the right orbital floor *(arrow).* The discontinuity of the right orbital floor can be seen, as can displacement of the fractured fragment inferiorly. In addition, there is an air-fluid level in the right maxillary sinus, as well as soft tissue density, projecting inferiorly from the orbital floor. *C,* A Caldwell view in a third patient demonstrates a right orbital floor fracture. The discontinuity of the orbital floor *(arrow)* is appreciated, as is opacification of the right maxillary sinus.

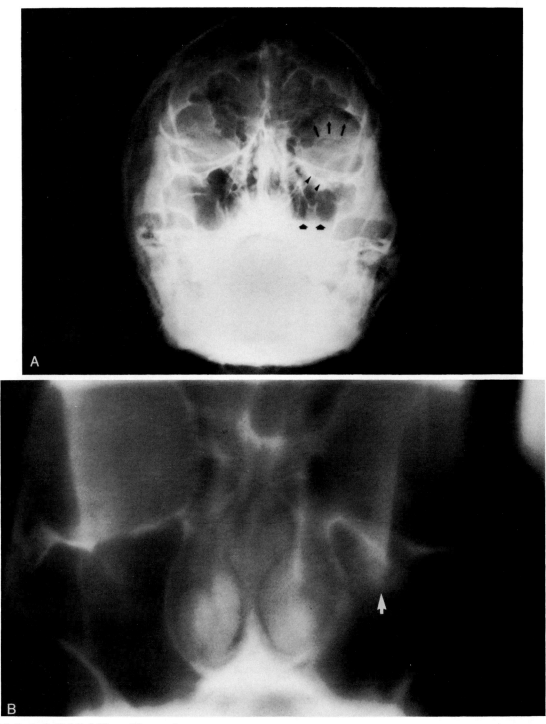

FIGURE 5–2. Left Orbital Floor Blow-out
• • • •
A, A Waters view demonstrates the classic radiographic findings. The orbital floor is discontinuous *(arrowheads).* Orbital emphysema is seen near the orbital roof *(small arrows).* A polypoid soft tissue mass is prolapsing into the superior aspect of the left maxillary sinus, and there is an air-fluid level in the lower part of the sinus *(large arrows).* This view is an upright film, which is useful to demonstrate such air-fluid levels. *B,* A single cut from a polytomographic study demonstrates both the bone discontinuity and the prolapsed orbital soft tissue mass *(arrow).*

Illustration continued on following page

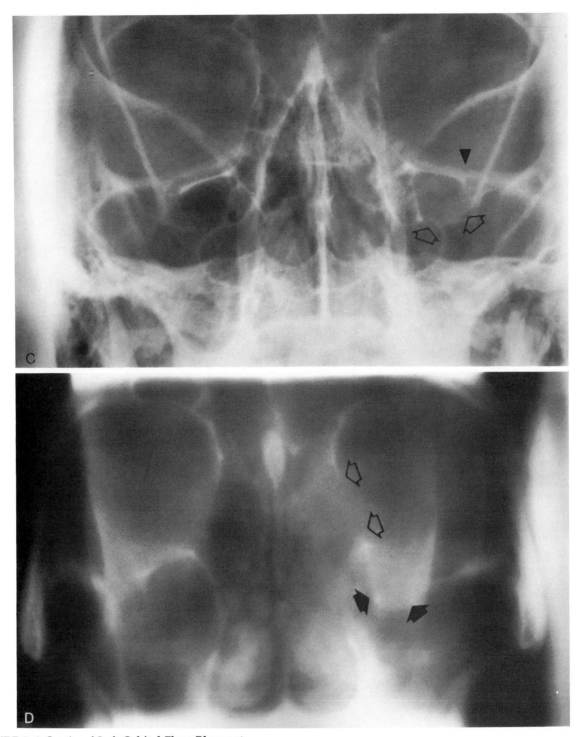

FIGURE 5–2 *Continued* **Left Orbital Floor Blow-out**

• • • •

C, A second patient has a soft tissue mass protruding into the left maxillary antrum *(open arrows)*; it is easily seen on the Waters view, but the fracture itself is very subtle *(arrowhead)*. D, A tomographic section in the Waters position demonstrates discontinuity of the orbital floor and the medial orbital wall. Soft tissue protrudes into the ethmoid air cells *(open arrows)* and into the maxillary sinus *(arrows)*.

bone and soft tissue windows. Axial sections do not depict the orbital floor well, but may provide additional diagnostic information. If the patient is unable to extend his or her neck to assume the coronal position, a flexed-neck CT projection can be obtained. The patient must flex the neck fully, and the gantry must be angled backward. This produces a projection at approximately 45 degrees to the canthomeatal line and is similar to that of a plain radiographic Waters view. Semisagittal or oblique sagittal CT views of the orbital floor can be performed, but these are not ideal projections of the orbital floor and are quite difficult to reproduce. CT provides excellent resolution of the fractures (Fig. 5–3), hematoma, and the orbital contents that have prolapsed into the maxillary sinus (Fig. 5–4).

Prolapse of the orbital soft tissue through the fracture often produces diplopia by causing traction on an ocular muscle, which is then unable to move normally (Fig. 5–5). It is relatively unusual to have entrapment of the inferior rectus muscle itself; however, this does occur and certainly produces diplopia. Gross enophthalmos and entrapment often require surgery to correct the diplopia. Other causes of diplopia with decreased eye movement following

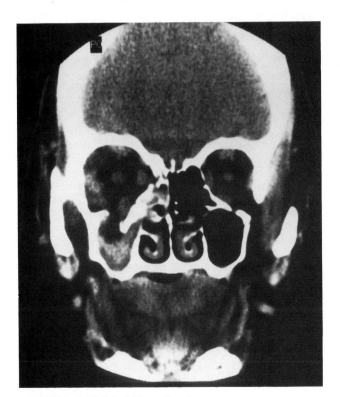

FIGURE 5–3. Orbital Floor Fracture

• • • •

This coronal computed tomography scan of the orbit demonstrates an orbital floor blow-out fracture, with the fracture fragment displaced into the opacified maxillary sinus. There is in addition a blow-out fracture of the medial orbital wall, with opacification of the ethmoid air cells.

trauma include edema and oculomotor nerve palsy. A delayed complication of blow-out fracture is the formation of scar tissue within the orbital connective tissue; scarring fixes the inferior rectus muscle to the orbital floor, impairing its function. These conditions are all readily amenable to diagnosis with high-resolution CT.

MR imaging of the orbit has a number of advantages over CT. These include the absence of ionizing radiation, high soft tissue contrast resolution, excellent evaluation of prolapsed orbital fat, and the lack of artifact from any dental prosthesis. Scanning in the oblique sagittal plane along the axis of the inferior rectus muscle provides valuable information about the relationship between the muscle and the orbital floor. Entrapment or kinking of the muscle due to tethering by prolapsed fat is clearly seen with coronal or oblique sagittal MR imaging (Fig. 5–6). Discontinuity of muscle at the bone defect is highly suggestive of muscle entrapment. The oblique sagittal plane also demonstrates the entire course of the optic nerve to good advantage, and optic nerve injury can be evaluated with a high degree of sensitivity (Fig. 5–7).

MR imaging should be performed using 3–5-mm thick cuts, a 256 × 256 or 512 × 512 matrix, and 2–4 acquisitions. The use of a surface coil dramatically increases the signal-to-noise ratio, making it possible to do thinner sections and thus achieve better spatial resolution that is comparable with that of CT. T_1-weighted images should be obtained in the coronal and in the axial or the oblique sagittal planes, using the spin-echo technique. Oblique sagittal plane imaging may not be available on all MR scanners; in such a case coronal and axial plane imaging suffices. The axial images provide excellent visualization of the medial rectus muscle and of medial fractures, whereas the oblique sagittal projection is ideal for evaluating orbital floor fractures and inferior rectus prolapse (Fig. 5–8). T_1-weighted images are useful for the detection and the localization of a fracture site, but both T_1- and T_2-weighted sequences are usually necessary for evaluating and characterizing soft tissue lesions. Short tau inversion recovery (STIR) sequences are useful adjuncts for orbital evaluation with MR imaging and should be utilized frequently. STIR suppresses fat and enhances visualization of inflammatory or post-traumatic changes within the orbit, and acquisition times are shorter than standard T_2-weighted imaging.

In order to avoid motion artifact, patients should be instructed to keep their eyes closed and to refrain from moving their eyes during the examination.

MR imaging does have certain disadvantages with respect to CT. The actual fracture is not demonstrated on MR images because of the signal void from the

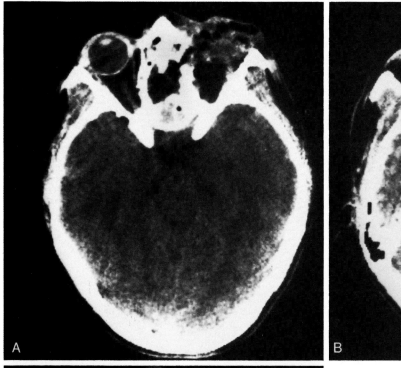

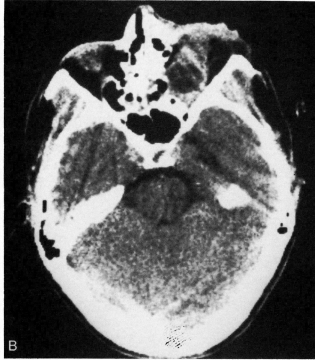

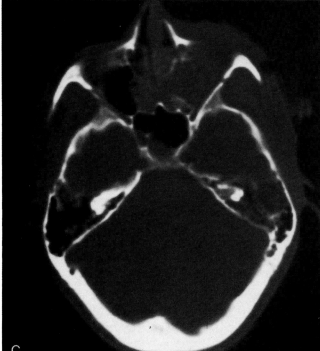

FIGURE 5–4. Left Orbital Floor and Medial Wall Fractures with Prolapse of the Orbital Contents into the Left Maxillary Sinus

• • • •

A, A 5-mm section at the level of the right globe demonstrates soft tissue swelling on the left; air is visible in the soft tissues, but no globe is seen. The left medial orbital wall fracture is demonstrated. *B,* A second section taken 10 mm caudal to the first demonstrates the left globe, which is both more dorsal and caudal to the right because it has prolapsed into the maxillary sinus. The axial plane of these computed tomography (CT) sections makes visualization of the orbital floor fracture very difficult. *C,* A CT section displayed at the bone window demonstrates opacification of the ethmoid air cells, the presence of fluid in the sphenoid sinus, and the fracture of the left medial orbital wall.

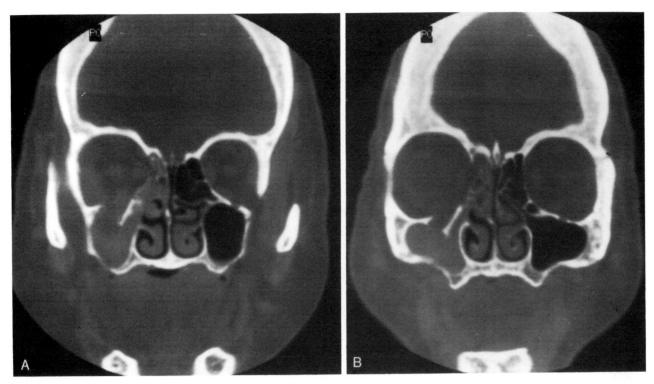

FIGURE 5–5. Orbital Floor Fracture with Prolapsed Orbital Contents

• • • •

A and *B*, These coronal computed tomography sections through the orbit demonstrate a right orbital floor fracture, with the fragment displaced into the maxillary sinus. In addition, orbital fat that has prolapsed through the defect into the superior portion of the maxillary sinus can be seen. The inferior rectus has partially prolapsed into the defect. Note also the high-density blood within the maxillary sinus as well as the high-density contusion in the lateral orbit. In addition, there is a medial wall blow-out fracture, with prolapse of orbital fat into the ethmoid sinuses, and slight medial deviation of the medial rectus.

FIGURE 5–6. Coronal Magnetic Resonance Imaging of Orbital Floor Blow-out Fracture

• • • •

A coronal magnetic resonance section (700 msec/40 msec) demonstrates herniation of high signal intensity orbital fat into the maxillary antrum through an orbital floor fracture. Within the fat, the lower signal intensity inferior rectus muscle is easily seen *(arrows)*. The comma configuration of the muscle indicates that it is "hooked" by the bone fracture edge. The patient did have diplopia (see also Fig. 5–7).

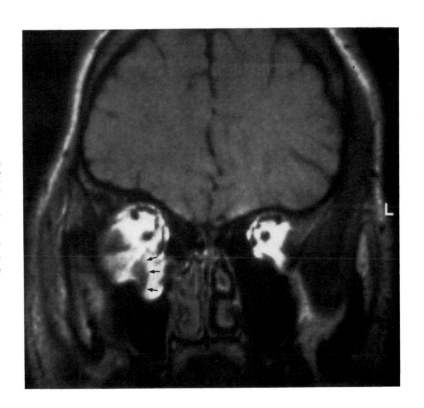

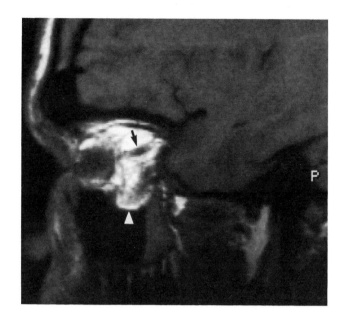

FIGURE 5–7. Oblique Sagittal Magnetic Resonance Image of an Orbital Floor Fracture with Soft Tissue Prolapse into the Maxillary Antrum

• • • •

The optic nerve *(arrow)* is well displayed as contrasted against the very high signal from the orbital fat. The prolapse of fat and the inferior rectus muscle into the maxillary sinus is also very well seen *(arrowhead)* (see also Fig. 5–6). There is an air-fluid level in the posterior maxillary sinus.

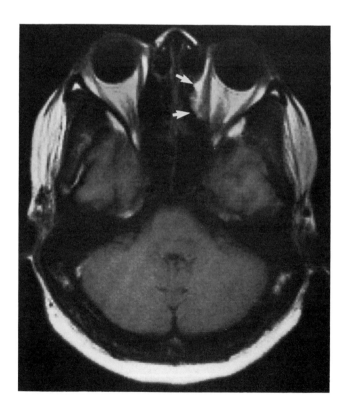

FIGURE 5–8. Medial Wall Blow-out Fracture

• • • •

This T_1-weighted axial image taken through the orbits demonstrates a fracture of the left medial orbital wall, manifested by opacification of some of the left ethmoid air cells with herniated orbital fat *(arrows)*. There is slight medial deviation of the medial rectus muscle. This magnetic resonance image provides excellent visualization of both the medial orbital wall and the medial rectus muscle.

cortical bone. Its presence is inferred by the prolapse of fat. A nondisplaced fracture or a fracture in which there is no prolapsed tissue may not be detected by MR imaging. Second, blood may not be visualized on T_1-weighted images, and STIR or T_2-weighted images are required to evaluate the extent of orbital hematoma.

Good plain films are adequate as a screen for orbital floor blow-out fractures. However, they may be very difficult to obtain in the acutely injured patient. CT is recommended if there is severe enophthalmos, if there is a large fracture seen on plain films, or if there is clinical evidence of entrapment, manifested by diplopia or a positive forced duction test. A positive forced duction test can occur without actual muscular entrapment if the muscle is temporarily anchored or hooked to the fracture site. Acutely injured patients demonstrate diplopia or a positive forced duction test acutely, but the findings resolve without operative therapy. CT is useful in distinguishing this group of patients from those who actually have entrapped inferior rectus muscles, which require surgical intervention to avoid long-term diplopia.

The appearance and the position of the inferior rectus muscle and its relationship to the fracture site should be studied. Three distinct categories occur: (1) a free inferior rectus muscle (the muscle is seen to be separate from bone density throughout its course), (2) a hooked inferior rectus (the majority of the muscle is continuous with soft tissue or fat density; however, the inferior rectus is in continuity with the bone along one side [Figs. 5–9 and 5–10]), and (3) an entrapped inferior rectus (the inferior rectus is seen to be adjacent to the bone, both nasally and temporally [Fig 5–11; see also Fig. 5–10]). Patients in the first two categories may have temporary diplopia related to the acute injury, which usually resolves. Conversely, those patients with entrapped muscles will have long-term diplopia and usually require surgical intervention.

Coronal high-resolution CT can evaluate the degree of orbital expansion and soft tissue prolapse (see Fig. 5–10). Prolapse is classified as grade 1 (mild), grade 2 (moderate), or grade 3 (severe). The entire globe may be prolapsed into the maxillary antrum. Mild or moderate orbital expansion and soft tissue prolapse is usually managed conservatively, but grade 3 orbital expansion and soft tissue prolapse usually require surgical management to avoid cosmetically unacceptable enophthalmos or persistent diplopia.

The indications for surgery remain somewhat controversial but include (1) significant enophthalmos, (2) a large bone defect demonstrated on CT or on plain radiographs (such a defect would most proba-

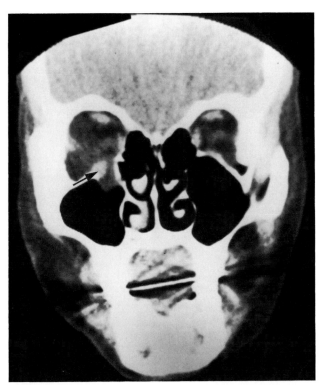

FIGURE 5–9. Coronal Computed Tomography Section Demonstrates a Blow-out Fracture of the Right Orbital Floor

• • • •

The fracture defect has allowed prolapse of orbital fat into the maxillary sinus. The inferior rectus muscle is also partially prolapsed and is "hooked" by the edge of the fracture (*arrow*).

bly result in long-term enophthalmos if not surgically corrected), (3) persistent diplopia, and (4) diplopia in the primary position.

Diplopia in the primary position suggests a possible compartment syndrome involving the inferior rectus that can result in Volkmann's ischemic necrosis. Patients at higher risk for this complication include the elderly, those with small fractures, hypotensive patients, and patients with high inferior rectus compartment pressures.

As previously mentioned, blow-out fractures of the orbital floor characteristically exclude fractures of the orbital rim. However, direct trauma to the orbit may cause a fracture of the orbital rim itself that can extend for a variable distance into the adjacent orbital floor. Depending on the intensity and the direction of the force, a spectrum of injuries can occur, ranging from a simple linear fracture of the orbital rim and the floor to extensive disruption, comminution, and displacement of the orbital rim, the floor, and the adjacent bones.

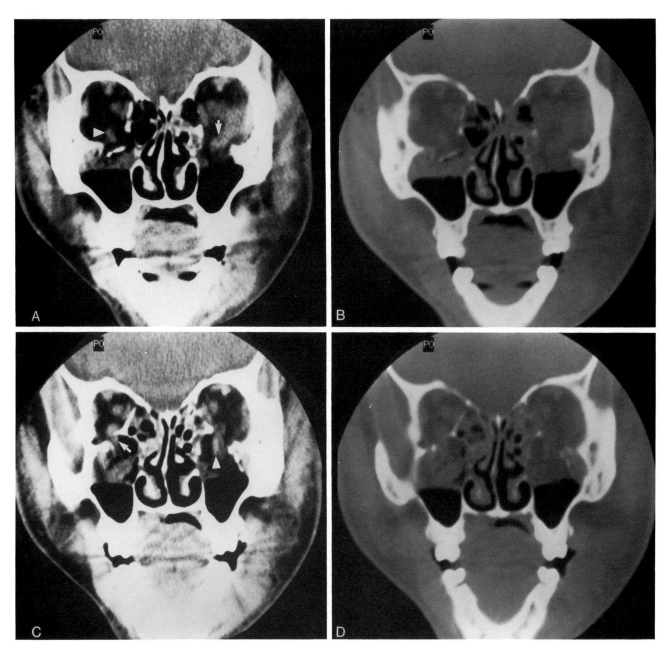

FIGURE 5–10. Coronal Computed Tomography of Extensive Bilateral Orbital Floor and Medial Wall Fractures

• • • •

These sections are 3 mm thick and were performed at 3-mm intervals in order to obtain high resolution. *A* and *B,* Bone and soft tissue displays demonstrate both orbital floor fractures. The left medial wall fracture is extensive, and fluid is present in the ethmoid air cells. The right medial wall fracture is less extensive. Soft tissue is seen prolapsing through both orbital floors, and fluid levels are present in the maxillary antra. It should be remembered that the patient is hyperextended for this coronal view. Notice that the right inferior rectus muscle is partially prolapsed *(arrowhead)* and that the left is completely prolapsed *(arrow)*. *C* and *D,* Bone and soft tissue displays of another section again demonstrate the fractures. The right inferior rectus muscle is "hooked" by the free margin of the orbital floor fracture *(arrow)*. The completely prolapsed left fracture *(arrowhead)* is clearly demonstrated.

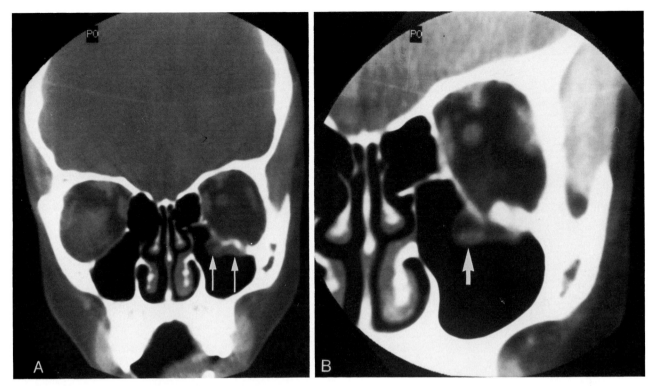

FIGURE 5–11. Coronal Sections of a Computed Tomography Scan Demonstrating a Blow-out Fracture of the Left Orbital Floor with Inferior Rectus Entrapment

• • • •

A, The comminuted fracture is well seen, and there is soft tissue protruding into the maxillary sinus *(arrows).* The soft tissue has both fat and muscle characteristics. *B,* A coned-down section 5 mm ventral to the first section clearly demonstrates the entrapped inferior rectus muscle *(arrow).*

Medial Wall Blow-out Fractures

Historically, isolated medial wall blow-out fractures of the orbit have been described as an unusual result of orbital trauma. More frequently, they have been seen in association with orbital floor blow-out fractures or other, more complex facial fractures. Since the development of CT and MR imaging, it is apparent that isolated medial wall fractures are in fact fairly common (Fig. 5–12). Muscular entrapment, a common sequela of orbital floor blow-out fractures, is rarely seen with medial wall fractures. The clinical presentation of medial rectus entrapment is similar to the inferior rectus entrapment seen with orbital floor fractures, but the diplopia is more pronounced in the horizontal plane. However, since entrapment is uncommon, most patients with medial wall blow-out fractures do not have diplopia and may not even seek medical advice. Radiographic findings of these fractures include opacification of the ethmoid air cells, orbital emphysema, and visualization of the fracture itself. High-resolution CT can be performed in both the axial and the coronal planes, providing excellent visualization of the medial wall and detailed evaluation of both the osseous and the soft tissue abnormalities. Coronal MR imaging provides excellent definition of the soft tissue abnormalities. Diplopia, when present, can be produced by a number of different soft tissue sequelae that CT can easily differentiate. They include (1) herniation or entrapment of the medial rectus muscle (Fig. 5–13), (2) laceration of the medial rectus, (3) hematoma or edema of the medial rectus, and (4) orbital hematoma, which displaces the medial rectus or impedes orbital motion.

Surgical intervention with medial orbital decompression and limited ethmoidectomy is indicated if there is medial rectus entrapment, if there is a large medial wall defect, or if bone fragments are identified adjacent to vital structures, such as the globe, the optic nerve, or the ocular muscles.

Orbital Roof Fractures

Orbital roof blow-out fractures are the rarest type of ocular blow-out injury. They imply the presence of an intact superior orbital rim (Fig. 5–14). The fracture generally occurs upward into the frontal

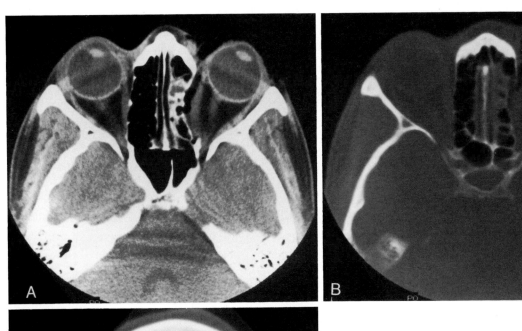

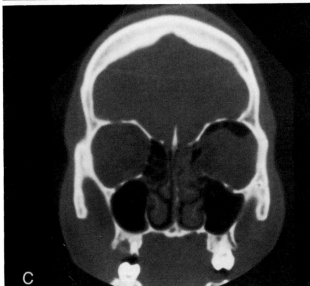

FIGURE 5–12. Medial Orbital Wall Blow-out Fracture Caused by Blunt Trauma to the Left Eye—Axial and Coronal Computed Tomography Scans

• • • •

A, An axial view displayed at a soft tissue window demonstrates medial displacement of the medial wall of the left orbit. The left medial rectus muscle is somewhat swollen, and fluid is seen in the ethmoid air cells. There is some air between the ethmoid air cells and the medial rectus muscle. *B,* The same computed tomography (CT) section displayed at a bone window demonstrates the orbital emphysema to better advantage and also well demonstrates the fluid in the compressed air cells. *C,* A coronal CT section displayed at a bone window also demonstrates the medial wall fracture to good advantage.

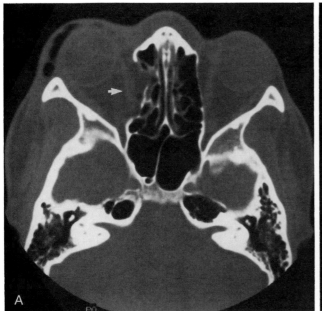

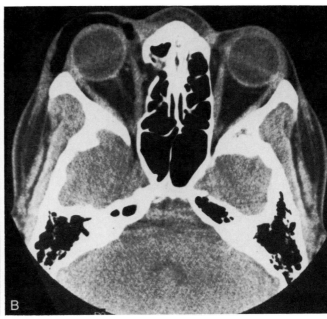

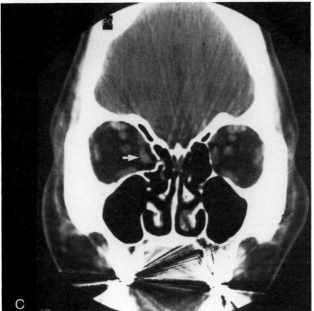

FIGURE 5–13. Medial Orbital Wall Blow-out Fracture with Herniation of the Medial Rectus Muscle

• • • •

A, This axial computed tomography (CT) section displayed at a bone window demonstrates the medial orbital wall fracture to advantage. The ethmoid air cells are disrupted, and a few of these cells are fluid-filled. The medial rectus muscle *(arrow)* is thickened and bowed medially. Orbital emphysema is present. *B,* Another axial CT section displayed at a soft tissue window demonstrates both the thickening and medial bowing or herniation of the medial rectus muscle. There is no evidence of bone entrapment. *C,* A coronal CT section also demonstrates the medial wall fracture. The medial rectus muscle *(arrow)* has moved medially but is not entrapped. There is a clear separation between the bone and the muscle. Note also the massive spray artifact generated by dental work.

Illustration continued on following page

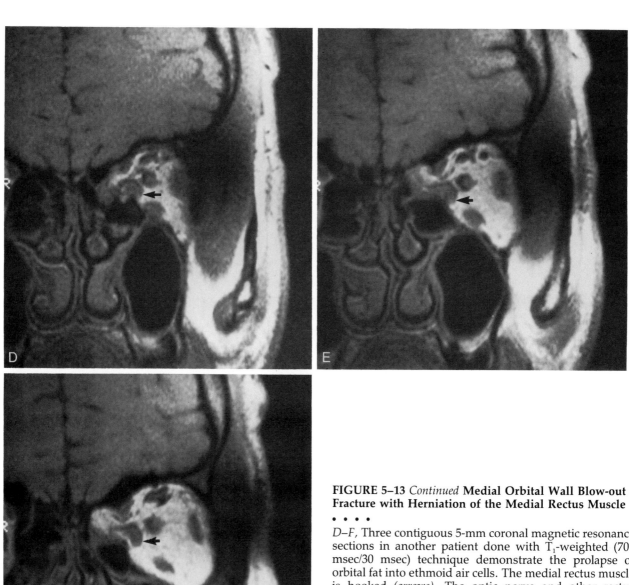

FIGURE 5–13 *Continued* **Medial Orbital Wall Blow-out Fracture with Herniation of the Medial Rectus Muscle**

• • • •

D–F, Three contiguous 5-mm coronal magnetic resonance sections in another patient done with T_1-weighted (700 msec/30 msec) technique demonstrate the prolapse of orbital fat into ethmoid air cells. The medial rectus muscle is hooked *(arrows)*. The optic nerve and other rectus muscles are well defined.

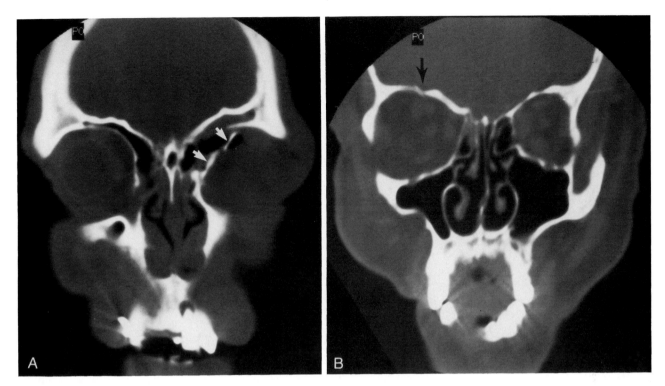

FIGURE 5–14. Orbital Roof Fracture

• • • •

A, A coronal computed tomography (CT) section of a more typical orbital roof fracture. The frontal sinuses are very large and extend over the orbital roofs bilaterally. The left orbital roof has a comminuted fracture. The fragments are displaced into the orbit *(arrows),* and the frontal sinus is largely opacified. There is also a subperiosteal hematoma (see also Fig. 5–37). *B,* A coronal CT section demonstrates a minimally displaced orbital roof fracture *(arrow).* This case is an exception to the general rule for orbital roof fractures because the frontal sinus is not involved.

sinus but rarely produces entrapment of the superior orbital muscles. Blow-out fractures of the orbital roof are usually seen in patients who have large frontal sinuses extending posteriorly into the roof of the orbits. It is thought that enlargement of the frontal sinuses results in the thinning of the bone of the orbital roof, which increases the susceptibility of the orbital roof to blow-out fracture.

Radiographic evaluation of orbital roof fractures should include plain radiographs of the face and the skull and a coronal high-resolution CT scan. The coronal plane is preferable to the axial plane because the orbital roof is oriented in the axial plane, and fractures therefore may not be detected with axial scans. More commonly, orbital roof fractures are part of a complex craniofacial fracture caused by severe craniofacial injury (Fig. 5–15). Under these circumstances, CT in both the axial and the coronal planes is required for adequate evaluation of the entire injury.

"Blow-in" fractures of the orbital roof are seen predominantly in children who have sustained direct trauma to the forehead. Fracture fragments may be found intracranially or intraorbitally with this injury. Soft tissue sequelae of orbital roof blow-in fractures include meningeal entrapment within the orbit with subsequent development of an intraorbital pseudo-meningocele or even encephalocele.

Tripod Fractures

A tripod fracture occurs when force is directed at the malar eminence. It is a separation of the zygoma from the rest of the face at all three struts, hence the term *tripod fracture.* It is essentially a facial fracture, and is therefore more extensively dealt with in Chapter 4. As it involves the orbital skeleton, a brief description is included.

The tripod fracture classically comprises zygomaticofrontal suture separation with a fracture extending through the lateral orbital wall, the orbital floor, the lateral wall of the maxillary sinus, and the zygomatic arch (Fig. 5–16). More extensive fractures may occur depending on the direction and the intensity of the applied force. These fractures include involvement of the orbital apex and the optic canal, extensive involvement of the lateral orbital wall, the orbital floor, and the orbital roof (with marked comminution and displacement of fragments), extension into the glenoid fossa, and even involvement of the coronoid process of the mandible.

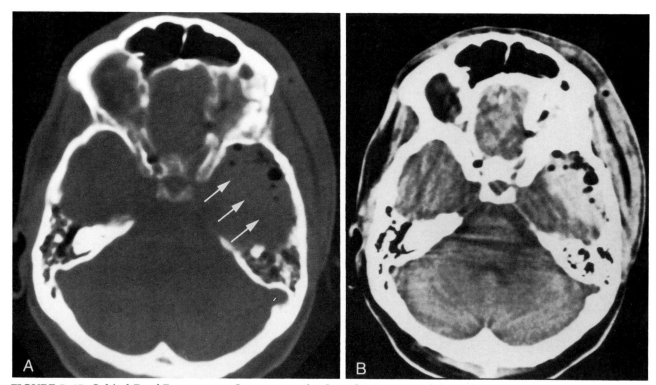

FIGURE 5–15. Orbital Roof Fracture as a Component of a Complex Fracture of the Left Craniofacial Bones

• • • •

The left side of the face is crushed, exploding the orbital roof and the sphenoid wing. Lower sections demonstrate proptosis and orbital emphysema. *A,* The crush fracture is seen. There is some orbital emphysema. Air is seen in the middle cranial fossa, and careful observation reveals a large temporal hematoma *(arrows),* emphasizing the need to routinely use both bone and soft tissue windows in studies performed for trauma. *B,* A soft tissue window display clearly and easily demonstrates the large left temporal hematoma.

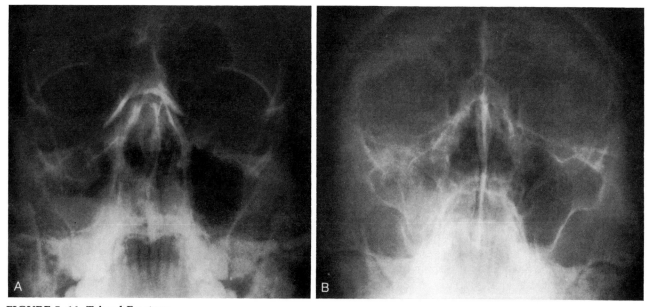

FIGURE 5–16. Tripod Fracture

• • • •

A and *B,* Waters's and Caldwell views of the face demonstrate a right tripod fracture. Components of the tripod fracture include fractures of the lateral wall of the maxillary sinus, fractures of the orbital floor and the lateral orbital wall, as well as the separation of the zygomaticofrontal suture and the fracture of the zygomatic arch. The orbital contents have prolapsed into the right maxillary antrum, and there is marked soft tissue swelling of the right cheek.

Orbital Apex Fractures

The orbital apex is the most posterior portion of the conical orbit and is formed entirely by the sphenoid bone. The sphenoid struts define two neurovascular channels, the optic canal and foramen, which transmits the ophthalmic artery and the optic nerve, and the superior orbital fissure, which contains the third and the fourth cranial nerves, the ophthalmic division of the fifth and the sixth cranial nerves, the superior ophthalmic vein, and a meningeal branch of the lacrimal artery.

Orbital apical fractures rarely occur in isolation, but instead are part of a complex craniofacial injury, including facial, skull base, and other orbital fractures. The majority of fractures are comminuted rather than simple; they are bilateral in approximately one third of patients.

Three types of apical fractures are recognized. There may be a simple linear fracture (Fig. 5–17), a comminuted fracture (Fig. 5–18), or an avulsion of the extreme orbital apex with an intact optic foramen. The third type is exceedingly rare.

The clinical importance of orbital apical fractures centers around the possible sequelae, including damage to the optic nerve, the superior orbital fissure syndrome, and the orbital apex syndrome, in which the neurovascular structures transmitted by these foramina are often injured.

Imaging of the orbital apex can be performed with plain radiographs, polytomography, or CT. Plain film radiography should include an angled anteroposterior view, which provides excellent visualization of the superior orbital fissure, an oblique view through which the optic foramen can be identified, a Caldwell view, and a Reese view. A submentovertex view may be hazardous in patients who have had severe trauma and have marked craniofacial and possible spinal injuries. Polytomography provides excellent visualization of the orbital apex, but CT is far superior for the definition of both osseous and soft tissue structures. The majority of these patients need to undergo an emergency CT scan to evaluate the intracranial contents for significant head trauma. Ideally, evaluation of the orbital apex should be performed in both the axial and the coronal planes using thin sections, and the images should be evaluated with both soft tissue and bone windows. Practically, this is not always possible as many patients, because of their injuries, are unable to assume the hyperextended position required for coronal scans. In such situations, coronal reconstructions from thin axial sections may be helpful.

CT of the orbital apex produces accurate identification and characterization of fractures. The optic canal and the superior orbital fissure are well seen, and fractures involving these neurovascular conduits can be delineated (Fig. 5–19). Associated soft tissue injury such as a soft tissue hematoma or injury to the optic nerve or the other neurovascular structures is demonstrated, and an appropriate plan of therapy can be instituted. Other injuries involving the craniofacial skeleton, the soft tissues, and the intracranial structures may be evaluated during the same examination.

In the past, orbital apical fractures were rarely diagnosed acutely with plain radiographs and polytomography. CT permits the orbital apex to be imaged to good advantage, conveniently and acutely, so that a diagnosis can now be made with confidence.

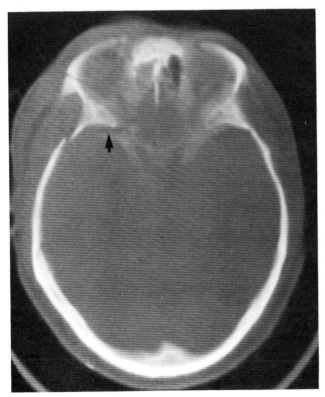

FIGURE 5–17. Linear Orbital Apex Fracture

• • • •

This computed tomography section through the orbital apex demonstrates a linear fracture (*arrow*) with slight separation of the fracture fragments. Fractures of the lateral orbital wall and temporal bone are also seen. Orbital emphysema is present in the right orbit.

Other Fractures

Numerous orbital fractures, such as Le Fort fractures, occur as part of more complex craniofacial or

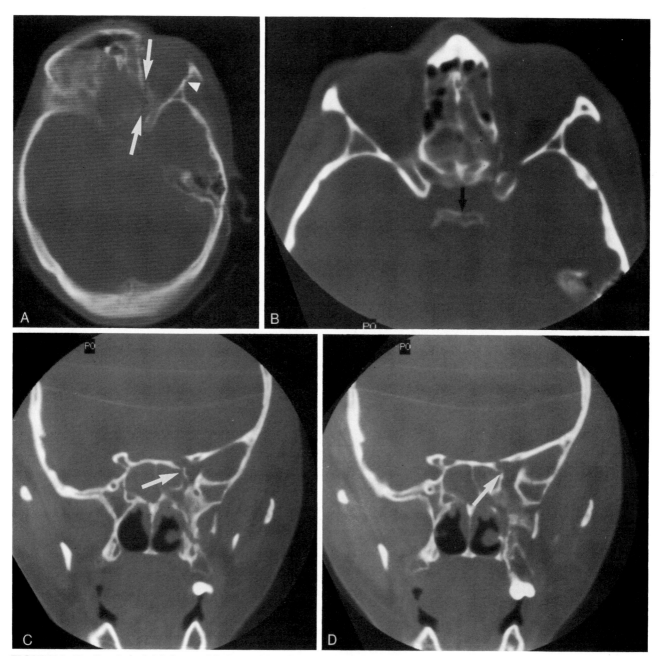

FIGURE 5–18. Craniofacial Injury with Comminuted Fracture of the Orbital Apex

• • • •

A, An axial computed tomography section demonstrates the extensive fracture. The lateral orbital wall *(arrowhead),* the medial orbital wall, and the orbital apex *(arrows)* are all fractured. The ethmoid air cells on the left are opacified. *B,* A coned-down axial section demonstrates the fractures at the orbital apex as well as a fracture of the dorsum sella *(arrow).* *C* and *D,* Coronal sections detail the numerous fractures and the involvement of the optic canal *(arrows).*

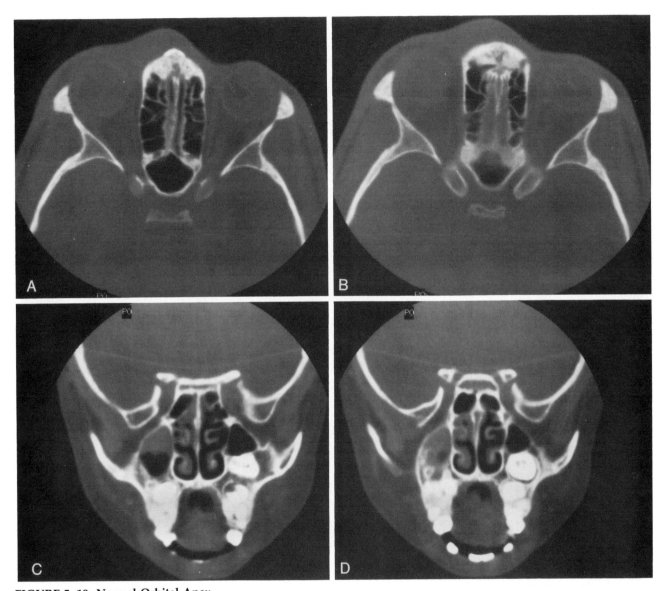

FIGURE 5–19. Normal Orbital Apex

• • • •

A and *B*, A computed tomography scan in the axial and coronal planes through the orbital apex demonstrates the anterior clinoid process, which separates the optic canal, medially, from the superior orbital fissure, laterally. *C* and *D*, The inferior orbital fissure is also well seen on the coronal image. A right maxillary fluid level is seen on the coronal views.

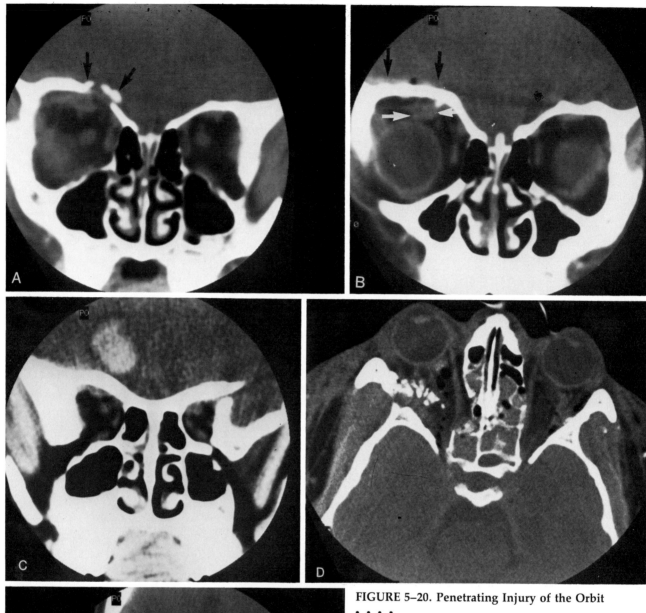

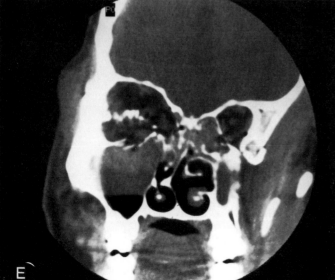

FIGURE 5–20. Penetrating Injury of the Orbit

• • • •

A 6-year-old child fell on scissors, which penetrated the orbit, fractured the orbital roof, and caused injury to the right frontal lobe. *A,* There is a comminuted fracture of the right orbital roof with displacement of the fracture fragments *(arrows).* *B,* Another section demonstrates a small epidural hematoma *(black arrows)* located at the floor of the anterior cranial fossa that contains a small air bubble. In addition, the superior rectus muscle is thickened *(white arrows).* *C,* A section near the orbital apex demonstrates a right frontal lobe hematoma. *D,* This axial computed tomography section of the right orbit after a self-inflicted gunshot wound demonstrates multiple metallic fragments as well as lateral and medial orbital wall fractures. The ethmoid air cells are opacified, and there is orbital emphysema. *E,* The coronal section demonstrates an orbital floor fracture. Between the two planes, precise localization of the fragments is achieved, and the fractures are identified.

facial injuries. They are more fully discussed by specific fracture type in Chapters 2–4.

Orbital fractures also may result from penetrating injuries, most commonly gunshot or stab wounds. These, too, are usually associated with other craniofacial injuries. The specific fracture that results is determined by the entrance, the direction, and the velocity of the missile (Fig. 5–20).

• • • •
INJURIES TO THE SOFT TISSUES OF THE ORBIT

Penetrating Injuries and Foreign Bodies

Penetrating wounds of the orbit occur under numerous circumstances and involve many types of penetrating objects. Most commonly, metal or glass missiles are involved (Fig. 5–21), but injuries with other substances, such as plastic and wood (Fig. 5–22), frequently occur. Organic foreign bodies, especially wood, incite more inflammatory and fibrotic local reaction than inorganic metal or glass, and thus have the potential for greater long-term morbidity if left untreated (Fig. 5–23).

Large superficially obvious wounds may cause surprisingly little damage to the vital structures of the eye. However, penetration of the globe or the orbit by a small missile may produce an inapparent entrance wound but cause significant orbital or even intracranial injuries. These injuries may not be detectable clinically and may go unnoticed by the patient. Accurate identification of injury, whether orbital, craniofacial, or intracranial, requires clinical and ophthalmologic evaluation as well as radiographic investigation.

Associated injuries of the paranasal sinuses, the facial bones, and the intracranial structures necessitate a team approach to penetrating orbital trauma, and such a professional team should include an ophthalmologist, a neurosurgeon, a head and neck surgeon, a neurologist, and a neuroradiologist.

Methods of foreign body identification and localization include (1) ophthalmoscopy, (2) plain film radiography, (3) ultrasound scanning, (4) CT, and (5) MR imaging.

Meticulous ophthalmoscopy detects and locates a large proportion of intraocular foreign bodies. The ophthalmologist is unable to visualize the extraocular tissues, and the presence of corneal or lens opacity or vitreous hemorrhage may obscure visualization of the intraocular foreign body.

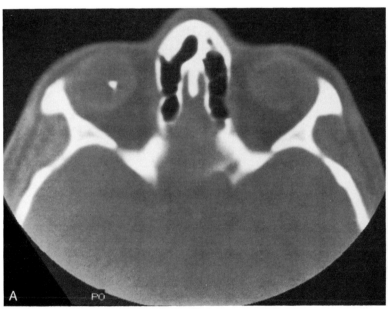 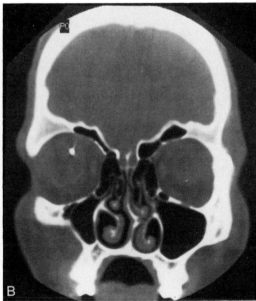

FIGURE 5–21. Intraorbital Metallic Foreign Body
• • • •
Axial and coronal computed tomography (CT) scans provide precise localization of the metallic pellet. *A,* In the first patient, the axial section demonstrates that the pellet is in the medial section of the globe just behind the equator. *B,* The coronal view shows that the pellet is in the upper medial quadrant. Both sections have a prominent star artifact caused by the high-density metallic foreign body.

Illustration continued on following page

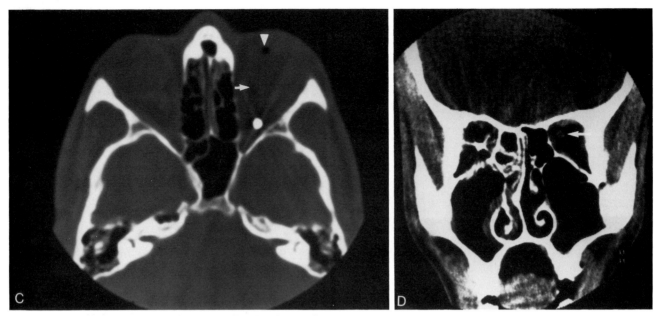

FIGURE 5–21 *Continued* **Intraorbital Metallic Foreign Body**

• • • •

C, The axial CT section on the second patient demonstrates the metallic pellet near the orbital apex. The artifacts radiating from the pellet obscure the optic nerve at the pellet, but the course of the pellet from the globe suggests that the optic nerve may also be injured *(arrow)*. Also note the air in the globe *(arrowhead)*. D, The coronal section demonstrates that the pellet in the right orbit lies slightly inferior to the position of the left optic nerve *(arrow)*. The metallic artifact obscures the right optic nerve, but clinically it was not injured.

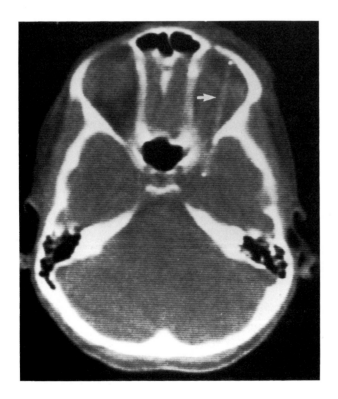

FIGURE 5–22. Wooden Splinter in the Left Eye

• • • •

A linear, moderately high-density foreign body *(arrow)* transverses the superior aspect of the orbit, passing through the superior orbital fissure into the medial aspect of the temporal lobe.

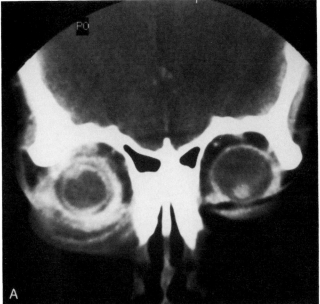
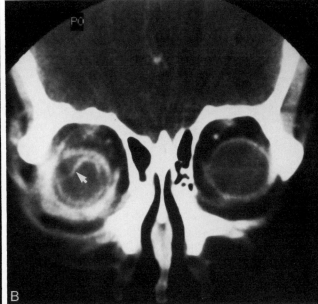
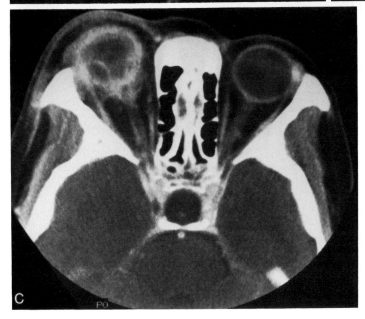

FIGURE 5–23. Panophthalmitis Following Penetrating Injury to the Right Eye with a Wooden Twig

• • • •

One week before coming to the emergency room, the patient had run into a low branch, and a twig from the branch entered her right eye. Her eye was red and swollen at the time of the scan. *A*, A coronal section demonstrates marked enhancement and thickening of the sclera on the right as compared with the left. The orbital fat also has inflammatory changes. *B*, A coronal section 5 mm dorsal to the first one reveals serous scleral separation *(arrow)*. *C*, An axial section demonstrates the generalized swelling of the orbital contents with exophthalmos as well as the inflammatory changes. No section demonstrates a foreign body. Since wood is nearly isodense, the possible presence of residual foreign material cannot be excluded in this study.

Plain film radiographs are useful in the identification of radiopaque foreign bodies (Fig. 5–24). With the use of orthogonal views one can identify intraorbital foreign bodies. However, accurate localization is somewhat difficult. Numerous methods using plain radiographs have been developed for more precise localization, but they have been replaced by newer imaging techniques, such as ultrasound scanning, CT, or MR imaging, which are vastly superior for both the identification and the localization of intraorbital foreign bodies.

As previously mentioned, orbital foreign bodies may be either intraocular or extraocular in location.

The extraocular category is further subdivided into the preseptal, postseptal extraconal, and postseptal intraconal subcategories. Preseptal foreign bodies usually have low penetrating power and therefore do not penetrate deeply into the orbit. Intraocular foreign bodies usually gravitate toward the dependent portion of the globe and are commonly found posteriorly or inferiorly.

Ultrasound scanning of the orbit is an excellent tool for the diagnosis of intraorbital foreign bodies because the intraorbital contents are largely sonolucent, whereas foreign bodies are generally hyperechoic and reflective, and do not permit the

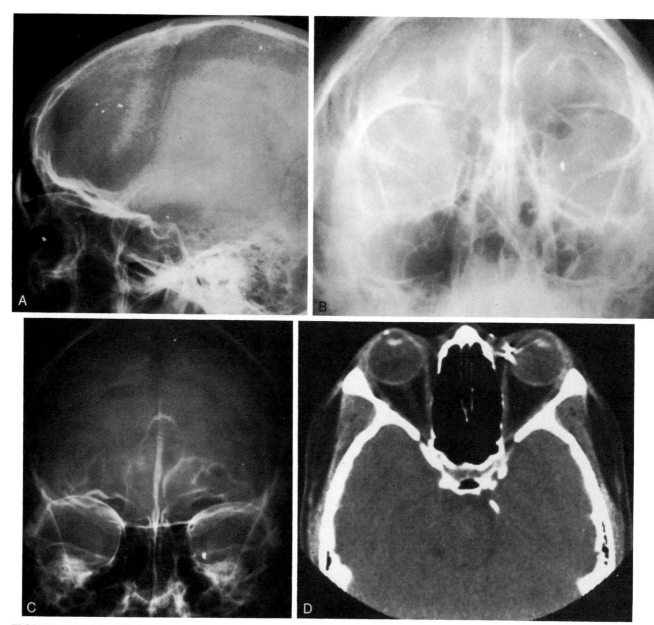

FIGURE 5–24. Metallic Foreign Bodies in and Around the Orbit

• • • •

A, A lateral skull film demonstrates one sizable metallic foreign body and two minute ones that could be within the orbit. Several other metallic fragments are seen. *B*, A Waters view demonstrates two metallic fragments over the left orbit and three small ones over the right orbit. *C*, A Caldwell view demonstrates two foreign bodies over the right orbit, which could be two of the three seen on the Waters view. On the left only one large fragment is seen. *D*, This computed tomography section demonstrates the large left metallic fragment at the medial edge of the globe. The artifact makes it difficult to locate this fragment precisely, but it appears to be adjacent to the scleral insertion of the medial rectus muscle. Smaller fragments are seen in the right cornea and in the skin of the nose on the left.

transmission of ultrasonic waves. Thus, detection of intraorbital foreign bodies is usually accomplished with a high level of accuracy. Ultrasound scanning has several disadvantages when compared to CT or MR imaging. These include the need for actual contact between the sonographic transducer and the eye via a link medium for the ultrasound examination.

This procedure can worsen the injury and introduce infection when there is an open injury to the eye. In addition, pressure is applied directly to the eye during the examination, and this can be extremely uncomfortable or even intolerable for the patient. There is also technical difficulty in detecting anteriorly situated foreign bodies because the most anterior structures of the eye are not well resolved with ultrasound scanning. Multiple small foreign bodies are difficult to detect sonographically, and those lying immediately adjacent to the sclera or retina may be missed. The advantages of ultrasound scanning over the other imaging modalities include the ability to detect retinal detachment more easily than CT and to detect wooden foreign bodies, which may be isodense on CT scans.

Currently, CT is the preferred method for identifying and localizing intraocular foreign bodies. CT is relatively quick and noninvasive, and no pressure or direct contact with the eye is necessary. Not only is CT exquisitely sensitive for the detection and localization of foreign bodies, but the various types of foreign body can often be differentiated. Metallic foreign bodies are easily distinguished from those that are nonmetallic by virtue of a very high CT Hounsfield (H) number (typically greater than 3000). Distinction between different metals is, however, not possible. Glass (300–600 H) is generally of much higher density than plastic (0 to +20 H) or wood (−199 to −50H). It may be difficult to distinguish between the latter two. Plastic or wooden foreign bodies are most easily detected when the CT scan is viewed at a narrow window width, which maximizes the contrast between the orbital tissues and the relatively isodense foreign body.

CT is also useful in identifying bone fragments associated with orbital or craniofacial fractures and in documenting their relationship to the vital orbital structures. Several patients have been described in whom intraorbital bone fragments were not demonstrated on plain films but were well seen on CT scans.

The soft tissue contrast and resolution seen on CT scans enable accurate delineation of the various complications that may be caused by an intraorbital foreign body. The ideal CT scan includes high-resolution (1–2-mm sections) scanning in both the axial and the coronal planes. Practically, however, axial scans with 3- or 5-mm-thick cuts are utilized most frequently. Axial scans are usually adequate for the detection of a single foreign body, but multiple foreign bodies may require coronal scanning, and precise localization requires scanning in both projections. Artifacts caused by a single large metallic body may obscure other smaller foreign bodies, making coronal scanning necessary. Even then, streak artifacts may interfere with the study (Fig. 5–25). A useful CT protocol includes a screening axial scan of the orbits utilizing 3–5-mm contiguous axial cuts in order to identify the presence of a foreign body. The scan can be performed at the same time as the cranial CT scan for acute head trauma. Coronal CT scans may not be feasible acutely because of associated

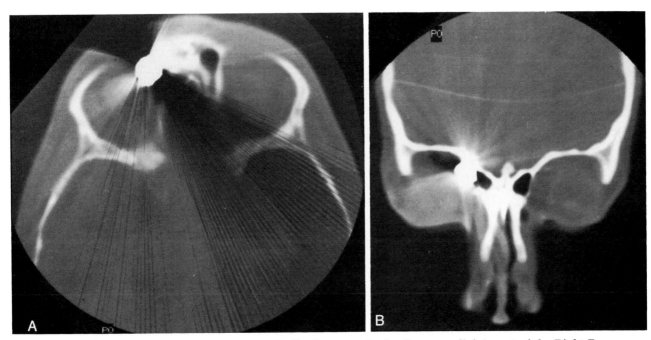

FIGURE 5–25. Streak Artifact Caused by a Large Bullet Fragment in the Superomedial Aspect of the Right Eye Precludes Adequate Evaluation by Computed Tomography

• • • •

A, An axial section displayed with a soft tissue window is impossible to interpret because of the extensive streak artifact. B, A coronal section displayed using a bone window provides more useful information, but small metallic fragments would be obscured by the residual artifact.

injuries. If a foreign body is identified, then biplane, axial and coronal high-resolution, and thin-section CT scans can be performed for precise localization of the foreign body and identification of any additional foreign bodies. The definitive biplane CT scan should be performed just prior to surgical removal because there is the potential for movement of the foreign body between the time of the scan and the surgery. Technical features that improve identification and localization include targeting of the images and utilization of a superimposed grid.

There are certain instances in which detection and precise localization of the foreign body may be difficult even with CT. Foreign bodies smaller than 0.5 mm in size may be below the spatial resolution of the CT scan, especially if they are isodense or relatively isodense with the soft tissues. Certainly metallic foreign bodies greater than 1 mm in size should be detected. Wooden foreign bodies may be isodense with the orbital soft tissues, and if small they are difficult to detect. Foreign bodies intimately related to the sclera may be difficult or even impossible to localize accurately as to intraocular or extraocular location. Volume averaging, streak artifact, and computer malreconstruction secondary to a metallic foreign body impede precise localization in these circumstances. Scleral foreign bodies may appear to project predominantly intraglobally or extraglobally, or both, if large enough, but in this circumstance a CT scan often cannot localize the foreign body accurately. This differentiation is important because intraocular foreign bodies require surgery, whereas extraocular foreign bodies may not; in addition, the surgical technique used when the location is intraocular differs from that employed when it is extraocular.

CT is able to define both the bone anatomy and the soft tissue structures of the orbit with exquisite definition of the optic nerve, the extraocular muscles, the orbital vessels, and the globe (Fig. 5–26). Multiplanar CT can provide precise localization of the foreign body as well as define its relationship to the vital structures, and identify any damage to these structures. Foreign bodies may cause orbital fractures, which are readily identified by CT. A number of intraorbital soft tissue complications of orbital foreign bodies may also be evaluated. Dislocation of the lens can be identified, either with CT or ultrasound scanning, by malposition of the lens. A traumatic cataract has a different CT density than that of the contralateral lens. Vitreous hemorrhage is manifested by a diffuse or focal increase in the CT density of the vitreous fluid (Fig. 5–27). Subchoroidal hemorrhage presents as a high-density collection in the subchoroidal region (Fig. 5–28). Scleral rupture is usually easily identified as discontinuity of the sclera with or without collapse of the globe. Retinal detachment, however, is more readily diagnosed with ultrasound scanning than with CT.

CT has the added advantage over ultrasound in that an evaluation of associated intracranial or craniofacial injuries can be performed simultaneously with an examination of the orbit. When planning surgery, the orbit cannot be treated in isolation but

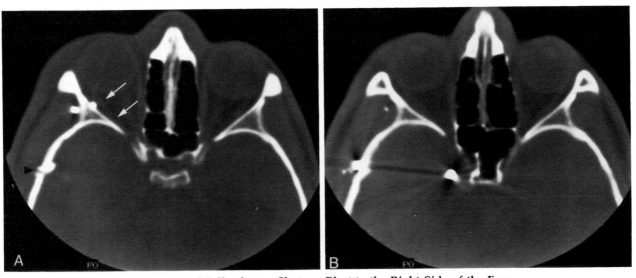

FIGURE 5–26. Intraorbital, Extraconal Pellet from a Shotgun Blast to the Right Side of the Face
• • • •
A, A pellet lies immediately lateral to the lateral rectus muscle *(arrows).* A second pellet lies immediately outside the orbit in the masseter muscle. A comminuted fracture of the temporal bone is also seen *(arrowhead). B,* A computed tomography section 5 mm caudal demonstrates a pellet in the region of the cavernous sinus as well as one just lateral to the temporal bone fracture.

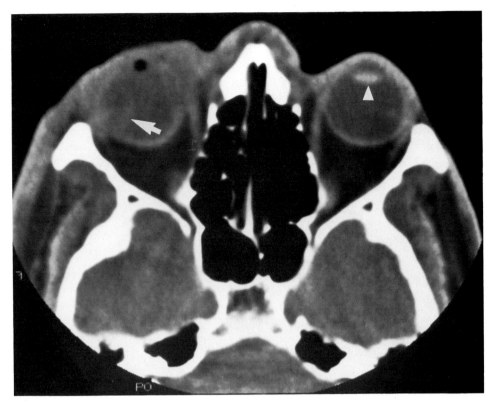

FIGURE 5–27. Penetrating Injury of the Right Globe Caused by a Stab Wound

• • • •

No foreign body is seen on this section. However, there is air in the anterior chamber of the right globe and increased density in the vitreous *(arrow)* caused by hemorrhage. In addition, the lens is not seen, suggesting the presence of a traumatic cataract or lenticular dislocation. A normal lens *(arrowhead)* is present in the left globe as a comparison.

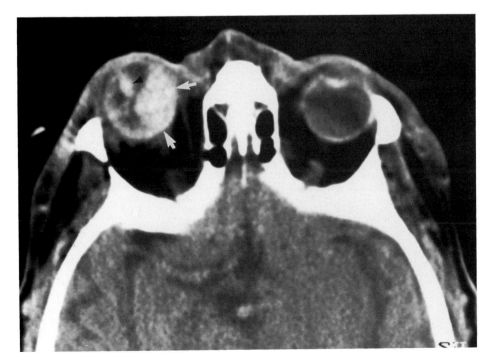

FIGURE 5–28. Subchoroidal Hemorrhage in a Young Man with a Large Corneal Laceration Preventing Ophthalmologic Examination

• • • •

A large, hyperdense, well-defined subchoroidal hemorrhage is seen medially within the globe *(white arrows)*. In addition, the lens has been dislocated posterolaterally *(arrowhead)*, and there is some vitreous hemorrhage.

needs to be treated in conjunction with the associated injuries.

If a major or even a minor vascular injury is suspected, arteriography may be required to demonstrate the presence and the location of the vascular injury (Fig. 5–29). CT may suggest vascular injury on the basis of extensive hematoma but is unable to localize the specific site of injury.

Finally, metallic foreign bodies should not be evaluated with MR imaging unless they are known to be nonferrous. The metallic foreign bodies may be moved by the magnetic field, increasing the injury.

Rupture of the Globe

Perforations of the globe may be caused by either penetrating or blunt injury. Penetrating injuries most commonly occur from industrial accidents and are caused by metallic foreign bodies. Attention must be

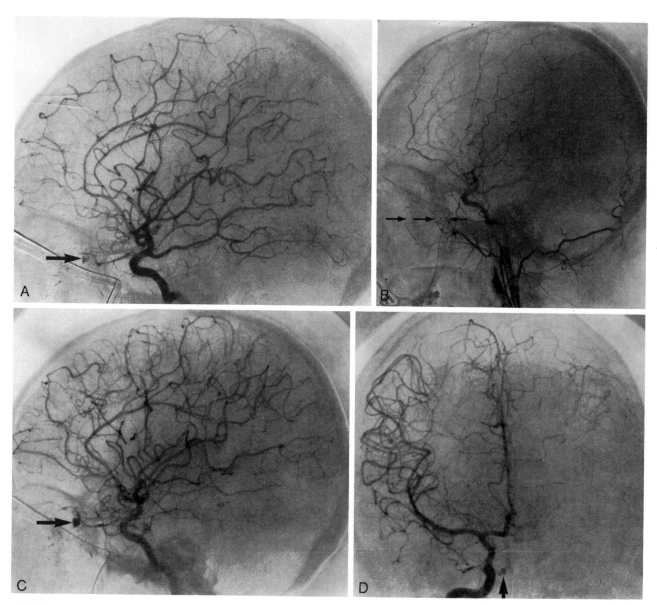

FIGURE 5–29. Acute Bleeding from Both Ophthalmic Arteries

• • • •

The patient was shot through the head from left to right just behind the eyes. *A,* An angiogram of the left internal carotid artery with a lateral projection demonstrates extravasation *(arrow)* from the left ophthalmic artery. *B,* An angiogram of the left external carotid artery with a lateral projection demonstrates several injured arteries *(arrows)* but no evident extravasation. *C,* This angiogram of the right internal carotid artery with a lateral projection demonstrates extravasation *(arrow)* from the right ophthalmic artery. *D,* An anteroposterior projection of the right internal carotid artery demonstrates extravasation from the right ophthalmic artery *(arrow).*

paid to the possibility of more than one perforation, namely an exit wound as well as an entrance wound.

Blunt orbital trauma may cause globe rupture owing to acutely increased pressure or to the perforation of the globe by a bone fragment. A direct compressive force to the eye causes a sudden increase in intraocular pressure combined with deformation of the globe. Decompression occurs by a blow-out fracture of the orbit, a rupture of the globe itself, or both, which happens in about 9% of these injuries. Ocular rupture secondary to blunt trauma usually occurs at the corneoscleral limbus in the superior nasal sclera, where there is some potential weakening caused by Schlemm's canal perforating vessels, and the trochlea. The next most frequent site of rupture is immediately posterior to the insertion of the rectus muscles.

The diagnosis of rupture of the globe is usually established clinically. Not infrequently, occult perforations are present, and it is incumbent upon the radiologist to make this diagnosis. Clinical signs of rupture include actual visualization of the traumatic defect in the sclera, the presence of a foreign body in the globe, chemosis, decreased intraocular pressure, associated soft tissue bruising and swelling, ocular pain, decreased vision, and intraocular hemorrhage. The radiologist usually makes the diagnosis by CT, which may be performed specifically for evaluation of the orbital contents or as part of a screening head CT in a patient with multiple trauma. MR imaging may also be used to evaluate the orbital contents. Apparent CT and MR imaging signs of a ruptured globe include obvious collapse or distortion of the globe with flattening of the posterior sclera (Fig. 5–30), an intraocular foreign body or gas, the *flat tire sign* (Fig. 5–31), frank scleral discontinuity or vitreous herniation (Fig. 5–32), thickening of the posterior sclera, and indistinctness and irregularity of the sclera or cornea, which results from buckling of the sclera (Fig. 5–33). Other suggestive but not diagnostic CT features include a blood-vitreous fluid-fluid level and an ill-defined inner scleral margin resulting from blood within the globe.

Optic Nerve Avulsion or Hematoma

The normal optic nerve is 3–4 mm wide, is thickest at its insertion into the globe, and gradually tapers as it approaches the optic canal. Optic nerve injury is more commonly due to penetrating than blunt trauma and is frequently associated with orbital apex fractures. Optic nerve avulsion usually occurs at the nerve's junction with the globe at the lamina cribrosa. CT findings include marked proptosis, retrobulbar hematoma, which is often localized to the point of

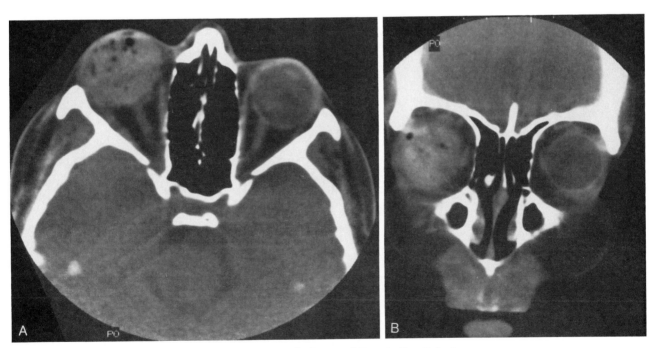

FIGURE 5–30. Ruptured Globe Caused by Combined Blunt and Penetrating Injuries

• • • •

A, The axial computed tomography (CT) scan demonstrates deformity of the globe with flattening. Air is present in the globe (an unequivocal sign of rupture). The vitreous has increased density, which is indicative of hemorrhage. The lens is not seen. *B,* The coronal CT scan demonstrates these abnormalities and also suggests herniation of the vitreous laterally.

Illustration continued on following page

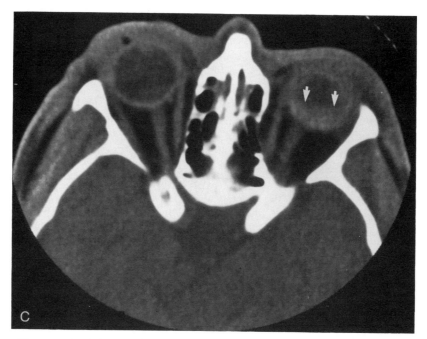

FIGURE 5–30 *Continued* **Ruptured Globe Caused by Combined Blunt and Penetrating Injuries**
• • • •
C, This single section through the orbits of a second patient demonstrates some posterior globe flattening on the left. More interesting is the blood-vitreous fluid-fluid level *(arrows)*. Air is seen anterior to the right globe.

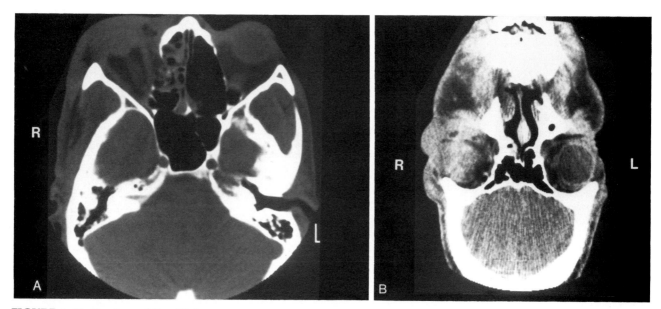

FIGURE 5–31. Rupture of the Globe
• • • •
A, The axial computed tomography section reveals collapse of the right globe. The high density within the collapsed globe is caused by blood. B, A coronal section demonstrates the marked deformity of the globe as well as the associated soft tissue injury.

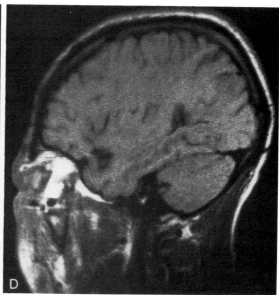

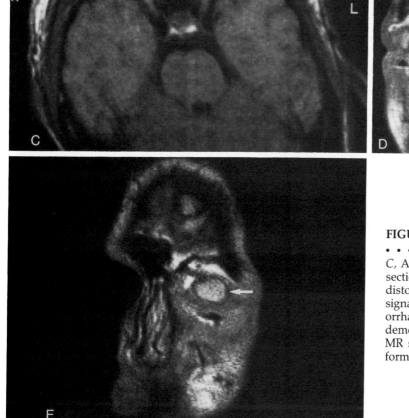

FIGURE 5–31 *Continued* **Rupture of the Globe**

• • • •

C, An axial T$_1$-weighted magnetic resonance (MR) section in another patient demonstrates similar distortion of the left globe, with the high-intensity signal from the globe indicative of vitreous hemorrhage. *D,* A sagittal MR view of the left eye demonstrates the collapsed globe. *E,* A coronal MR section also demonstrates the collapsed, deformed globe *(arrow).*

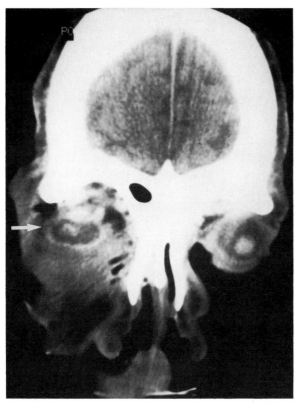

FIGURE 5–32. Ruptured Globe Following a Penetrating Injury to the Orbit

• • • •

Scleral discontinuity *(arrow)* is seen in a collapsed globe that has a typical *flat tire sign* configuration. Also see Figure 5–33, which shows a scan of same patient.

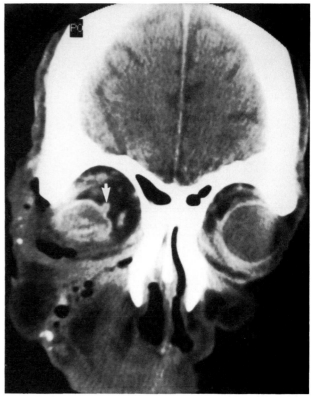

FIGURE 5–33. Ruptured Globe Following a Penetrating Injury to the Orbit

• • • •

A coronal scan demonstrates scleral buckling *(arrow)* medially in a collapsed globe. The globe is displaced, and there is air in the soft tissues of the face and orbits.

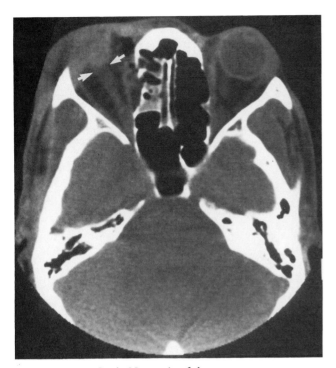

FIGURE 5–34. Optic Nerve Avulsion

• • • •

The patient had no light perception. There is discontinuity of the optic nerve at the posterior pole of the globe *(arrows).* In addition, the globe is ruptured and collapsed (see also Fig. 5–31A), and there is a medial orbital wall fracture.

the avulsion, and discontinuity of the optic nerve (Fig. 5–34). Incomplete disruption may cause subtle or obvious CT changes in the optic nerve, including an irregular contour, a high-density optic nerve hematoma, and abnormalities in the surrounding tissue (Fig. 5–35). There may also be a retrobulbar hemorrhage. Traumatic hematoma of the optic nerve causes an enlargement of the optic nerve or the sheath near the orbital apex and may be associated with high CT density due to the recently extravasated blood (Fig. 5–36). A "stretch injury" to the optic nerve causes damage to the nutrient vessels as well as subsequent hemorrhage, edema, and contusion of the nerve.

Retrobulbar hematoma is not a specific finding for optic nerve injury and may occur without such an injury, usually as a result of penetrating trauma. These isolated retrobulbar hematomas are often eccentrically located rather than being intimately related to the optic nerve.

Subperiosteal Hematomas of the Orbit

Subperiosteal hematoma of the orbit is a distinct clinical entity that differs in mechanism, presentation, and treatment from other periorbital hemato-

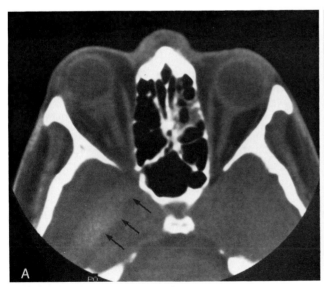
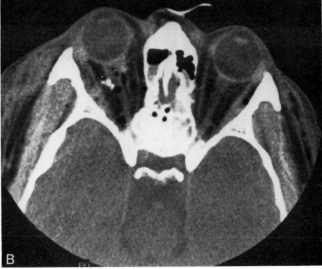

FIGURE 5–35. Optic Nerve Injury

• • • •

A, Partial disruption of the right optic nerve caused by a stab wound to the orbit. The optic nerve is thickened near the globe, and there is hemorrhage in the intraconal fat lateral to the optic nerve. In this patient, thickening of the optic nerve is the primary finding; in others, hemorrhage or irregular contour may be seen. Note also the hematoma in the right temporal lobe *(arrows).* B, Injury to the optic nerve caused by a gunshot injury is shown. Metallic fragments and air abut the thickened right optic nerve.

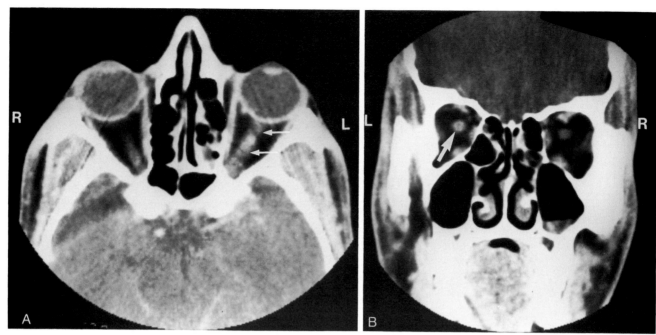

FIGURE 5–36. Optic Nerve Contusion and Hematoma

• • • •

A, An axial computed tomography section demonstrates that the left optic nerve *(arrows)* is thicker than the right optic nerve and that it has increased density compared with that on the right. Swelling and bleeding are the cause. *B,* The coronal view, which was performed with left-to-right reversal, also demonstrates the enlarged dense left optic nerve *(arrow).*

mas. Typically, subperiosteal hematomas result from relatively trivial trauma to the face or head in young white males. They occur in the frontal bone of the orbital roof. Clinical features include orbital pain, exophthalmos, and diplopia, which may develop a few days after the injury. Usually no associated eyelid hematoma is present. The diagnosis is easily established at CT or MR imaging because a typical subperiosteal collection is seen under the roof of the orbit (Fig. 5–37). This is best demonstrated on coronal CT or MR imaging cuts and may not be seen on the axial images. The density or the signal intensity of the collection depends upon the stage at which imaging is performed, because the CT density and the MR imaging intensity of a hematoma vary with age. Acute hematomas have a high density on CT scans and a low or intermediate signal intensity on T_1- and T_2-weighted MR images, whereas subacute or chronic subperiosteal hematomas have a low density on CT scans and a high signal intensity on T_1- and T_2-weighted MR images.

The treatment of a subperiosteal hematoma is percutaneous aspiration through the eyelid. Typically 3.5–4 ml of fluid are aspirated. The prognosis is excellent.

Vitreous Hemorrhage

The normal vitreous fluid should be homogeneous, uniform, and bilaterally similar with a CT density (H) and MR signal characteristics approximately that of simple fluid. Vitreous hemorrhage causes the density of the vitreous fluid to increase; this is manifested by a homogeneous increase in density on CT scans and an increased signal intensity on MR images (Fig. 5–38). This can be readily seen by comparing the injured eye with the normal eye. Streak artifacts from the bone of the orbital roof can produce linear streaks of opacity through the vitreous and must not be mistaken for the diffuse increased density of vitreous hemorrhage (Fig. 5–39).

Subconjunctival Hemorrhage

The normal cornea and conjunctiva have a uniform thickness on CT that should not be greater than 1–2 mm. Thickening or irregularity of the corneal or conjunctival margins can be seen with subconjunc-

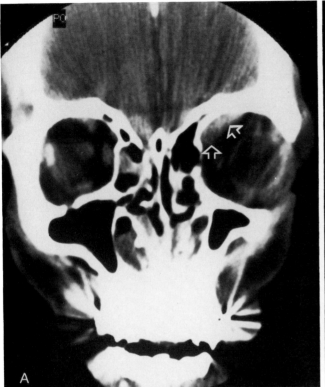

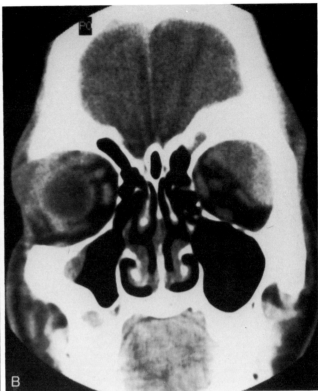

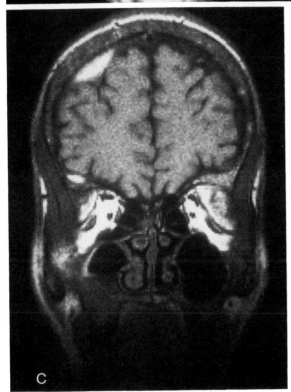

FIGURE 5–37. Subperiosteal Hematoma

• • • •

A, The superomedial hematoma has an increased attenuation and is sharply defined *(arrows).* The globe is displaced inferolaterally. *B,* A coronal computed tomography scan in another patient shows a left subperiosteal hematoma in the upper outer quadrant of the orbit. The conal structures are all displaced inferomedially by the hematoma. *C,* A coronal magnetic resonance image on a third patient who had bilateral orbital subperiosteal hematomas as well as a small right subdural hematoma after falling downstairs. On this T₁-weighted image, the hematomas are still partly isointense, indicating that they are acute.

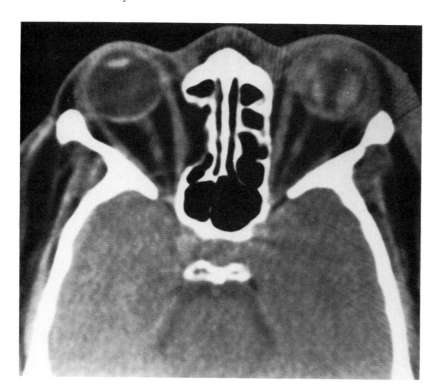

FIGURE 5–38. Facial Injuries (Including Decreased Vision in the Left Eye) Caused by a Motor Vehicle Accident

• • • •

An axial computed tomography scan demonstrates patchy high density within the globe, which is indicative of vitreous hemorrhage. In addition, there is scleral thickening, and the lens is obscured. The medial wall of the right orbit has a blowout fracture, and the right medial rectus muscle is slightly bowed and thickened.

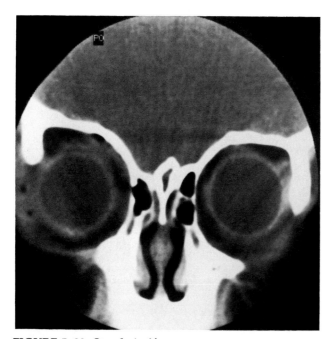

FIGURE 5–39. Streak Artifacts

• • • •

The soft tissues in and around the right orbit are swollen, and there is orbital emphysema. There are bilateral streak artifacts from the orbital roof; they cross the inferolateral aspect of both globes and simulate the increased density seen in vitreous hemorrhage. The very linear nature of the streaks should alert the radiologist to their true nature.

tival hemorrhage on CT scans (Fig. 5–40). However, this is not a specific finding because chemosis or simple lid edema can produce a very similar CT picture.

Proptosis/Enophthalmos

Proptosis is often the result of periorbital edema or contusion, but its presence should alert both the clinician and the radiologist to the possibility of a more serious ocular injury. High-resolution CT of the orbit is appropriate to detect clinically silent retrobulbar lesions.

Enophthalmos in the setting of trauma is usually due to orbital fracture and prolapse of the orbital contents into the maxillary sinus or the ethmoid air cells.

Lens Injury

The lens is suspended from the ciliary body and is separated from it by a symmetric circumferential space of 0.5 mm. It lies immediately posterior to the iris. Gross dislocation of the lens is usually obvious both clinically and on CT scans (Fig. 5–41). However,

FIGURE 5–40.
Subconjunctival
Hemorrhage

• • • •

Performed following an aggravated assault, this computed tomography (CT) scan shows thickening of the left conjunctiva caused by hemorrhage. There is an associated medial wall fracture on the left as well as orbital emphysema. This diagnosis is more accurately made clinically. Edema and chemosis would produce an identical CT picture.

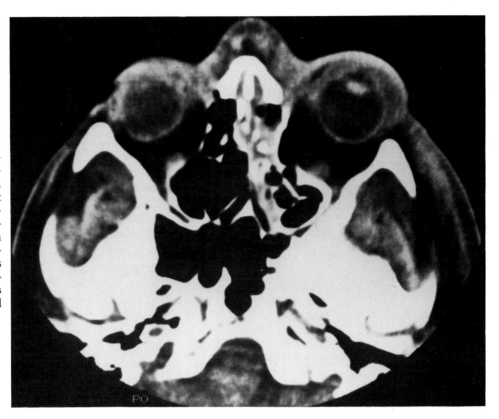

more subtle injuries may be inapparent clinically, and the position of the lens should be carefully evaluated on CT scans because mild asymmetry may be the only indication of a subtle dislocation.

Traumatic cataract may be diagnosed on CT scans as hypodensity of the abnormal lens, which can be readily seen when it is compared with the lens on the normal side. The abnormal lens density ap-

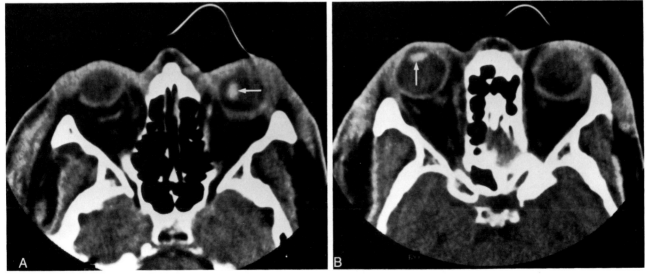

FIGURE 5–41. Lens Dislocation

• • • •

A, The first axial section demonstrates the left lens in an abnormal position *(arrow)*. *B*, The normal right lens *(arrow)* is seen on adjacent cut. Note also the deformity and thickening of the wall of the left orbit on both sections.

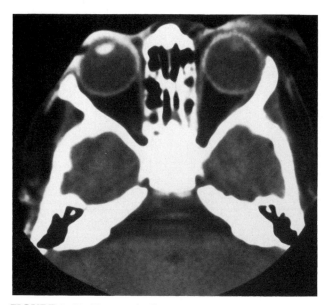

FIGURE 5–42. Traumatic Cataract

• • • •

A single axial computed tomography section demonstrates marked difference in the attenuation of the normal right and the abnormal left lens. Care must be taken to be certain that this difference is not due to partial volume defects. The asymmetric lens density must be seen on all sections that include the lens. Thin sections are necessary.

proaches that of the surrounding fluid, making it less visible than the normal lens (Fig. 5–42; see also Fig. 5–28).

Choroidal Detachment

Hemorrhagic choroidal detachment may be caused by either blunt or penetrating injury to the eye. In the acute setting, the suprachoroidal collection appears on CT scans as a uniformly hyperdense, localized collection that does not change when patient position is altered. With time, the mound-like collection becomes inhomogeneous and hypodense, thereby mimicking a serous choroidal detachment. This is seen more commonly following surgery or in association with inflammatory lesions. Ultrasound scanning demonstrates numerous echogenic foci within a hemorrhagic detachment, whereas a serous detachment is uniformly sonolucent. Multiplanar MR imaging demonstrates choroidal detachments beautifully and shows varying signal characteristics depending on the composition of the collection and the age of the hemorrhage (Fig. 5–43).

Penetrating injuries to the globe may produce ocular hypotonia, which predisposes to serous cho-

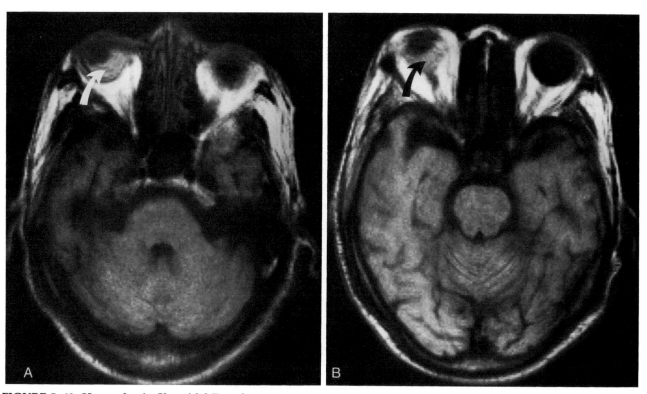

FIGURE 5–43. Hemorrhagic Choroidal Detachment

• • • •

A and *B,* Axial T$_1$-weighted images through the orbit demonstrate abnormal high-signal intensity, peripherally and posteriorly in the right globe *(arrow),* representing a hemorrhagic choroidal detachment. The high signal on the T$_1$-weighted images corresponds to subacute hemorrhage.

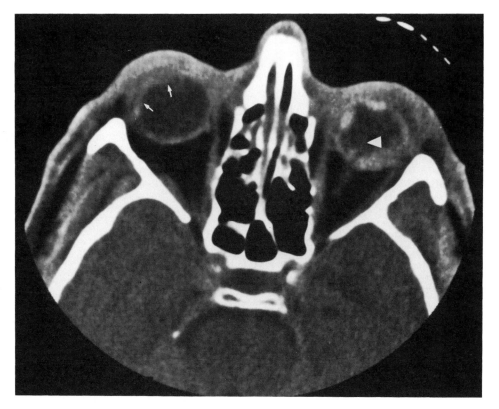

FIGURE 5–44. Hyphema

• • • •

There is thickening of the anterior aspect of the right globe *(arrows)*, which is caused by hemorrhage into the anterior chamber of the eye. Hyphema is a clinical diagnosis, but this is an excellent computed tomography demonstration. The left globe is collapsed with scleral buckling. A small bomb fragment *(arrowhead)* is seen at the origin of the optic nerve.

roidal detachment by upsetting ocular and choroidal pressure homeostasis. With egress of fluid into the choroid and the suprachoroidal space, serous choroidal detachment may form wherever the choroid is not attached to the sclera by nerves or vessels. Scleral infolding, which often indicates a ruptured globe, may simulate a choroidal detachment as it can produce focal choroidal thickening on CT scans.

Retinal Detachment

Retinal detachment cannot be reliably diagnosed by CT. Fundoscopy and ultrasound scanning remain the primary diagnostic tools for this diagnosis.

Hyphema

Hyphema is hemorrhage into the anterior chamber of the eye. It is obvious clinically and rarely detectable on CT scans (Fig. 5–44). Thus, hyphema remains a clinical diagnosis, and the radiologist does not take part in the evaluation of this abnormality.

Bibliography

Avrahami E, Sperber F, Cohn DF. Computerized tomographic demonstration of intraorbital bone fragments caused by penetrating trauma. Ophthalmic Surg 1986; 17:41–43.

Berkowitz RA, Putterman AM, Patel DB. Prolapse of the globe into the maxillary sinus after orbital floor fracture. Am J Ophthalmol 1981; 91:253–257.

Bhimani S, Virapongse C, Sarwar M, Twist JF. Computed tomography in penetrating injury to the eye. Am J Ophthalmol 1984; 97:583–586.

Brinkley JR, Acomb T. Simulated blowout fracture of the orbit. Ophthalmic Surg 1983; 14:499–500.

Cobb SR, Yeakley JW, Lee KF, et al. Computed tomographic evaluation of ocular trauma. Comput Radiol 1985; 9:1–10.

Coker NJ, Brooks BS, El Gammal T. Computed tomography of orbital medial wall fractures. Head Neck Surg 1983; 5:383–389.

Converse JM, Smith B. On the treatment of blowout fractures of the orbit. Plast Reconstr Surg 1978; 62:100–104.

Crow W, Guinto FC Jr, Amparo E, Stewart K. Normal in vivo eye dimensions by computed tomography. J Comput Assist Tomogr 1982; 6:708–710.

Curtin HD, Wolfe P, Schramm V. Orbital roof blow-out fractures. AJR 1982; 139:969–972.

Fujino T. Experimental "blowout" fracture of the orbit. Plast Reconstr Surg 1974; 54:81–82.

Fujino T, Makino K. Entrapment mechanism and ocular injury in orbital blowout fracture. Plast Reconstr Surg 1980; 65:571–574.

Gilbard SM, Mafee MF, Lagouros PA, Langer BG. Orbital blowout fractures. The prognostic significance of computed tomography. Ophthalmology 1985; 92:1523–1528.

Greenwald MJ, Lissner GS, Tomita T, Naidich TP. Isolated orbital roof fracture with traumatic encephalocele. J Pediatr Ophthalmol Strabismus 1987; 24:141–143.

Grove AS Jr. Orbital trauma and computed tomography. Ophthalmology 1980; 87:403–410.

Hammerschlag S, Hughes S, O'Reilly G, et al. Another look at blow-out fractures of the orbit. AJR 1982; 139:133–137.

Hammerschlag S, Hughes S, O'Reilly G, et al. Blow-out fractures of the orbit: A comparison of computed tomography and conventional radiography with anatomical correlation. Radiology 1982; 143:487–492.

Henrikson GC, Mafee MF, Flanders AE, et al. CT evaluation of plastic intraocular foreign bodies. AJNR 1987; 8:378–379.

Keene J, Doris PE. A simple radiographic diagnosis of occult blow-out fractures. Ann Emerg Med 1985; 14:335–338.

Kersten RC. Blowout fracture of the orbital floor with entrapment caused by isolated trauma to the orbital rim. Am J Ophthalmol 1987; 103:215–220.

Koornneef L, Zonneveld FW. The role of direct multiplanar high resolution CT in the assessment and management of orbital trauma. Radiol Clin North Am 1987; 25:753–766.

Kulwin DR, Leadbetter MG. Orbital rim trauma causing a blowout fracture. Plast Reconstr Surg 1984; 73:969–971.

Laurin S, Johansen CC. Oblique lateral projection of the orbital floor. Acta Radiol [Diagn] (Stockh) 1982; 23:423–431.

Lindahl S. Computed tomography of intraorbital foreign bodies. Acta Radiol 1987; 28:235–240.

Lins M, Kopietz L. Foreign body masquerading as a ruptured globe. Ophthalmic Surg 1985; 16:586–588.

Lipkin AF, Woodson GE, Miller RH. Visual loss due to orbital fracture. Arch Otolaryngol Head Neck Surg 1987; 113:81–83.

Lobes LA Jr, Grand MG, Reece J, Penkrot RJ. Computerized axial tomography in the detection of intraocular foreign bodies. Ophthalmology 1981; 88:26–29.

Mafee MF, Peyman GA. Choroidal detachment and ocular hypotony: CT evaluation. Radiology 1984; 153:697–703.

McArdle CB, Amparo EG, Mirfakhraee M. MR imaging of orbital blow-out fractures. J Comput Assist Tomogr 1986; 10:116–119.

Putterman AM, Stevens T, Urist MJ. Nonsurgical management of blow-out fractures of the orbital floor. Am J Ophthalmol 1974; 77:232–239.

Rauch SD. Medial orbital blow-out fracture with entrapment. Arch Otolaryngol 1985; 111:53–55.

Risco JM, Stratas BA, Knott RH. Prolapse of the globe into the ethmoid sinus. Am J Ophthalmol 1984; 97:659–660.

Sassani JW, Peart RE, Haak NW, Hodes BL. Combined use of A-scan ultrasound, plain roentgenograms, and computerized axial tomography in the evaluation of a pseudo-intraocular foreign body. J Clin Ultrasound 1984; 12:171–173.

Sevel D, Krausz H, Ponder T, Centeno R. Value of computed tomography for the diagnosis of a ruptured eye. J Comput Assist Tomogr 1983; 7:870–875.

Sibony PA, Anand AK, Keuskamp A, Zippen AG. Post-traumatic cerebrospinal fluid cyst of the orbit. J Neurosurg 1985; 62:922–924.

Smith B, Lisman RD, Simonton J, Della Rocca R. Volkmann's contracture of the extraocular muscles following blowout fracture. Plast Reconstr Surg 1984; 74:200–208.

Smith B, Regan WF Jr. Blow-out fractures of the orbit. Mechanism and correction of inferior orbital fracture. Am J Ophthalmol 1957; 44:733–739.

Spierer A, Tadmor R, Treister G, et al. Diagnosis and localization of intraocular foreign bodies by computed tomography. Ophthalmic Surg 1985; 16:571–576.

Tonami H, Nakagawa T, Ohguchi M, et al. Surface coil MR imaging of orbital blowout fractures: A comparison with reformatted CT. AJNR 1987; 8:445–449.

Tonami H, Yamamoto I, Matsuda M, et al. Orbital fractures: Surface coil MR imaging. Radiology 1991; 179:789–794.

Topilow HW, Ackerman AL, Zimmerman RD. Limitations of computerized tomography in the localization of intraocular foreign bodies. Ophthalmology 1984; 91:1086–1091.

Unger JM. Orbital apex fractures: The contribution of computed tomography. Radiology 1984; 150:713–717.

Watson A, Hartley DE. Alternative method of intraocular foreign-body localization. AJR 1984; 142:789–790.

Weisman RA, Savino PJ, Schut L, Schatz NJ. Computed tomography in penetrating wounds of the orbit with retained foreign bodies. Arch Otolaryngol 1983; 109:265–268.

Wolter JR. Subperiosteal hematomas of the orbit in young males: A serious complication of trauma or surgery in the eye region. J Pediatr Ophthalmol Strabismus 1979; 16:291–296.

Yamamoto Y, Sakurai M, Asari S. Towne (half-axial) and semisagittal computed tomography in the evaluation of blowout fractures of the orbit. J Comput Assist Tomogr 1983; 7:306–309.

Zinreich SJ, Miller NR, Aguayo JB, et al. Computed tomographic three-dimensional localization and compositional evaluation of intraocular and orbital foreign bodies. Arch Ophthalmol 1986; 104:1477–1482.

SECTION TWO

The Spine

Overview of the Spine*

• • • • • • • •

RICHARD A. SUSS, M.D.

• • • •

ANATOMY

The functional spinal column includes not only the vertebrae, the discs, and numerous other intervertebral linkages, but also the spinal cord and the nerve roots, the meninges and their adjacent fluid and soft tissue compartments, blood circulation, and innervation. Whether imaged directly or evaluated indirectly, these components have diagnostic significance.

Vertebrae

The basic vertebral configuration is a horizontal ring thickened anteriorly, except in the atlas vertebra. The anterior thickening is the vertebral body. The remainder of the ring is the neural arch. The typical hemiarch consists of a pedicle, a superior articular process, an interarticular part (the *pars interarticularis*, which is incorporated with the facets into the cervical articular pillar), an inferior articular process, and a plate-like lamina. In addition to the facet-bearing articular processes, the typical vertebral ring bears a spinous process, which is based at the junction of the laminae, and two transverse processes, which project laterally from the arch near the superior facet. The cervical transverse process also includes an anterior strut that projects from the vertebral body and gives it a more anterior position than that of the lower transverse processes. The sacral transverse processes are fused as the alae.

Most of the vertebral body derives from an ossification center called the *centrum*. Superior and inferior ring apophyses contribute to the vertebral end plate margins. Each hemiarch ossifies from a single primary center that also contributes to the posterolateral portion of the vertebral body as well as from a

variable number of secondary ossification centers. The major synchondroses are those between the primary ossification centers, namely the neurocentral synchondroses, located anterolaterally and slightly within the vertebral body, and the median posterior interlaminar synchondrosis. Most of the spinous process develops from the two arch centers. The only midline ossification centers are the centra, ring apophyses, spinous process tip apophyses, anterior C1 arch, and dens apex.

The vertebrae have several important "holes." The large vertical hole in the vertebral ring is the *vertebral foramen*, the bony wall of the spinal canal. The intervertebral (neural) foramina transmit blood vessels and the spinal nerves. Only the cervical vertebrae have transverse foramina; these foramina pass vertically through the transverse processes. After skipping those of C7, the vertebral arteries pass through those of C6–C1.

Most of the free vertebrae are more similar in shape to each other than to the first two cervical vertebrae. The following divisions differ systematically in their anatomy, their motions, and their injuries:

1. The upper cervical spine, which comprises the atypical first two cervical vertebrae and their craniad articulations
2. The lower cervical spine, which comprises the five typical cervical vertebrae and their six associated discs
3. The thoracic spine
4. The lumbar spine
5. The sacrum and the coccyx

In trauma, however, groups 1 and 2 are evaluated together.

Intervertebral Linkages

The intervertebral disc is a symphysis with a fluid cushion at its center. The fibrocartilaginous annulus

---

*References for the Overview of the Spine may be found at the end of Chapter 6.

169

confines the partly gelatinous and partly fibrocartilaginous nucleus pulposus. With age or degeneration the nucleus becomes more fibrous and less fluid.

Anterior and posterior longitudinal ligaments run along the vertebral column and attach to the annuli and to the vertebrae. The anterior longitudinal ligament extends to the anterior base of C2, continues as the anterior atlantoaxial ligament to attach to the anterior arch of the atlas, and from there continues as the anterior atlanto-occipital membrane to attach to the inferior surface of the occipital bone. The posterior longitudinal ligament continues above the body of C2 as the tectorial membrane, which extends behind the odontoid process and attaches to the clivus of the occipital bone. Both longitudinal ligaments extend down to the sacrum.

The neural arches are linked by several accessory ligaments. The elastic flaval ligaments connect adjacent laminae. Interspinous ligaments connect adjacent spinous processes. The supraspinous ligament runs over the tips of the spinous processes and continues as the nuchal ligament up to the external occipital crest. Intertransverse muscles link consecutive cervical and lumbar transverse processes. In the lumbar spine there are also intertransverse ligaments. The principal articulations of the thoracic transverse processes are with the ribs. The ligaments and the annuli are the major stabilizers of the vertebrae.[118]

The diarthrodial facet (zygapophyseal) joints from C2–3 downward link the articular processes. The orientation of the facet joint surface controls the mobility of the vertebrae. The facet surfaces are imbricated and overlap like roofing shingles; at each joint the inferior facet of the higher vertebra overlaps posteriorly the superior facet of the lower vertebra. This arrangement permits oblique vertical sliding for flexion and extension while it restrains direct anterior movement of a vertebra on the one below. Seen from above, the cervical and the thoracic facet joint planes are coronally oriented, whereas the lumbar facet joint planes are oblique, curved, or nearly sagittal.

The linkages at an intervertebral level constitute the functional spinal unit in studies of motion and injuries. Therefore, instead of thinking of the vertebrae as the segments of primary interest, it is often useful to shift attention to the "motion segments." The upper cervical spine thus consists of two motion segments (C0–1 and C1–2), and the lower cervical spine consists of six (C2–3 through C7–T1). This "frame shift" simplifies the analysis of many injuries.

Spinal Canal Contents

The spinal canal is bounded by the inner bony walls of the vertebral foramina, the disc annuli, the posterior longitudinal ligament, the facet joint capsules, and the flaval ligaments. It is lined by epidural fat and veins and by the dura and the arachnoid mater. Internal to the arachnoid are the cerebrospinal fluid (CSF), the spinal cord, and the proximal portions of the spinal nerve roots.

The organization of the spinal cord is the inverse of that of the brain. Thick tracts of myelinated and unmyelinated axons surround a central column of gray matter. Within the central gray matter is a narrow central canal that cannot yet be normally visualized with medical imaging. The anterior and the posterior white matter columns are each divided by ventral and dorsal median fissures. The ventral median fissure is often visible on intrathecally enhanced CT, but the dorsal median fissure usually is not. Sometimes posterolateral sulci are opacified indistinctly between the dorsal columns and the dorsal root entry zones.

Motor cell bodies and sensory fiber connections associated with the brachial and the lumbosacral plexes produce regional enlargements. The cervical enlargement expands primarily the transverse diameter of the cord from C3 to C7, relatively flattening it without narrowing the anterior and the posterior subarachnoid space. The lumbar enlargement above the conus medullaris is rounder. At other levels the cord is flattened slightly.

The spinal cord has numerous transverse attachments in addition to its attachments to the medulla oblongata and to the sacrum by the filum terminale. The ventral and the dorsal nerve roots are the most obvious. The denticulate (dentate) ligaments attach the dura mater (or dura) through the spinal arachnoid to the pia mater of the cord laterally; this restricts longitudinal motion of the cord.[106] Thus, vertebral distraction does not simply stretch the entire length of the cord evenly but can also lacerate it locally. Posteriorly in the lower cervical and the thoracic segments, a fenestrated median subarachnoid septum (septum posticum) and numerous paramedian subarachnoid trabeculae connect the pia mater with the spinal arachnoid.[23] These affect CSF flow and often cause irregular signal patterns behind the thoracic spinal cord on MR images.

During fetal development the body outgrows the cord, so that by the time of birth the conus medullaris has "risen" into the upper lumbar spinal canal. During childhood the conus tip rises to between T12 and L2. Most of the lumbar spinal canal contains the cauda equina, which consists of long lumbar, sacral, and coccygeal sensory and motor nerve roots. The spinal cord does have lumbar, sacral, and coccygeal portions, but they lie near the thoracolumbar junction of the spine. Likewise, thoracic cord levels lie higher than the like-numbered vertebrae, with a smaller upward one half to one segment shift in the cervical spine. The level of cord injury should *not* be denoted by the vertebral level but instead by either the lowest intact or the highest damaged *cord* level. Physicians must be clear about which of the latter two systems they use.

Although there are only seven cervical vertebrae, the cervical cord and root levels are numbered from one through eight. The first through seventh roots exit the neural foramina just *above* the like-numbered vertebral pedicles, whereas the eighth roots exit at C7–T1. Thus, there can be a "C8 injury," but only to the cord or to the nerve root. The thoracic, the lumbar, and the sacral roots exit the foramina just *below* the like-numbered pedicles.

Arterial supply to the spine is multiple. Much is derived from the vertebral arteries, which anastomose with other branches of the subclavian arteries and with branches of the external carotid arteries. Other supply comes from intercostal, lumbar, and sacral arteries. Cord circulation is divided into three territories: the cervicothoracic, the midthoracic, and the thoracolumbar. The arteries along the cord are arranged in three longitudinal axes: one anterior and two posterolateral. These axes can be discontinuous, particularly at upper and lower thoracic border zones. Paired anterior spinal arteries arise from the intracranial vertebral arteries, descend and fuse in the midline, and contribute the major supply to the median medulla and the cervical cord. The fused "anterior spinal artery" runs in the ventral median fissure and supplies the anterior 80% of the cord. The lower cervical cord is supplemented by a dominant radicular artery called the *artery of the cervical enlargement*. The midthoracic territory is supplied principally by a dominant midthoracic radicular artery. The thoracolumbar territory, including the conus, is supplied principally by a dominant lower thoracic or high lumbar radicular artery called the *artery of Adamkiewicz*. Paired posterior spinal arteries arise from the posterior inferior cerebellar arteries or from the intracranial vertebral arteries and descend as "posterolateral arteries." These arteries receive numerous small collateral feeders and supplement the supply to the posterior columns and gray posterior horns.

• • • •
CHARACTERIZATION OF SPINAL INJURIES

Spinal injuries are characterized by numerous features along several conceptual "dimensions" that must be integrated into the reader's search and analysis skills.

Spinal Region

The regional divisions of the spine serve as a simple scheme to organize discussion. In clinical practice, precise vertebral localization is required. How many regions are injured? Within each region, which vertebrae and motion segments are injured?

Type of Tissue Injured

Bone injury can be a contusion, ischemic necrosis (rare in vertebrae), an initially microscopic stress fracture, or an overt fracture. Injuries to intervertebral linkages can be ligamentous sprain or rupture, annular tearing or nuclear herniation, capsular tearing or articular cartilage contusion, or muscle strain or rupture. There may be a momentary or a persistent dislocation, either isolated or as a part of a fracture-dislocation.

Several different pathologic states can underlie disc protrusion. An annular bulge is an exaggeration of the convexity of the annulus in its vertical profile that is not due to predominantly focal degeneration or to overt rupture. Bulges tend to be centered in the midline posteriorly and usually also create or exaggerate posterior annular convexity in the axial profile. Seen after acute trauma, a bulge often is a pre-existing abnormality, but it can be transiently accentuated and can contribute to spinal stenosis and cord injury. A herniation is a focal annular protrusion resulting from locally accentuated weakening, with penetration of nuclear material through part or all of the thickness of the annulus. A complete annular tear can lead to the extrusion of nuclear material, which may then remain at the disc level or migrate away and become sequestered. Not all protrusions can be easily determined to be bulges or herniations. Even an annular tear can be seen with little or no bulging and without focal herniation.

Spinal epidural hematomas are venous but can cause cord compression.[81, 124] Significant subdural hematomas are rare. Paraspinal or prevertebral hematomas result from soft tissue injury or from fracture and periosteal tearing, for which they are occasional sentinels. The vertebral arteries, the anterior spinal artery, and the intercostal arteries supplying the cord are vulnerable to occlusion and to laceration. Of ultimate concern are the spinal cord and its nerve roots. The cord can be compressed or torn by bone spurs, fracture fragments, chronic or acute disc protrusions, buckled ligaments, meningeal hematomas, or penetrating missiles. It can be infarcted by arterial injury. Fixed by its numerous transverse attachments, the cord is subject to localized stretching at the level of an intervertebral distraction. Permanent cord injury is common even without transection. Nerve roots can be compressed or avulsed.

Age Group of the Patient

Injuries and normal radiographic anatomy differ in the immature, the mature, and the senile spine. Infants have tiny, incompletely ossified vertebrae that contain synchondroses of variable thickness and that are interconnected by relatively lax ligaments. Demineralization weakens elderly bones, and together with spondylosis increases the likelihood of cord and root injury while hampering radiologic diagnosis. Apparent "minor degenerative changes" may really be avulsions or compressions (see Figs. 6–35B and 6–52B); when such findings seem inappropriate for the age of the patient and a realistic suspicion of injury exists, they must not be accepted as degenerative without confirmation by computed tomography (CT) or by comparison with old films.

Clinical Stability

Based on a definition developed by White and colleagues,[113, 120] the spine is "clinically stable" if, under *physiologic* loads, it maintains intervertebral relationships that prevent cord and root damage, incapacitating deformity, and excessive pain. Thus, clinical instability is not limited to major trauma. Preexisting spinal stenosis, deformity, and structural weakness enter into the evaluation of injuries. The definition derived by White and colleagues does not address decreased resistance to pathologic loads, but when "dangerous loading" is anticipated the criteria for instability can be made more inclusive.[120]

It is often unclear whether derivatives of the word "stable" as commonly used are intended to conform to this definition, just as it is often difficult to apply this definition or any other in clinical practice. An intuitive assessment of mechanical stability may not correlate with that of clinical stability. A few millimeters of abnormal offset or abnormal motion does not imply clinical instability. In this chapter, unmodified terms related to "stable" describe "clinical stability." Spinal stability is distinct from general medical stability.

Specific named fractures and dislocations have sometimes been classified as "stable" or "unstable." This can be misleading because of the variety of complex injuries and anatomic circumstances subsumed under the limited number of injury names. The literature is replete with diverse opinions about the stability of specific injuries. In an initial assessment, if a component commonly classified as "unstable" is present, then the injury at that level should be considered clinically unstable until demonstrated otherwise. Ultimately, stability is a *clinical* judgment that is based on radiologic evidence and clinical knowledge. In a treatment context, an unstable spine can be "stabilized" in a position that opposes a dominant traumatic force. For example, flexion injuries may be unstable in flexion but stable in extension, and vice versa.

Mechanism of Injury

The normal cardinal spinal motions are flexion, extension, lateral bending, and rotation. Compression, distraction, and shearing are additional cardinal *traumatic* forces. Some injuries, often the common simple ones, can be described by one or two of these terms; however, many cannot. Simple mechanistic terms are clinically acceptable terminology, but their use should not be mistaken for a real understanding of the dynamics and the pathology of spinal injuries.

Even approximate and tentative conclusions about the mechanism of injury are clinically useful. Any information from the patient, from emergency medical personnel, from other injuries, and from damage to the patient's skin or clothing may guide initial stabilization and imaging. An index of suspicion based on a documented mechanism may influence interpretation of questionable radiologic findings, although every attempt must be made to evaluate the findings objectively. The inferred mechanism may then determine the method of reduction and stabilization.

Radiographic Appearance

This is a heuristic classification based on the radiologic findings. Its purpose is to guide the search pattern and to describe the observations that are fundamental to inferences about the pathologic anatomy, the injury mechanism, and the prognosis.

No Signs of Acute Trauma

The first question is whether the spine is radiographically normal or at least at "baseline" on the plain x-ray films. Technical artifacts, anatomic superimpositions ("pseudofractures"), normal developmental anatomy in the immature spine, anatomic variations, congenital abnormalities, old fractures and deformities, and other nontraumatic abnormalities must be distinguished from acute injury. Some of these findings may still be significant in the acute evaluation of an injury with pain or neurologic deficit and may suggest further imaging. For example, spinal stenosis, whether congenital or spondylotic, limits the safety margin around the cord and the nerve roots during rapid spinal motion. Degenerative loss of elasticity in the ligamenta flava causes buckling during hyperextension and contributes to cord injury in the elderly. Concussive and permanent injuries to the cord can occur without any detectable acute vertebral column injury—with or without any predisposing anatomic condition—following extension, axial compression, and flexion injuries.[112, 114, 125]

Genuine acute spinal column injury may be undetectable on the best initial radiographs. Disc herniations and intraspinal hematomas are invisible on plain films. An "occult" fracture is truly invisible on standard films of good quality. A strong clinical index of suspicion, with or without findings of stenosis or other chronic structural defects, is a cue for additional imaging.

Telltale Hints of Injury

These direct and indirect signs of injury are typically small or subtle and are often hard to distinguish from normal or insignificant findings. They may indicate little about the type and the extent of injury but often are the first radiographic clues to significant and even unstable injuries. Signs that individually would be of doubtful significance are more incriminating when present in combination and may be appreciated only after a conscious search has been made.

Mild vertebral wedging could indicate new or old injury or normal variation. Small marginal avulsions and chip fractures often accompany a variety of major injuries, sometimes as the only fracture associated with a limited ligamentous avulsion or a major transient dislocation. Small osteophytes, degenerative calcifications (see Fig. 6–29), or accessory ossicles can be confused with chips near end plates or facets. Some of these osseous findings are objectively recognizable as fractures on close inspection (see Figs. 6–35B and 6–52B). Others require an appropriate index of suspicion, comparison with old films, consideration of accompanying signs, or CT study.

Subtle malalignment of juxtaposition or curvature may indicate muscular guarding or spasm, sprain or subluxation, or a misleadingly small residuum of a major dislocation. Particularly in younger patients, a focal malalignment or an alteration of disc height clearly distinguishing one motion segment from the others is suspicious (see Fig. 6–53A and B), although minimal offsets and curve changes are commonly normal. In older patients, malalignments and alterations of disc height become common in spondylosis but may deserve further work-up as possible signs of structural and neurologic vulnerability. When circumstances permit, flexion-extension lateral films can be obtained under voluntary patient control.

Soft tissue swelling is also notoriously difficult to evaluate. Some bleeding always accompanies a fracture because bone and periosteum are highly vascular, but small fractures of thin bony plates often do not produce large hematomas or visible soft tissue swelling. Soft tissue swelling is most apparent when it displaces airways or fat planes on x-ray films. CT scans or magnetic resonance (MR) images can show smaller hematomas adjacent to questionable fractures or may verify the absence of hematoma adjacent to a larger lesion of questionable nature or age.

Obvious Fracture or Dislocation

These "component" and "entity" injuries are the primary subjects of the following sections. The descriptions deal mostly with the recognized "simple" injuries as a kind of "vocabulary." In practice these are often encountered in combination at a given vertebral level, at multiple vertebral levels, and in complex atypical forms. The purposes of the analytic approach are to organize the subject in order to make it tractable, to train the reader to search for and to recognize individual signs of injury, and to familiarize the reader with the common patterns and mechanisms of injuries.

• • • •
PRINCIPLES OF IMAGING

The emergency physician must decide which areas of the spine need to be radiographed for possible unstable injury. Cervical spine films are probably indicated for patients who have lost consciousness, even if only transiently, have neck tenderness or deformity, neurologic deficit consistent with cord or root injury, or fracture or soft tissue injury in the head or the neck.[10, 93] The remainder of the spine may also need to be "cleared." Total spine "clearance" has been recommended in severely injured patients with skull fractures or altered consciousness, in any high-energy injury, and when any spinal fracture is detected.[80, 85]

Plain Film

For each spinal area there are several standard projections. Some are the basic minimum projections.

Others are supplemental projections obtained because of specific clinical indications, limitations of the basic projections, or issues raised by the basic projections. Filming protocols are described in their respective sections.

Geometric Tomography

Geometric tomography blurs the transmission x-ray image progressively in the directions away from one infinitesimally thin, theoretically unblurred, tomographic plane. Even structures centered in the tomographic plane are perceptibly blurred. There is no true "section thickness." In order to narrow the apparent thickness of tissue in focus, the tomographic arc is widened. The anatomic interval between sections is chosen arbitrarily and is preferably 2–3 mm in the cervical spine and 3–5 mm at lower levels. The only useful function of tomography is to blur confusing overlying structures, thus removing camouflage. Tomography does not improve the intrinsic contrast resolution beyond the standard radiographic scale of gas/fat/water/bone/metal.

Only rarely should tomography be selected instead of or in addition to state-of-the-art CT. A sagittal, a coronal, or an oblique orientation may be needed to answer a single well-defined question. The patient may be too big or too heavy for the available CT or may refuse CT. Tomography should not be preferred simply because of cost or minor factors. High-resolution CT with modern reconstructive algorithms renders tomography obsolete in most cases.

The preferred type of tomography for spine imaging is multidirectional "complex motion" tomography and is commonly hypocycloidal polytomography. Ghost (false) images are less common and less confusing than those that occur with linear or circular tomography. The x-ray beam is vertical at the middle of the tomographic arc, yielding a coronal (frontal) image plane from a supine patient. The patient must be turned on his or her side for a sagittal (lateral) plane.

Tomography may fail to achieve adequate x-ray penetration and tissue contrast through thick body parts of big patients, such as lateral views of the cervicothoracic and the lumbosacral junctions. Provided the patient fits on the CT scanner, CT still yields useful bone information at these levels and helps to assess vertebral alignment.

Computed Tomography

CT has become the primary supplement to plain x-ray filming. CT is more tomographic than geometric tomography because it defines a section more sharply and eliminates interference from outside the section. State-of-the-art CT has superior sharpness, resolution, and interpretability. These advantages must be complemented by an understanding of the geometry of sectionally imaged structures.

To best see small structures, fractures, and disc protrusions, spatial resolution must be optimized in all three dimensions. Volume averaging is reduced by limiting section thickness to 1.5–2.0 mm in the cervical spine and 1.5–3.0 mm at lower levels. Pixel (picture element) size is reduced by limiting the field of view (FOV) for *primary* image reconstruction from the raw data to about 8.0–10.0 cm in the cervical spine, 10.0–12.0 cm in the thoracic spine, 12.0–15.0 cm in the lumbar spine, and 15.0–20.0 cm in the sacrum.

A high-resolution "bone" algorithm increases image sharpness and spatial resolution in bone on a well-performed CT scan, but it cannot correct anatomically large pixels (from too large an FOV) or thick sections. The bone algorithm sacrifices low-contrast resolution, making the soft tissues appear very flat and grainy at narrow window widths. This limits or prevents visualization of disc protrusion, epidural hematoma, the spinal cord, and paravertebral hematoma. Since small voxel (volume element = pixel × section thickness) size is the more important factor in resolution, a more standard algorithm is optimal for trauma screening. Before deletion, the raw data can be re-reconstructed with a bone algorithm and printed separately. When fracture delineation is the only issue, the bone algorithm can be used initially. A specific bone algorithm is *disadvantageous* at levels that are degraded by artifacts from metal, motion, shoulders, or obesity because it sharpens the appearance of the artifacts and further obscures the anatomy. The applicability of these considerations varies with different high-resolution algorithms and must be determined individually for each CT model.

Table incrementation—the center-to-center interval of consecutive sections—need not equal the section thickness. Fracture screening may include small "gaps" of 0.5–2.0 mm. The increased sharpness of a fracture more than compensates for any hypothetic "loss of a fracture into a gap." Thus, for instance, 1.5-mm sections may be obtained at 2.0-mm intervals. For screening a long region of the spine, 1.5–2.0-mm sections at 2.0–3.0-mm intervals are optimal in the cervical spine, and 1.5–3.0-mm sections at 3.0–5.0-mm intervals are optimal in the thoracic, the lumbar, and the sacral spine. In obese patients, thicker and perhaps overlapping sections with the same table increments may be chosen to obtain sufficient x-ray flux at the cost of more volume averaging while maintaining the desired close spacing. For intensive examination of one or two vertebrae in a cooperative patient, close spacing (1.0–2.0-mm contiguous sections in the cervical spine, 1.5–2.0-mm sections with 2.0–3.0-mm increments at lower levels), an FOV barely larger than the greatest vertebral diameter, and use of a bone algorithm significantly increases resolution. For missile injuries and other foreign body examinations, the "gaps" should be closed by using contiguous and usually slightly thicker sections.

Stacked CT sections can be reformatted into sagittal, coronal, and oblique "reconstructions." Sagittal reconstructions offer a convenient view of vertebral alignment. Good reformations require patient cooperation and sections that are thin and closely spaced, although not necessarily contiguous. The reader must be wary for misregistration artifacts (patient motion between sections) and for loss of longitudinal spatial resolution due to volume averaging. It is instead sometimes possible to obtain *direct*, nearly coronal sections of the craniocervical junction or seated coronals of the lumbosacral spine in stable patients.

If a fracture is large or obviously displaced, even a suboptimal scan shows it. But crude technique misses some subtle fractures and can lead to misdiagnosis or endless discussion about small lines and odd shapes. With major injuries or unstable patients, however, examination time must be limited, technical parameters may need to be compromised, and reformatted images may be useless.

Magnetic Resonance Imaging

MR imaging has several advantages in spinal trauma. In addition to evaluating the cord contour, MR imaging shows edema, hemorrhage, myelomalacia, and cysts. MR imaging usually differentiates hemorrhage from disc protrusion and can also show directly the discontinuity of some ruptured ligaments and disc annuli. It demonstrates vertebral and disc contours and alignment at the cervicothoracic and the lumbosacral junctions in large patients, sometimes an impossible problem with swimmer's views, tomography, and CT. Although MR imaging often misses vertebral arch fractures, it usually shows major fractures of the vertebral bodies and the pillars. It may demonstrate a variety of signal changes (increased or decreased on T_1-weighted and usually increased on T_2-weighted and short time to inversion recovery [STIR] sequences) in subtle fractures (see Fig. 6–53H–J.[9, 29, 61, 65]

The basic indication for MR imaging (or for myelography) in acute spinal trauma is to examine the spinal canal contents. Cord compression by soft tissues is suspected when a neurologic deficit is delayed, progressive, or poorly correlated with x-ray findings. Treatment of incomplete cord syndromes, particularly the acute anterior cord syndrome, may depend on cord imaging. Whereas myelography can show extradural compression, MR imaging more readily differentiates among disc protrusion, hematoma, and pre-existing thick epidural fat, particularly in combination. Myelography can show anatomic cord transection or swelling, but MR imaging is the only means of differentiating edema from hematoma or of detecting these lesions in a cord with a normal or a minimally abnormal contour. MR imaging does not necessarily distinguish between edema and pre-existing gliosis in the absence of swelling, particularly in areas of spondylotic narrowing.

Contraindications to MR imaging include the presence of a cardiac pacemaker, neurosurgical aneurysm clips (except for specific types known to be safe), an intraocular metallic foreign body, certain other implants, and external spinal supports that are not sufficiently compact and nonferromagnetic to permit imaging. Orthopedic implants are usually safe for MR imaging, but rods and wires located *in the spinal region being examined* usually prevent useful imaging.

The very indications for MR imaging of acute spinal trauma constitute relative contraindications and present technical difficulties. Progression or extension of the deficit is a concern in the setting of an injury that could be unstable. Continuous stabilization of the spine is critical but is nowhere more difficult than in the MR scanner. If traction is necessary, the tension on the equipment must be adjusted carefully as the patient is positioned in the long magnet bore. The structural apparatus and weights must be proved to be nonferromagnetic before they are allowed to approach the magnet. Basic cardiorespiratory support must already be secure. Mechanical ventilation and blood pressure monitoring are especially difficult, and other monitoring is likely to be impaired. Emergency MR imaging of acute spinal trauma probably is practical only if the compatible equipment for stabilization and monitoring has been acquired and tested in advance.[60, 74, 80]

The usefulness of MR imaging depends on the characteristics of the specific unit and of its surface coils and on the size and cooperation of the patient. Surface coils may not fit with an external spinal support or it may not be possible for them to be safely positioned under a patient with an unstable injury. Use of the body coil alone may be necessary and may be adequate.[88] These considerations must be assessed for the individual institution and patient.

Almost any sequence parameters (repetition time [TR], echotime [TE], and flip angle) can show useful cord and spinal column contours. The FOV should be optimized for the required anatomic coverage as well as for the pixel size and the signal-to-noise ratio (SNR) that permit adequate spatial and contrast resolution. Acquisition times must be limited to minimize patient motion. Sagittal plane imaging is essential and may be all that is needed, although an axial sequence may be helpful if pathology is found. At least two of the following three types of sequences should be attempted: T_1-weighted (short TR), T_2^*-weighted (gradient-echo with small flip angle), and T_2-weighted (long TR of about 2000 msec with at least two echoes). The sagittal sections should be 5 mm or less in thickness.

The T_1-weighted sequence demonstrates the contours of the cord and of the discs outlined against the dark CSF. It also demonstrates the dark patches of marked chronic myelomalacia or distinct cysts, and the bright signal of methemoglobin in subacute hemorrhage. Higher spatial resolution is more feasible with this than with any other sequence, and therefore the FOV can be reduced to 20 cm or less (depending on the machine) if a level of interest is known.

The T_2^*-weighted sequence shows the cord, the annuli, and the intraspinal ligaments against bright CSF. Disadvantages are a decreased tolerance for small FOVs on some machines, increased artifact and signal loss in areas near tissue boundaries with changes in magnetic susceptibility, and poorer detection of edema as compared with T_2-weighted images. But the signal loss from magnetic susceptibility inhomogeneity can be exploited to detect acute hemorrhage in the cord, even on medium-field machines.[36, 64, 65]

Long TR multiple-spin-echo imaging provides two different sequences that may suffice if the examination must be ended. The first echo is preferably at 20 msec but no longer than about 45 msec. This sequence is sometimes called "proton- (spin-) density weighted," but it maintains enough T_1 effect to keep the CSF dark and show the cord contour, while at the same time having enough proton-density and T_2 effect to show edema in the cord. Either echo may fail to differentiate between edema and methemoglobin, as both are bright. The second, more strongly T_2-weighted echo is more sensitive to cord edema and, at least on high-field machines (1 or 1.5 Tesla), may differentiate acute cord hemorrhage as a dark area caused by the T_2 shortening effect of deoxyhemoglobin.[42, 65, 95]

A STIR sagittal sequence may be added to elucidate signal properties of confusing areas in identified lesions or in questionably normal muscles or adipose regions. STIR suppresses fat signal, making lesions stand out in fat and marrow. It also shows lesions in muscle better. It may demonstrate an epidural he-

matoma or ligament damage that is obscure on other sequences.[61] Disadvantages of STIR include poor SNR and difficulty in obtaining uniform fat suppression. The sequence parameters must be selected according to the field strength.

Cord swelling accompanies marked edema or hemorrhage but may not be detectable in milder cases. Edema (bright on the second and perhaps on the first echo T_2-weighted sequences, and dark or isointense compared with the cord on the T_1-weighted sequence) has been associated with some subsequent neurologic improvement, whereas hemorrhage (acute [dark on T_2 at high field or on T_2^*] or subacute [bright on T_1]) has not.[65] The cord may be narrowed by pre-existing atrophy, particularly in spondylosis even without overt compression, by continued compression (whether acute or chronic), or by partial anatomic transection (which is likely to be clinically "complete"). Extradural pathology is recognized primarily by its shape, with some help from signal, and includes disc bulges and contained herniations beneath the dark annular rim, nuclear extrusions, osteophytes, epidural hematomas, and thickened ligamenta flava.

Myelography

Myelography is the established means of imaging the spinal cord emergently, and it remains valuable when MR imaging is unavailable or impractical. It can sometimes be completed more quickly and more predictably than MR imaging, especially when traction and other life support systems must be maintained or when respiratory or other motion is likely to degrade MR images. The acute clinical indications are the same as for MR imaging. Later, myelography is preferred for demonstration of nerve root compression or avulsion. CT following myelography with water-soluble media may be the only means of showing a dural tear.[88]

In the potentially unstable patient, cervical or thoracic myelography is performed by lateral C1–2 puncture with the patient in the supine position. Cervical puncture should be performed by or under the direct supervision of a physician who is trained and experienced in the technique and requires lateral fluoroscopy.

Lateral filming is paramount for emergency myelography, but frontal films should also be obtained if time permits. Diagnostic filming should be attempted even if immediate CT is planned (in case the patient or the CT scanner is unable to complete the intended study). Sufficient contrast material should be instilled and tilting performed to opacify the subarachnoid space at the level of interest. The required supine position is not ideal for imaging because most compressive pathology is ventral and because cervical pooling is usually impossible. However, visualization is facilitated if subarachnoid block is present, and CT should complete the study whenever feasible.

Vascular Imaging

Vascular imaging is no longer limited to contrast angiography. MR imaging shows major blood vessels as signal blackout (flow voids) even without special MR angiography (MRA) software. Spinal arterial imaging in trauma is limited to the vertebral arteries in the cervical spine. This topic is discussed in detail in Chapter 6. The intraspinal arterial supply to the cord and to the nerve roots is too small for MRA, whereas classic spinal angiography has no clinical role and is impractical in trauma. Venous imaging is not performed deliberately. Visualization of the epidural venous plexus on CT scans and MR images must not be confused with disc protrusion or with hemorrhage.

CHAPTER 6

Cervical Spine

RICHARD A. SUSS, M.D.

Topics that pertain to the entire cervical spine, such as the selection and the technique of emergency plain film projections, initial clearance of the lateral view, soft tissue swelling, and the vertebral arteries, are discussed in this section. Topics that pertain predominantly to the upper or to the lower cervical spine, such as anatomic features, detailed analysis of the films, and specific injuries, are discussed in the following sections.

Plain Film Projections

Numerous projections can be used to evaluate possible cervical spine injury. The examination is not complete without successful anteroposterior (AP) and lateral projections of the entire cervical spine, which require at least three or four films. Additional imaging may be indicated by the findings and the limitations of these films or by clinical evidence of radiographically occult injury.

Lateral filming must include all eight cervical motion segments, from C0–1 through C7–T1 (Figs. 6–1 to 6–3). When possible, the lateral film is taken with the patient in a seated or a standing position and with enough extension to keep the mandibular rami off the upper cervical vertebrae. The shoulders are lowered by weights in the hands or by traction on

the hands and by exposing at full exhalation. If refilming of the upper cervical spine is desired, detail can be improved by placing a smaller cassette against the ear and collimating tightly. If the standard lateral film fails to demonstrate the entire lower cervical spine, it must be supplemented by a swimmer's view.

The swimmer's view distributes the bulk of the shoulders more evenly by elevating one arm above the head (see Fig. 6–3C). This displaces the ipsilateral pectoral girdle cranially as well as slightly anteriorly or posteriorly. The opposite shoulder is deviated as far caudally as feasible and is rotated slightly posteriorly or anteriorly, opposite the first. The patient can be in a supine, prone, decubitus, seated, or standing position. The x-ray beam is positioned nearly parallel to the coronal plane of the spine but is angled a few degrees craniocaudally as if to "shoot over" (and thus project more inferiorly) the caudally deviated shoulder. In horizontal beam shots, a full intravenous bag placed beside the neck on this side further evens out the film density. AP collimation should be tight. For accurate vertebral counting, the swimmer's view must include C2 unless a lower cervical vertebra is uniquely identifiable.

The alignment and the contours of the vertebral bodies down to the upper part of T1 must be visible. Otherwise external cervical support must be maintained, and CT, MR imaging, or another swimmer's

---

•••• *APPROPRIATE RADIOGRAPHIC STUDIES*

I. **Plain Films**
  A. Lateral cervical spine view
    1. Must be a true lateral view.
    2. Must include the base of the skull to the upper portion of the T1 vertebral body.
    3. Severe injury should be ruled out before the patient is moved.
  B. Swimmer's view
    1. This angled lateral view is designed to demonstrate the lower cervical vertebral bodies and the C7–T1 interspace. It is frequently needed in patients with large shoulders and in the presence of extensive injury.
  C. Anteroposterior cervical spine view
  D. Odontoid view
  E. Oblique view

II. **Geometric Tomography**
  A. Generally has been replaced by computed tomography (CT).
  B. Used if a specific question needs to be answered or if a patient is too large for CT. Multidirectional tomography is preferable to linear tomography.

III. **Computed Tomography**
  A. CT for trauma should generally be performed using a standard algorithm rather than a bone algorithm, which can obscure soft tissue abnormalities.
  B. Reconstructions in multiple planes may demonstrate vertebral body alignment.

IV. **Magnetic Resonance Imaging**
  A. Especially useful for evaluation of the spinal cord in trauma patients.
  B. Less accurate than CT for evaluation of bone injury but does demonstrate many bone abnormalities.

V. **Myelography**
  A. Can demonstrate the spinal cord and subarachnoid blockage.
  B. Provides less information than magnetic resonance (MR) imaging but may be needed when MR imaging is not possible.

---

view are necessary. Bilateral oblique views have poor sensitivity and cannot substitute for an adequate examination by lateral projection, CT, or MR imaging. Even on a good swimmer's view, x-ray scatter and the elevated pectoral girdle often obscure the C7–T1 articular pillars. Clinical assessment helps to determine whether CT is warranted to examine the C7–T1 facet joints.

In the seriously injured patient the cervical spine must be "cleared" for further positioning or removal of a brace by obtaining a supine cross-table lateral view, supplemented as needed by a supine swimmer's view. The shoulders should be lowered voluntarily when feasible, and an alert patient may cooperate with gentle traction on the arms. No cra-

niospinal traction can be applied before clearance. During positioning for a swimmer's view, extreme care must be taken in the acutely injured, potentially unstable patient, because transient vertebral subluxation can occur (see Fig. 6–53A and B).[21] The full and open-mouth AP views can be made supine at the time of initial lateral filming or supine or upright after "clearance" of the lateral. Emergency room films made with portable equipment are acceptable only when absolutely necessary and should be supplemented by definitive films when feasible.

"Clearance" of the cervical spine to rule out an unstable injury depends primarily on the alignment and on the contours of the vertebrae in the lateral view or views. Prevertebral swelling; compression,

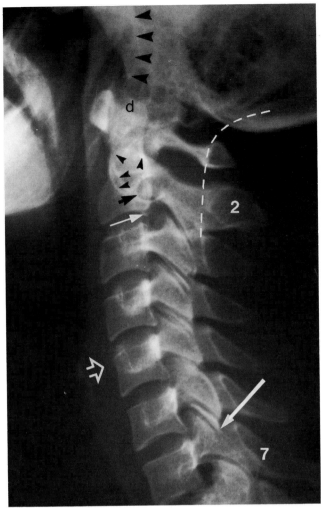

FIGURE 6–1. Ideal Normal Lateral Cervical Spine Film of a 27-Year-Old Woman

• • • •

Note the curved clival slope *(row of arrowheads)* leading to the tip of the dens *(d)*, the interpolated spinolaminar line *(dashed line)* passing anterior to the C2 spinolaminar line, the Harris rings *(arrowheads)* seen slightly asymmetrically in C2, one subarticular vertebral artery canal *(black arrow)* in C2, the bulky C2 and long C7 spinous processes, and the C7 posterior pillar lines with bilateral concavities *(long arrow)* and frequently indistinct visualization below the concavity. The dens contour is visible inside the superimposed C1 lateral masses; it aligns with the portion of Harris's ring that represents the upper C2 body cortex. The persistent unfused inferior C2 apophysis *(small white arrow)* and the prominent anterior tubercle on the C5 transverse process(es) *(open arrow)* are variations. The parallelism of facet surfaces is less precise than that of some cervical alignments and vertebral body parallelisms.

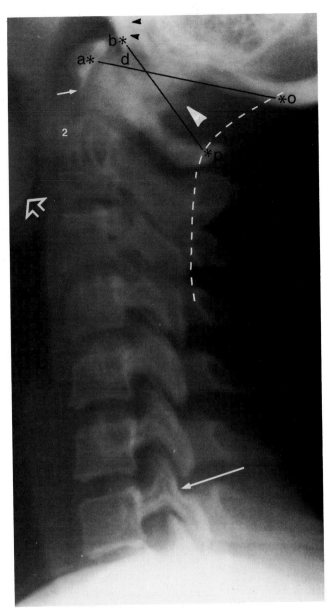

FIGURE 6–2. Nonspecific Post-traumatic Neck in an 11-Year-Old Girl with Head and Neck Pain After a Motor Vehicle Accident

• • • •

A true lateral view of the lower cervical spine, C1 (superimposed posterosuperior margins at the white arrowhead), and the head (superimposed mandibular angles at the open arrow) are shown. Rotation is present at C2–C4; note the anterior rotation of one side of the C2 articular plateau *(2)* and the double projections of the pedicles and the pillars. (The anteroposterior open mouth view also showed mild C1–2 rotation. The significance of such common, minor degrees of apparent C1–2 rotary restriction is not known.) The proximity of the basion *(b,* with the dorsal clival surface marked by arrowheads) to the dens *(d)* is closer than average. As is normal, *ao > bp* ("Powers ratio": bp/ao <1[57]). The location of the opisthion *(o)* is approximate. Note the normal variants: the "hockey-stick" C1 posterior arch *(p)* and the lordotic dens. Ring apophyses are visible anteriorly and posteriorly in the inferior end plates from C2 to C7. Note the overlay shadow, probably from the lateral mass attachment, that appears to extend the anterior C1 arch posteroinferiorly *(small arrow)*. The posterior C7 pillar margin has a normal notch *(long arrow)*. The upper part of T1 was visible on the original film.

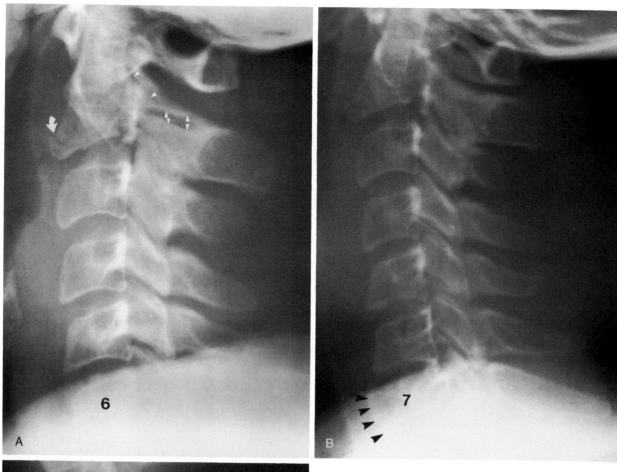

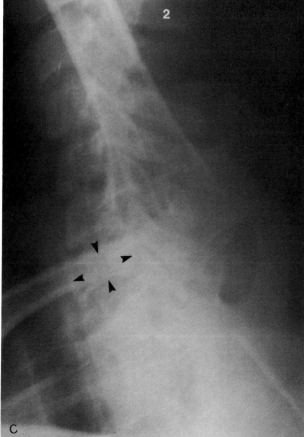

FIGURE 6–3. C2 and C7 Fractures in a 37-Year-Old Woman Who Struck the Top of Her Head in a Motor Vehicle Accident and Had No Neurologic Deficit

• • • •

A, The initial lateral film. Extensive fractures of the upper surfaces of the C2 arch *(arrowheads)* and the posterior body wall avulsion *(straight arrow)*, probably equivalent to hangman's fracture, can be seen. An anteroinferior avulsion *(curved arrow)* supports the extension mechanism (the extension teardrop). Caudal visualization is inadequate. An extension of 10–15 mm in prevertebral thickness as high as C3 suggests lower cervical injury. Focal swelling just above the acute C2 fracture outweighs the normal 5-mm thickness adjacent to the fragment. *B,* A subsequent lateral film shows a C7 burst fracture *(arrowheads)*. *C,* A swimmer's view shows biconcavity of the end plates and biconvexity of the anteroposterior walls of C7. C2 is recognizable by its prominent spinous process *(2)*, confirming C7 as the burst vertebra. Arrowheads outline the compressed body of C7.

expansion, or chipping of vertebral bodies; discontinuities in the many cortical lines; a possible fragment in the spinal canal; abnormal angulation of the bodies, the pillars, or the spinous processes; and a loss of imbrication and parallelism among the facets and among the spinolaminar lines should be sought. Normal anterior and posterior vertebral offsets might reach 3.0 mm in size[116] but are usually less, and they must be appropriate to the degree of flexion or extension, respectively, at the motion segment. Instead of having a normal lordosis, the spine is commonly straight or has a localized mild kyphosis.[58, 116] This is not necessarily a sign of spasm or of any other abnormality, but it may warrant flexion and extension films.

Flexion and extension lateral views are useful elective views in the stable patient who is symptomatic or has a peculiar cervical curvature. The flexion and the extension motion must be *active and voluntary on the part of the patient*; the physician or the technologist must *not* assist motion except by verbal instruction or by self-demonstration. When subtle clinical instability is suspected, flexion and extension can be performed by the patient under fluoroscopic observation by a physician. The flexion or the extension should involve the upper and the lower cervical spine together. Flexion or extension of the head, limited to the craniocervical junction, can produce minimal or contrary effects in the spine. When the symptomatic patient cannot cooperate, this limitation must be accepted. Any motion that reveals an injury is helpful, even if full flexion and extension are prevented by spasm or external support. Commonly, however, the flexion-extension study can wait until spasm subsides.

The AP open-mouth view is required to assess the C1–2 articular surfaces and their relationships as well as dens integrity (Fig. 6–4). Inclusion of the occipital condyles is desirable but often unattainable. The x-ray beam is directed through the widely opened mouth, initially perpendicular to the film and parallel to a plane extending from the upper central incisor edges to the mastoid tips. Considerable anthropologic variation in this region makes filming and interpretation challenging. The extension that would be required for a submental odontoid projection is contraindicated in suspected acute trauma. A straight transfacial projection parallel to the orbitomeatal line, preferably posteroanterior in order to demagnify the nasal complex, may show lateral C1–2 joint alignment. Forty-five–degree AP oblique transfacial projections may show the occipital condyles, the lateral masses, and the base of the dens if the patient can turn his or her head voluntarily, but they are not sufficient to exclude a dens fracture without tomography or CT.

The full AP view combines mild extension and 15–20-degree cephalad beam angulation to project the mandible upward and to uncover the lower border of C2. A second film can be made with a 20–30-degree caudal beam angulation for better demonstration of the arches and the pillars. Oblique projections and special arch and pillar projections can help evaluate the posterior elements, but scrupulous attention to detail on good lateral and AP films suffices in most cases. When the history is suggestive or when the standard plain films inadequately evaluate or raise questions about the cervical spine, CT or MR imaging is preferred for supplemental imaging.

Prevertebral Soft Tissue Swelling

The evaluation of prevertebral soft tissue swelling is difficult and unreliable except when it is marked. Yet this evaluation may be necessary in the comatose or the symptomatic patient and in patients with ambiguous osseous signs of acute trauma along the anterior vertebral and disc margins. Swelling should be evaluated on all lateral films even when vertebrae are hidden by the shoulders, although swelling limited to the lowest cervical levels is uncommon. The specific terms *retropharyngeal* and *retrotracheal* are preferable to *prevertebral* when discussing specific measurements; in addition, *retropharyngeal thickness* is more sensitive and specific than *retrotracheal thickness*.

There is no single clinically decisive measurement at any level (Tables 6–1 to 6–5). A range of normal measurements leaves many indeterminate cases. Published series give various ranges and are contradictory, possibly owing to different patient populations or unrecognized technical or methodologic differences. For example, Ardran's and Kemp's means[6] exceeded Hay's maximums[50] (see Table 6–3). Measurements for young children are even more variable than those for adults and are also subject to marked respiratory variation. Oon[77] and Weir[116] found no normal adults with a thickness greater than 5.0 mm at C3, but both Wholey and associates[21] (at C2) and Templeton and coworkers[110] (at C2–C4) allowed a retropharyngeal thickness up to 7.0 mm before recommending further investigation. Templeton and coworkers laid stronger emphasis on a retropharyngeal thickness of 10.0 mm or greater. Wholey and associates selected a retrotracheal thickness of 22.0 mm in adults and 14.0 mm in "children" under 15 years of age as warranting further investigation. Paakkala[79] suggested using the mean plus one standard deviation as an "alarm limit." The differences among levels within the retropharyngeal and the retrotracheal ranges are as great as the differences between the maximums of the ranges and the means plus one standard deviations. Without access to detailed tables, the easiest rule to remember might

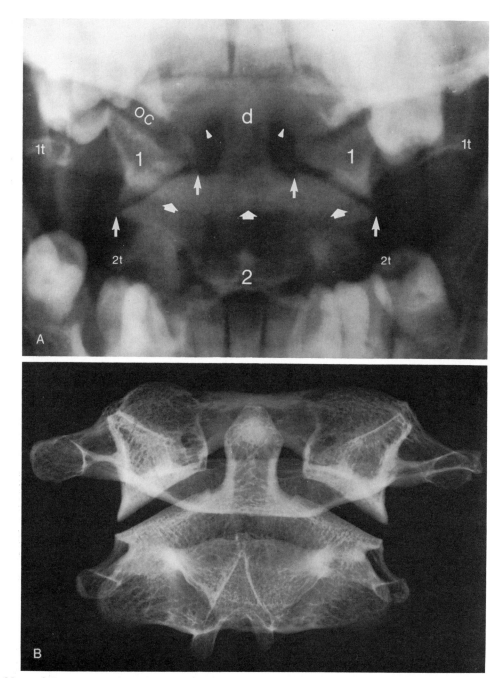

FIGURE 6–4. Normal Anteroposterior View of C1–2 in a 51-Year-Old Man

• • • •

A, The lateral C1 masses *(1)* are symmetric wedges with precise vertical alignment *(narrow arrows)* at the lateral and, when defined by notches on C2, the medial margins of the lateral C1–C2 joints. Minimal shifts of the median gaps between the upper and the lower central incisors to the right and the slightly greater overlap of the left molars over C1 and C2 indicate minimal head rotation and are insignificant. The vertical alignment of the dens *(d)* with the inverted "V" of the C2 spinous process *(2)* indicates that C2 is *not* rotated. Beam angulation typically projects the posterior arches of C1 (the lower border is marked by fat arrows) and C2 *(2)* downward. The posterior arch margins and the Mach lines adjacent to them sometimes simulate fractures. The upwardly projected anterior arch of C1 is rarely visible as it is here (the lower border is marked by arrowheads; compare *A* with *B*). The C1 and C2 transverse processes *(1t, 2t)* may be difficult to discern. The right occipital condyle *(OC)* articulates with the upper three fifths of the superior slope of C1, whereas the left is obscured. This is the same patient as shown in Figure 6–14. *B,* A specimen radiograph.

TABLE 6–1. Normal Retropharyngeal Soft Tissue Thickness in the Adult

Source	Total No. of Patients	TFD	Level*	Mean (mm)(†)	Mean + 1SD (mm)(†)	Maximum (mm)(†)
Hay[49]						
Males	50	‡	C2–C4§	0.2 × C5 ‖		0.3 × C5 ‖
Females				0.19 × C5		0.3 × C5
Wholey and associates[121]	480	60 in.	C2	3.4 (3.8)		7.0 (7.8)
Oon[77]	150	72 in.	C3¶	3.1 (3.6)		4.5 (5.2)
Weir[116]	360	60 in.	C3	3.7** (4.1)		4.8 (5.4)
Penning[83]	50	47 in.	C1	4.6 (4.8)		10.0 (10.5)
			C2	3.2 (3.4)		5.0 (5.3)
			C3	3.4 (3.6)		7.0 (7.4)
			C4††	5.1 (5.4)		7.0 (7.4)
Paakkala[79]	70	47 in.	C1	4.7 (4.9)	6.1 (6.4)	8.0 (8.4)
			C2	3.5 (3.7)	4.5 (4.7)	6.0 (6.3)
			C3	4.0 (4.2)	5.0 (5.3)	7.0 (7.5)
			C4††	5.4 (5.7)	7.2 (7.6)	11 (11.6)
Templeton and coworkers[110]	236‡‡	40 in.				
Males			C2	5.0	6.7	
			C3	5.1	6.6	
			C4	6.6	8.7	
Females			C2	4.4	5.6	
			C3	4.8	6.2	
			C4	6.2	8.0	

*Measured at the anteroinferior vertebral margin except as noted.
†"De-corrected" to correspond to a 40 in. TFD, assuming adult shoulders of average width.
‡Irrelevant.
§Where the posterior wall of the pharynx runs parallel to the vertebrae.
‖ Anteroposterior diameter of the middle portion of the C5 vertebral body; Templeton and coworkers[110] found 0.3 × C5 to measure 6.0 ± 0.6 mm in males and 5.3 ± 0.7 mm in females (± 1 SD, 40-in. TFD).
¶Measured at the midbody level.
††Measured at the anterosuperior margin.
**Midpoint of the range.
‡‡Total in the study; not every subject was measured at each level.
TFD: Target-film distance.

TABLE 6–2. Normal Retrotracheal Soft Tissue Thickness in the Adult

Source	Total No. of Patients	TFD	Level*	Mean (mm)(†)	Mean + 1SD (mm)(†)	Maximum (mm)(†)
Hay[49]						
Males	50	‡	C5§	0.54 × C5 ‖		0.7 × C5 ‖ ¶
Females				0.5 × C5		0.6 × C5‖**
Wholey and associates[121]	480	60 in.	C6	14.0 (15.7)		22 (25)
Oon[77]	150	72 in.	C6††	12.4 (14.4)		17 (20)
Penning[83]	150	47 in.	C5	14.9 (15.7)		20 (21)
			C6	15.1 (15.9)		20 (21)
			C7	13.9 (14.7)		20 (21)
Paakkala[79]	70	47 in.	C5	13.6 (14.3)	17.5 (18.4)	20 (21)
			C6	15.9 (16.7)	19.1 (20.1)	22 (23)
			C7	15.2 (16.0)	18.8 (19.7)	23 (24)

*Measured at the anteroinferior vertebral margin except as noted.
†"De-corrected" to correspond to a 40 in. TFD, assuming adult shoulders of average width.
‡Irrelevant.
§Postcricoid soft tissue at approximately C5 measured "between the posterior surface of the cricoid cartilage and the anterior surface of the adjacent cervical vertebra."
‖ Anteroposterior diameter of the middle portion of the C5 vertebral body.
¶Calculating from Table 6–1, note ‖, Hay's maximum measurement in males would correspond to about 14 mm (TFD = 40 in.).
**Calculating from Table 6–1, note ‖, Hay's maximum measurement in females would correspond to about 10.6 mm (TFD = 40 in.).
††Approximately C6, more precisely " . . . from a point immediately below the inferior horns of the thyroid cartilage to the anterior border . . . of the adjacent vertebra (or, if coinciding with a disc) a line joining the midpoints on the anterior borders of the two corresponding vertebrae."
TFD: Target-film distance.

TABLE 6–3. Normal Retropharyngeal Soft Tissue Thickness in the Child

Source	No. of Patients	TFD	Age (yr)	Mean (mm)(*)		Maximum (mm)(*)	
Hay[49]	25	†	0–1			1.5 × C5‡	
			1–2			0.5 × C5	
			2–3			0.5 × C5	
			3–6			0.4 × C5	
			6–14			0.3 × C5	
Wholey and associates[121]	120	60 in.	?–15	3.5§	(3.8)	7§	(7.5)
Ardran and Kemp[6]	100	†	½–5	0.75 × C ‖			

*"De-corrected" to correspond to a 40-in. TFD, assuming child shoulders of average width.
†Irrelevant.
‡At the level of the epiglottic valleculae; compared with the anteroposterior diameter of the ossified part of the C5 vertebral body.
§At C2.
‖ ". . . about three quarters of the anteroposterior diameter of the adjacent vertebra."
TFD: Target-film distance.

TABLE 6–4. Normal Postventricular or Retrotracheal Soft Tissue Thickness in the Child

Source	No. of Patients	TFD	Age (yr)	Mean (mm)(*)		Maximum (mm)(*)	
Hay[49]	25	†	0–1			2.0 × C5‡	
			1–2			1.5 × C5	
			2–3			1.2 × C5	
			3–6			1.2 × C5	
			6–14			1.2 × C5	
Wholey and associates[121]	120	60 in.	up to 15	7.9§	(8.5)	14§	(15)

*"De-corrected" to correspond to a 40-in. TFD, assuming child shoulders of average width.
†Irrelevant.
‡Postventricular "distance between the posterior commissure of the larynx and the nearest osseous portion of the cervical spine"; compared with the anteroposterior diameter of the ossified part of the C5 vertebral body.
§Retrotracheal at C6.
TFD: Target-film distance.

TABLE 6–5. Technical Factors Contributing to Variation of the Magnification Factor

TFD	Magnification Factor Range*	
	Adult†	Child‡
40 in. (Templeton and coworkers[110])	1.29–1.43	1.18–1.29
47 in. (Penning[83], Paakkala[79])	1.24–1.34	1.15–1.24
60 in. (Wholey and associates[121], Weir[161])	1.18–1.25	1.11–1.18
72 in. (Oon[77])	1.14–1.20	1.09–1.14

*Approximate ranges calculated as MF (magnification factor) = TFD/(TFD − SFD), assuming SFD (subject-film distance, i.e., from the vertebrae to the film cassette at the shoulder[77, 83, 116] to measure †9–12 in. in most adults and ‡6–9 in most "children."
TFD: Target-film distance.

be a "rule of sevens"; that is, 7.0 mm retropharyngeal, 14.0 mm retrotracheal in the child and 21.0 mm retrotracheal in the adult. The choice of thresholds determines the sensitivity and the specificity, and these can be intelligently adjusted, albeit only intuitively, according to the patient's body habitus and the index of suspicion.

Retropharyngeal measurements in *flexion* increase at C1–C3 by averages of 0.1–1.0 mm; those in *extension* decrease at C1 and increase at C4 by averages of 0.9–1.2 mm. Retrotracheal measurements in *flexion* increase at C7 by an average of 0.5–0.8 mm; those in *extension* decrease at C6 and C7 by averages of 0.9–

2.0 mm.[79, 83] Expiration increases the adult retropharyngeal space by an average of 1.5 mm.[79]

Many additional caveats must be observed. Endotracheal and nasogastric tubes invalidate abnormal measurements. Anterior osteophytes limit the value of nearby measurements. Many patients have increased prevertebral thickness for reasons unrelated to trauma or for no apparent reason. Localization of swelling does not necessarily match the injury level. Injuries limited to the posterior elements and even those involving posterior portions of the vertebral bodies and the discs often do not cause prevertebral swelling. Even some injuries involving anterior vertebral borders have normal prevertebral soft tissues initially but develop swelling hours to days later. Swelling can remit within 3 days of injury or can last 1 month.[79, 110] Published figures are direct, uncorrected film measurements, but differences among magnifications are only a minor practical issue (see Table 6–5).

When it is visible, the prevertebral fat stripe (the retropharyngeal and the retroesophageal spaces) can be more sensitive and specific as a sign of swelling than total soft tissue thickness. This thin stripe runs closely parallel the anterior longitudinal ligament down to C6, whereupon it curves anteriorly and loses its usefulness. Anterior deviation of the stripe indicates pathology behind it, whereas posterior deviation or lack of deviation behind real swelling indicates a primary soft tissue process without cervical spine injury.[117] The stripe usually requires an excellent film for visualization,[79] is rarely visible in abnormal patients,[110] is less frequently seen in children than in adults,[117] and may be invisible even in normal noninjury adults.[79]

CT and MR imaging show the prevertebral tissues more directly. Using the standard or the soft tissue technique (as opposed to a specific bone algorithm), CT can evaluate the prevertebral fat for displacement or edema in the absence of fracture. MR imaging is the modality of choice for soft tissue evaluation, particularly in symptomatic patients who have no fractures. Prevertebral edema or hemorrhage has been directly visualized as T_2-weighted hyperintensity even with minimal swelling (see Fig. 6–53H and I).[59] In the extraspinal tissues MR imaging may not distinguish between edema and hemorrhage, which are probably mixed in most patients. Ligamentous and annular tears are directly imaged.[9, 22, 37, 61, 65, 76, 123] A diagonal band of edema has been described crossing the neck in several patients and suggests the plane of greatest injury stress.[9, 61]

Vertebral Arteries

An index of suspicion for vertebral artery injury arises when a vertebral fracture crosses a transverse foramen (see Fig. 6–21) or when there are signs of posterior fossa ischemia. Positional occlusion, dissection, thrombosis, embolization, laceration, pseudoaneurysm, and arteriovenous fistula may occur. There is a poor correlation, however, between vertebral bone injuries and arterial injuries. Vertebral artery injury, particularly dissection, has occurred after vertebral displacements in the absence of fracture or dislocation, even outside of the acute trauma setting. Most fractures through transverse foramina do not significantly injure the artery.

Angiography is generally required for definitive diagnosis. Endovascular occlusion may be contemplated for treatment of vertebral artery injury but should be performed by those trained in such techniques. Although MR imaging can demonstrate vertebral artery flow and sometimes suggest occlusion, sufficient detail is not yet available to exclude injury.

• • • •
UPPER CERVICAL SPINE

Structural and Radiologic Anatomy

The highest two cervical vertebrae, the atlas (C1) and the axis (C2), are specialized for head rotation. Because their structure, articulations, and injuries differ so markedly from those of the remainder of the spine, they are called the "upper cervical" vertebrae. In the context of cervical spine articulations, the occiput is called *C0*. The functional upper cervical spine therefore comprises C1, C2, and the atlantooccipital (C0–1), atlantoaxial (C1–2), and occipitoaxial (C0–2) joints (see Figs. 6–1, 6–2, and 6–4).

The convex occipital condyles articulate with concave superior facets on the lateral masses of the atlas. These two lateral joints function together as a hinge joint that permits anteroposterior nodding of the head. Axial rotation at C0–1 in maximum voluntary head rotation is typically 1 degree and rarely more than 5 degrees.[53, 84] The craniovertebral junction also includes several ligaments and a pair of suboccipital muscles that link C2 directly to the occipital bone. The strongest component of this C0–C2 joint is a pair of alar ligaments. Each passes from near the tip of the dens in a lateral and slightly superior direction to the medial base of each occipital condyle. The alar ligaments are the primary restraint on excessive head rotation and are a secondary restraint on AP translation of the skull with respect to the spine.

The atlas ring comprises a short anterior arch, two lateral masses, and a long posterior arch. The anterior arch is not homologous with any structure in the lower vertebrae. The primary unique feature of the atlas is the loss of its centrum to C2, which leaves it without a unified vertebral body but with "lateral masses" instead. The posterior arch consists of two halves that arc posteromedially and are usually fused in the midline. Absence of a spinous process suggests a more general term, *inner laminar line*, to name the anterior vertical midline cortex at the junction of the laminae (as seen in lateral projection) which is homologous to the spinolaminar line seen at the lower levels. Zygapophyses have been completely lost.

Each hemiarch is horizontally broadened and superiorly flattened to form a broad sulcus for the vertebral artery.

The lateral masses combine the principal functions of weight-bearing and mobility, whereas stability depends on the anterior arch and the transverse ligament. Each lateral mass has broad superior and inferior articular facets. The superior facets are concave, receive the occipital condyles, and may be partially or completely divided into anterior and posterior areas. Whereas the inferior bone facets also are concave, their centrally thickened cartilaginous surfaces are convex. Their articulation with the AP convex C2 articular surfaces allows the head to descend with rotation and prevents premature tightening of the alar ligaments. Lying anterior to the first and the second cervical nerves, the C0–1 and the lateral C1–2 articulations evolved by modification of uncovertebral (Luschka) joints.[15]

The superior and the inferior lateral mass surfaces slope transversely and converge into the medial tubercles. The medial tubercles are yoked by the strong transverse ligament, a component of the cruciate ligament passing immediately behind the dens. Each lateral mass is trapezoidal or almost triangular in frontal projection. Long transverse processes extend from their lateral surfaces. Each consists of two struts supporting one lateral tubercle. Between the struts is the foramen transversarium, which passes the vertebral arteries vertically until they turn posteriorly over the posterior strut.

The atlas has numerous congenital variations. The most common variation is persistence of a thin posterior median synchondrosis, which eliminates the inner laminar line (see Fig. 6–15). A wider midline gap is sometimes present; this is an asymptomatic normal variation that is of importance only to a surgeon contemplating a C0–1 fusion. Uncommonly an anterior midline synchondrosis persists into adulthood. It is usually accompanied by a persistent posterior midline synchondrosis forming a *bipartite atlas*,[13, 17, 70] which is a sort of congenital Jefferson fracture. Such an atlas ring may be weaker than normal. A wide gap in or the absence of the anterior arch is rare. A gap may occur laterally in one or both posterior hemiarches. Radiologically this is distinguished from acute or chronic fracture by its tapering margins and its larger hiatus. There is sometimes a bony arch over the vertebral artery sulcus that converts it into a foramen. A complete bridging arch is called a *ponticulus posticus* (see Figs. 6–14A and 6–16A), but frequently only incomplete and asymmetric portions are present.

Occipitalization of the atlas is a partial assimilation of the atlas into the occipital bone. Commonly one or two atlantal synchondroses persist. The fusion to the occiput can involve almost any combination of separate components of a complete or anomalous atlas. The appearance may be confusing and on lateral projection may lead to erroneous counting of the axis vertebra as "the first" cervical vertebra. Commonly the atlas-dens interval is widened, which does not signify an old injury but potentially increases risk to the cord in an injury.

"Occipital vertebra" refers to a very small partial mimic of the atlas that is sometimes seen between the atlas and the occiput. It is unlikely to confuse vertebral counting but could be mistaken for a fracture fragment. Its appearance is highly variable.

The atlantoaxial (C1–2) joint is the main pivot of the neck and accounts for about one half of all maximum cervical rotation as well as for some flexion-extension. Each of the synovial components of the C1–2 joint moves in two directions to permit rotation, nodding, and tilting of the head, but the dominant motion is rotation. AP stability of the C1–2 joint results from the tight sandwiching of the odontoid process between the anterior arch of C1 and the transverse ligament of C1. There is not a single obvious mechanism stabilizing this joint transversely, but the same sandwich mechanism favors bilateral symmetry as do the slopes of the lateral C1–2 joint surfaces and several tensional forces within and around the upper cervical spine. For vertical stability, C1 is held between the occiput and C2 by the alar and apical ligaments, the vertical fibers of the cruciform ligament, and the muscles of the upper neck.

The axis is the tallest vertebra by virtue of its odontoid process or dens. In lateral projection the dens may be straight (see Fig. 6–1) or may look like an extended thumb with a variable degree of backward curve or tilt to its upper portion (see Fig. 6–2). The body of C2 is broadened to include superolateral articular surfaces (the articular plateau) for the lateral atlantoaxial joints. The inferior end plate of C2 is the smallest in the spine. The pedicles tie the articular plateau and the entire rostral axial skeleton to the C2–3 facet joints, which resist forward translation. Superior zygapophyses have been completely lost. Behind the inferior facets are broad laminae that unite under a stout spinous process. This is not the longest or necessarily the most massive cervical spinous process, but it has the "blockiest" shape in all imaging planes and it is larger than those of C3 through C5 or C6.

C2 is an easily discernible landmark on imaging studies. On CT scans the broad articular plateau is instantly recognizable, the lower portion of the body is rounder than other cervical vertebral bodies, and the spinous process is disproportionately wider and more broadly bifid than are those of the other cervical

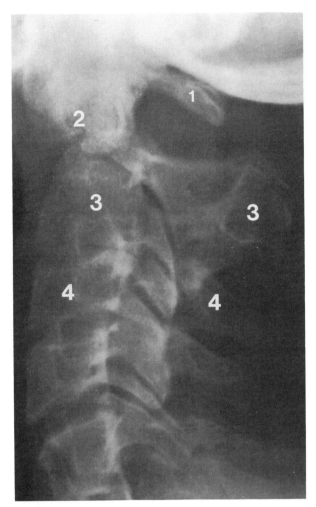

FIGURE 6–5. Congenital Anomaly Simulating a Hangman's Fracture

• • • •

A tilted lateral projection of a congenitally anomalous cervical spine simulates a Type IIa hangman's fracture in a 31-year-old man. The C1 posterior arch is hypoplastic and downsloping, and C3–4 and C6–7 discs are hypoplastic in block vertebrae. An untilted lateral film and computed tomography proved that the stout spinous process was part of C3.

vertebrae. The lateral profile can be recognized on a standard film or a swimmer's lateral film, on a lateral CT localizer scanogram, or on a low-resolution sagittal body-coil MR image used for the numbering of thoracic vertebrae. Identification of C2 is essential to the accurate counting of vertebrae.

The most important and controversial variations of C2 are the os odontoideum and spondylolisthesis. Some cases of each have been caused by perinatal or infantile trauma. An os odontoideum may have perfectly smooth, symmetric margins that would be unusual following fracture. Some examples have a short dens and an os odontoideum of intermediate size, making both trauma and simple ununited apical center unlikely. Some spondylolistheses have such

smooth and symmetric margins that injury seems unlikely.

The horizontal portion of the subdental synchondrosis can persist, simulating part of a Type III dens fracture. This gap is symmetric, smooth, and unconnected to the upper surfaces. On lateral view it is a short, horizontal lucency located surprisingly low within the body of C2 (slightly above its midlevel).

The neural arch may be altered by persistence of its midline synchondrosis or by its complete absence,[7] both anomalies being much rarer than their counterparts at C1. Absence of the arch is associated with a modified C3 spinous process resembling that of a normal C2, apparently to conserve attachment of the rectus capitis posterior major and the obliquus capitis inferior muscles that help rotate the head. The combination of the deficient C2 and the large C3 spinous process can simulate a hangman's fracture (Fig. 6–5).

Analysis of Films

Lateral View

The foramen magnum must be included on the lateral view. If the basion is not visible, its position can often be approximated as the intersection of lines along the anterior and the posterior clival surfaces. The angle of the clivus varies, but it should "point toward" the tip of the dens or the predens space (see Figs. 6–1 and 6–2) and not directly to the anterior arch of the atlas. The opisthion is harder to see, and its position cannot be reliably approximated; however, if it is visible it should continue and exaggerate the curve set by the cervical inner laminar lines.

The anterior arch of C1 resembles a (backward) "D" or a triangle. The anterior C1–2 joint space need not have a uniform thickness and commonly forms a "V." The atlas-dens interval (ADI) is measured at the closest approach of the opposing cortices, usually inferiorly. The primary measurement is made in the neutral position, and any change with flexion or extension should be only a fraction of a millimeter.[52, 55] The normal maximum ADI in adults has been reported to be 2.0 mm,[20] 2.5 mm,[55] or 3.0 mm.[105] In children, maximums of 4.5 mm[55] and 5.0 mm[71] have been reported. Locke and associates studied 200 children from 3 to 15 years of age; they found no significant difference with sex or age, found only one measurement of 5.0 mm (in a 13-year-old boy), and recommended further investigation of any measurement greater than *4.0 mm*.[71]

An increased ADI can be caused by acute or old trauma that has damaged the transverse ligament of the atlas (see Fig. 6–17B). Other causes are rheumatoid arthritis and related diseases, acute and subacute inflammations of the face and the neck, and various congenital disorders, including occipitalization of the atlas and Down's syndrome. In the setting of trauma, an increased ADI requires further imaging, particularly because isolated traumatic disruption of the transverse ligament is rare. CT is indicated to evaluate the atlas and the axis for fractures, particularly a Jefferson fracture of the atlas. Flexion-extension films help gauge the mechanical stability of the C1–2 joint.

Both sides of the posterior arches of the atlas and the axis may be visible separately or they may be superimposed on a lateral film (see Fig. 6–14). They should be inspected carefully for fracture on all available cervical spine and skull films, including rejected films. A posterior arch fracture may be isolated or may be part of a more complex C1–2 injury.

The inner laminar line of C1 lies 1–2 mm anterior to a smooth curve continued upward from the curve of the C2 and the lower cervical spinolaminar lines or interpolated between this spinolaminar line curve and the opisthion. Conversely, the spinolaminar line of C2 stays up to 2.0 mm behind a curve drawn from the opisthion through the inner laminar line of C1 and continuing through the C3 and the lower spinolaminar lines (see Figs. 6–1 and 6–2). Reversal of this normal "misalignment" indicates posterior displacement of the atlas, usually due to odontoid fracture; exaggeration indicates anterior C1–2 subluxation with or without odontoid fracture (see Figs. 6–13A, 6–17B, 6–20B, and 6–25D) or hangman's fracture or variant (see Figs. 6–3, 6–23A, and 6–26A).

The anterior cortex of the dens is a smooth upward continuation of the anterior cortex of the body of the axis as shown on a true lateral view (see Fig. 6–1). With slight rotation, one side of the C2 articular plateau projects forward as a "shelf" (see Figs. 6–2, 6–15A, and 6–38C), interrupting this continuity and perhaps suggesting retrodisplacement of the dens. A common normal variation sometimes mistaken for a post-traumatic deformity is the *lordotic dens* (see Fig. 6–2), which has its own prominent lordotic curve that resembles a strongly extended thumb.

Anteroposterior Open-mouth (Transoral Odontoid) View

On this one small film several alignments and measurements should be studied for evidence of rotation, shift, or fracture (see Fig. 6–4). The lateral C1–2 joints should have symmetric, precise vertical alignments at their sharp lateral margins. Care may need to be taken in order to avoid confusing a C2 transverse process with part of the articular plateau. Sometimes there are notches on each side of the base

of the dens such that the lateral border of the notch is the medial border of the C2 articular surface; this border should then align with the medial tubercle of the lateral mass. The C0–1 alignments are not as sharply defined.

The distances between the medial tubercles and the dens are usually equal. The literature has been contradictory on whether spasm alone can induce asymmetry of this distance (i.e., unilateral shift of C1 on C2) in the absence of rotation. Such shift definitely can occur without rotation (Fig. 6–6) and is of doubtful clinical significance by itself.[53]

Rotation is more specifically assessed with other signs. The following structures should be aligned in the midline: the chin and the lower central incisors (provided there is no displaced mandibular injury or deformity), the upper central incisors, the dens, the C2 spinous process (an inverted cortical "V"), the middle of the fusiform thickening of the C1 posterior

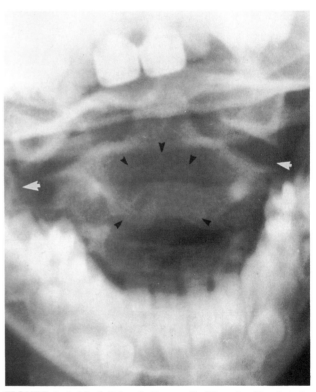

FIGURE 6–6. Neck Muscle Spasm Pulling the Head and C1 to One Side

• • • •

A 4-year-old boy fell 4½ ft. onto the left side of his neck and head, and was transferred with a diagnosis of "rotary fixation." The asymmetry of the lateral atlantodental intervals is striking, but the head is not rotated around the vertical (z-) axis. At the level of the anteroposterior (x-) axis of head tilt (i.e., at the base of the dens), the line (not drawn) connecting the median gaps between the upper and the lower central incisors is negligibly shifted from the midline. The C2 spinous process is midline (faintly outlined, *arrowheads*). The C1 offset on the right (*arrow*), 4 mm on film, slightly exceeds the 3-mm inset on the left (*arrow*) owing to "pseudospread." The spasm and tilt remitted overnight.

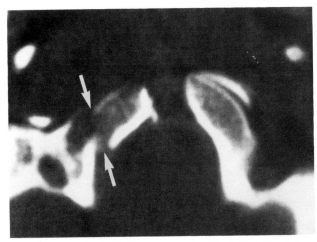

FIGURE 6–7. Type II Fracture of the Occipital Condyle

• • • •

A linear, predominantly vertical fracture through the base of the occipital condyle (Type II) in a 20-year-old woman is shown *(arrows)*.

arch, and the median occipital crest. C2 rotation is excluded if its spinous process is aligned vertically with the dens and is projected midway between the pedicles. The other listed structures attest to the position of the head and presumably of C1 but do not rule out *pathologic* rotation of the head at C0–1. Precise assessment of C1 rotation requires CT, but an indication of gross rotation is given by measuring the widths of the inferior portions of the lateral masses; the wider mass is rotated forward.

Specific Injury Components and Patterns

Atlanto-occipital (C0–1) Injuries

OCCIPITAL CONDYLE FRACTURES

Fractures of the occipital condyles are classified into one of three types. Type I is a comminuted impaction fracture caused by axial compression. Type II (Fig. 6–7) is a linear basilar skull fracture through the occipital condyle. Type III (Fig. 6–8B and C) is

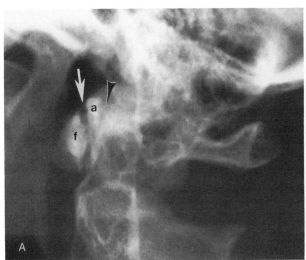

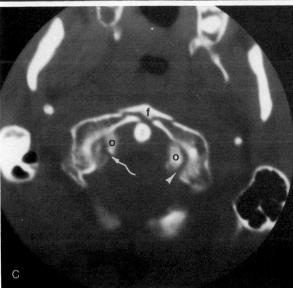

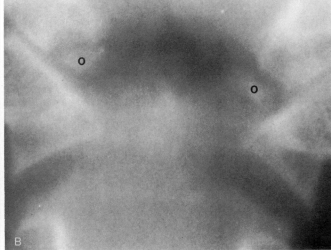

FIGURE 6–8. Combined Bilateral Type III Occipital Condyle Fractures and a C1 Anterior Arch Fracture in a 21-Year-Old-Man

• • • •

A, A false "atlas-dens space" *(white arrow)* separates the midline anterior fragment *(f)* from the residual anterior arch *(a)* and is distinct from the true atlas-dens space *(black arrowhead). B,* A tomogram showing occipital condyle avulsions *(o). C,* A symmetric midline C1 fragment *(f)* was apparently split out by an impact against the dens. The gap between the remaining sides of the anterior arch was wider on lower sections and narrowed to a minimal line on higher sections, giving this fracture combined horizontal and vertical features. Occipital condyle fracture lines were visible *(wavy arrow)* on this and other sections but should not be confused with the normal C0–1 joint space *(arrowhead).*

an avulsion by the alar ligament due to rotation or lateral bending; it is the fracture most likely to be unstable and may accompany atlanto-occipital dislocation.[12] All of these fractures are difficult to diagnose on plain films.[4] They may be isolated or may accompany massive craniocervical injury. Diagnosis usually requires a high index of suspicion and high-resolution thin-section axial CT or AP tomography, although Type I or Type III fracture may be visible on an AP open-mouth view.

ATLANTO-OCCIPITAL DISLOCATION

Dislocation of the skull from the spine is usually fatal, but some long-term survivals have occurred (Fig. 6–9), and rare survival without permanent neurologic deficit is known. This unstable injury makes the patient especially vulnerable to disaster during intubation, which therefore requires very careful technique in any trauma victim. Radiologic diagnosis is difficult because the osseous landmarks are poorly defined.

Bilateral atlanto-occipital dislocation requires a powerful distractive hyperextension.[12] The occipitoatlantal and occipitoaxial ligaments, including the alar ligaments, must be ruptured or severely stretched. Most commonly the head is dislocated anterosuperiorly. A lateral component and pure anterior, vertical, and posterior dislocations are less common. Transection or at least contusion of the neuraxis at the foramen magnum is virtually certain and may produce central apnea and total spinal paralysis.

The dislocation may be clinically obvious, but the more subtle cases require prompt, accurate diagnosis. Use of a simple dens-basion distance is unreliable. The anterior vector of displacement can be detected by finding a reversed Powers ratio,[86] provided that the opisthion and the basion as well as the inner midline surfaces of the anterior and the posterior C1

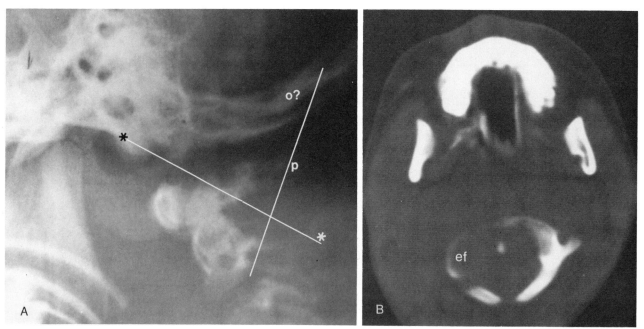

FIGURE 6–9. Atlanto-occipital Dislocation in a 6-Year-Old Boy Who Survived as a Quadriplegic
• • • •
There are three signs: Lee's X, clival-C2 misalignment, and an empty C1 facet.

A, This lateral film shows marked retropharyngeal swelling but is otherwise difficult to interpret, only partly owing to the obscurity of the C1 and C2 arches. The application of Lee's X method is possible after modification. The basion-C2 line (**) of Lee's X is tangential to the dens, which is normal or consistent with an anterosuperior dislocation. The opisthion is not precisely defined radiographically *(o?),* and no C1 inner laminar line exists because the arch is unfused. Extrapolating an inner laminar line *(p)* permits the extension of a line from the body of C2 that passes posterior to any reasonable estimate of the opisthion. This means that the opisthion-C2 line would pass anterior to the C1 inner laminar line, thereby confirming anterosuperior dislocation. Considering that the apical and the alar ligaments normally tie the basion to the dens, the elevation of the basion above the C1 plane and the alignment of the clivus closer to the anterior C1 arch (clival-C2 misalignment) imply their disruption. *B,* This computed tomography scan of the head (an 8-mm section) shows an empty right C1 condylar facet *(ef).* As a result of tilt, the section passed mainly through the condyle-facet gap on the right, whereas the condyle or the facet filled part of each adjacent section on the left so that the sign was not apparent (the volume-averaging effect of thick sections).

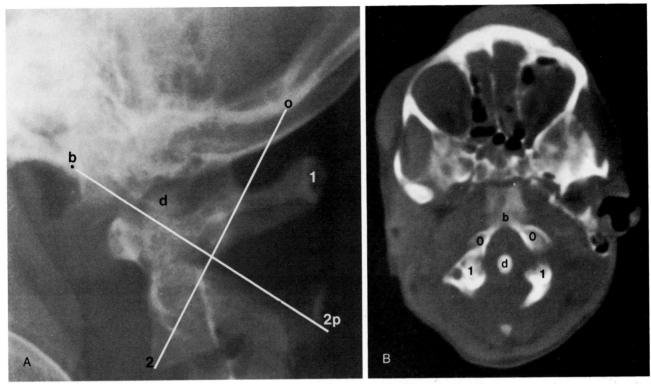

FIGURE 6–10. Atlanto-occipital Dislocation in an 8-Year-Old Girl Who Subsequently Died

• • • •

A, Marked retropharyngeal swelling can be seen. No abnormal vertical C0–1 gap is obvious. Lee's X (basion: dot at *b;* opisthion: *o;* posteroinferior body C2: *2;* anteroinferior C2 spinolaminar line tangent: *2p*) crosses the dens *(d)* and misses the C1 posterior arch *(1)* to a similar extent, indicating relatively pure anterior dislocation. *B,* A thick (8-mm) computed tomography section shows anterior displacement of the occipital condyles *(O)* compared with the C1 lateral masses *(1).* Note the wide anteroposterior gap between the basion of the clivus *(b)* and the dens *(d).*

arches are visualized on a lateral film (see Fig. 6–2). A clever diagrammatic way to diagnose any direction of dislocation (other than lateral) was reported by Lee and coworkers,[68] but this method still requires visualization of the opisthion and the basion (Figs. 6–10*A* and 6–11; see also Fig. 6–9*A*). Rarely, a Type I dens fracture resulting from alar ligament avulsion may be visible.[101]

ROTARY ATLANTO-OCCIPITAL (C0–1) DISPLACEMENT

Unilateral, or rotary, C0–1 subluxation or dislocation has been reported as an apparently compensatory component in some cases of C1–2 rotary fixation or subluxation.[3, 18, 28, 63, 115] There may be cranial nerve deficits or no neurologic deficit. This unusual subluxation can be diagnosed on lateral, AP, or axial views when C1 is rotated with respect to both the head and C2 while the latter are aligned nearly normally with each other.

Atlas (C1) Fractures

ANTERIOR ARCH FRACTURES

Anterior arch fractures come in two fundamental configurations, each with two possible mechanisms. An unusual example with combined features of both types is shown in Figure 6–8.

A "vertical" fracture interrupts the continuity of the anterior arch between the lateral masses. It can be unilateral or bilateral but generally not midline. The majority are components of Jefferson fractures, which are usually produced by axial compression. Isolated anterior arch fractures are thought to result from hyperextension with impact of the anterior arch against the dens. When isolated, a single anterior arch fracture is usually stable. A double vertical anterior arch fracture (Fig. 6–12) removes a major restraint against posterior dislocation of C1 and the head on C2 and may permit the transverse ligament of C1 to compress the spinal cord against the posterior arch of C2.

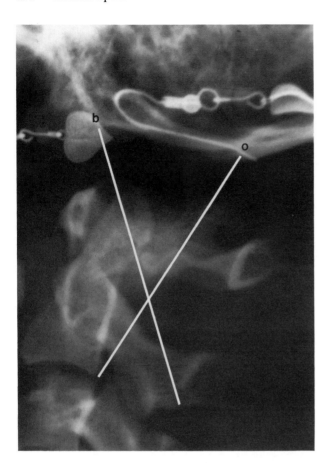

FIGURE 6–11. Atlanto-occipital Dislocation in a 17-Year-Old Woman Who Subsequently Died

• • • •

The basion and the opisthion are difficult to define on the rotated skull, but points *b* and *o* are perhaps the best approximations. Lee's X crosses the dens, and by a greater amount passes anterior to the C1 arch, indicating antero-superior displacement of the head. The opisthion is clearly anterior to an extension of the line (not drawn) connecting the inner laminar lines of C2 and C1. An obvious gap between C1 and the skull is usually sufficient for diagnosis.

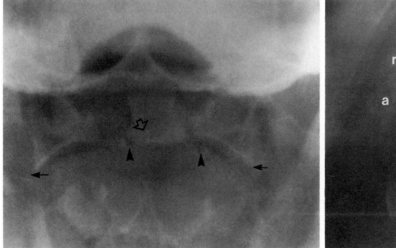
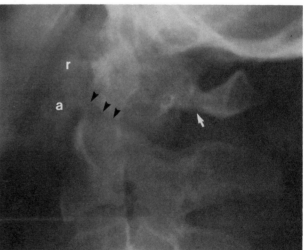

FIGURE 6–12. Double Vertical Anterior Arch C1 Fracture with a Hairline Single Posterior Arch Fracture and a Displaced Dens Fracture in a 51-Year-Old Man

• • • •

A, An anteroposterior open-mouth view shows C1–2 asymmetry and a tilted dens fracture. The net spreading of C1 is minimal (a total articular surface span of 62 mm for C1 and 61 mm for C2 as measured on film) because the 5-mm offset of C1 on the right is nearly balanced by the 4-mm inset on the left *(arrows)*. The dens is tilted 13 degrees and is displaced to the right with respect to notches marking its base *(arrowheads)*. The base of the dens is deformed and widened and has a faint diagonal fracture line *(open arrow)*. *B*, A lateral view shows a Jefferson and a dens fracture. A major portion of the anterior arch of C1 *(a)* is displaced downward, whereas a remnant *(r)* marks its normal level. An inferior cortical step-off *(arrow)* and a faint diagonal line mark the posterior arch fracture. The dens is slightly elevated and tilted backward *(arrowheads* along the fracture), but it is not posteriorly displaced at its base. The inner laminar line of C1 is retrodisplaced with respect to the spinolaminar line of C2; because the posterior arch fracture is not displaced (and unilateral), this indicates retrodisplacement of most of C1 on C2 due to the combination of dens tilt and the effective loss of the C1 anterior arch. Note also the marked retropharyngeal swelling.

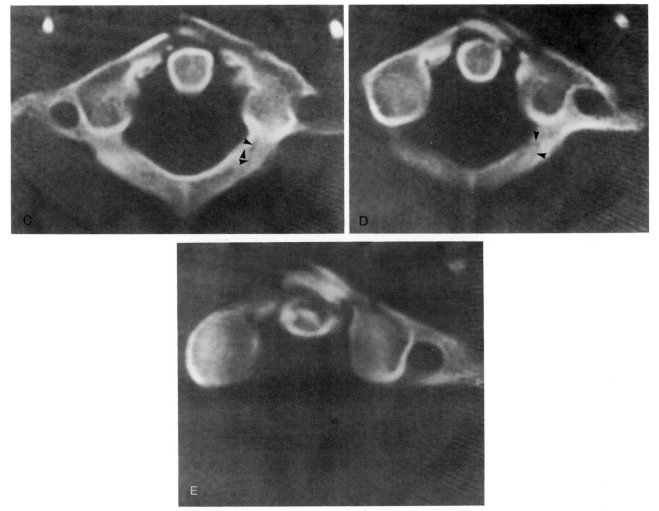

FIGURE 6–12 *Continued* **Double Vertical Anterior Arch C1 Fracture with a Hairline Single Posterior Arch Fracture and a Displaced Dens Fracture in a 51-Year-Old Man**

• • • •

C–E, Consecutive computed tomography sections 5 mm thick obtained at 3-mm table increments with a high-resolution algorithm are shown. The opening of the anterior arch is obvious, and the dens fracture (incomplete cortex in *D* and *E*) is apparent despite the thick sections. A posterior arch fracture is suggested in *C* and *D* *(arrowheads)*. This may be a "save" by the high-resolution algorithm, but the fracture would have been clearer on thinner sections. The addition of a posterior arch fracture to the anterior arch fracture suggests a Jefferson fracture. However, it is not clear whether the posterior arch fracture is complete or greenstick, whereas the lack of spreading and the configuration and displacements of the anterior fractures indicate a hyperextension rather than a classic Jefferson axial compression mechanism.

A "horizontal" fracture leaves a continuous but attenuated anterior arch after downward avulsion of part of its inferior margin (Fig. 6–13). The mechanism is thought to be hyperextension, with either a tension avulsion by the anterior atlantoaxial membrane (anterior longitudinal ligament) and longus colli muscle or a shearing avulsion by the tip of the dens (see Fig. 6–8). In the lateral view, the inferiorly displaced fragment may echo the profile of the anterior arch. Ligamentous ossifications and earlobe shadows are common in the same region and simulate this injury.

POSTERIOR ARCH FRACTURES

The most common atlas fracture is a bilateral or unilateral posterior arch fracture. This fracture usu-ally occurs through or slightly posterior to the vertebral artery sulcus. The mechanism is hyperextension of the head on the upper cervical spine, which levers the posterior arch upward or downward with respect to the lateral masses as the latter are compressed between the head and C2. One side of the arch may fail first. This interrupts the arch and allows a local displacement that reorients the larger arch component and relieves some of the angular strain at its base. The second side may fracture after sufficient further deflection.[107] Isolated fractures of the posterior arch ordinarily do not produce clinical instability even with moderate angulation and displacement. Suboccipital neuralgia has been reported as a long-term complication.

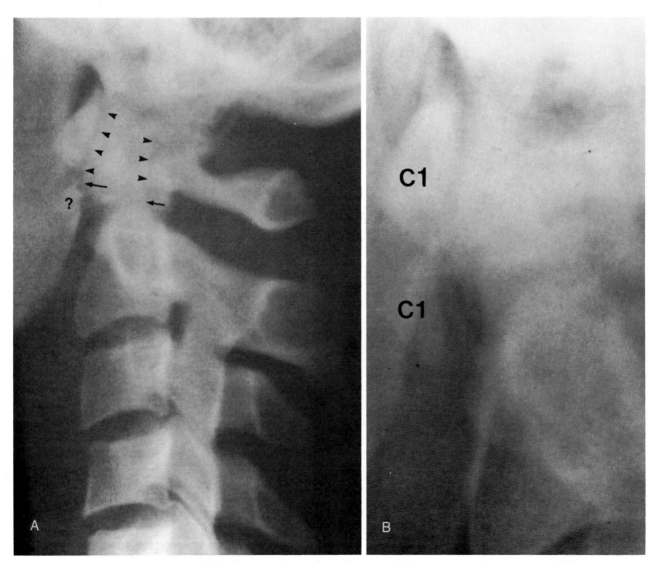

FIGURE 6–13. Horizontal Fracture of the C1 Anterior Arch and a Type II Dens Fracture in a 26-Year-Old Man
• • • •
A, Preatlantal swelling measures 15 mm in this lateral film. The dens *(arrowheads)* is displaced anteriorly *(arrows).* An unexplained shadow *(?)* beneath the anterior arch is sometimes ligament calcification. *B,* Detail from a lateral skull film shows a subatlantal shadow with a contour resembling the anterior arch. The anterior arch of the atlas is marked C1.

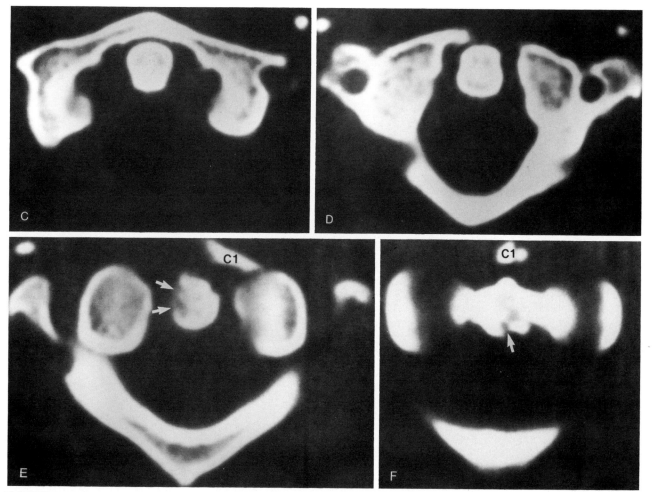

FIGURE 6–13 *Continued* **Horizontal Fracture of the C1 Anterior Arch and a Type II Dens Fracture in a 26-Year-Old Man**

• • • •

C–F, Computed tomography sections (1.5-mm). The anterior arch is continuous in *C* but has a large gap in *D*. In *E* and *F,* the missing fragment *(C1)* appears lower, explaining the inferiorly displaced anterior arch ghost on the lateral films. These thin sections detect a fracture in the base of the dens as a faintness or a defect of the cortex *(arrows).*

The lateral view is the key for this laterally located fracture (Figs. 6–14 to 6–17; see also Fig. 6–12B). Good films with slight tilt easily show both fractures or show a unilateral fracture with the opposite side intact. The atlas-dens distance should be normal; if it is increased then a Jefferson fracture is probably present (see Fig. 6–17). A hyperextension dens fracture may coexist with a posterior arch atlas fracture, but an anterior arch fracture is likely to be present as well (see Fig. 6–12).

JEFFERSON FRACTURE

Any combination of at least one vertical anterior arch fracture and at least one complete posterior arch fracture is called a *Jefferson fracture*. The essence is the loss of a bony connection between the lateral masses of the atlas. In most fractures of this type, a vertical compressive force along the craniospinal axis is modified by the sloping surfaces of the lateral C1 masses into a lateral spreading force. The anterior and the posterior arches snap under sudden tension

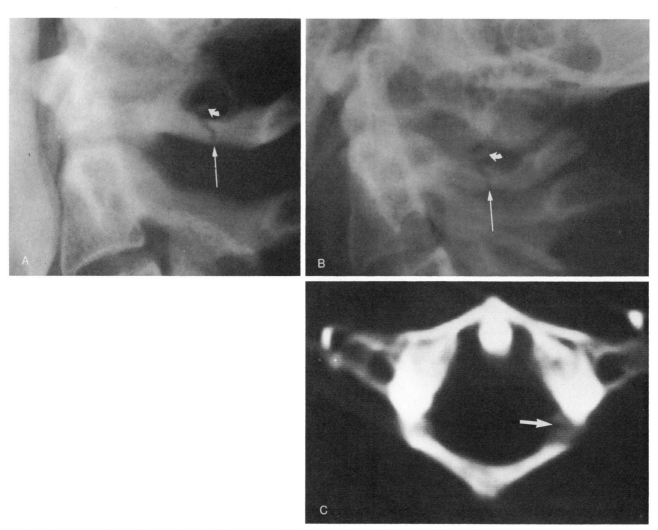

FIGURE 6–14. Unilateral Posterior Arch Fracture of C1 in a 51-Year-Old Man with Neck Pain and Right Upper Posterior Neck Tenderness After a Fall

• • • •

A and *B*, Two of four lateral films at various degrees of tilt show a unilateral (right) fracture *(straight arrows)*. A separate small fragment is displaced upward *(curved arrows)*, but there was no clinical suspicion of vertebral artery injury. In *A* the fracture line interrupts the cortical surfaces of one hemiarch, whereas the surfaces of the nearly superimposed opposite hemiarch are continuous. Note the intact ponticulus posticus continuous with the intact hemiarch. In *B*, the tilt separates the fractured right from the intact left hemiarch. Note the absence of the ponticulus posticus from the superior profile of the fractured hemiarch, indicating that it is on the intact side. *C*, Computed tomography shows a fracture *(arrow)* on the right on an EMI 5005 ''topview'' orientation. This is the same patient as in Figure 6–4 and as in Case 1 of Reference No. 107.

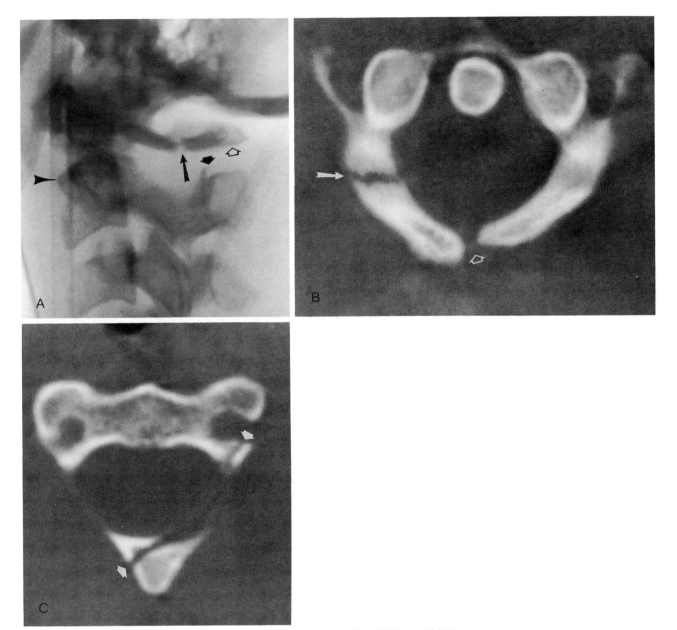

FIGURE 6–15. Combined Posterior Arch C1 and C2 Fractures in a 32-Year-Old Woman

• • • •

A, An overpenetrated lateral film reversed on a subtraction film. *B* and *C,* High-resolution 1.5-mm computed tomography (CT) sections. Persistent C1 midline posterior synchondrosis is apparent (*open arrows* in *A* and *B*); note the double-pronged appearance of the posterior arch and the absence of the C1 inner laminar line, as well as incidental anterior rotation of one side of the C2 articular plateau (*arrowhead*), in *A.* The unilateral C1 posterior arch fracture passes through the sulcus for the vertebral artery (*long arrows* in *A* and *B*). In *B,* note the jagged, complementary, noncorticated fracture margins through the right vertebral artery sulcus (the broader, subtle lucency) on a 1.5-mm CT section reconstructed with a bone algorithm; note also the normal left vertebral artery sulcus. The fracture of the C2 lamina extends from the transverse foramen to the base of the spinous process (*short solid arrows* in *A* and *C*).

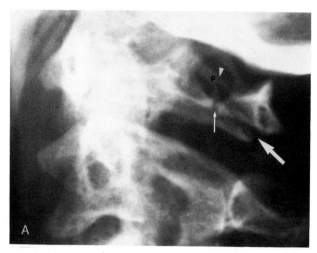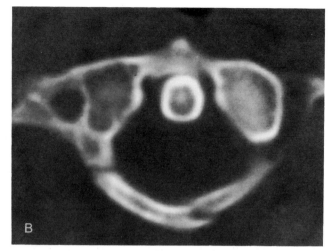

FIGURE 6–16. Bilateral Fracture of the Posterior C1 Arch

• • • •

A, Detail from a lateral skull film. The oblique left posterior fracture line *(large arrow)* indicates impact against C2, which deflected the C1 arch upward. An apparent gap *(arrowhead)* is a fortuitous juxtaposition of the edge of the arch fragment with the intact left ponticulus posticus *(p).* The ponticulus apparently reinforced the arch and shifted the fracture more posteriorly than usual. The right ponticulus appeared intact on this and another film. Slight posteroinferior displacement of the right margin of the arch fragment *(small arrow)* also suggests the effect of the intact right ponticulus. *B,* Computed tomography (a 5-mm section) shows fractures through the sulcus for the vertebral artery on the right and more posteriorly than usual on the left.

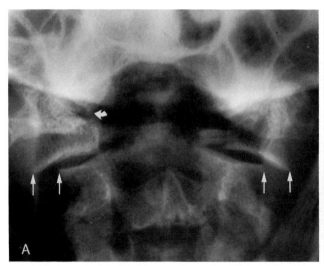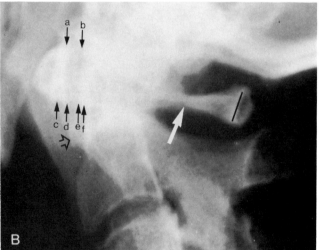

FIGURE 6–17. Jefferson Fracture in a 68-Year-Old Man

• • • •

A, An anteroposterior open-mouth view. Marked bilateral lateral offset of the C1 lateral masses is evident *(arrows).* The offset on *each* side measures 7 mm. (A *sum* of ≥7 mm suggests instability.) Although no precise alignment standards are established, the occipital condyle *(curved arrow)* extends farther than usual down the upper slope of the lateral mass, which is consistent with the lateral displacement of the mass and the descent of the head toward C2. *B,* A lateral view. A subtle and probably single posterior arch fracture is shown *(white arrow).* The atlanto-dens interval (ADI) is widened, but an exact measurement is uncertain. Landmarks for the usual measurement inferiorly are ambiguous. Judging from the form of the atlas, *c* should be the posteroinferior margin of the anterior arch; *d* is probably an overlay shadow equivalent to that in Figure 6–2. Disregarding the anteriorly rotated articular plateau *(open arrow),* the curve of the midline anterior cortex of C2 continues upward as *f,* but sometimes there is a slight anterior jog at *e* where the anterior subarticular cortex of the dens becomes thicker. Thus, *ce* is probably the actual interosseous space, which measures 5 mm. The distance *de* measures 3 mm but is too small for the observed posterior arch displacement (see below); *df* measures 4 mm, and *cf* 6 mm. Distance *ab* (4 mm) is also a valid interosseous distance; the minimal ADI occurs superiorly in this patient because the head and the atlas are extended, and because the dens is not "lordotic," thus avoiding the normal V-shaped pre-dens space. Although the C1 inner laminar line *(black line)* normally is slightly anterior to the C2 spinolaminar line, here it is abnormally far forward by 4 or 5 mm.

as the ring bursts.[56] Under continuing axial compression, spreading proceeds until it is resisted by the transverse ligament of the atlas. This ligament may then rupture, permitting even further spreading. The classic radiologic finding is lateral spreading of the lateral masses of the atlas so that they overhang the articular plateau of the axis (Fig. 6–18; see also Fig. 6–17). Lateral offset may be bilaterally symmetric or asymmetric, or it may be unilateral with the other lateral mass apparently normally aligned or displaced medially to a lesser extent.

An alternative mechanism to pure axial compression is a combination of hyperextension fractures of the posterior and the anterior arches, generally accompanied by a Type II dens fracture (see Fig. 6–12). This combination of fractures can also result from pure axial compression, however. Extension-type "Jefferson" fractures are seen commonly in elderly patients, may have minimal C1 spreading or dens displacement, and may require CT for diagnosis.

When the lateral atlantoaxial joints are obscured by teeth, the superolateral margins of the atlas are usually visible. Spreading of the lateral masses can be estimated using the ratio of the intertubercular width to the outer width of the lateral masses at their superolateral margins. The maximum of this "atlas spread index" is 0.58 at 0.5–6 months of age, 0.56 at 0.5–2 years of age, 0.53 at 2–4 years of age, and 0.36 in teenagers and adults (mean + 2 SD).[108] A normal ratio does not necessarily exclude mild spreading,

but an abnormally high ratio should lead to further investigation. The ratios are not valid for a dysmorphic, a rotated, or an osteophytic atlas.

As little as 1.0 mm of spread can be pathologic, whereas measurements under 1.0 mm are not reliable. Film rotation can create an appearance of a 1.0–2.0-mm spread. Children up to about 7 years of age often show normal growth-related "pseudospread" of the ossified portions of C1 compared with C2, commonly by 2.0 or 3.0 mm and rarely up to 10.0 mm (combined bilateral offsets).[13, 108] A real spread of 1.0–2.0 mm may result from persistence of normal or normal-variant synchondroses.[13, 17, 31] A Jefferson fracture is virtually certain if true spreading exceeds 2.0 mm. Because the anterior arch is difficult to evaluate for vertical fracture on plain films, an apparently isolated posterior arch fracture, whether unilateral or bilateral, may be part of a Jefferson fracture unless it is excluded by CT.

The lateral film typically shows a unilateral or a bilateral posterior arch fracture, but the anterior arch component is not seen unless there is an unusual vertical displacement of fragments (see Fig. 6–12). A common clue that a posterior arch fracture is really a Jefferson fracture is the presence of an increase in the ADI above 3.0 mm due to the stretching of the transverse ligament of the atlas (see Fig. 6–17).

CT is the ideal diagnostic modality for complete evaluation of a suspected Jefferson fracture, although plain AP tomography of the anterior arch and lateral tomography of the posterior arch can be used. Of at

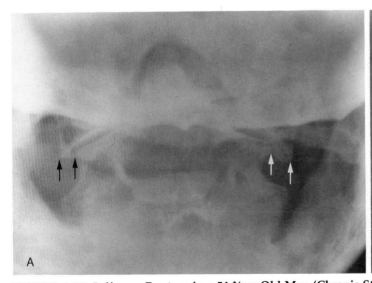 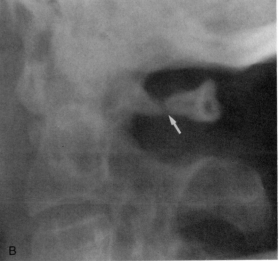

FIGURE 6–18. Jefferson Fracture in a 54-Year-Old Man (Chronic Stage)

• • • •

A, A suboptimal anteroposterior open-mouth view showing marked bilateral lateral offset of the C1 lateral masses. The offset measured 3 mm on the right (*black arrows*) and 5 mm on the left (*white arrows*), indicating mechanical instability. *B*, A lateral view. A posterior arch fracture (*arrow*) is visible, but neither widening of the atlanto-dens interval nor anterior displacement of the C1 posterior arch is apparent.

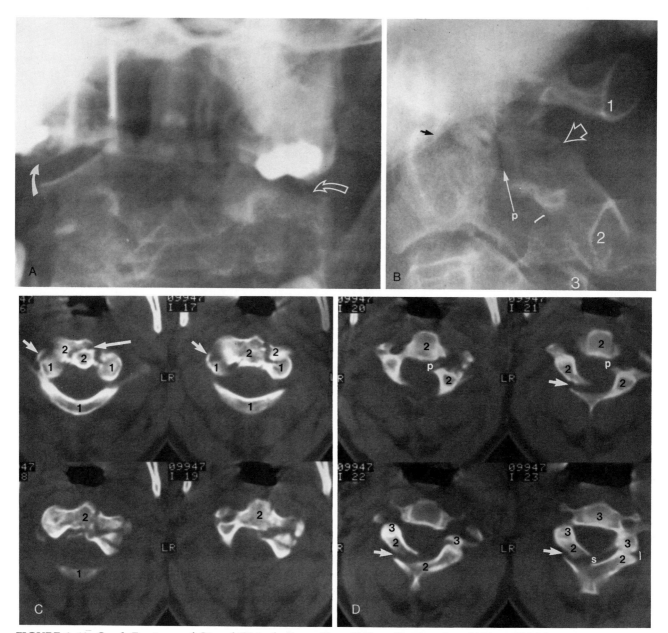

FIGURE 6–19. Crush Fractures of C1 and C2 Including a Type II Dens Fracture in a 34-Year-Old Man

• • • •

A, An anteroposterior open-mouth film. Noncongruence of the right lateral C1–2 joint surfaces is not entirely pathologic because both surfaces may be concave; however, lateral gaping indicates major compression on the left. The inferior surface of the right C1 lateral mass is fractured laterally *(solid arrow).* C1 is shifted to the right (with lateral offset on the right, and inset behind the tooth on the left). The left C2 articular surface is crushed *(open arrow).* The lines at the base of the dens cannot be distinguished from anatomic overlays and Mach lines. *B,* A rotated and tilted lateral film. An articular plateau fracture *(open arrow)* identifies the posterosuperiorly projected hemiarch as the left; this is consistent with the left pedicle fracture *(long arrow)* confirmed by computed tomography (CT) in *D.* With retrodisplacement of the anterior cortex of the base of the dens *(short arrow)* and a normal atlanto-dens interval (2 mm), the C1 inner laminar line *(1)* should be retrodisplaced with respect to the C2 spinolaminar line *(2).* Instead, the latter is retrodisplaced with respect to C3 *(retouched line* anterior to *3)* because of the extensive C2 arch fractures that are underrepresented by the visualized fracture lines. (Because of obliquity, these "spinolaminar" lines are actually the left paramedian inner laminar lines; however, their displacements have the same significance.) The left C2–3 facet joint is widened *(angled bracket). C,* CT sections at the C1–2 joint and upper C2 body. Portions of C1 and C2 are numbered *(1, 2).* Note the dens fracture *(long arrow),* the inferolateral right C1 fragment *(short arrows),* and the extensive left C2 crush. Opposing surfaces are apparently unfractured (left C1 is also shown well on another film). *D,* CT sections at the C2–3 level. Portions of C2 and C3 are numbered *(2, 3).* On the left, note completion of the pedicle transection *(p)* downward from the crushed plateau, and note the widened C2–3 facet joint *(angled bracket).* The right lamina fracture *(arrows)* is occult on film; it accounts for the spinolaminar line displacement *(s).*

least equal importance is the search for coexisting "occult" injuries elsewhere in the cervical spine. Therefore, thin-section high-resolution CT is preferable, and CT scanning should extend from the foramen magnum through any level not adequately cleared by plain films.

Mechanical stability of a Jefferson fracture depends on the transverse ligament of the atlas. A medial C1 tubercle avulsion may signal a ligament rupture. A spread of 7.0 mm or more indicates complete rupture of the transverse ligament.[104] As the lateral masses slide apart, either acutely or with chronic stretching of the transverse ligament, the head descends toward the axis vertebra. Cranial settling can cause odontoid protrusion into the foramen magnum.

LATERAL MASS AND TRANSVERSE PROCESS FRACTURES

Sometimes vertical compression crushes a lateral mass, which may have an irregular inferior surface on the AP open-mouth view (Fig. 6–19). A C2 articular crush should also be sought, with CT if necessary. These injuries presumably result from an oblique compressive vector or an asymmetric patient posture.

Avulsion of the medial tubercle is an important diagnostic sign of transverse ligament injury, provided it is not confused with the normal irregularity or with a gap between teeth on the odontoid view. Marked compressive comminution of a lateral mass has the same effect as a complete avulsion.

Transverse process fractures are uncommon. Reports have attributed them to forced lateral flexion of the head.[1, 19]

Atlantoaxial (C1–2) Injuries

C1–2 injuries include various malpositions of C1 on 2, without or with odontoid fracture. Odontoid fractures are discussed with C2 fractures.

ATLANTOAXIAL SUBLUXATION

Forward subluxation of C1 on C2 demands inspection both of the ADI and of the base of the dens. Widening of the ADI should first lead to suspicion of a Jefferson fracture (see Fig. 6–17), then to any other atlas fracture that can involve the attachment of the ligament to the lateral mass, and finally to chronic post-traumatic, inflammatory, or malformative conditions. Jefferson fractures are sometimes associated with odontoid fractures. Patients with chronic subluxations are at heightened risk in deceleration or flexion trauma. Purely traumatic, isolated transverse atlantal ligament injuries are unusual because the dens usually fails first.

ROTARY ATLANTOAXIAL FIXATION AND DISPLACEMENTS

Fielding and Hawkins defined four types of "atlantoaxial rotatory fixation."[27] Type I has no net anterior displacement on the atlas, and its ADI is less than 3.0 mm. The degree of rotation does not exceed the normal range. Type II has a net anterior displacement of the atlas up to an ADI of 50 mm. Type III has further anterior atlas displacement with the ADI exceeding 50 mm. Type IV is a posterior displacement with an eroded or a separated dens. All types have an abnormal restriction of rotation, generally assumed to be a complete fixation. The head is commonly rotated or tilted, but actual C1–2 rotation, rather than mere lateral shifting or tilting, must be present in order to diagnose rotary fixation or subluxation (compare with Fig. 6–6). Types II and III are also called "atlantoaxial rotary subluxation," and Type III may have a true dislocation on one side. Up to 90 degrees of rotational dislocation has been reported.[38]

An AP open-mouth view shows a rotation of C1 on C2. In the simplest case of rotary fixation, with the patient able to bring his or her head to the neutral position, the head, C1, and the chest are aligned anteroposteriorly while C2 is rotated. Alternatively, the C1 anterior arch and the mandible are paradoxically rotated toward the same side as the C2 spinous process, so that the latter is shifted to the side opposite the anteriorly rotated (wider) C1 lateral mass. The head is commonly rotated to one side, tilted to the other, and flexed.[27]

It is necessary to rule out a primary lower cervical rotational abnormality of any sort for which C1–2 rotation might be compensatory. A full AP view with the head and chest in AP position (with or without head tilt) shows that the C3 and lower spinous processes progressively return to the midline. A lateral view of the same position also shows a gradual derotation from C2–3 downward. Thus, C1–2 is the only level of rotational discontinuity. These conditions document a pathologic restriction of C1–2 rotation that prevents return to a neutral position. Absolute fixation may be present and can be documented by two series of CT sections through the C1–2 region with maximum voluntary head rotation to each side.[63] Significant restriction without absolute fixation is also possible, as in a case of the author's in which rotation of C1 was restricted to the range between 20 degrees left and 43 degrees left with respect to C2.

Because of the possibility of coexisting pathologic C0–1 rotation[3, 18, 28, 63, 115] C0–1 relations should be assessed either by confirming C1 lateral mass symmetry when the head is not rotated or by CT.

In pure C1–2 rotary subluxation or dislocation the rotational signs are the same as in rotary fixation, but the crucial finding is an ADI of 3.0 mm or greater. The anterior displacement of the posterior C1 arch narrows the spinal canal against the dens, but in addition the posteriorly displaced lateral mass and the ipsilateral lamina may further narrow the spinal canal from the side. A thick CT section or a sagittal reformation of thin sections shows the presence or absence of interlocking at the edges of the articular surfaces.

Axis (C2) Fractures

ODONTOID FRACTURES

The odontoid process is one of the most commonly fractured structures in the spine. The mechanism is usually hyperextension, with impact by the anterior arch of the atlas, and less commonly hyperflexion with impact by the transverse ligament of the atlas. Regardless of the direction of impact, once the odontoid process is detached from the ring of the axis vertebra it is free to move in any direction except downward. The observed displacement may reflect the fracture mechanism, but it can be reversed by subsequent forces.

Odontoid fractures are classified into three types.[74] Type III fractures have a "U" shape and dip distinctly into the body of C2. They occur in younger patients and are most likely to heal with union.

Type II fractures are horizontal or oblique short fractures at the base of the odontoid process. They constitute about one half of all odontoid fractures, are proportionally more common in the elderly, and are the most susceptible to nonunion. Type II fractures have the most unstable configuration, but many occur with little displacement and no neurologic injury, suggesting effective stabilization by soft tissues. This fracture may be accompanied by fractures of one or both atlas arches (see Fig. 6–12; see also Jefferson Fracture). A subtype called Type IIa has been described as having additional chip fragments at the base of the odontoid process that increase the instability and the likelihood of nonunion (Fig. 6–20).[43]

The rare Type I fractures are located near the top of the odontoid process and are steeply oblique. Most probably result from avulsion by an alar ligament in rotation. As such, they may be associated with C0–1 dislocation.[101] An atypical case of a coronally oriented fracture extending downward from the tip of the odontoid process[57] suggests an alternative mechanism of axial compression with impact against the basion.

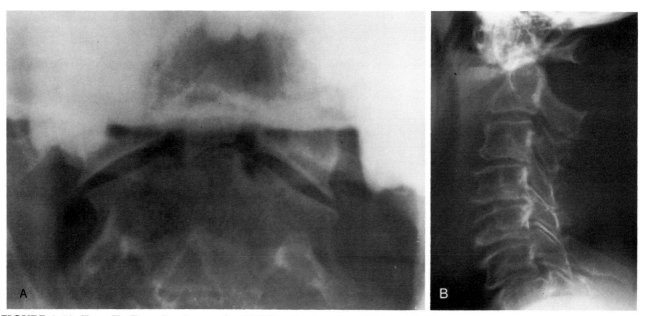

FIGURE 6–20. Type IIa Dens Fracture and a C6 Pillar Fracture in a 62-Year-Old Woman Presenting Several Days After a Fall

• • • •

A, This anteroposterior open-mouth view shows an oblique fracture line at the base of the dens. *B,* A lateral view shows marked anterior C1–C2 subluxation. The dens is obscured by mastoids. Retropharyngeal thickness at C1 measures 8–13 mm on the film (the shortest diagonal distance), depending on the choice of landmarks (double pharyngeal border, questionable anteroinferior tubercle on C1). Diffuse spondylosis is marked and masks the detail of the bone contours; this could explain the retrolisthesis of C3 and the anterolisthesis of C6.

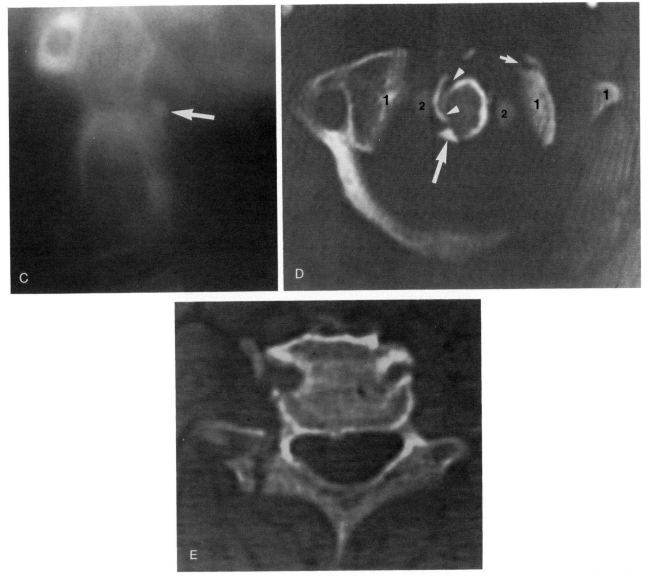

FIGURE 6–20 *Continued* **Type IIa Dens Fracture and a C6 Pillar Fracture in a 62-Year-Old Woman Presenting Several Days After a Fall**

• • • •

C, This lateral tomogram reveals a third fragment from the dens fracture *(arrow)*. *D*, A high-resolution 2-mm computed tomography (CT) section shows the Type II fracture *(large arrow)*, other cortical dens fractures *(arrowheads)*, and an anteroinferior left C1 lateral mass chip fracture *(small arrow)*. Other portions of C1 and C2 are numbered *(1, 2)*. *E*, A 4-mm CT section is shown; it is one of several showing a sagittal plane fracture with acute features passing through the right pillar of C6. The pillar fracture suggests an extension mechanism, whereas the residual dens position does not reliably indicate the direction of the initial force.

The lateral view often shows a fracture line or wedge-shaped gap (see Fig. 6–12B) at the base of the odontoid process in a Type II fracture. A gap may be invisible because it is minimal or because of poor positioning. It is then helpful that most odontoid fractures are anteriorly or posteriorly displaced, but CT or tomography may be necessary if displacement is minimal.

If displacement is substantial it is evident on even a poor lateral film with rotation, tilt, or osteoarthrosis. The C1 anterior arch may be obviously too anterior with respect to the anterior surface of the body of C2 without a visible ADI (see Fig. 6–20B). There may be an obvious step-off of the anterior or the posterior cortex near the odontoid-body junction (Fig. 6–21B). A true lateral projection increases sensitivity for a small step-off without interference from a rotated articular plateau, but it may also show a small normal anterior step-off of the anterior dens surface. The curve described by the inner laminar lines should be studied carefully for abnormal C1–2 alignment (see The Upper Cervical Spine, Analysis of Films, Lateral View). A lateral film sign of a Type III fracture is a horizontal interruption of the oval cortical ring that is normally superimposed on the upper half of the body of C2 (see Fig. 6–1).[45, 111]

A good AP odontoid view shows most odontoid fractures (see Figs. 6–12A and 6–20A). If the odontoid process is better centered with respect to C1 than to C2, and especially if it is off-center with respect to the notches at the medial margins of the superior C2 articular surfaces, then a new or an old fracture is likely. A lateral tilt of more than 3 degrees suggests fracture and may be the only AP film abnormality in a Type III fracture.[111]

High-resolution CT can diagnose odontoid fracture at least as well as geometric tomography and adds additional information (see Figs. 6–12D and E, and 6–20D). One to two-millimeter sections, preferably contiguous and using all high-resolution parameters, should be obtained through the odontoid process and down into at least the upper part of the body of C2. Cortical displacement and at least some areas of interrupted cortical and trabecular bone are found and may be accompanied by comminuted fragments and soft tissue swelling. Tomography is used if CT is not available.

HANGMAN'S AND OTHER FRACTURES OF THE ARCH

Pedicle fractures are another common group of axis fractures. The fracture plane often slopes anteroinferiorly and may pass through the posteroinferior portion of the C2 vertebral body, producing an apparent triangular fragment.[67] Regardless of its exact course, the effect of bilateral pedicle fracture is to separate an anterior fragment (primarily the body, which bears the atlas and the head) from a posterior fragment (primarily the arch, which is linked through

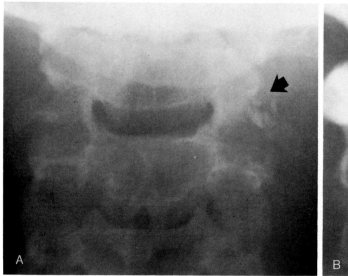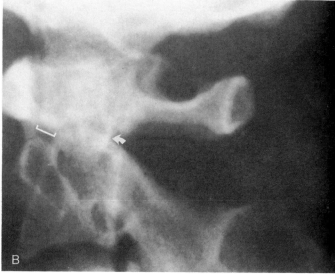

FIGURE 6–21. Fractures of the Dens and the Left Transverse Process of C2 in an Adult Male
• • • •

A, An anteroposterior (AP) view. A transverse process fracture (arrow) is shown. B, A lateral view. Anterior displacement (angled bracket) and slight anterior angulation of the dens, with a fracture gap visible posteriorly (arrow). The anterior contour of the C2 body is probably explained by rotation. No AP open-mouth view or computed tomography view was available.

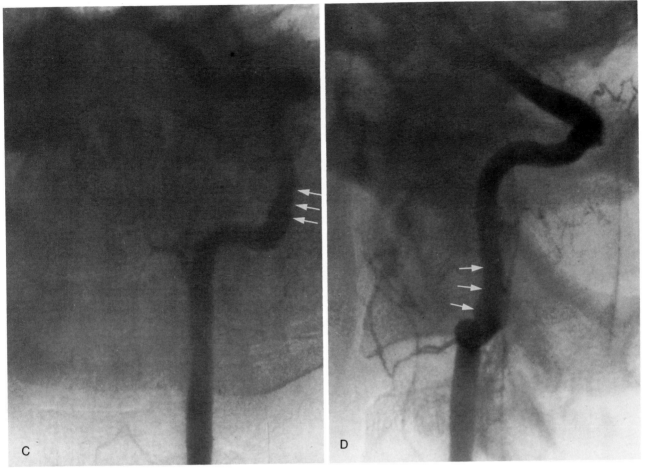

FIGURE 6–21 *Continued* **Fractures of the Dens and the Left Transverse Process of C2 in an Adult Male**

• • • •

C and *D*, This angiogram shows caliber irregularities in a segment of the left vertebral artery near the transverse process *(arrows).*

the facet joints with the rest of the spine). This separation is analogous to the lumbar isthmic spondylolysis, although the fracture sites are not homologous.

Effendi and associates[25] have classified ring fractures by the type of C2–3 displacement. Type I consists of bilateral, or rarely unilateral (Fig. 6–22), pedicle fracture without displacement. These comprised 65% of their series and were stable. Type II includes C2–3 disc damage and displacement of the body of C2, which may be in flexed, neutral, or extended angulation with C3 (Fig. 6–23). These are potentially unstable. Type III is a marked flexion angulation complicated by unilateral or by bilateral C2–3 facet locking and is unstable. These injuries are most commonly caused by compressive hyperextension but can also result from hyperflexion. Levine and Edwards[69] added a fourth group, called Type IIa, which is characterized by anterior angulation hinging on the anterior longitudinal ligament without anterior displacement (Fig. 6–24). Whereas

extension is considered the dominant mechanism in the majority of hangman's fractures, flexion is implicated as the primary mechanism in Types IIa and III and as a secondary mechanism in Type II.[69]

When uncomplicated, ring fractures tend to preserve or widen the spinal canal. But the advanced types of hangman's fracture are readily complicated and are common in traffic fatalities.[11] The judicial "hangman's fracture" is complicated by lethal distraction and angulation of the cord.[41, 100, 122]

The neural arch of C2 is otherwise similar to those of the lower cervical vertebrae except for its higher location and its stouter architecture and is subject to the same injuries (see Fig. 6–15).

AXIS BODY AND TRANSVERSE PROCESS FRACTURES

The articular plateau can be crushed unilaterally by a vertical compressive force that is biased to one side at C1–2 (Fig. 6–25; see also Fig. 6–19). This may

Text continued on page 213

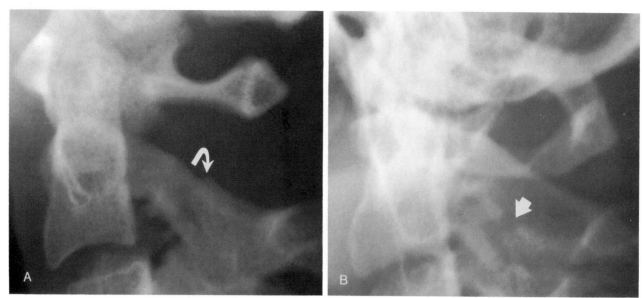

FIGURE 6–22. Unilateral Hangman's Fracture in a 30-Year-Old Woman
• • • •
A, A well-positioned lateral view barely shows the fracture with a broad gap and a single visible posterior margin *(arrow).*
B, This tilted view separates the laminae (the lower one with the fracture *[arrow],* and the upper one that is intact).

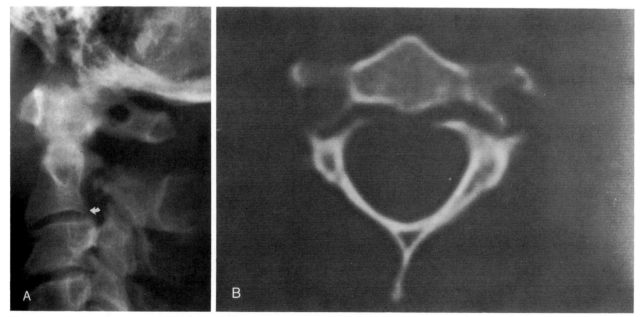

FIGURE 6–23. Benign Type II Hangman's Fracture in a 60-Year-Old Man with Neck Stiffness 5 Days After an Assault
• • • •
A, A true lateral view. Bilateral symmetric pedicle fractures with superimposed cortical interruptions are shown. Bilaterality is also implied by anterolisthesis *(arrow). B,* This computed tomography scan shows the extension of the fracture planes into the posterior body cortex.

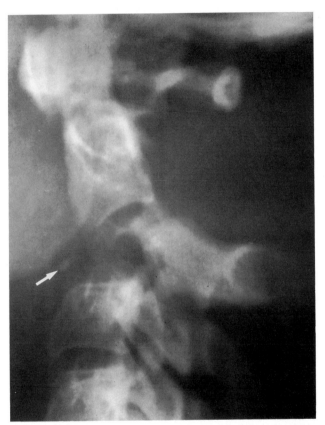

FIGURE 6–24. Fatal Type II (IIa?) Hangman's Fracture in a 30-Year-Old Woman

• • • •

Marked angulation and longitudinal distraction are visible. A lack of anterior displacement would suggest reclassification as Type IIa, but with the anteroinferior avulsion *(arrow)* and the distraction, the anterior longitudinal ligament must be ruptured. The mechanism was probably hyperextension followed by flexion (Type II).

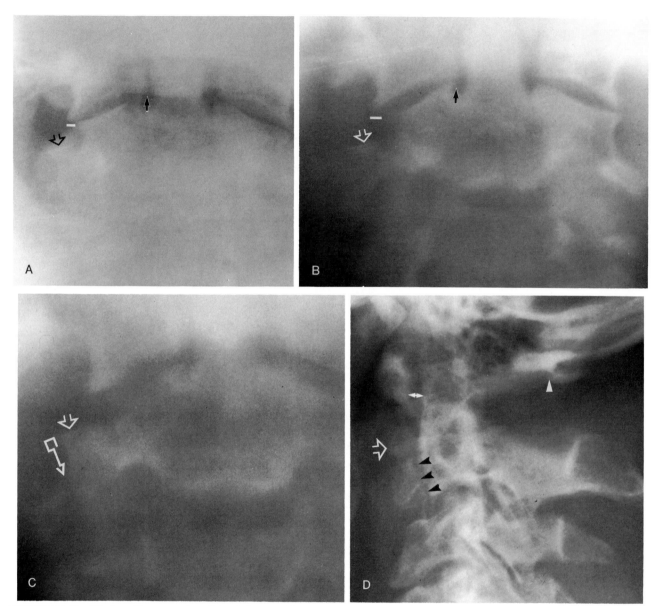

FIGURE 6–25. Flexion-Compression C1–2 Injury with Fractures of the Articular Plateau, Lower Body, and Transverse Process of C2, and C1–2 Subluxation in an 80-Year-Old Man

• • • •

A, An anteroposterior (AP) open-mouth view. *B* and *C*, AP tomograms. An apparent "supernumerary" right articular facet on C2 *(open arrows)* is shown. False lateral offset of C1 *(white bar)* without lateral displacement of the medial tubercle *(small arrow)* is present. The small medial spur in *B* indicates that the apparent slight medial offset is normal and that the asymmetry of widths of the lateral atlantodental intervals is developmental. Note the transverse process fracture *(box arrow)* in *C. D*, A plain lateral view. An anteroinferiorly displaced plateau fragment *(open arrow)* is visible. The diagonal anteroinferior body fracture *(arrowheads)* resembles an extension teardrop, but in this compression injury it must be a shear avulsion due to a flexion component (possibly a C2 "flexion-teardrop"). The atlanto-dens interval *(double-headed arrow)*, difficult to define precisely, measured at least 3 mm on the film. The C1 inner laminar line *(white arrowhead)* is anteriorly displaced.

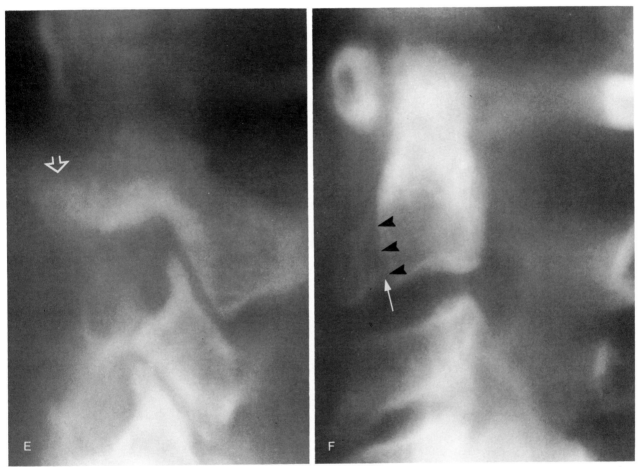

FIGURE 6–25 *Continued* **Flexion-Compression C1–2 Injury with Fractures of the Articular Plateau, Lower Body, and Transverse Process of C2, and C1–2 Subluxation in an 80-Year-Old Man**

• • • •

E, A right lateral tomogram. The anteroinferiorly displaced plateau fragment *(open arrow)* is shown. *F*, A midline lateral tomogram. Slight upward displacement of the anteroinferior fragment suggests upward shear due to flexion-compression (similar to the flexion-teardrop mechanism, although no retrolisthesis is evident). C1–2 subluxation, if acute, would support the flexion mechanism.

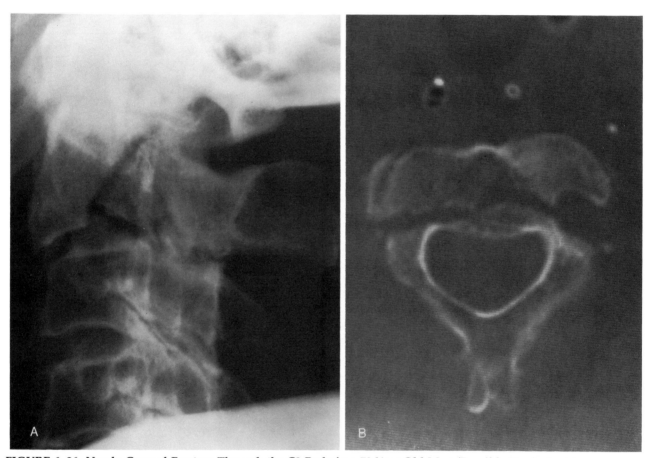

FIGURE 6–26. Nearly Coronal Fracture Through the C2 Body in a 78-Year-Old Man (Possibly Equivalent to a Hangman's Fracture)

• • • •

Effective spondylolisthesis is shown by anterior displacement of the posterior C1 arch with a normal atlanto-dens interval (ADI) and an atraumatic dens. (The ADI is not discernible on reproduction, but the anterior arch is appropriately aligned with the anterior margin of the C2 body in *A*; a 1.5-mm high-resolution computed tomography scan showed normal ADI and arthritic changes of the dens.) Note the extension of the fracture to the vertebral artery canal in *B* (lower sections showed extension also to the right canal).

accompany a crush injury of the impacting C1 lateral mass. The articular surface appears irregular on an AP open-mouth view, whereas CT scans may show more extensive fine fracture lines in the upper lateral C2 body that extend into the transverse process. The small C2 transverse process is seldom broken in isolation. C2 is the level of the most intimate involvement of the vertebral artery with the vertebrae, as the transverse foramen lies partly within the lateral portion of the body under the plateau. Plateau fractures with or without specific (or visible) transverse process fracture may injure this artery, or associated hematoma may narrow it (see Fig. 6–21).

Other fractures of the C2 body include Type III odontoid fractures, variants of the hangman's fracture that pass broadly through the body (Fig. 6–26) or separate its posteroinferior margin, and anteroinferior margin fractures (Fig. 6–27; see also Figs. 6–3A, 6–24, and 6–25). The latter are discussed in the following section on the lower cervical spine.

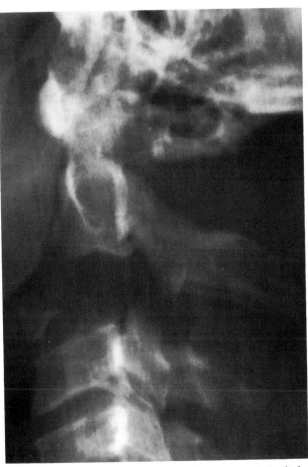

FIGURE 6–27. Extension Teardrop Fracture with Lethal C2–3 Longitudinal Distraction in a 43-Year-Old Man

• • • •

• • • •
LOWER CERVICAL SPINE

Structural and Radiologic Anatomy

The lower cervical spine comprises the five "typical" cervical vertebrae, the six "typical" motion segments from C2–3 through C7–T1, and associated structures. There are a number of practical anatomic considerations peculiar to the lower cervical spine that are important to ensure an adequate examination and an accurate description.

The "uncovertebral (uncinate) joint" or "neurocentral lip articulation"[2] of Luschka occurs only at the lower cervical articulations, from C2–3 through C7–T1. Von Luschka's original description of these as synovial joints is controversial. Each consists of a lateral or a posterolateral ridge rising from a superior end plate and a complementary bevel on the inferior end plate above. The disc annulus is excluded from the intervening gap, which is filled by loose fibrous tissue and blood vessels in the fetus and later develops a cleft filled with serum transudate that can simulate a synovial space.[51, 78, 90] The process and the joint space are oriented almost sagittally from C2–3 through C5–6 but become more oblique at C6–7 and C7–T1.

Vertebra prominens is a name applied to C7 because its spinous process is the one felt most prominently at the base of the neck. It is almost as long and as thick as that of T1, but it tapers to a smaller tubercle. The C6 spinous process has the most variable length, sometimes barely longer than that of C5 and sometimes closer in length to that of C7. The spinous processes of C3, C4, and C5 are about the same size and are shorter and less massive than that of C2.

In the AP projection C7 is distinguished from T1 by its usual lack of ribs and by the downward slope and rounded or pointed ends of its smaller transverse processes. The transverse processes of T1 are more rectangular and slope upward. On AP projections, the relation of the first ribs with the vertebrae can be confusing. The transverse processes are easier to use as landmarks. Even when cervical ribs are well developed and the C7 transverse processes are unusually prominent, they project laterally rather than superolaterally and are thinner than those of T1. Direct identification of C7 and T1 on the AP film may be helpful because the mandible can prevent reliable counting downward from C2 (Fig. 6–28).

Another distinction among the lower cervical vertebrae occurs in the sagittal profile of the articular pillar. The pillars of C3 through C6 have outlines that are basically parallelograms (extending an im-

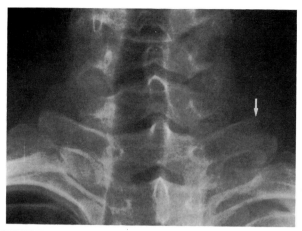

FIGURE 6–28. T1 Transverse Process Fracture in a 27-Year-Old Man

• • • •

Fracture margins *(arrow)* are not corticated. The distal fragment is inferiorly displaced (with the first rib), unlike the normal location of an unfused apophysis.

aginary line across the junction with the pedicle as part of the outline). This contour absorbs the equivalent of the lumbar pars interarticularis into the stout pillar and places each superior facet directly above the inferior. The C7 pillars have a more complex shape with a posterosuperior concavity producing a subtle isthmus that suggests a pars interarticularis as the inferior facets "reach" backward to articulate with the superior facets of T1 (see Figs. 6–1, 6–2, 6–44C, 6–49, and 6–50B). Smaller posterosuperior concavities may occur on the higher pillars, most often C6. The "stretched" C7 pillar can be visualized on an adequate lateral film or, frequently without the apparent concavity, on MR images (see Fig. 6–53J), but the reader should preferably count from above and should not be misled if the C6 pillar approaches this shape.

Recognition of the transition from C7 to T1 on axial sections is the only way to be certain of adequate coverage on CT scans. The lateral localizer may not show the lowest cervical vertebrae through the shoulders, or the patient may move and invalidate the section lines on the localizer. The ribs can be confusing, but even with well-developed cervical ribs the difference in the shapes and the slopes of the transverse processes can be appreciated across several adjacent sections. With a cooperative patient it is possible to count the vertebrae from above if the scan begins at least as high as C3–4 and continues through C7–T1. The C2–3 level is recognizable by the more nearly round shape of the inferior end plate of C2 compared with all other cervical end plates and by

the unusually broad C2 spinous process that may be seen overhanging C3 even if the C2–3 disc is excluded from the scan.

MR imaging on a cooperative patient obviates many of the problems of visualization at the cervicothoracic junction. Accurate counting of the vertebrae usually depends on including and recognizing C2 or the skull base.

Analysis of Films

Lateral Film

The heights and the proportions of the vertebral bodies are evaluated primarily on the lateral film. The majority of the vertebrae serve as "normal controls." There should not be a sudden discrepancy in height or shape. An exception to this rule is that C3, C4, or C5 can have a "wilted" profile, with smooth concavity of three or all four sides, that may differ distinctly from that of an adjacent vertebra. Even with this profile the differences in anterior and in posterior height among the vertebrae should be minimal.

The four corners of each vertebral body must be inspected for avulsions. The common mimics are osteophytes, ossifications in ligaments and annuli (Fig. 6–29), and ring apophyses (see Figs. 6–1 and 6–2). Osteophytosis makes the vertebral margins harder to evaluate for trauma. A degenerative ossification can simulate a chip fracture, possibly even with a simulated donor site. Ring apophyses are usually seen at the inferior end plates of multiple vertebrae and indicate their normality. However, avulsion of a portion of a ring apophysis, with abnormal angulation and displacement, is a significant fracture.

Normally the spinal canal in the lateral projection is bounded by the posterior vertebral body and disc margins and by the laminae. The laminae are usually visible only at their midline junction at the base of the spinous process as an "inner laminar" or "spinolaminar" line. In spinal cord or root injury, any abnormal spinal canal boundaries are relevant. Osteophytes and ligamentous ossifications narrow the spinal canal and may be accompanied by unossified disc protrusion and by flaval ligament hypertrophy or buckling.

Congenital or degenerative stenosis can cause neurologic injury in trauma without a cervical fracture or dislocation. The AP diameter of the cervical spinal canal, between the posterior vertebral body surfaces at the midvertebral levels and the spinolaminar lines, normally approximates the midvertebral body diameter, which is usually about 18.0 mm. A ratio of less

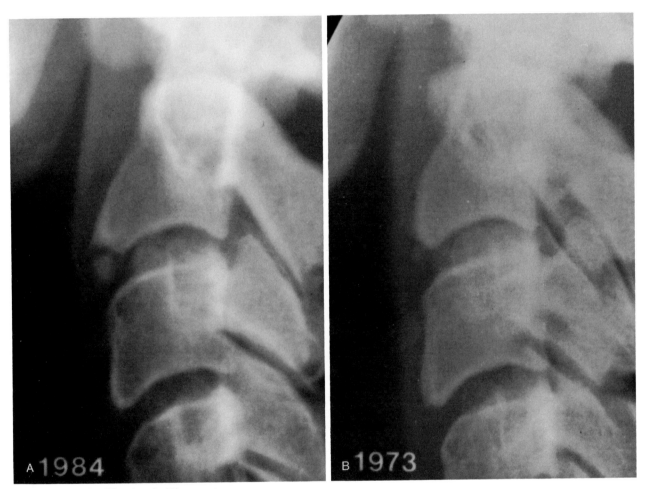

FIGURE 6–29. Ossification in Ligaments

• • • •

A, Degenerative ossification simulating a hyperextension avulsion in a 54-year-old man. Note the simulation of the donor site (by the cortical spur or the anterior longitudinal ligament ossification) and of the anterior rotation of the fragment (common with hyperextension avulsion). However, the hypothetic fracture margins are not congruent or matched in length. *B,* Ossification had begun 9 years earlier. (Trauma might still have been an initiating factor.)

than 80–82% is stenotic.[82, 112] In a true lateral projection the pillars should project entirely over the spinal canal, and both posterior pillar lines should project a few millimeters anterior to the spinolaminar lines. In congenital stenosis, flattening of the laminae projects the spinolaminar lines close to the posterior pillar lines, and short, widely spread pedicles project the anterior pillar lines over the vertebral bodies. Degenerative stenosis results from osteophytes, disc protrusions, and flaval ligament thickening.

The five principal vertical alignments in the lateral view of the lower cervical spine involve the anterior and the posterior vertebral body cortices, the two columns of pillars, and the spinolaminar lines. Their evaluation depends on comparison throughout the cervical spine, allowing for the AP slope of the cervical spine at the given level (see Figs. 6–1 and 6–2). They are not obscured by moderate craniocaudal beam angulation or by scoliosis.

The anterior and the posterior cortices of the vertebral bodies are the most nearly vertical and join with the end plates at distinct angles. The anterior cortex often curves posteroinferiorly slightly above its junction with the inferior end plate. The longitudinal alignments based on the positions of these angles are usually precise to within 1.0–2.0 mm. Experienced evaluation is essential in the presence of osteophytes or normal juvenile laxity. With spondylosis, the alignment becomes less precise, often by different amounts at different levels, without signifying injury or clinical instability. Yet an anterolisthesis of two to several millimeters is sometimes the most visible sign of a fracture or a dislocation involving the facet-pillar-pedicle complex. A retrolisthesis without degenerative changes suggests a serious injury, either by a flexion-compression mechanism (see Figs. 6–33B, 6–34B, and 6–35B) or by hyperextension dislocation (see Specific Injury Components and Patterns, Injuries of the Vertebral Bodies and the Discs, Acute Disc Injury). A burst fracture can displace the anterior cortex anteriorly and the posterior cortex posteriorly without obvious compression (see Figs. 6–3B and 6–31B).

The normal cervical lordosis is so variable that its loss has limited meaning. A smooth or slightly angulated kyphosis can occur normally in the supine or the standing position with the chin tucked (military position). The angle between two vertebrae can be measured using any comparable landmarks, usually the inferior end plates. A difference of more than 11 degrees between the intervertebral angle at the motion segment in question and that of either of the adjacent motion segments is abnormal.[118] Focally decreased lordosis or increased kyphosis of this de-

gree indicates a hyperflexion sprain either in isolation or as a component of a more extensive flexion injury. Focally increased lordosis indicates hyperextensive anterior ligament disruption. Sometimes an angular difference of less than 11 degrees is suspicious and merits investigation with flexion-extension films.

In studying the pillars, the superposition of right and left is very useful. Asymmetry of the pillars is suspicious, but even an excellent lateral film does not necessarily superimpose exactly the cortical lines of a symmetric pair of pillars. Beware of an apparently perfect superposition; sometimes there is such a marked degree of pathologic rotation at a motion segment that the pillars on one side above this level have rotated forward and have become superimposed on the vertebral bodies, where they are not noticed. The lateral film must be reasonably lateral, and both posterior pillar lines at each level must be visible within very few millimeters of each other. The horizontal distance between these two lines for each vertebra must not change much from one vertebra to the next; changes that are present must progress smoothly along the length of the cervical spine. Small changes in this distance indicate minor degrees of rotation without definite significance, but an abrupt change suggests an injury to the facet-pillar-pedicle complex.

The fully imbricated, diagonally oriented facet joint surfaces are highly characteristic, although they vary in their visibility depending on tilt and rotation. Superposition of the two sides is sometimes confusingly out-of-phase vertically, but even if the two pillar columns are hard to separate and the joint planes are hard to count, they still assist in the evaluation of rotation. The "stacks" of these two columns of diagonal joint planes should align vertically and be superimposed on the spinal canal or, in spinal stenosis, be partially superimposed on the vertebral bodies. If facet joint planes suddenly are fully superimposed on the vertebral bodies above or below a motion segment, a facet injury is present (usually a unilateral facet dislocation) at that motion segment. In slightly rotated projections, the two joint spaces at each level, or at least three of the four cortical facet lines, should be visible. At each level the joint planes are almost always parallel to each other.

The curved spinolaminar line is the anterior cortex of the midline junction of the laminae. Except for the normal 1.0–2.0-mm deviation at C1–2, the spinolaminar lines are arranged in a smooth curve that serves as a guide to the normal alignment of the laminae and the spinous processes in the lateral projection. Each individual line is slanted so that if it were extended it would be imbricated with its neighbors (see Figs. 6–1 and 6–2). This "near-imbrication" is exaggerated by a retrolisthesis and diminished or reversed by an anterolisthesis unless the arch is avulsed. Isolated reversal at a motion segment without vertebral body anterolisthesis suggests a flexion injury with avulsion of the caudal spinous process and portions of the laminae (see Fig. 6–39A).

Anteroposterior Film

The AP projection provides limited information about the vertebral body. Lateral wedging or other end plate irregularities, an uncinate process fracture or uncovertebral joint widening, interuncinate widening, and lucencies overlying the vertebral bodies that are not part of the laryngotracheal airway should be sought. The oblique cervical pedicles are not seen precisely, but the medial pillar cortex at the pedicle-lamina junction may (see Figs. 6–32A and 6–33A) or may not (see Figs. 6–34A and 6–35A) be visualized to permit an estimation of "interpediculate" widening.

The vertebral body component visualized as a rectangle on the AP view is primarily the posterior surface. This can appear normal even after fairly marked anterior wedging. Because of the anteroposterior curvatures of the end plates and the posterior fanning of the AP x-ray beam, few if any end plates are profiled, especially in a normally lordotic cervical spine. Horizontal "end plate" lines are more likely end plate margins, and they may reflect body fractures (see Fig. 6–34A).

Lucent clefts may be superimposed on but distinguishable from the airway. Midline vertical clefts, whether sharp and thin or wide and irregular, indicate sagittal or flexion-teardrop fractures (see Figs. 6–32A, 6–33A, 6–34A, and 6–35A). Parasagittal clefts, especially if paired, suggest the borders of a retro-displaced burst fragment (see Fig. 6–31A). An inverted "V" lucency centered in the midline indicates a fracture at the base of the spinous process through the laminae (see Figs. 6–56A and 6–57A).

The articular pillars must be examined in AP projection. The lateral pillar margins should form smoothly undulating lines that are bilaterally symmetric and reasonably uniform from level to level. A sharp angulation or the shortening of a segment of this undulation indicates a pillar or facet fracture. A concordant jog of both undulating lines to one side indicates a facet subluxation or dislocation, with or without fracture (see Fig. 6–44), unless there is degenerative laxity. A unilateral or bilateral outward jog indicates either a pillar fracture or, with "inter-

pediculate" and interuncinate widening, a comminuted burst fracture or a sagittal fracture (see Figs. 6–32A, 6–33A, 6–34A, and 6–35A). The transverse processes should be inspected, including T1 (see Fig. 6–28).

Specific Injury Components and Patterns

Injuries of the Vertebral Bodies and the Discs

There is considerable overlap of the morphologic, the mechanistic, and the clinical features among the variously named vertebral body fractures. The key anatomic distinctions to be made radiologically concern (1) whether the posterior vertebral body surface is involved and, if so, whether this is by a sagittal fracture or by multiple fracture lines isolating a comminuted burst fragment, (2) whether the spinal canal is narrowed by vertebral body encroachment and, if so, whether this is by a central comminuted fragment ("piston stenosis") or by the entire posterior vertebral body with respect to the next higher or lower vertebral lamina ("shearing stenosis"), and (3) whether the neural arch is involved and, if so, whether primarily by fracture or by distractive disruption of the posterior ligamentous complex. Although these characteristics could distinguish many different injury complexes, only three or four categories are usually recognized as major entities. Neurologic involvement is not a component of the definitions of these morphologic entities, despite its historical importance in the development of this classification and its correlation with certain features of these injuries.

CT has made these anatomic distinctions much easier, so that some of the descriptive vagueness and omissions in the literature can be improved upon by our present diagnostic capability. However, considerable inconsistency and some genuine uncertainty remain regarding conceptual matters such as definitions and mechanisms. The terms "wedge" and "compression" are most commonly applied to fractures that do not disrupt the posterior wall of the vertebral body. But "compression" is a particularly ambiguous term that also describes (1) a force component present throughout this family of injuries and (2) chronic fractures due to osteoporosis, infection, or neoplasm that sometimes do disrupt the posterior vertebral body surface. Posterior body disruption is a neurologically damaging feature in "burst," "sagittal," and "flexion-teardrop" fractures. But any of these fractures, especially the flexion-teardrop fractures, can have a "wedge" component in its appearance. In traumatology, three categories are most useful: the "wedge compression" or simply "wedge" fracture, which does not have posterior surface involvement; the "burst" fracture, which has random comminution; and the "flexion-teardrop" or simply "teardrop" fracture. A fourth, partial category that overlaps the latter two (especially the last) is the "sagittal" fracture.

WEDGE FRACTURE

The wedge fracture assumes this configuration in the lateral view apparently because the compressive strain is concentrated anteriorly, perhaps either by a preceding flexion of the neck or by greater resistance of the posterior portions of the vertebra. The posterior vertebral body wall remains intact and the spinal canal and the neural foramina are not narrowed or contiguous to fractures. Clinical stability is usual because of preservation of the posterior longitudinal ligament, the posterior annulus and disc, and the posterior two thirds of the vertebra. Reciprocal disruption of the posterior ligamentous complex can occur, become reduced and inapparent on the lateral film, and produce delayed instability.[47]

Diagnosis may be possible initially only on the lateral film because the wedging can be difficult to detect on oblique views and impossible to see or infer on the AP film. The spinous processes may be spread apart on the AP as well as on the lateral views, but the variations of their lengths and shapes can make AP interpretation of interspinous distances unreliable. Careful inspection of all films and the performance of CT are essential because many fractures with wedging are more complex, having burst and arch components (Fig. 6–30), whereas pure wedge fractures are not common.

In both acute and old traumatic wedge fractures, usually only the superior end plate and the anterosuperior trabecular portion of the body collapse, whereas the inferior half of the vertebra appears normal. In other pathologic forms of collapse, the process tends to span the height of the body more uniformly. Pre-existing neoplastic collapse can present clinically after minor trauma. Careful inspection of the regions of the pedicles, optimally on oblique views but often on the AP film, may show the lytic process.

Lateral wedging is unilateral or very asymmetric compression of the right or the left side of the

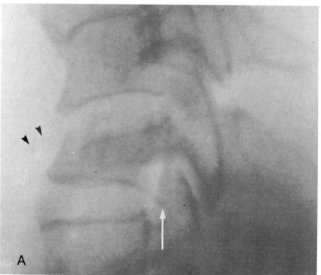 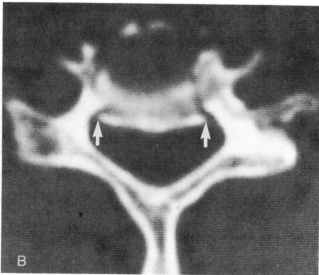

FIGURE 6–30. Wedge-like Burst Fracture of C6 in a 52-Year-Old Man Who Hit the Back of His Head in a Fall and Was Briefly Paralyzed

• • • •

A, An overpenetrated lateral film reversed on a subtraction film. The shape of C6, with its anterior superior end plate collapse, resembles a wedge compression fracture. The anterior end plate rim is avulsed and thrust forward (shown faintly at the arrowheads and partially obscured by white artifacts). A vertical gas-like overlay (possibly an artifact) extending posteroinferiorly across the C6–7 disc is unexplained because computed tomography (CT) was performed a day later. The retrodisplaced posterior C6 vertebral margin *(arrow)* and the interruption of the inferior end plate indicate the retrodisplaced burst fragment. *B,* This CT scan at the top of C6 shows a typical, broad, piston-like fragment bounded by sagittal-plane fracture lines *(arrows)* at the medial bases of the pedicles.

vertebral body. Careful assessment of vertebral body symmetry on the AP view is required because no discrete fracture lines may be visible. Contralateral lateral flexion injuries, such as distraction[92] and perhaps a transverse process fracture, may be found. The diagnosis must lead to a search for other injuries because this fracture usually occurs as a component of predominantly hyperextension or flexion injuries.[34]

BURST FRACTURE

Burst fractures result from direct axial compression that shatters the vertebral body, including its posterior wall (see Figs. 6–3 and 6–30). There is typically a chaotic pattern of seemingly randomly arrayed fracture lines through the vertebral body. Some component of transverse spreading, absent in wedge fractures, is present in burst fractures and may be apparent as "interpediculate" and interuncinate widening on the AP film. This spreading usually causes arch fractures.

A burst fracture may be detected on the lateral film by AP expansion or vertical compression of the vertebral body (Fig. 6–31B; see also Fig. 6–3C) or by changes at the vertebral margins (see Fig. 6–30A). Some of the random fracture lines may be visible within the body (see Fig. 6–31A). A retropulsed ("piston") fragment may be seen with its cortex still parallel to its normal orientation (see Figs. 6–30 and 6–31), but the displaced fragment may be small or rotated or the films may be rotated; in such cases lateral tomography or preferably CT is required for detection. Maximum fragment displacement during the peak traumatic deformation is not demonstrated on the CT scan; therefore, the neurologic deficit may be disproportionate to the visible narrowing. Complete and incomplete (central[75, 98] or anterior[73]) cord syndromes are common. The posterior longitudinal ligament may retain enough integrity to pull the fragment partially back into place with the immediate rebound or in traction. Burst fractures have sometimes been classified as stable owing to preserved posterior support, but many are clinically unstable and should be regarded as such until proved to be otherwise.

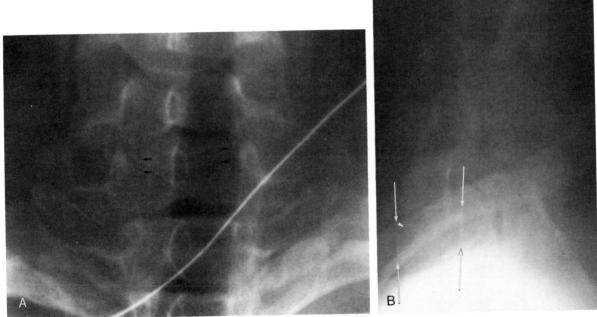

FIGURE 6–31. C7 Burst Fracture and a C6 Sagittal Fracture in an 18-Year-Old Man

••••

A, This anteroposterior film shows vertical lucencies *(arrowheads)* overlying lateral portions of the C7 body, suggesting the presence of a "piston" fragment in a burst fracture (see *E* and *F*). *B,* This suboptimal swimmer's view faintly shows outwardly displaced cortical lines (between the opposing arrows), mainly posteriorly, confirming the burst fracture. The C6–7 disc is narrow (see *D*). The posteroinferior displacement of the anterosuperior body margin *(arrowhead;* see *F)* suggests a flexion component.

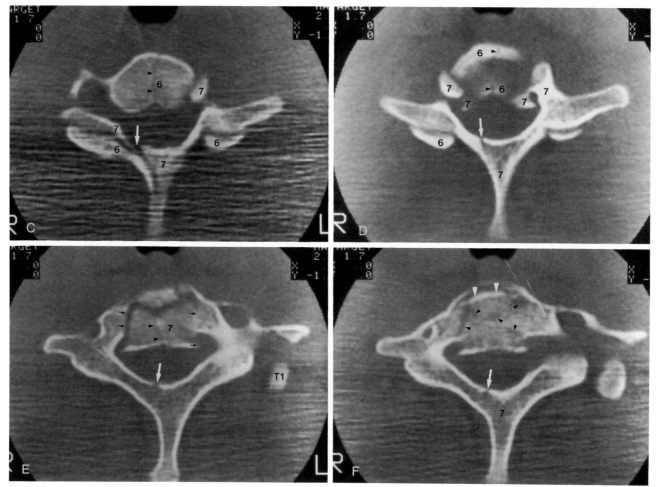

FIGURE 6–31 *Continued* **C7 Burst Fracture and a C6 Sagittal Fracture in an 18-Year-Old Man**

• • • •

C–F, High-resolution 1.5-mm computed tomography sections.

C, The lower level of C6 has an undisplaced sagittal fracture *(arrowheads)* that is not suggested on the films. A lamina fracture *(arrow)* is in C7, and the left uncovertebral joint is widened by C7 spreading. C6 has no evidence of an arch fracture, and its sagittal fracture is limited to the lower four sections through C6. This compression injury is probably related to the gaping, flexion type of sagittal fracture only in name and orientation, despite evidence of a flexion component present here as well (in *B* and *F*). *D,* Substantial portions of the C6 and C7 end plates are volume-averaged into this 1.5-mm section, confirming disc narrowing (see *B*). The C6 sagittal fracture *(arrowheads)* may have resulted from the disc being driven against C6 (i.e., *nuclear intrusion,* one hypothesis to explain sagittal fractures), or from tension created by the transverse spreading of C7, which is consistent with the C7 lamina fracture *(arrow)*. *E,* Random comminution with a displaced "piston" fragment bounded by nearly parasagittal fracture lines *(black arrows; see A)* is shown. The vertical cortical defect in the right lamina *(white arrow)* continues downward. An undisplaced sagittal fracture *(arrowheads)* within the "piston" (also on the next two higher sections, which are not shown) matches the C6 fracture; therefore, explanation by the nuclear intrusion hypothesis is favored in this instance. *F,* This C7 section shows the central "piston," a posteriorly displaced upper anterior cortex *(white arrowheads; see B),* irregular intrabody fracture lines *(black arrowheads),* and a faint lamina fracture *(arrow)*.

FLEXION-TEARDROP FRACTURE

A vertebral body compression with a large anteroinferior or anterior fragment generally results from flexion and is called a *flexion-teardrop fracture* or a *fracture-dislocation* (Figs. 6–32 to 6–34). The term "teardrop" refers less to the shape of the separated fragment than to the prognosis of the cord injury present in most cases.[99] This mechanistic morphologic entity was first described in connection with the anterior cord syndrome,[97, 99] but complete tetraplegia, the central cord syndrome, paraplegia, the Brown-Séquard syndrome, and an absence of any neurologic deficit have also been reported.[67] Conversely, the fundamental injury components, including an anterior cord syndrome, have resulted from the same basic mechanism even without formation of an anterior fragment.[97, 99]

The teardrop fragment can be sheared off as the vertebra is pressed in flexion against the one below ("shearing avulsion") or can be excised by the anteroinferior margin of the vertebra above. The anterior fragment need not be partially rounded like a teardrop. It may be triangular or rectangular, comminuted or highly irregular, or not visible as fully separated from the major portion of the body. The greatest compression may be in the most anterior portion or in the anterior middle portion of the vertebra.

This injury is really a fracture-dislocation because it produces a retrodisplacement of the posteroinferior vertebral body margin, either exclusively or to a

Text continued on page 228

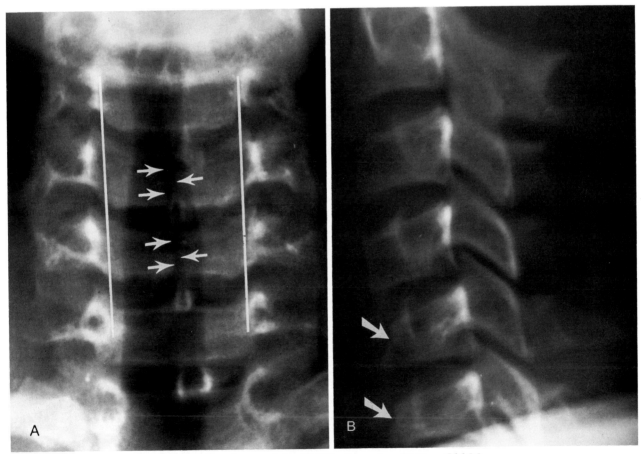

FIGURE 6–32. Double-Level Flexion-Teardrop and Sagittal Fractures in a 16-Year-Old Man

• • • •

A, This anteroposterior (AP) film shows sagittal fractures superimposed on the airway at C5 and C6 *(arrows)*. Widening of the interpediculate and interuncinate distances is indicated by lateral deviations at C5 and C6 on the right. *B,* This lateral film shows small flexion-teardrop fragments at the anteroinferior C5 and C6 margins *(arrows)* and mildly wedged bodies. The anterosuperior margin of C5 has been driven posteriorly as well. There is no obvious violation of the spinal canal, but the posterior C5 and C6 body margins have lost their normal concavities.

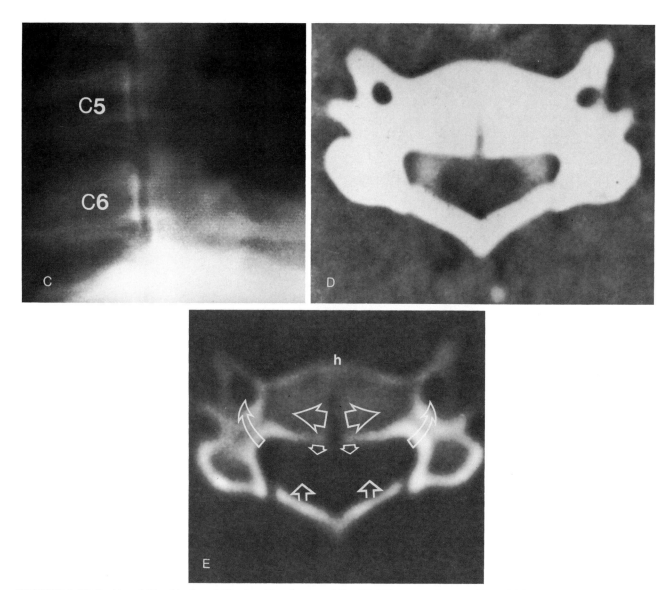

FIGURE 6–32 *Continued* **Double-Level Flexion-Teardrop and Sagittal Fractures in a 16-Year-Old Man**

• • • •

C, A lateral myelographic film shows an effaced ventral subarachnoid space at C5 and C6, due to a yet unexplained fullness or retrodisplacement of the posterior vertebral body contours. *D*, This computed tomography section shows a widened spinal cord filling the AP diameter of the canal and containing a right ventrolateral density, which is suspicious for blood or a contrast material in a contusion. The wider posterior part of a sagittal fracture is visible. *E*, A bone window of same section shows a sagittal fracture gaping posteriorly, but the fracture is closed and apparently "hinged" anteriorly *(h)*. Bilateral laminar fractures have separated the entire laminar complex from the pillars. The hypothesized mechanism includes an earlier stage during which vertical tension on interlaminar ligaments during flexion pulls the unfractured laminae forward, widens the obtuse interlaminar angle, pushes the pillars apart, and rips the vertebral body open from behind. With continued displacements in the directions indicated *(open arrows)*, the flattened laminae are broken by the angular strain at their junctions with the pillars; this frees the laminar complex to sink into the flexed spinal canal and compress the cord against the protruding posterior margins of the sagittal fracture. Tissue relaxation following maximum injury displacement can restore structures nearly to normal locations (as seen on imaging).

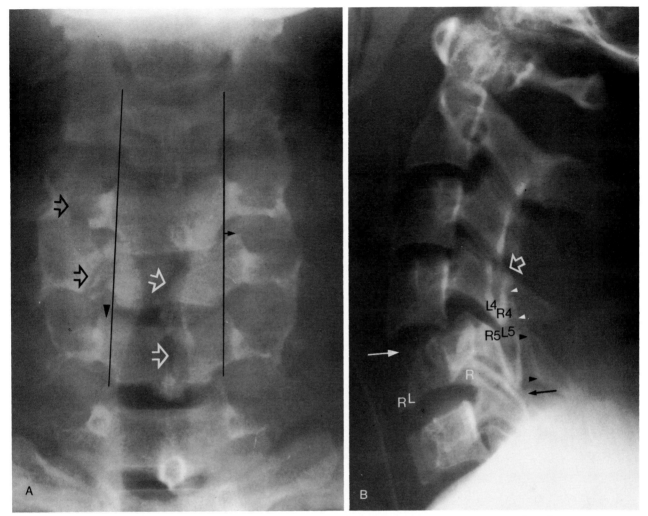

FIGURE 6–33. Complex Multivertebral Fracture-Dislocation Including Flexion-Teardrop, Sagittal Body, Transverse Process, Pedicle, Pillar, Facet Margin, Lamina, and Sagittal Spinous Process Fractures as Well as Unilateral Facet Dislocation in a 22-Year-Old Man

• • • •

This case is a microcosm of almost every major class of lower cervical spine fracture except wedge-compression, comminuted burst, and clay-shoveler's fractures. *A,* This anteroposterior film shows the increased width of three vertebrae (C4–C6). Coarse vertical lucent bands *(black open arrows)* through C4 and C5 indicate pillar/pedicle fractures. Delicate vertical lucencies *(white open arrows)* through the bodies of C5 and C6 superimposed on the airway indicate sagittal fractures. "Interpediculate" widening and deviations of the left C5 *(small arrow)* and right C6 *(arrowhead)* uncinate processes (compared with the vertical lines aligning the other uncinate processes) confirm the component of spreading due to the sagittal fractures and not attributable to the pillar/pedicle fractures. *B,* This lateral film shows a flexion-teardrop fracture-dislocation of C5. A pair of teardrop fragments (anterior *R* and *L*) is present. (Right-left determinations required computed tomography [CT].) The overall anterior C5 vertebral body height (the anterosuperior margin is shown faintly at the white arrow) is not reduced compared with the expected height of C5. At the posterior vertebral body margins, C4 anterolisthesis exceeds C5 retrolisthesis, which is the opposite of the usual appearance in flexion-teardrop fractures; this suggests additional C4–5 injury. Correct right-left labeling of the four facets benefited from CT, but the superposition of the parts of the R4 and L5 facet surfaces indicates that they are on opposite sides (crossed obliquity) even without proof by CT. Reversal of the imbrication of the C4 and C5 spinolaminar lines *(arrowheads)* and the crossed obliquity of the C4 and C5 pillars indicate C4–5 facet joint injury. The left C4–5 facet relationship (*L4* and *L5*) indicates that they are at least perched. Approximation of the posterior margin of the right C4 pillar (from the *open arrow* to *R4*) toward the C4 spinolaminar line indicates pillar retrodisplacement and therefore fracture of the right C4 pillar or pedicle. The C3 facets are too far anterior for the deformed and partially naked right superior C4 facet surface *(open arrow)* but not far enough or elevated enough to be jumped; this indicates fracture of at least the C4 facet even though there is no C3–4 body anterolisthesis.

Illustration continued on following page

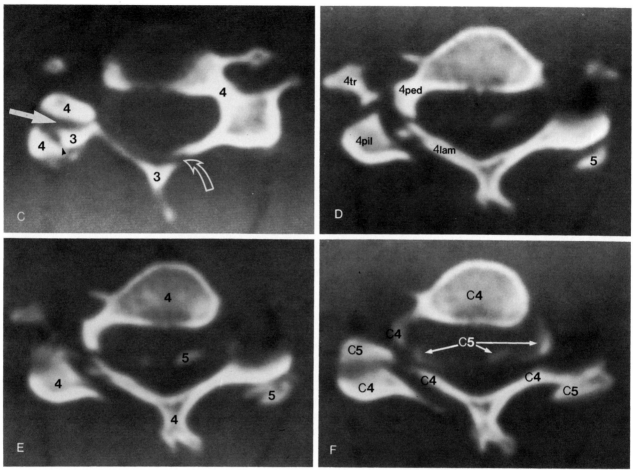

FIGURE 6–33 *Continued* **Complex Multivertebral Fracture-Dislocation Including Flexion-Teardrop, Sagittal Body, Transverse Process, Pedicle, Pillar, Facet Margin, Lamina, and Sagittal Spinous Process Fractures as Well as Unilateral Facet Dislocation in a 22-Year-Old Man**

• • • •

C–J, Selected 1.5-mm CT sections, from cranial to caudal levels. The vertebral fragments are numbered.

C, Most of the right inferior C3 facet has a nearly normal relationship with part of the superior C4 facet, except for slight joint space widening *(solid arrow).* Behind the C3 facet, fragments are displaced upward from the C4 pillar, and the inferolateral margin of C3 is chipped off *(arrowhead).* Note the laminar pseudofracture (interlaminar space) on the left *(open arrow;* compare with *F* and *H*). *D,* A comminuted fracture mutually separates the right C4 transverse process (4tr), pedicle (4ped), pillar (4pil), and lamina (4lam). The *left* inferior C4 facet is dislocated anterior to C5 *(5).* *E,* The left superior C5 facet margin is irregular in this section (it has been chipped). *F,* The back-to-back configuration of a jumped left C4–5 facet joint is shown. The combination of a left unilateral facet dislocation and a right C4 pillar fracture permits marked anterolisthesis (about 50% with respect even to the more "conservative" left half of C5, and much more than in *B*) and shearing stenosis of the spinal canal. Note the oblique fracture of the right C4 lamina (compare with *C* and *H*).

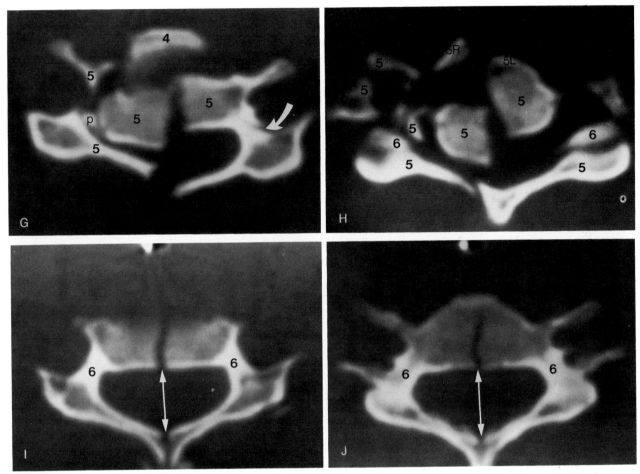

FIGURE 6–33 *Continued* **Complex Multivertebral Fracture-Dislocation Including Flexion-Teardrop, Sagittal Body, Transverse Process, Pedicle, Pillar, Facet Margin, Lamina, and Sagittal Spinous Process Fractures as Well as Unilateral Facet Dislocation in a 22-Year-Old Man**

• • • •

G, This sagittal fracture of C5 gapes widely posteriorly; the right half is fully mobilized. Note the comminuted right pedicle fracture fragment *(p)* and the greenstick left pedicle fracture *(curved arrow)*. The lateral tension fracture of the left pedicle supports the sagittal fracture mechanism described in the text and in Figure 6–32E. Note the unfractured anteroinferior margin of C4, which is not to be mistaken for the common, single, crescentic anteroinferior "teardrop" fragment from a sagittally fractured body. H, The pairing of teardrop fragments *(5R and 5L)* indicates that they formed after the sagittal fracture (compare with Fig. 6–34E). Note the right lamina fracture (compare with C and F) and the comminuted right pedicle and transverse process fractures. I, J, C6 has sagittal body and spinous process fractures *(double-headed arrows)* along its full height, which extend from the spinal canal but remain incomplete peripherally.

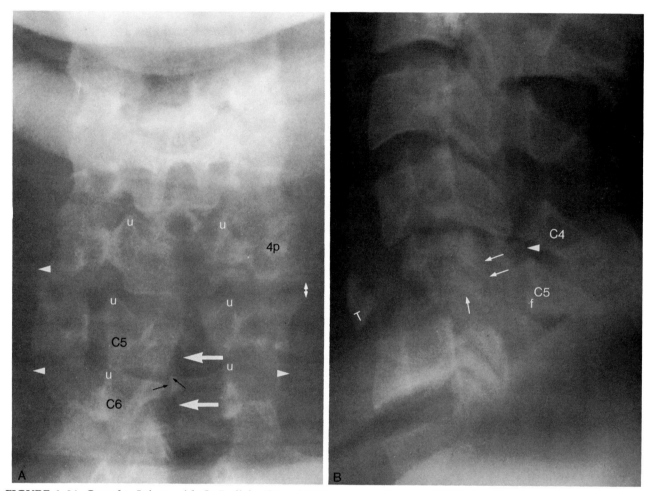

FIGURE 6–34. Complex Injury with C4 Pedicle, C4 and C5 Transverse Process, C5 Flexion-Teardrop, C5 and C6 Sagittal, and C4–C6 Laminar Fractures in a 25-Year-Old Man with Complete Tetraplegia

• • • •

A, This anteroposterior (AP) film shows widening of vertebrae C4–C6. Interuncinate *(u-u)* widening of C5 and C6 is present compared with C4. The widening of C4 is due to a comminuted pedicle fracture visible medial to the pillar *(4p).* C5 is the most widened and has step-offs *(white arrowheads).* The mobilized left C4 pillar is rotated; it does not have adjacent step-offs but does have lateral widening of the C4–5 facet joint *(double-headed arrow).* Sagittal fractures are seen as indistinct lucencies added to the airway *(white arrows)* and as a step-off in the superior C6 end plate *(black arrows).* *B,* A lateral film shows disintegration of the C5 body with a rotated teardrop fragment *(T).* The vague density *(arrows)* superimposed on the anterior spinal canal and the pillars is the retrolisthetic C5 body (fragments). Laminar avulsion is obvious at C4 (it is retrodisplaced) and is suggested at C5 by fragments *(arrowhead* and *f; see also E).*

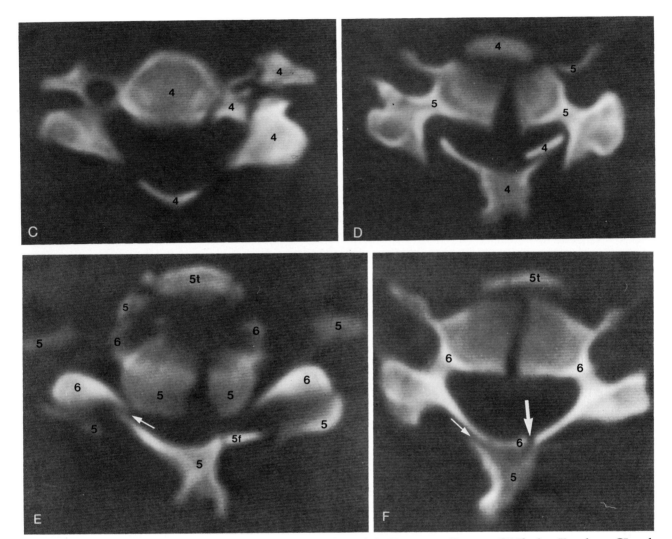

FIGURE 6–34 *Continued* **Complex Injury with C4 Pedicle, C4 and C5 Transverse Process, C5 Flexion-Teardrop, C5 and C6 Sagittal, and C4–C6 Laminar Fractures in a 25-Year-Old Man with Complete Tetraplegia**

• • • •

C–F, 5-mm computed tomography sections.

C, Left C4 transverse process and pedicle fractures are visible. The upper edge of the laminar arch is caudally and slightly posteriorly displaced. *D,* A widely gaping sagittal fracture of C5. Splaying of the pedicles eliminates landmarks for determining the "interpediculate" distance on an AP film. Bilaminar C5 avulsion is present, but here the cord is pinched against the caudally and anteriorly displaced lower edge of the avulsed C4 arch. Note the left C5 transverse process fracture. The unfractured anteroinferior margin of C4 should not be mistaken for the crescentic anteroinferior "teardrop" fragment from C5.

E, The C5–6 intervertebral level, volume-averaged by thick section. The dominant crescentic teardrop *(5t)* and the lateral fragments seem to complete a ring with the uncinate processes and the posterosuperior margin of C6. The failure of the sagittal fracture to penetrate the teardrop indicates that the teardrop formed first (compare with Fig. 6–33H). Note the comminuted C5 intralaminar fracture on the left *(5f,* seen on a lateral film) and the interlaminar space on the right *(arrow).* F, A narrow C6 sagittal body fracture combined with a narrow inner laminar fracture *(short arrow).* The interlaminar space *(thin arrow)* distinguishes the caudally displaced C5 spinous process from the C6 arch.

greater degree than the posterosuperior margin (Fig. 6–35B; see also Fig. 6–34B [compare with Fig. 6–33B]),[62, 99] and a reciprocal distractive disruption of the posterior ligamentous complex. The retrodisplacement is the fundamental feature that injures the cord. In its fully developed form this injury leaves no stabilizing support between the fractured vertebra and the one below. Often two or three contiguous levels have fractures, particularly sagittal fractures, sometimes with multiple levels of gross instability.

The increased AP diameter and further fracturing of the vertebral body may simulate a burst fracture, and typical flexion-teardrop fractures have sometimes been implicitly classified as subtypes of burst fractures. The flexion-compression mechanism and the distractive posterior ligamentous disruption exclude them from the category of burst fractures. Instead of the random comminution typical of burst fractures, sagittal vertebral body fractures occur in many if not most patients.[62, 66]

SAGITTAL FRACTURE

The sagittal or "vertical" fracture splits the vertebral body into lateral halves (see Figs. 6–31C and D, 6–32 to 6–35). The cleavage is usually midline and reasonably planar. In common with burst fractures, the arch is usually split, the interuncinate and the "interpediculate" distances are widened, the posterior vertebral body surface is involved, and the spinal cord is injured. Coexisting (see Fig. 6–31) and transitional (see Fig. 6–35; however, this may represent a minimal flexion-teardrop fragment rather than "random comminution") examples exist, and some sagittal fractures may arise from an axial compression burst mechanism (see Fig. 6–31). However, most sagittal fractures result from a flexion mechanism.

Other differences between burst fractures and sagittal fractures include a higher rate of tetraplegia, the frequent presence of sagittal fractures in two or three consecutive vertebrae, a strong association with flexion-teardrop fractures, a normal AP vertebral body diameter in cases without a teardrop, and other evidence of hyperflexion instead of direct axial compression. The sagittal fracture often gapes posteriorly and can be incomplete anteriorly.

Skold explained these features by a "re-entry" or a "rear entry" mechanism (see Fig. 6–32E).[103] Marked hyperflexion, with or without a flexion-teardrop fracture and retrolisthesis, tightens the interlaminar ligaments. In a deformation similar to a kink in bent tubing, one or more arches are drawn forward to be in a straighter line with those above and below and are flattened, and as a result they push the pillars

apart. The spreading pillars act through the pedicles to rip open the posterior surface of the vertebral body ("re-entry" of fracturing into the body following a flexion-teardrop fracture). The splitting halves hinge anteriorly and increase the divergence of the pedicles. Prior to laminar separation, bending of the pedicles may initiate tension fractures along their lateral surfaces (see Fig. 6–33G). Laminar flattening may initiate a sagittal arch fracture in the base of the spinous process (see Fig. 6–33I) or bilateral laminar avulsions from the pillars (see Figs. 6–32, 6–34, and 6–35). The latter event permits continuing interlaminar tension to pull the laminar arch deeper into the spinal canal. At the same time, the spinal canal is narrowed by the posterolaterally rotating posterior margins of the sagittal fracture. The cord is crushed from anterior and posterior directions. With the relief of hyperflexion, these displacements and angulations are variably reduced, and the cause of cord injury may be obscured.

Radiographic detection of sagittal fractures is difficult, and in the absence of a flexion-teardrop fracture the osseous injury can be overlooked on plain films (see C6 in Figs. 6–31B, 6–33B, and 6–34A). The lateral film may show subtle distortion of the vertebral body, with slight wedging or an anterosuperior[66, 67] or anteroinferior (see Fig. 6–35B) marginal compression or avulsion. Visualization of the fracture requires frontal or transaxial imaging. On the AP film an irregular but basically vertical median or paramedian lucency is often visible superimposed on or near the airway and coinciding with the vertical span of a vertebral body. The interuncinate and the "interpediculate" distances are widened and the facets are laterally offset (see Figs. 6–32A, 6–33A, 6–34A, and 6–35A). CT shows even an incomplete hairline fracture on multiple sections through the vertebra, whereas a prominent but normal vascular channel crosses the body on only one or two sections.

MARGIN FRACTURES IN THE LATERAL PROJECTION

As much as radiologists are responsible for "the four corners of the film," they must study the four margins of each vertebral body on the lateral view. By themselves, margin fractures are not entities, but rather are signs. A variety of injury complexes, mechanisms, and prognoses may be signaled by margin fractures.[67] A margin fracture may be the most definite or even the only sign of one of these injuries on the supine lateral "clearance" film.

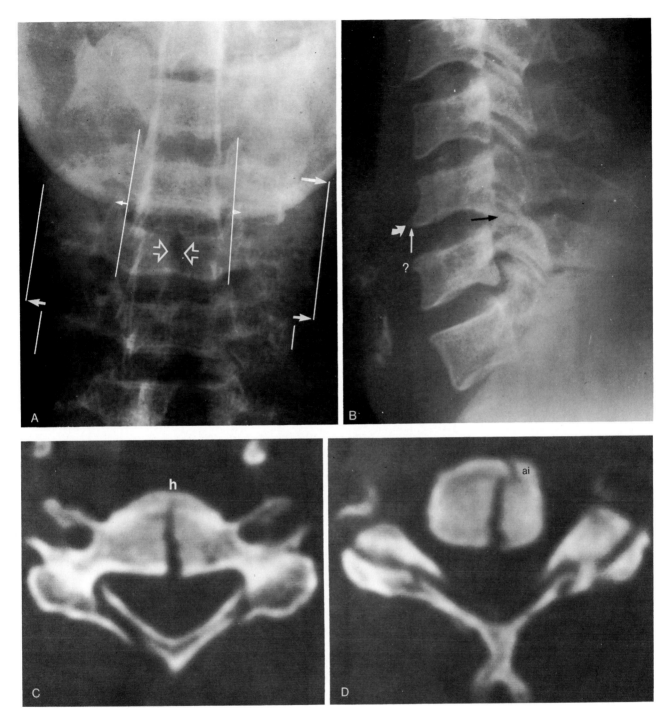

FIGURE 6–35. Sagittal Fracture of C5 in a 38-Year-Old Man

• • • •

A, This anteroposterior film (from a myelogram) shows lateral spreading of C5. Bilateral spreading of the C5 pillars is shown with respect to C6 at the lower arrows, whereas the relationship with C4 is asymmetric *(upper arrow on left).* The C5 uncinate processes are also spread *(small arrow on right, arrowhead on left;* the medial pedicle-lamina junctional cortices are not visible for the assessment of "interpediculate" distances). The anterior "hinging" of the vertebral body exaggerates the spreading of the pillars as compared with that of the uncinate processes. The sagittal fracture is visible *(open arrows).* *B,* This lateral view shows retrolisthesis at the posteroinferior C5 body margin *(black arrow)* akin to a flexion-teardrop injury; a minimal anteroinferior fragment is also present *(curved arrow).* A distinct density difference marks the apparent "spur" as a fragment from just part of the margin; this fragment corresponds to the anteroinferior fragment in *D.* Incomplete computed tomography (CT) failed to document the nature of the anterosuperior prominence on C6 (marked on *B* by "?"). *C* and *D,* Sagittal fracture is shown gaping posteriorly on 1.5-mm CT sections through C5; it is hinged at the anterior vertebral cortex *(h* in *C)* and accompanied by bilateral laminar avulsions. Laminae are depressed into the spinal canal in *C.* Note the slightly displaced anteroinferior fragment *(ai)* in *D.*

Anteroinferior Margin Fracture, Hyperextension Dislocation, and "Extension Teardrop" Fracture

The flexion-teardrop fracture discussed earlier is the most obvious margin fracture, produces the largest and most variable fragments, and was the only one intended by the original metaphor, "teardrop."[99] The other margin fractures tend to preserve their triangular shapes, although they may be so small that their shapes are not clear.

In addition to compressive flexion, distractive extension also can avulse anteroinferior vertebral margins. Traction by the anterior longitudinal ligament and by the anterior disc annulus avulses the anteroinferior margin of the upper vertebra at the motion segment, apparently in preference to the anterosuperior margin of the lower vertebra.

Hyperextension dislocation (HED) is the primary injury suggested by a small, predominantly horizontal avulsion fragment from the anteroinferior margin of an otherwise intact lower cervical vertebral body. This fracture is not required in HED. Because HED is sometimes a momentary dislocation reduced by elastic anterior neck structures and because of the tendency of the supine position for radiography to reduce it, the anteroinferior margin fragment with diffuse prevertebral swelling is a key and reasonably specific sign, even with normal vertebral alignment. A hyperextension sprain need not result in a complete rupture with dislocation and can be suggested by the history, prevertebral swelling, or MR imaging (see Fig. 6–53H and I). Other signs are discussed later (page 231).

The lower body of C2 is nearly typical of the lower cervical vertebrae but is the usual site of an anteroinferior fragment that differs from the typical fragment in HED in that it is larger and taller and nearly has the shape of an equilateral triangle. This has been called an "extension teardrop" fracture (ETF), possibly because of its relative plumpness as compared with the usually flatter fragments in HED.[46] Clinical status is usually better than that with HED, although not always (see Fig. 6–27). ETF is unrelated to the classic (flexion-) teardrop fracture in mechanism, prognosis, and vertebral level. (Compare with Fig. 6–25D and F.)

The existence of a relationship between ETF and HED is uncertain. They are both tension avulsions. A typical HED with an acute central cord syndrome and a (late) retrolisthesis has been described at C2,[24] whereas a more benign apparent ETF was reported at C3 (Fig. 6–36).[67] Equilateral fragments have been illustrated at C4 and C5 in a patient with an injury described as "disruptive hyperextension,"[32] and it is

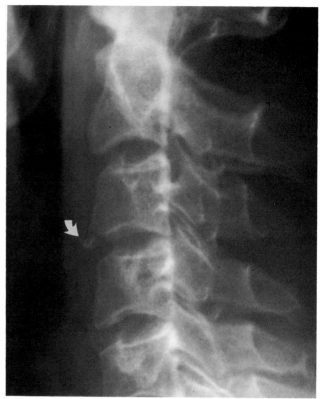

FIGURE 6–36. Hyperextension Avulsion ("Extension Teardrop Fracture") of C3 in a 45-Year-Old Man
• • • •
Note the approximately equilateral triangular shape and the anterior rotation of the fragment (arrow).

not clear whether these fragments were low ETFs or plump HED fragments. Either configuration can be associated with a hangman's fracture or variant (see Figs. 6–3A and 6–24). Thus, the vertebral level alone does not determine the configuration and the prognosis, but a clear mechanistic difference between HED and ETF has not been thoroughly defined.

Anteroinferior avulsions have been associated with facet dislocation, usually not at the same motion segment but one or two segments lower. In this setting, sagittal fractures are common and neurologic injury is even more common,[67] suggesting that the association of anteroinferior avulsions with facet dislocation is indirect, being a part of a severe, multilevel flexion injury with flexion-teardrop fractures (see Fig. 6–33).

Anterosuperior, Posteroinferior, and Posterosuperior Margins

Avulsion of the anterosuperior margin has accompanied a variety of injuries and mechanisms and is associated with a high rate of cord injury.[67] Flexion injuries have included wedge fracture,[47] sagittal fracture, hyperflexion sprain, spinous process fracture, and facet dislocations, with some of the last group having additional posteroinferior margin avulsions from the anterolisthetic craniad vertebra. An anterosuperior fragment has also been associated with pillar fractures (extension injury with anterolisthesis, see Fig. 6–50), other arch fractures,[67] and hyperextension dislocation.[35] Such fragments can be mimicked by a prominent anterior tubercle on a lower cervical transverse process (see Figs. 6–1 and 6–47C).

Posteroinferior avulsions in the lower cervical spine are associated with facet dislocations or pillar fractures, are usually unilateral (see Figs. 6–52 and 6–53), and sometimes have an anterosuperior avulsion from or compression of the caudad vertebra (see Fig. 6–37).[67] At C2 a posteroinferior fragment is often seen when the plane of a hangman's fracture passes slightly anterior to one or both pedicles to enter the posteroinferior vertebral body.[67]

Posterosuperior avulsions are rare. One has been reported with a unilateral facet dislocation.[67] Thus, avulsion of any of the four margins of the vertebral body in the lateral projection can be associated with facet dislocation.

UNCINATE PROCESS FRACTURE

Uncinate process (uncus) fracture is an uncommon fracture that is produced by lateral hyperflexion. It may cause a radiculopathy as well as neck pain. The articulating inferolateral surface of the craniad vertebra can also be fractured.[2, 33] A discrete fracture line across the base of the process may be suggested, but this line must be differentiated from a Mach band and from a persistent synchondrosis under a secondary ossification center.[33] The uncovertebral joint space may be widened in the absence of a posteriorly distractive disc injury (e.g., a facet dislocation) by a combination of a reduction or an apparent absence of the process and an increase in the beveling of the craniad surface, which indicates fractures of both surfaces.[2] The uncus may be developmentally hypoplastic; in such a case no complementary bevel is present on the craniad vertebra.[33] These fractures are difficult to detect on plain film and may require meticulous thin-section CT or tomography.

ACUTE DISC INJURY

Some degree of disc disruption and protrusion is common and may be the rule with any injury involving intervertebral translation or vertebral compression. Whereas large acute disc herniations are relatively uncommon with vertebral fractures and dislocations, the occurrence of acute neurocompressive disc herniations outside of the setting of major trauma suggests they may be found along with major trauma and with or without any other traumatic lesion. Any degree of annular protrusion, even modest diffuse bulging, whether acute or chronic, limits the tolerance of the spinal cord and roots for vertebral displacement, ligament swelling, and hematomas. Herniations are occult on plain film examination unless accompanied by a marginal avulsion or gross acute disc narrowing and require an index of suspicion leading to CT, MR imaging, or myelography for detection. CT is already likely to be performed for other reasons in these cases. MR imaging is the optimal technique to show the disc contour, other soft tissue swellings, and their effect on the spinal cord. MR imaging has been recommended to search for disc injury in the presence of an incomplete neurologic lesion, or in the presence of a complete lesion if the deficit is worsening or poorly correlated with the bone injuries or if decompression is contemplated for root salvage.[91] In some MR imaging series the prevalence of disc protrusions has reached 30–50%, although many protrusions have been small and of unclear significance.[9, 22, 29, 44, 61, 76, 87, 95]

When focally narrowed spondylotic disc is present, acute herniation often occurs at an adjacent level.[22] Bone spurs within a disc protrusion, better distinguished by CT, indicate chronicity of at least part of the protrusion. Acutely injured discs show T_2-weighted hyperintensity on MR images (see Fig. 6–53H and I).[22, 29] Otherwise, it is difficult to determine the age of disc protrusions, even if they are extruded.

Distractive disc injury results from a variety of partial and complete intervertebral distraction mechanisms. In flexion injuries obvious posterior element injuries are usually present, although pure hyperflexion sprain can be subtle. Hyperextension sprain or dislocation may be difficult to recognize if there is no fracture (see p. 230) because the supine filming position tends to reduce the dislocation. The most common sign is marked diffuse prevertebral swelling. Prevertebral edema on MR images with or without swelling suggests a hyperextension sprain, and disc or annular injury may be directly visualized (see Fig. 6–53 H and I). An acute central cord syndrome can be produced by a transient retrolisthesis that pinches the cord against the arch of the subjacent vertebra or against the ligamenta flava, and some retrolisthesis may remain.[35, 72] Other signs include residual anterior widening of the disc space, a gas cleft in the disc, a spinous process fracture as a manifestation of a reciprocal posterior compressive component, and fractures of the mandible, the face, or the forehead as manifestations of the primary mechanism.[24]

Injuries of the Neural Arch

HYPERFLEXION SPRAIN (ANTERIOR SUBLUXATION)

Hyperflexion sprain is a bilateral subluxation whose definition excludes persistent dislocation; as a result, it has sometimes been called simply "subluxation." The pathology consists of disruption or sprain of the supraspinous and the interspinous ligaments, the flaval ligaments, the facet joint capsules, the posterior longitudinal ligament, and at least the posterior portion of the disc and the annulus. Contrary to an earlier belief that this injury is improbable (the force required to disrupt all these ligaments would then easily dislocate the facets bilaterally), it is not rare and can be subtle. Its features, however, are more commonly present as components of more complex injuries (Figs. 6–37, 6–38A, and 6–39B). Even in pure form, hyperflexion sprain can be mechanically or clinically unstable, and either type of instability can develop late.

The diagnosis depends on several positional signs.[40] The localized kyphosis that is present has pathologic features distinguishing it from the smooth or slightly angulated normal kyphosis seen in the "military" position. The interspinous space is distinctly the widest ("fanning"). Facet subluxation is directly visible because the inferior facets of the higher vertebra have ridden up on the superior facets

of the lower. Additionally, the facet joint space may gape posteroinferiorly (see Fig. 6–37). The space between the posteroinferior margin of the higher vertebral body and the anterosuperior margin of the lower vertebra's superior facet on a true lateral view may exceed the normal limit of 3.5 mm. These features are absent in the normal kyphosis even when locally angulated. Anterior vertebral rotation and anterior narrowing or posterior widening of the disc space may be present, but when mild these signs are nonspecific. The localized kyphotic angulation is significant when the *difference* in angulation between the segment in question and the adjacent segments exceeds 11 degrees. A flexion view may be required for a convincing demonstration of hyperflexion sprain.

Extension of the disruption through the disc to the anterior annulus and the anterior longitudinal ligament permits an anterolisthesis to develop. The same slip leads to the use of the term *dislocation* in hyperextension fracture-dislocation, but anterolisthetic hyperflexion sprain continues to be called *anterior cervical subluxation* in order to emphasize its differentiation from facet dislocation. A slip of up to 30% has been illustrated without facet perching.[96] Such cases are diagnostically more obvious and have little or no protection from developing bilateral dislocation. The same appearance may be seen with reduced bilateral facet dislocation, which is likely to recur. However, even without a slip there may be great disruption and instability, and complete tetraplegia has resulted from radiologically subtle injury.[96]

FACET-PILLAR-PEDICLE COMPLEX

Often the first diagnostic feature noticed in facet, pillar, and pedicle (FPP) injuries is abnormal vertebral alignment on the lateral film—that is, the superior vertebra usually slips a few millimeters forward when the FPP complex is damaged. In the absence of obvious spondylosis, an anterolisthesis usually implies either an FPP fracture or a dislocation, or both. In the setting of trauma, even with spondylosis, any anterolisthesis can indicate a fracture or dislocation. However, some pure fractures (see Fig. 6–53A) and perhaps a unilateral dislocation with contralateral joint space widening may fail to show this sign.

Facet Dislocations

A variety of terms are applied to various degrees of facet displacement along the plane of normal motion. Such displacements are flexion injuries, presumably with a distractive component. Subluxation, usually bilateral, is equivalent to hyperflexion sprain (see Fig. 6–38A). The inferior facet(s) of the higher vertebra may "jump" forward over the superior

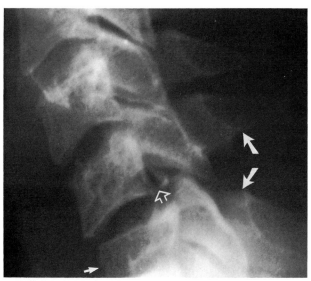

FIGURE 6–37. Fracture-Subluxation of C6–7 (Complicated Hyperflexion Sprain, Bilateral Facet Subluxation) in a 23-Year-Old Man
• • • •
Note fanning *(paired arrows)*, opening of the facet joints, and moderate anterolisthesis. The posteroinferior margin of the C6 body is avulsed *(open arrow)*, and the anterosuperior margin of C7 is compressed *(small arrow)*.

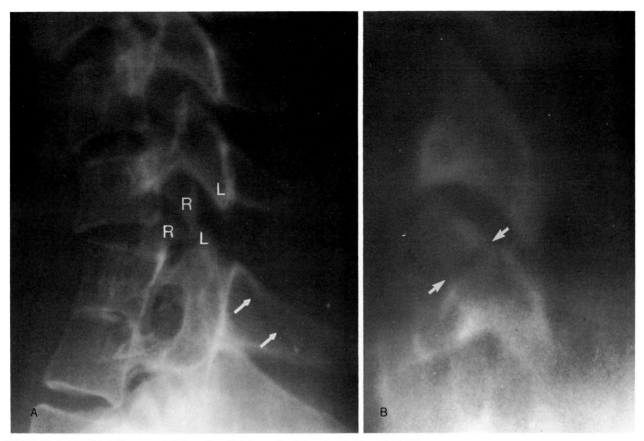

FIGURE 6–38. C5–6 Fracture-Dislocation Without Locking in 32-Year-Old Woman

• • • •

A, This oblique lateral film shows fanning of the spinous processes, vertical distraction of the left facet joint (*L, L*) with retained contact between the right facets (*R, R*), anterolisthesis, a congenital block C6–7 vertebra, and a fracture line within the C6 spinous process. The obliquity is equal above and below the injury, so there is no pathologic rotation around the vertical axis. *B,* This lateral tomogram shows a superior C6 facet fracture (*arrows*), which indicates a component of shear or compression on this side.

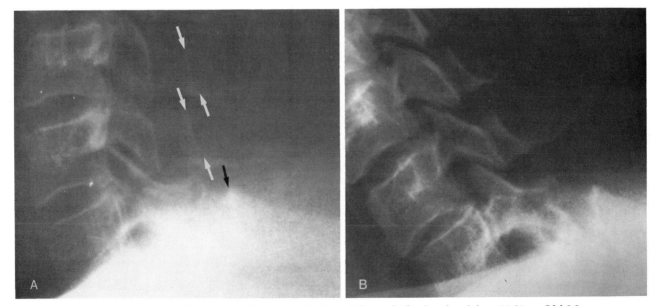

FIGURE 6–39. Avulsion of the C7 Spinous Process at Its Base (Through the Laminae) in a 35-Year-Old Man

• • • •

A, An initial lateral film does not show convincing fanning of the spinous processes. If the spinolaminar lines of C5 and C6 are extended (*white arrows*) they may be thought of as imbricated. This relationship is interrupted at C7 (*black arrow*).
B, This flexion lateral film confirms the C6–7 fanning and the complete avulsion of the C7 spinous process.

facet(s) of the lower vertebra and become "locked" in unilateral facet dislocation (UFD, Figs. 6–40 and 6–41; see also Fig. 6–33) or bilateral facet dislocation (BFD, Figs. 6–42 to 6–44). A lesser jump or an incomplete reduction of a lock may leave the facet joint(s) "perched" in point-to-point contact of the

acute facet angles in a status intermediate between a subluxation and a dislocation (see Fig. 6–43B). Dislocations, with or without marginal fractures, are distinguished from pure fractures by a reversal of imbrication between the two adjacent pillars on the dislocated side(s) (see Figs. 6–40 and 6–42B). UFD

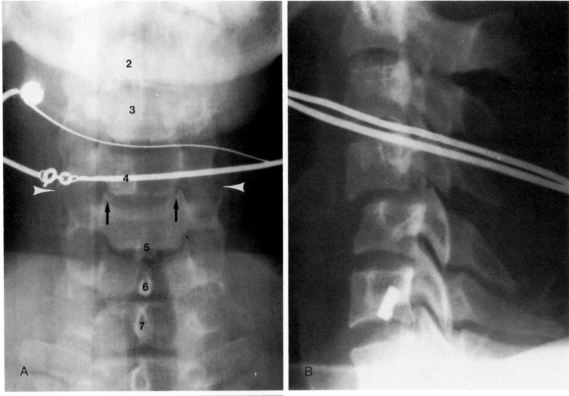

FIGURE 6–40. Unilateral Right C4–5 Facet Dislocation with Complete Tetraplegia in a 20-Year-Old Man

• • • •

A, Numbers mark the positions of the spinous processes on this anteroposterior film. Those of C4 and above are displaced to the right compared with those of C5 and below. The vertical interval between those of C4 and C5 is increased. The lateral margins of the pillar columns are interrupted (arrowheads), with C4 pillars deviated to the right on C5, whereas the uncovertebral joints remain aligned (arrows). B and C, A lateral film without and with annotation. Thick lines outline the normally aligned left pillars. Rotational discrepancy is present: thin and dashed lines outline the anteriorly rotated right pillars above C4–5 seen in oblique projection, whereas the right pillars below C4–5 are almost perfectly superimposed on the left in true lateral projection. Mild fanning of the C4 and C5 spinous processes is present, as are subluxation and mild posterior widening of the nondislocated left C4–5 facet joint. Note the normal posterosuperior concavity of the C7 pillar (arrow).

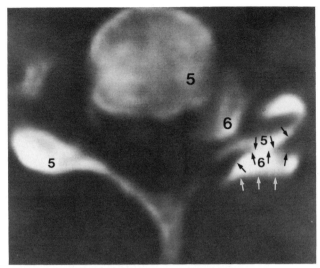

FIGURE 6–41. Back-to-Back Facet Sign in Facet Dislocation-Locking in a 35-Year-Old Man

• • • •

The convex nonarticular surfaces of C5 and C6 *(black arrows)* meet like the backs of hands. The concave superior articular facet of C6 faces posteriorly *(white arrows)*. The lucent band across the inferior right C5 pillar results from trabecular (noncortical) bone lucency, which is exaggerated by a narrow window setting. The C5–6 uncovertebral joint is necessarily dislocated by the anterolisthesis.

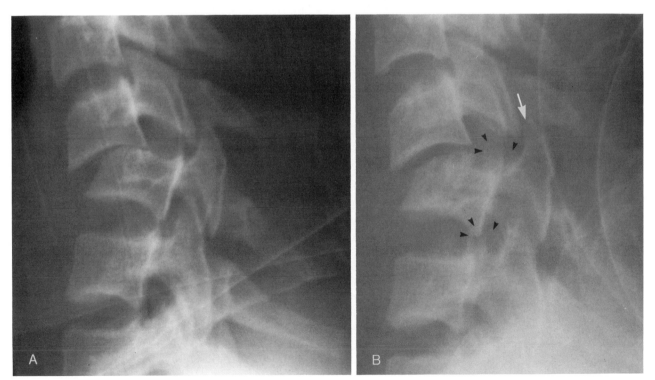

FIGURE 6–42. Bilateral C5–6 Facet Dislocation in a 15-Year-Old Man with Complete Tetraplegia

• • • •

A, There is little right-left rotation above or below the injury, both pairs of facets are visibly locked, the spinous processes are fanned, and the disc space is effaced. The anterolisthesis measures only 45% of the anteroposterior diameter of the inferior C5 or the superior C6 end plate. *B,* Reduction to unilateral facet dislocation is shown. Anterolisthesis decreased to 30–35%. The C6 and C7 pillars on one side are more anterior *(arrowheads around the superior facets)*. Note the blunt tip *(arrow)* of the superior C6 facet over which C5 remains dislocated.

Illustration continued on following page

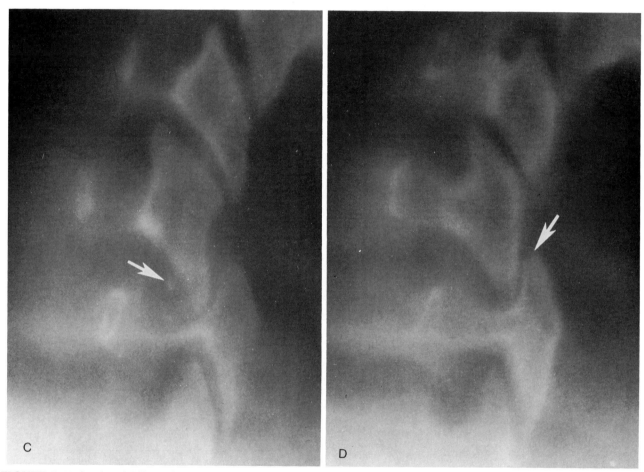

FIGURE 6–42 *Continued* **Bilateral C5–6 Facet Dislocation in a 15-Year-Old Man with Complete Tetraplegia**
• • • •
C and *D,* These tomograms of the right side show a small chip (*arrow* in *C*) from the superior C6 facet margin donor site (*arrow* in *D*). Tomograms on the left (not illustrated) confirmed the reduction and showed no fracture.

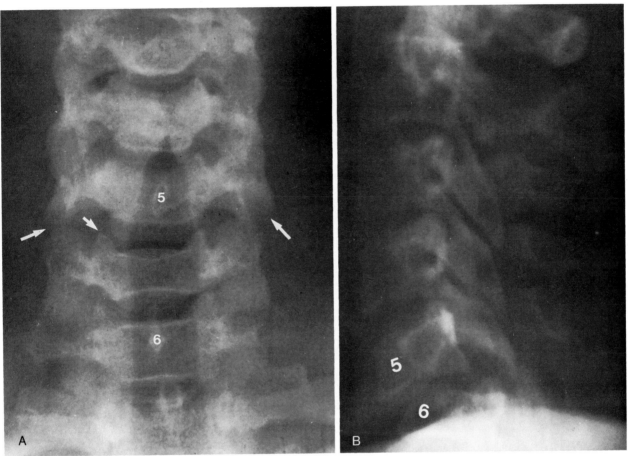

FIGURE 6–43. Bilateral C5–6 Facet Dislocation with Temporary Tetraparesis in a 32-Year-Old Woman

• • • •

A, This anteroposterior film shows vertical opening of C5–6 facet joints as diminished overlap of the articulating facets (compared with those seen at other levels) and as increased visibility of the rounded inferolateral facet margins *(long arrows).* Vertical interbody distraction is seen on the right as uncovertebral joint distraction *(short arrow).* Spinous process fanning is seen as a wide gap between the tips of C5 and C6 (without rotation). *B,* A lateral film shows the body of C5 to be "falling over" the anterosuperior margin of C6, but anterolisthesis measures only 38%. Facets are more nearly perched than tightly locked, but not much more anterolisthesis would be required for locking. The limited anterolisthesis contributed to a favorable outcome.

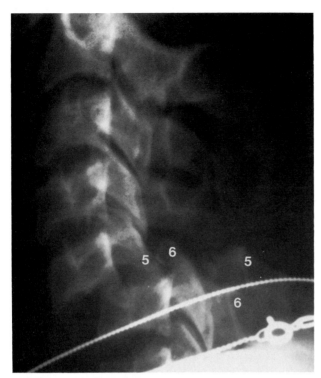

FIGURE 6–44. Bilateral Facet Dislocation with Marked Anterolisthesis, Avulsion of C5 Laminae from the Pillars, and Paralysis from C5 Downward in a 19-Year-Old Man

• • • •

Pillar columns both above and below the injury are bilaterally superimposed.

has a greater component of lateral flexion and rotation, although the opposite facet joint probably also subluxed or dislocated transiently (see Fig. 6–40C). Even in BFD some slight rotation may be required to rip the many posterior ligaments and jump the facets more or less in succession rather than exactly simultaneously.

A fundamental sign in unilateral FPP injuries is a rotational discrepancy above and below the level of injury (see Figs. 6–33B, 6–40C, 6–45B, 6–46C, 6–47D, and 6–54C), although this may be subtle or absent if fracture predominates over dislocation (see Figs. 6–37C, 6–48B, and 6–51B). Of all the FPP injuries, the rotational discrepancy is most marked with unilateral locked facets because the upper facet has moved forward by the full AP thickness of the pillar. In UFD and some FPP fractures, the vertebrae above the injured joint and those below it cannot all be lateral on the same film; as a result, no single true lateral view of the whole cervical spine can be produced. As a result, retakes may be required, all of which should be studied. The pillars may all be oblique, but careful analysis indicates a reversal of the obliquity ("crossed obliquity") at the injured level (see Figs. 6–33B and 6–47C). At least one film should show one group of vertebrae in true lateral projection with their pillars nearly superimposed pairwise (see

Fig. 6–40C). Deliberate inspection is often needed to discover the second column of parallellograms projected over the other vertebral bodies.

The diagnosis of UFD can usually be made unequivocally based on these lateral films by the unilateral reversed imbrication of the dislocated facet joint. Small fractures may occur in one or both of the dislocated facets and may require additional imaging to be detected (see Figs. 6–33E and 6–42B). Although the sagittal view available with tomography might seem the most logical, state-of-the-art CT is preferable for bone detail and for evaluation of the neural foramen, the disc, and the thecal sac. Jumped facets are obvious on CT scans because of their incongruous "back-to-back" (convex-to-convex) arrangement (see Figs. 6–33F and 6–41). Sagittal MR imaging or sagittal CT reconstructions demonstrate reversed imbrication.

The side of the unilateral injury, especially of a dislocation, must be determined to assist proper reduction. This can often be determined on an AP film. It is important to verify the accuracy of right-left labeling on all examinations for UFD. The upper vertebra moves forward on the affected side, rotating the spinous process of the upper vertebra toward that side (see Figs. 6–40 and 6–54). The offset must be convincing and the spinous processes must be symmetric in form and in alignment at the other levels (compare Figs. 6–40 and 6–47). This rotation also shifts the pillars above the injured motion segment to the same side (see Fig. 6–40A). The side of injury is also evident on oblique films, tomography, CT scans, and MR images.

UFD tends to be mechanically stable because anterior support and unilateral posterior support are nominally maintained. However, clinical stability is uncertain. During maximum displacement, the remaining anterior and posterior supports were stretched and their residual strengths are unknown. UFD can result after attempted reduction of BFD (see Fig. 6–42B), which tends to recur. The spinal canal is narrowed by the anterolisthesis, so tolerance for anteroposterior intervertebral motion is decreased. Any pre-existing spinal stenosis further reduces the likelihood of clinical stability in UFD.

Comparing BFD with UFD, the rotational component around the vertical axis is eliminated, but the anterior slip is increased. The distinction is best made directly by analysis of the vertical alignments of the two columns of pillars on lateral and nearly lateral films. In the presence of a significant anterolisthesis, an AP film showing anatomically typical spinous processes all in the midline ordinarily rules out UFD. If oblique films are available, they may show the bilateral dislocations. BFD entails a complete transverse disruption of all ligaments and joint capsules and is highly unstable. However, there have been patients with BFD who did not display permanent neurologic deficit (see Fig. 6–43).

The commonly stated rule evoked to distinguish BFD from UFD indirectly, based on whether the slip is more (BFD) or less (UFD) than 50%[8], is not reliable. The minimum slip that can result from BFD with solid locking depends on the ratio of the pillar thickness that must be jumped to the AP widths of the involved vertebral end plates. In many cases this requires a slip of greater than 50%, as inferred from the inspection of normal radiographs, but there have been exceptions that measured as little as 23% (see Figs. 6–42 and 6–43).[26, 48, 54] It has also been disputed that a slip *greater* than 50% would necessarily *indicate* BFD.[14]

Facet and Pillar Fractures, and Hyperextension Fracture-Dislocation

Facet and pillar fractures are, in a sense, two aspects of the same phenomenon. They can arise in flexion or in extension and are associated by either mechanism with anterolisthesis. A relatively pure marginal or surface fracture is called a *facet fracture* (Figs. 6–45 to 6–47; see also Figs. 6–33C and E, 6–38B, and 6–42B). A relatively pure compression or splitting of the pillar is called a *pillar fracture* (Figs. 6–20E, and 6–48 to 6–53), but the fracture usually still distorts or crosses a facet surface.

Flexion fractures are often recognized based on the presence of an accompanying facet dislocation, whose reduction these fractures make more difficult (See Fig. 6–42). Some flexion fractures are found without dislocation and must be recognized by their morphology or by the history. They tend to produce chips or slivers from the acute margins of one or both of the involved facets. Such fractures, especially when small, may be impossible to detect on plain films even when an obvious facet dislocation or subluxation is present. Therefore, CT or tomography is usually needed for complete evaluation of UFD, BFD, and any suspicious anterolisthesis.

Text continued on page 253

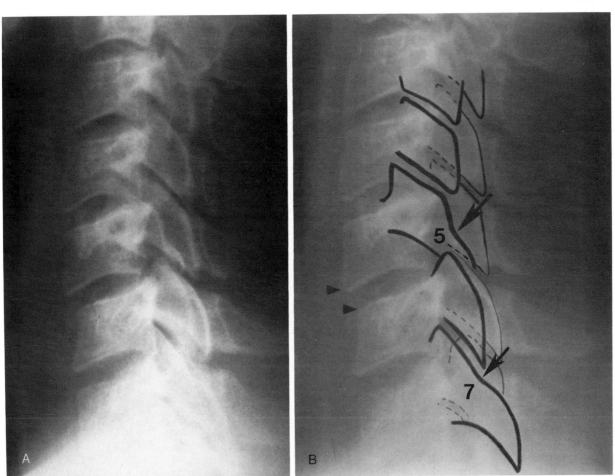

FIGURE 6–45. Left C5 and C6 Facet Fractures in a 24-Year-Old Man
• • • •
A and *B*, A lateral film is presented without and with annotation. The heavier lines are on the left side. Anterolisthesis *(arrowheads, B)* and mild rotational discrepancy occur at C5–6. Similar concave posterior pillar lines *(arrows, B)* are normal at C7 but pathologic at C5. A fracture is so far apparent only in the C5 facet.

Illustration continued on following page

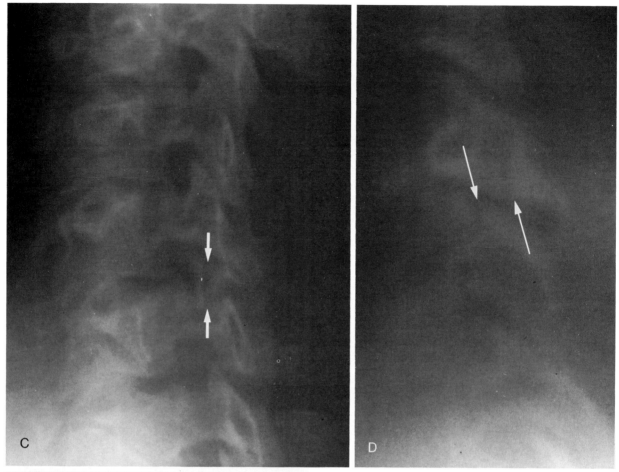

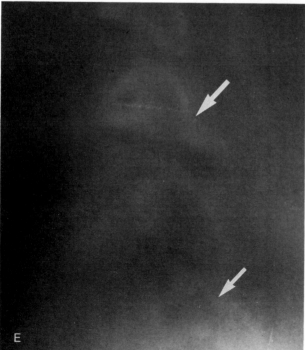

FIGURE 6–45 *Continued* **Left C5 and C6 Facet Fractures in a 24-Year-Old Man**

• • • •

C, An oblique film confirms the side of the injury and shows the superior C6 facet fracture *(arrows), D* and *E,* Lateral tomographic planes 3 mm apart show the posteroinferior portion of the inferior C5 facet to be displaced posterosuperiorly following compressive hyperextension. C5 and C6 facet fracture planes *(thin arrows)* may have lined up during injury. Concave posterior pillar surfaces *(heavy arrows)* indicate fracture at C5 but are normal at C7.

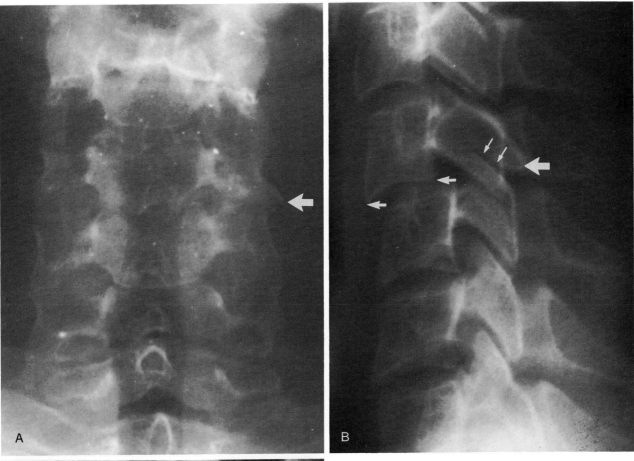

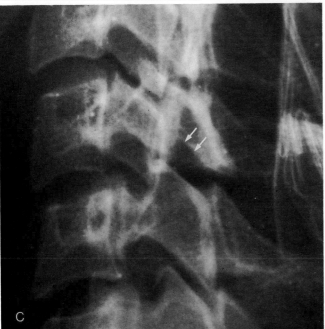

FIGURE 6–46. Left Inferior C4 Facet Fracture in a 21-Year-Old Man

• • • •

A, This anteroposterior film shows a wedge displaced laterally *(arrow)*, indicating a fracture. *B*, An acute lateral film shows the left superior C5 facet displaced into a concavity in the inferior C4 facet *(small arrows)*, an uplifted inferior C4 facet fragment pointing posteriorly *(large arrow)*, and anterolisthesis of C4 *(medium arrows)*. *C*, Two days later the C5 facet is reduced out of the C4 defect *(arrows)*, and anterolisthesis is diminished.

Illustration continued on following page

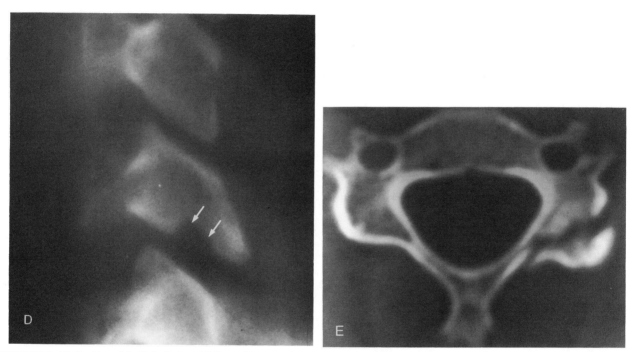

FIGURE 6–46 *Continued* **Left Inferior C4 Facet Fracture in a 21-Year-Old Man**

• • • •

D, A lateral tomogram shows the inferior C4 facet impression *(arrows)* from the compressive impact against the C5 pillar. There must also be a complete fracture plane to permit postero-supero-lateral displacement of the fragment, but this is seen only on a computed tomography scan *(E)*.

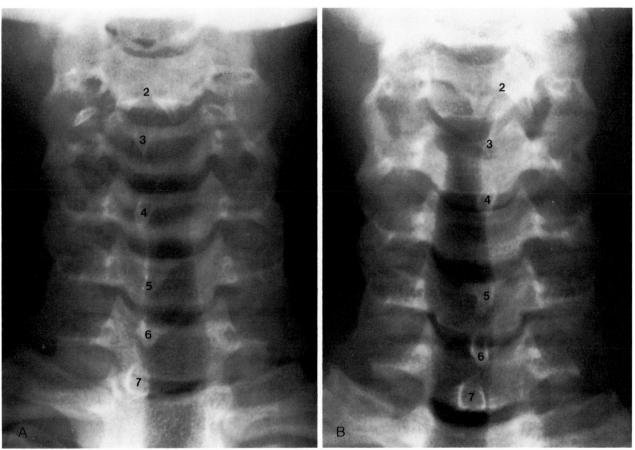

FIGURE 6–47. Left Inferior C4 Facet Fracture-Dislocation in a 22-Year-Old Man (Absence of a Spinous Process Deviation After Injury)

• • • •

A, This somewhat rotated anteroposterior (AP) film taken in 1979 shows crooked alignment of the spinous processes (*numbered*), with apparent right deviation of C4 on C5 and left deviation of C6 on C7. Variations in the symmetry of spinous processes can cause apparent or real deviations of their visualized portions. *B,* A 1984 AP injury film shows vertical spreading and "pseudoalignment" of the C4 and C5 spinous processes. This interval shift of the C4 spinous process to the left indicates that the injury is on the left (confirmed tomographically). The fracture is invisible and the lateral pillar lines fail to show deviations.

Illustration continued on following page

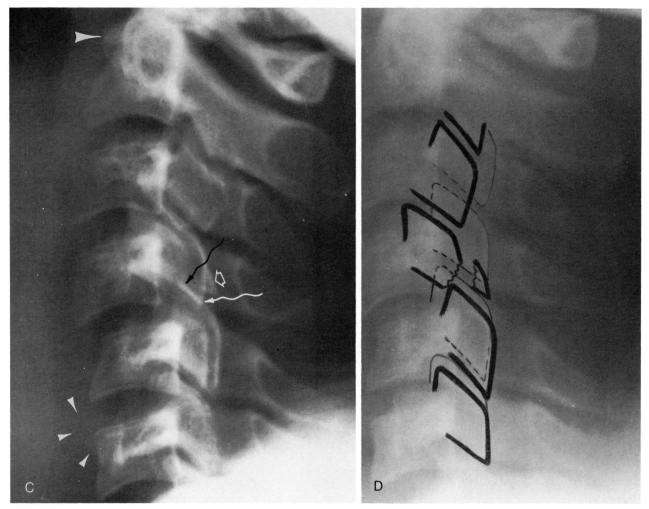

FIGURE 6–47 *Continued* **Left Inferior C4 Facet Fracture-Dislocation in a 22-Year-Old Man (Absence of a Spinous Process Deviation After Injury)**

• • • •

C and *D*, Two similarly projected lateral films show anterolisthesis, a posteriorly displaced and angulated fragment from the C4 inferior facet (*open arrow, C*), and crossed obliquity between C4 and C5. The overlap of normal C4 and C5 pillars (*long white arrow*) places them on opposite sides; the left C5 pillar is therefore impacted against the posterior fracture margin of the left C4 pillar (*long black arrow, C;* the heavy lines in *D* represent the left side). This fracture permits locking with less intervertebral rotation than in pure unilateral facet dislocation, thereby impeding the interpretation of rotation on the AP film. The rotational discrepancy at C4–5 is greater than might seem obvious; this is because on both films the left pillars are *anterior* above C4-5 but *posterior* below C4-5 ("crossed obliquity"). Note the anterior rotation of the left side of the C2 articular plateau (*single arrowhead, C*). Note also the prominent anterior tubercle of the C6 transverse process (*arrowheads, C*), which could have been mistaken for an anterosuperior margin avulsion if the facet injury had been at C5–6 (compare with Fig. 6–50*B*).

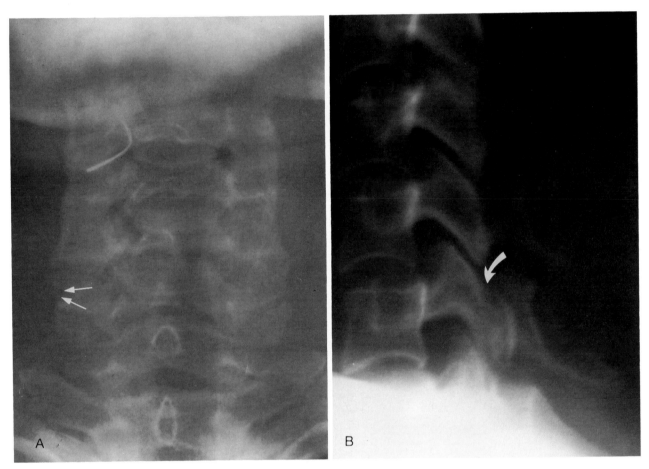

FIGURE 6–48. Right C6 Pillar Fracture in a 28-Year-Old Woman

••••

A, An anteroposterior film suggests double density at the lateral right C6 pillar border *(arrows).* The right pillar is not shortened compared with the left pillar. *B,* This lateral film shows a fracture posteriorly through the inferior facet *(arrow).* Even though the fragment is posteriorly displaced and the joint space may be narrowed, there is no anterolisthesis at C6–7 that is greater than the normal step-offs present at each of the other levels. *C,* A lateral tomogram confirms the fracture through the inferior facet and the pillar (compressive hyperextension).

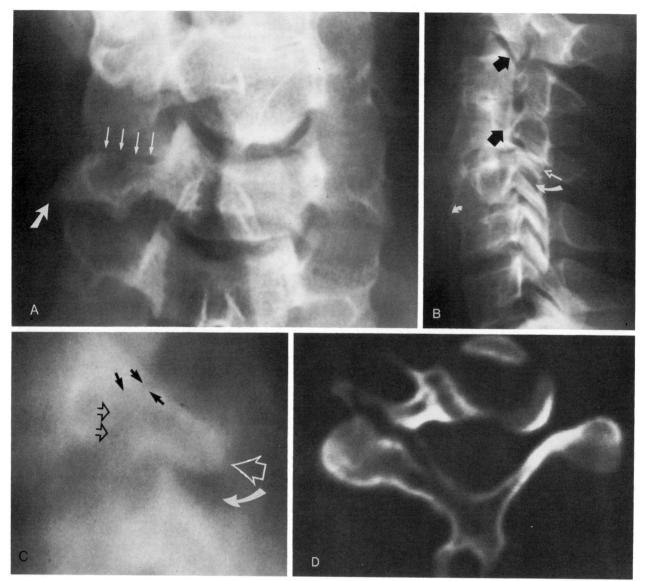

FIGURE 6–49. C5 Pillar Fracture Between the Superior and the Inferior Facets ("Traumatic Spondylolisthesis") in a 21-Year-Old Man

• • • •

A, This anteroposterior (AP) film shows a wedge of pillar projecting laterally *(large arrow)* and a horizontal fracture line *(small arrows).* *B,* A lateral film shows a congenital block C3–4 vertebra and a dysmorphic appearance that may mislead the viewer into believing the film is too complex to analyze rigorously. Slight anterolisthesis of C5 *(short curved arrow)* is visible. A rotational discrepancy occurs at C5–6; the C4–5 and C2–3 facet joints (right side) are rotated anteriorly *(black arrows),* but the C6 and C7 pillars are bilaterally superimposed (although tilted). Furthermore, only one normal C5 pillar is visible in line with these elements. The long curved arrow points to the middle of this (left) C5 pillar but also points to the empty space above the (right) C6 pillar. Although with difficulty, the deformed right C5 inferior facet can be seen uplifted above this widened joint space *(open arrow;* compare with *C).* *C,* A lateral tomogram. The horizontal component of the fracture *(solid black arrows)* was visible on the AP film *(A).* The vertical component of the fracture *(open black arrows)* is analogous to a displaced lumbar isthmic spondylolysis and permits forward slippage of C5. The curved arrow shows the joint space widening; the open white arrow shows the uplifted, deformed inferior facet seen in *B. D,* This 1.5-mm computed tomography section shows the fracture indistinctly owing to the excessively large field of view (20 cm) that was reconstructed.

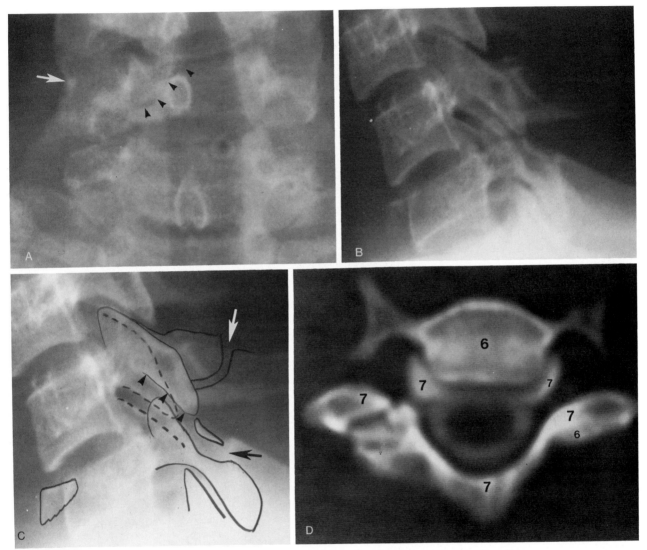

FIGURE 6–50. C6 and C7 Arch Fractures in a 20-Year-Old Woman with Right C7 Radiculopathy
• • • •
A, This anteroposterior film shows a diagonal fracture line overlying the right side of C6 *(arrowheads)* and subtle angulation and double density in the lateral right C6 pillar *(white arrow)*. *B* and *C*, A lateral film without and with annotation. The dashed lines are the normal left side. Fractures of the C6 and C7 laminae *(arrows)*, including the C7 pillar, and of the anterosuperior C7 margin (all confirmed by computed tomography [CT]) are obvious. The shortened height of the right C6 pillar indicates compression of its inferior facet *(arrowheads)*. This suggests a hyperextension fracture-dislocation mechanism and correlates with the abnormal lateral pillar margin shown in *A*. *D*, A thick (5-mm) postmyelographic CT section shows a fractured right C7 pillar. Note the anterolisthesis of C6 at the uncovertebral joints. A single section (not shown) through the C6 pillars failed to show a convincing fracture. Thick sections can easily fail to resolve the features of impacted undisplaced fractures.

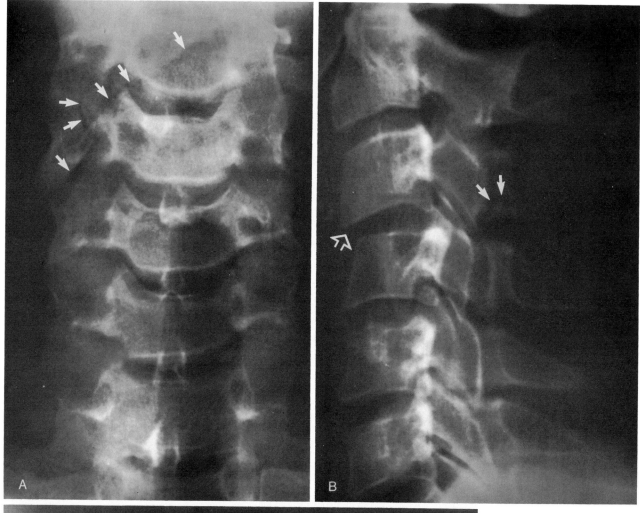

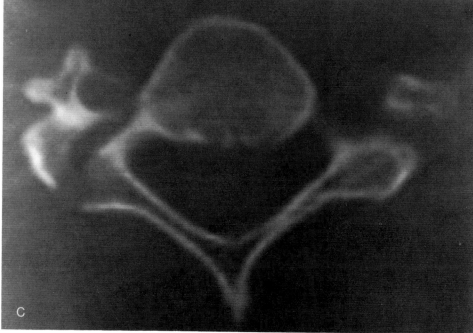

FIGURE 6–51. Fractures of the C3 Lamina and the C4 Pillar in a 35-Year-Old Man

• • • •

A, Complex fracture lines are shown crossing various vertebral elements (arrows). B, Anterolisthesis (open arrow); only C3 laminar fracture (arrows) is visible. Computed tomography confirmed the C3 laminar fracture (not illustrated) and shows a nearly sagittal C4 pillar fracture in C.

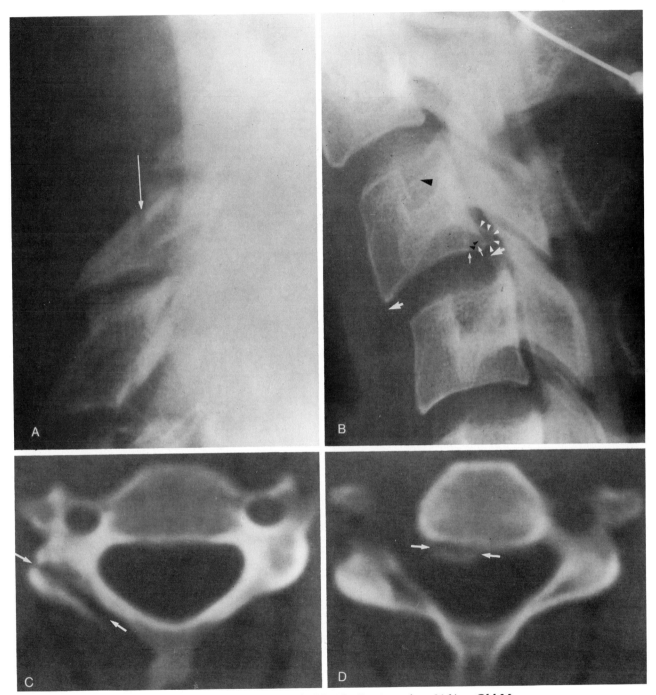

FIGURE 6–52. Right C3 Pillar and Posteroinferior Body Margin Fractures in a 21-Year-Old Man

• • • •

A, A direct-magnification left posterior oblique film (from a myelogram) shows a faint vertical fracture line in the pillar *(arrow). B,* A direct-magnification lateral film (from a myelogram) shows anterolisthesis *(fat arrows)* that leaves behind a nonanterolisthetic posteroinferior margin fragment *(white arrowheads)* simulating an osteophyte. The margins of the donor site are discernible *(black arrowheads,* parallel to the *small arrows). C,* This 5-mm computed tomography (CT) section shows a narrow, planar oblique fracture that would be visible only on left-posterior-oblique/right-anterior-oblique projections. *D,* A lower CT section shows a margin avulsion with a fracture line *(arrows)* that would be visible only on a lateral projection.

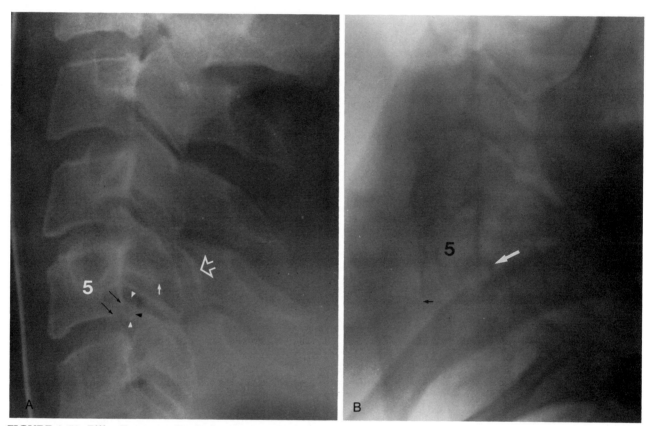

FIGURE 6–53. Pillar Fractures C5–C7 in a 31-Year-Old Man

• • • •

A, This lateral film shows nearly normal body alignment through the top of C7 (borderline at C3–4). The posterior surface of a C5 pillar is retrodisplaced *(open arrow),* and its inferior facet surface is interrupted *(small arrow).* C4–5 and C5–6 discs are mildly narrow (possible disc degeneration at age 31?). Not originally noticed, a fragment *(arrowheads)* is displaced from the interrupted posteroinferior C5 margin *(black arrows). B,* An overpenetrated swimmer's view reversed on subtraction film is shown. C5–6 anterolisthesis has developed *(black arrow).* A posteroinferior C5 chip is visible *(white arrow),* although it is hard to recognize. Slight anterolisthesis at C3–4 may be a sign of early spondylosis or it may be normal laxity.

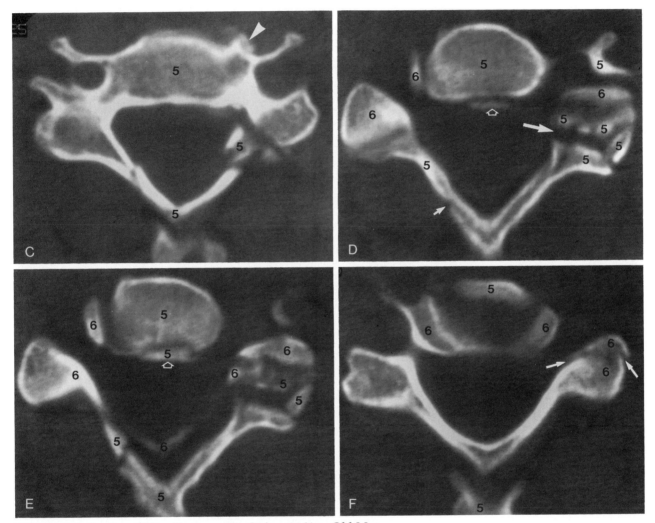

FIGURE 6–53 *Continued* **Pillar Fractures C5–C7 in a 31-Year-Old Man**

• • • •

C–G, Two-millimeter computed tomography sections.

C, This section shows bilateral comminuted C5 lamina fractures extending into the left pillar. C5 uncinate hypertrophy *(arrowhead)* confirms C4–5 disc degeneration. *D,* On this section a dominant coronal plane division of the left C5 pillar *(long arrow)* with comminution can be seen. The top of the posteroinferior C5 body margin fracture *(open arrow)* is also visible. The right lamina fracture is subtle *(short arrow)*. *E,* Some pillar fragments are difficult to attribute between C5 and C6. The right C5 lamina fracture is again obvious. The posteroinferior C5 body margin fracture *(open arrow)* corresponds well with that shown on the lateral film *(A)*. *F,* The left superior C6 facet fracture continues inferiorly *(arrows)*.

Illustration continued on following page

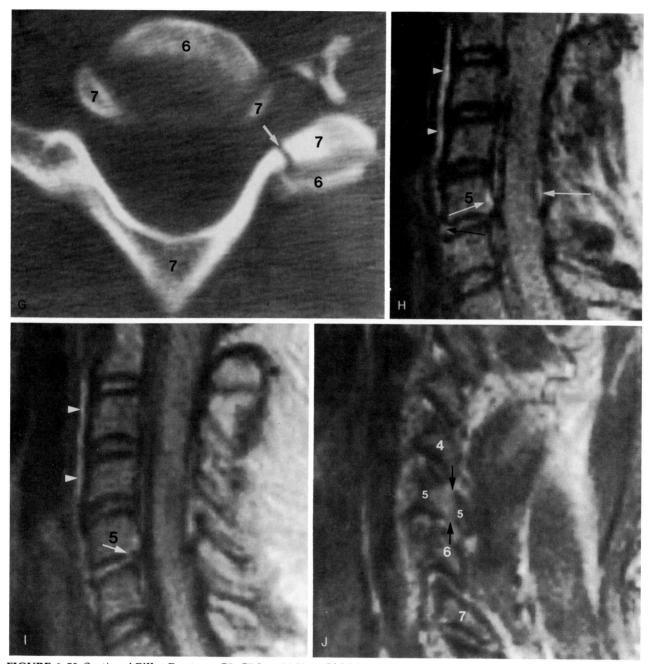

FIGURE 6–53 *Continued* **Pillar Fractures C5–C7 in a 31-Year-Old Man**
• • • •

G, A minimally displaced fracture *(arrow)* is visible at the lamina-pillar junction (extending downward into pillar).

H–J, Magnetic resonance images obtained at 0.35 Tesla (5-mm sections on a 32-cm field of view, 256 × 256 matrix).

H, SE (spin echo) 1500 msec/80 msec section through the right half of the spinal cord, and *I*, SE 1500 msec/40 msec section through the left half of the cord show a normal cord contour and signal at limited resolution. The patient was neurologically intact. An injured C5–6 disc, now with mild retrolisthesis, is narrow and abnormally bright and probably has a torn anterior anulus *(black arrow)*. The C5 margin fracture is visible, with associated bright signal *(short arrow)*. The hyperintense prevertebral stripe *(arrowheads)* probably represents edema from a reciprocal component of hyperextension sprain accompanying the posterior extension-compression mechanism indicated by the split pillar. The small posterior epidural hematoma *(long arrow)* is clinically insignificant. The C4–5 disc is dark and bulging (degenerated but uninjured). *J*, An SE 1500 msec/40 msec section farther left shows the coronal split of the C5 pillar *(arrows)*. The overall outline resembles the normal posteroinferior elongation of the C7 pillar.

Hyperextension fracture-dislocation was described by Forsyth and associates.[30] Like the flexion injury, this fracture can produce partial cord deficits and has been considered unstable. "Dislocation" refers not to the facets but to the anterolisthesis, which was previously misinterpreted as a sign of flexion. Compressive extension exaggerates the cervical lordosis (and may induce a reciprocal hyperextension sprain anteriorly; see Fig. 6–53H and I). The force vector, a straight line, is predominantly compressive in the upper cervical spine but, because of the lordosis, produces a component of anatomically anterior shear stress in the lower cervical spine. Compressive failure of a pillar permits this shear to cause an anterolisthesis. Often much of the inferior facet surface of the upper vertebra, sometimes the entire pillar, is distorted upward and backward (see Figs. 6–41C, 6–46, and 6–49), and in patients with a rotational component it is also distorted outward.[30] Compression or coronal splitting (see Fig. 6–53) of the middle trabecular portion of the pillar most closely resembles a traumatic spondylolisthesis of the lower cervical spine, albeit with unilateral impaction and backward rotation at the "pars interarticularis" rather than straight bilateral separation. The subjacent facet may also be fractured, more likely laterally in cases with a rotational component in the mechanism. The facet joint space typically is widened posteriorly as if to recall the transient hyperlordosis. Associated compressive fractures of the laminae and spinous processes may occur at multiple noncontiguous levels.

Thus, morphologic differences exist between the facet fractures from hyperextension and those from hyperflexion, whereas the anterolistheses are similar.

Careful inspection of the pillars, especially of their acute superior and inferior angles, may reveal a fracture line or angular deformity (see Fig. 6–47C), but many fractures are apparent only as distortions of the pillar outline (see Fig. 6–45). The contour of each pillar must be inspected on lateral and on AP films and compared with the expected contour at the given vertebral level. The posterior pillar lines at any level usually have similar shapes, although asymmetry can be normal. The posterior concavity and the elongated posteroinferior extension of the pillar that are normal at C7 may indicate an inferior facet fracture if present at a higher level, especially if unilateral (see Figs. 6–45B and 6–53J). On the AP view, fractures cause interruption, angulation, segmental shortening, or a double density (see Figs. 6–48A and 6–50A) of the undulating lateral margin of one or both pillar columns. A bone wedge jutting out (Fig. 6–54; see also Fig. 6–46A) almost certainly is a displaced pillar fragment, provided it is distinguished from a transverse process. A fracture line may be visible crossing the pillar column on an AP

or an oblique projection (see Figs. 6–33A, 6–34A, 6–49A, 6–51A, and 6–52A).

Pedicle Fracture

Unlike the C2 hangman's fracture, lower cervical pure pedicle fractures are uncommon because the pedicle is not the functional pars interarticularis. The injury probably is equivalent to hyperextension dislocation with displacement of the entire pillar.[30] The anterolisthesis may be distributed to two consecutive levels as the pillar rotates around its transverse axis (Fig. 6–54). The lamina may be bent or fractured. In complex injuries, pedicle fractures occur as components of arch fractures (see Figs. 6–33G and 6–34C).

LAMINA AND SPINOUS PROCESS FRACTURES

Lamina and spinous process fractures are closely associated because the fractures tend to be near the base of the spinous process and often extend into the laminae. Serious flexion, compression, and extension injuries commonly involve the laminae and the spinous processes, often at multiple levels. These include facet dislocations, flexion-teardrop fracture-dislocation, sagittal fractures, burst fractures, and hyperextension fracture-dislocation.

The common isolated spinous process fracture is called the *clay-shoveler's fracture* (Figs. 6–55 to 6–57). This usually affects C7 and sometimes C6 or T1. If truly isolated it is a stable injury. It can involve the spinal canal by extension into the laminae accompanied by hemorrhage. The mechanism involves sharp twisting forces at the shoulders and at the base of the neck, classically associated with the shoveling of heavy, sticky materials. Purer flexion strain can produce similar fractures, perhaps with a greater tendency to involve the laminae.

Detection of a defect in a spinous process on a lateral view is easy unless the entire process is avulsed at its base and shows only a deviation of its spinolaminar line (see Fig. 6–39). An interrupted spinous process can be an acute fracture, an old fracture, or an ununited apophysis, or can be simulated by an ossification in the nuchal ligament. A fracture usually occurs in the anterior half of the spinous process and is more diagonal (posterosuperior to anteroinferior), whereas a persistent synchondrosis is more posterior and more vertical. Only an acute fracture is truly sharp and jagged.

Translaminar fractures are hard to detect on a lateral film. A spinolaminar line may be fractured (see Fig. 6–15), or imbrication may be interrupted, but films of flexion-extension may be required. The

Text continued on page 258

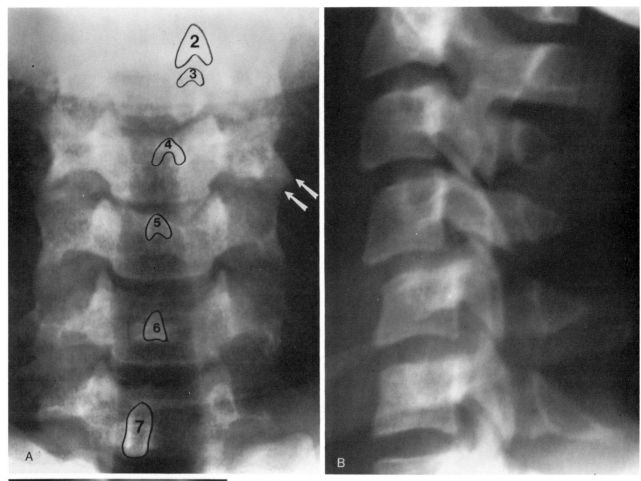

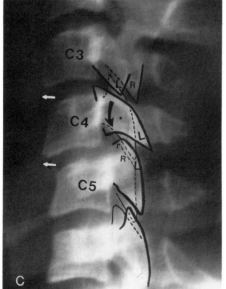

FIGURE 6–54. Left C4 Pedicle Fracture in a 19-Year-Old Man

• • • •

A, This anteroposterior (AP) film shows spinous process deviations: C3 to the left on C4, and C4 to the left on C5. A wedge juts inferolaterally from the left C4 pillar (arrows); this often indicates a pillar fracture, but in this case it probably represents a combination of lateral displacement and rotation of the pillar around its own AP axis. B and C, The same lateral film is shown without and with annotation. The thick lines delineate the injured left side; the thin solid and dashed lines delineate the right side. Note the right-left rotation: at C6 and C5 the left pillars are more posterior, but at C3 the left pillar is more anterior. The C4 pedicle has rotated around its own central x-axis, permitting anterolistheses of C3 and C4 (arrows) and indicating a coronal plane pedicle fracture.

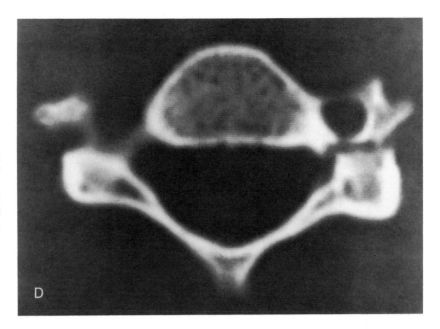

FIGURE 6–54 *Continued* **Left C4 Pedicle Fracture in a 19-Year-Old Man**

• • • •

D, A coronal fracture plane through the left C4 pedicle is confirmed as the only fracture in this 1.5-mm computed tomography section with bone algorithm. Note the lateral displacement of the pillar; the lamina must be slightly bent and twisted.

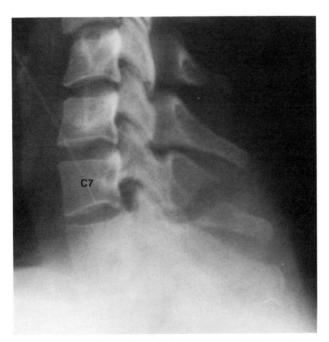

FIGURE 6–55. Clay-Shoveler's Fracture of C7 in a 16-Year-Old Woman

• • • •

A diagonal fracture line in the anterior half of the spinous process has sharp, complementary, and noncorticated borders. The distal fragment is displaced inferiorly but there is no abnormal flexion.

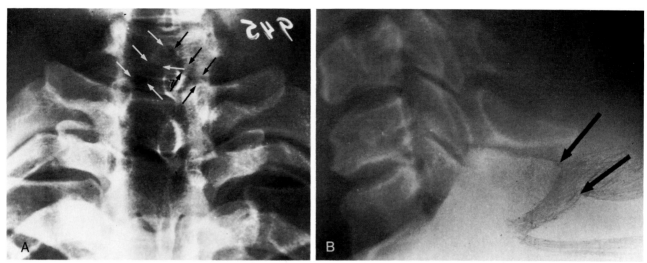

FIGURE 6–56. C7 Spinous Process Fracture in a 44-Year-Old Man with Intermittent Dull Cervicothoracic Pain 3 Days After a Direct Cervicothoracic Impact in a Fall

• • • •

A, An anteroposterior chest film shows an inverted "V" *(arrows)* slightly *above* the visible tip of the C7 spinous process *(7). B,* A lateral view of a classic clay-shoveler's fracture (retouched). The fracture slopes downward anteriorly and involves the middle and the anterior half of the process *(arrows).*

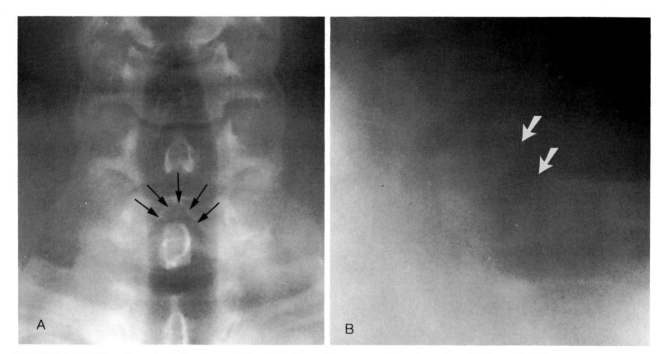

FIGURE 6–57. Clay-Shoveler's Fracture of the C7 Spinous Process and Laminae in a 28-Year-Old Man

• • • •

A, This anteroposterior film shows a faint inverted "V" lucency *(arrows)* just above the "spinous process" shadow (posterior portion of the spinous process). *B,* A lateral tomogram shows a typical clay-shoveler's fracture *(arrows)* within the anterior half of the spinous process.

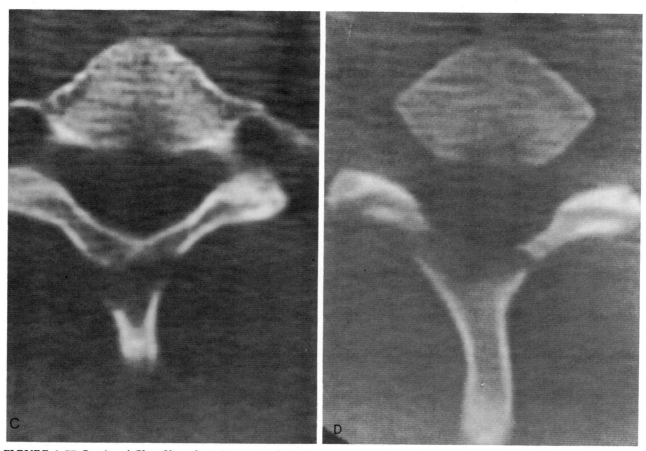

FIGURE 6–57 *Continued* **Clay-Shoveler's Fracture of the C7 Spinous Process and Laminae in a 28-Year-Old Man**

• • • •

C, This 1.5-mm computed tomography (CT) section taken at the inferior C7 pedicle level shows a(n) (oblique-) coronal spinous process fracture. *D,* This CT section at the C7–T1 facet joint level shows continuation of the fracture into the C7 laminae.

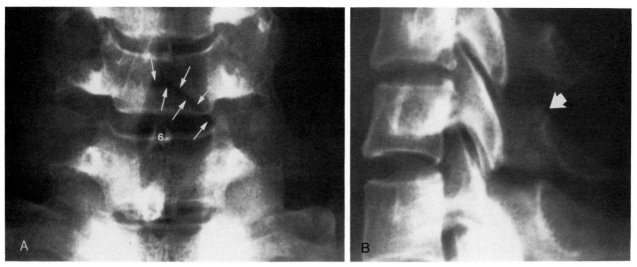

FIGURE 6–58. C6 Lamina Fracture in a 33-Year-Old Woman with Neck Pain 8 Weeks After a Motor Vehicle Accident
• • • •
A, This anteroposterior film shows an asymmetric partial inverted "V" *(arrows) well above* the visible tip of the C6 spinous process *(6)*. *B*, A lateral film shows a fracture *(arrow)* at the superior spinolaminar junction.

AP film may show a broad inverted "V" lucency with arms of uniform width positioned symmetrically in the arch (see Figs. 6–56*A* and 6–57*A*). The laminae may not be well outlined on an AP film, but the "V" is seen through a vertebral body or a disc region. An asymmetric inverted "V" (Fig. 6–58*A*) or a diagonal line (see Fig. 6–50*A*) may be seen instead.

TRANSVERSE PROCESS FRACTURE

Isolated fractures of the lower cervical transverse processes are uncommon. Sometimes pillar or complex body fractures are found on CT to extend into a transverse process (see Figs. 6–33*D*, and 6–34*C* and *D*), often crossing the transverse foramen and raising concern for the vertebral artery. Lateral hyperflexion transverse process fractures occur at one or two contiguous levels on the "convex" side (ipsilateral to the impact) due to avulsion by attachments; these fractures are frequently associated with other arch fractures at various levels and sometimes with brachial plexus injury. Most of the avulsions are at C7, whereas C6 and T1 are the next most frequent locations.[94] Aside from displaced avulsions, cervical transverse process fractures are very difficult to see on the AP film because of their fine, irregular configurations and owing to x-ray overpenetration. Fractures of the larger T1 transverse processes reflect first rib trauma and are easier to see (see Fig. 6–28) but must be distinguished from fully corticated unfused apophyses.

Whiplash

"Whiplash," or "acceleration injury," literally denotes a mechanism of injury and predominantly involves extension. By common usage it denotes a heterogeneous group of injuries to the soft tissues of the spinal column, other neck soft tissues, and even the head, that result from the mechanism. The term is typically applied in the absence of major cervical fracture or dislocation, but it can be applied in their presence. The essence of the mechanism is a force applied to the torso; the subsequent inertia of the head then strains the cervical spine and the neck muscles. Usually the body is accelerated forward, as in a rear-end motor vehicle collision, and the head is thrown into extension. A flexion component may develop when the head bounces off a headrest or is recoiled by spinal ligaments and neck muscles. Initial flexion with recoil extension and lateral flexion with contralateral recoil also correspond to the concept.

The pathology of the whiplash syndromes presumably involves sundry injuries to cervical ligaments and joints and also sometimes involves cervical muscle strains. MR imaging can demonstrate some of the soft tissue injuries, such as anterior annular tears, posterior disc herniations, longus colli strain, and fluid around a facet joint.[22] More significant hyperextension dislocation and disc protrusion must be ruled out, and small fractures may be sought with CT.

• • • •
NEUROLOGIC INJURY

Spinal Cord

Clinical Syndromes

Several clinical syndromes have been defined, although they often have incomplete expression or display a mixture of characteristics. Some, particularly certain incomplete cord syndromes, are most common or only fully expressed at the cervical level. These cervical cord syndromes suggest certain spinal injuries that must be sought if not already apparent.

Neurapraxia of the cervical spinal cord comprises sensory changes and almost always a motor deficit (usually tetraplagia) that resolve completely over several hours or a few days. This syndrome corresponds to a spinal cord concussion. It results from various injury vectors and typically occurs without radiologic signs of acute injury and with or without a predisposing anatomic condition such as stenosis.[112, 125]

The anterior cord syndrome comprises tetraplegia, hypesthesia, and hypalgesia below the lesion with preservation of most posterior column functions, particularly proprioception.[99] Partial loss of touch and vibratory sense indicates involvement of the deep portion of the posterior columns.[99, 113] Pain and temperature sensation, mediated through the spinothalamic tracts, may be abolished; the degree to which these are preserved suggests a better prognosis for functional motor recovery.[39] In addition to the severance of the descending motor tracts, upper extremity anterior horn cells and ventral roots at the level of the injury are destroyed. The proximate mechanism may be any combination of direct cord disruption and anterior spinal artery occlusion affecting the anterior two thirds of the cord. The precipitating spinal injuries typically are flexion-teardrop fractures and acute disc protrusions, but there can be others, such as unilateral or bilateral facet dislocation.[14, 97] Surgical decompression is considered if continuing compression may be a factor in the existing deficits or in possible progression as determined by CT, myelography, or MR imaging.

The central cord syndrome comprises tetraparesis that is worse in the upper extremities, especially in the small hand muscles, and that is often accompanied by urinary retention or other bladder dysfunction as well as by variable sensory deficits below the level of injury.[75, 98] The lesion is centered in the central gray matter and involves varying portions of the deeper white matter. Thus, there is a more severe lower motor neuron deficit in the upper extremities, due to anterior horn damage at the level of injury, combined with a milder upper motor neuron deficit in the lower extremities to whatever degree the deeper anterolateral white matter is involved. Considerable functional recovery is common. The most common injury mechanism is hyperextension in which the cord is squeezed from the front by osteophytes, by a transient annular bulge, or by a vertebral body margin (retrolisthesis in hyperextension dislocation, and anterolisthesis in hyperextension fracture-dislocation) at the same time as it is squeezed from behind by the buckling of thickened or normal ligamenta flava or by a neural arch. When there is little plain film or CT evidence of acute trauma, congenital or acquired spinal stenosis is usually present. The central cord syndrome is by no means limited to hyperextension injuries but also occurs with compressive injuries, such as burst fracture, with flexion injuries, such as facet dislocations, and with C1 and C2 fractures.[75] Surgery is usually not indicated.

The Brown-Séquard syndrome comprises ipsilateral anesthesia and lower motor neuron paralysis at the level of the lesion, an ipsilateral loss of proprioception and vibratory sense as well as upper motor neuron paralysis below the lesion, and a contralateral loss of pain and temperature sensation beginning a few segments below the lesion. Although it is typically due to penetrating injuries, variations on this syndrome can occur in closed spinal trauma with unilateral facet dislocation, lateralized epidural hematoma,[124] disc herniation, or spondylotic stenosis. In closed spinal trauma, the components *below* the level of injury often have a good prognosis for functional recovery.[39]

The pathogenetic difference among these syndromes lies in the direction and the intensity of the force. If anterior cord impact is very focal and rapid, as in many burst and flexion-teardrop fractures and acute disc herniations, tissue damage is predominantly localized anteriorly. With blunt compression, regardless of whether the offending protrusion is anterior or posterior, or both, the inherently greater susceptibility of the central cord leads to a central cord syndrome. More extreme injuries by any mechanism produce complete or nearly complete physiologic transections that are indistinguishable from each other.[89] In some cases of neurapraxia, particularly without stenosis, force may be transmitted to the cord without any direct impact.[125]

The presence of sacral sparing, consisting of persistent perianal sensation or voluntary sphincter contraction, classifies the syndrome as incomplete even if insufficient additional functions are preserved to qualify as one of the above syndromes. A complete cord syndrome shows no conscious sensory or voluntary motor function below the lesion, although reflex functions of the conus medullaris may persist. However, 4–5% of patients with clinically complete syndromes show significant neurologic improvement.[39]

Pathology

Concussion is a temporary functional disturbance without demonstrated anatomic changes. With increasing diagnostic sophistication, more injuries may be found to have subtle anatomic components and mild residual deficits. Contusion is equated with bruising and requires at least microscopic hemorrhage by definition. Necrosis and microhemorrhage occur early in cord injury and can be presumed to be present when edema is recognized by imaging after trauma. Contusion can result from cord compression with local ischemia and tissue disruption and can produce a physiologic transection. Primarily edematous lesions that are small may recover without clinically apparent deficit. Hematomyelia is macroscopic hemorrhage into the spinal cord. Marked hemorrhage and blood pooling indicate permanent cord damage. Laceration is a tearing of tissue that causes hemorrhage and various degrees of anatomic transection. Additional cord lesions that can develop in the chronic stage are atrophy and gliosis (myelomalacia), cavitation (syringomyelia), and an expanding cavity under pressure (progressive post-traumatic cystic myelopathy).

Cord Imaging

There are several possible significant findings at myelography. Subarachnoid block to contrast medium flow indicates cord compression (the deformed cord effaces the subarachnoid space at the level of the blockage). The degree of compression may be less and not result in complete block but still signify cord damage resulting from a greater transient compression during the injury. Subsequent edema may or may not be sufficient to swell the cord sufficiently to produce a complete block. If the contrast medium passes, it may enter the cord at a laceration or at a gross cavitation (see Fig. 6–32D). The cord shadow may disappear at the level of the injury, indicating anatomic transection. Myelographic findings can be refined by subsequent CT. CT often shows contrast medium passing a myelographically "complete" block.

MR imaging can show significant intramedullary pathology with or without swelling or laceration. Gross transection is shown, analogously with myelography, as a disappearance of cord signal contrasted against the (bloody) CSF. Finer pathologic-clinical correlations will likely develop as MR imaging technology improves. Prognostic evaluation with MR imaging may improve the clinical salvage rate from more restricted surgical selection.

At any field strength, edema prolongs relaxation times and thereby increases signal on T_2-weighted images and decreases it on T_1-weighted images. T_2-weighted images are most sensitive to edema, but their high signal does not distinguish between edema and necrosis,[42, 76] and at low and medium field strengths they do not distinguish between edema and hemorrhage.[37, 59, 60, 109, 123] T_2^*-weighted gradient-echo images may show increased signal with edema, but with less sensitivity.[29] STIR may show abnormal signal not shown on other sequences.[61] T_1-weighted sequences are less sensitive to edema and usually show isointensity with the cord. Edema is usually manifested on T_1-weighted images only as swelling. Lesions with T_1 hypointensity are more severe and show poor recovery.[123] The presence, the size, and the resolution of edema have correlated fairly well with clinical findings and improvement.[9, 22, 59, 61, 65, 95, 123] Exceptions have been noted, however. The cord has appeared normal in the presence of incomplete cord syndromes.[65, 95] Some patients with traumatic cord edema with little clinical deficit have been observed.[65] Clinical improvement has been seen despite evolution to myelomalacia or to worsening edema.[76]

Dominant hemorrhage is best distinguished from dominant edema at high field strength of at least 1 Tesla and usually 1.5 Tesla. The higher field strength accentuates the T_2-shortening effect of intracellular deoxyhemoglobin, which produces a signal void in acute hematomas.[42, 65, 95] A similar effect occurs on gradient-echo T_2^*-weighted images and may be visible at lower field strengths.[36, 65]

Imaging at 1.5 Tesla, Kulkarni and associates described two polar types of cord appearance and an intermediate type that correlated with prognosis.[65] One group had increased T_2-weighted signal that resolved on subsequent imaging. These patients had either normal neurologic status or incomplete cord syndromes that improved. The intermediate group had a zone of increased T_2-weighted signal containing a central hypointensity that turned bright on subsequent imaging. Of the two patients, one showed partial neurologic recovery. The third group showed T_2-weighted hypointensity relative to cord acutely; on subsequent imaging this persisted with peripheral hyperintensity resembling the acute stage of the intermediate group. These patients had complete and incomplete cord deficits. In other series most patients with a similar appearance had complete deficits[29, 95] that rarely if ever were accompanied by any neurologic recovery. The T_2-weighted hypointensity apparently indicated gross hemorrhage with permanent tissue destruction.

Axial T_2-weighted images may show a loss of internal cord detail [16] and have shown hemorrhagic foci bilaterally in the central gray matter at the gray matter–white matter junctions.[65]

MR imaging is the best means to demonstrate persistent cord compression by soft tissues. Increasing numbers of disc protrusions and epidural hematomas (EDHs; see Fig. 6–53H and I) are found, although their significance awaits quantitative evaluation. EDH may be difficult to distinguish from edema and engorged epidural vessels[9] for which a STIR sequence has been advocated.[61]

Root Injuries

Roots are commonly compressed by foraminal narrowing related to facet fractures and to other local injuries. Such injuries are best appreciated clinically and by myelography or CT. Nerve root avulsions result from extremity trauma rather than from spinal trauma; however, the cord can be injured by the avulsion. Avulsions more commonly involve the brachial than the lumbosacral plexus. One or several cervical roots may be avulsed with their dural sleeves. Myelography may opacify a rounded or an irregular pseudomeningocele within the spinal canal or extending through the neural foramen. When multiple, the pseudomeningoceles are unilateral and usually vary considerably in size and shape. They may superficially resemble lumbosacral root sleeve (Tarlov) cysts, but avulsed nerve roots are absent. The dura and the arachnoid mater usually tear before the roots, however, so roots within a pseudomeningocele may remain intact, whereas absence of a pseudomeningocele argues against a root avulsion.[102]

References

1. Abel MS. Occult Traumatic Lesions of the Cervical and Thoraco-Lumbar Vertebrae. 2nd ed. St. Louis: Warren H. Green, 1983, pp 44–49, 95, 106–109.
2. Abel MS. Occult Traumatic Lesions of the Cervical and Thoraco-Lumbar Vertebrae. 2nd ed. St. Louis: Warren H. Green, 1983, pp 47–49, 82, 90–92.
3. Altongy JF, Fielding JW. Combined atlanto-axial and occipito-atlantal rotary subluxation. J Bone Joint Surg 1990; 72:923–926.
4. Anderson LD, D'Alonzo RT. Fractures of the odontoid process of the axis. J Bone Joint Surg (Am) 1974; 56:1663–1674.
5. Anderson PA, Montesano PX. Morphology and treatment of occipital condyle fractures. Spine 1988; 13:731–736.
6. Ardran GM, Kemp FH. The mechanism of changes in form of the cervical airway in infancy. Med Radiogr Photogr 1968; 44:26–38, 54.
7. Barber-Riley WP. Agenesis of the neural arch of the axis. AJNR 1982; 3:75–76.
8. Beatson TR. Fractures and dislocations of the cervical spine. J Bone Joint Surg (Br) 1963; 45:21–35.
9. Beers GJ, Raque GH, Wagner GG, et al. MR imaging in acute cervical spine trauma. J Comput Assist Tomogr 1988; 12:755–761.
10. Bone L, Bucholz R. The management of fractures in the patient with multiple trauma. J Bone Joint Surg 1986; 68:945–949.
11. Bucholz RW. Unstable hangman's fractures. Clin Orthop 1981; 154:119–124.
12. Bucholz RW, Burkhead WZ. The pathological anatomy of fatal atlanto-occipital dislocations. J Bone Joint Surg (Am) 1979; 61:248–250.
13. Budin E, Sondheimer F. Lateral spread of the atlas without fracture. Radiology 1966; 87:1095–1098.
14. Burke DC, Berryman D. The place of closed manipulation in the management of flexion-rotation dislocations of the cervical spine. J Bone Joint Surg (Br) 1971; 53:165–182.
15. Cave AJE. The morphology of the mammalian cervical pleurapophysis. J Zoology (London) 1975; 177:377–393.
16. Chakeres DW, Flickinger F, Bresnahan JC, et al. MR imaging of acute spinal cord trauma. AJNR 1987; 8:5–10.
17. Childers JC, Wilson FC. Bipartite atlas. J Bone Joint Surg (Am) 1971; 53:578–582.
18. Clark CR, Kathol MH, Walsh T, El-Khoury GY. Atlanto-axial rotatory fixation with compensatory counter occipito-atlantal subluxation. Spine 1986; 11:1048–1050.
19. Clyburn TA, Lionberger DR, Tullos HS. Bilateral fracture of the transverse fracture of the atlas. J Bone Joint Surg (Am) 1982; 64:948.
20. Coutts MB. Atlanto-epistropheal subluxations. Arch Surg 1934; 29:297–311.
21. Davis JW. Cervical injuries: Perils of the swimmer's view: Case report. J Trauma 1989; 29:891–893.
22. Davis SJ, Teresi LM, Bradley WG Jr, et al. Cervical spine hyperextension injuries: MR findings. Radiology 1991; 180:245–251.
23. Di Chiro G, Timins EL. Supine myelography and the septum posticum. Radiology 1974; 111:319–327.
24. Edeiken-Monroe B, Wagner LK, Harris JH. Hyperextension dislocation of the cervical spine. AJNR 1986; 7:135–140, and AJR 1986; 146:803–808.
25. Effendi B, Roy D, Cornish B, et al. Fractures of the ring of the axis. J Bone Joint Surg (Am) 1981; 63:319–327.
26. Epstein BS. The Spine: A Radiological Text and Atlas. 4th ed. Philadelphia: Lea & Febiger, 1976, p 541.
27. Fielding JW, Hawkins RJ. Atlanto-axial rotary fixation (fixed rotary subluxation of the atlanto-axial joint). J Bone Joint Surg (Am) 1977; 59:37–44.
28. Fielding JW, Stillwell WT, Chynn KY, Spyropoulos EC. Use of computed tomography for the diagnosis of atlanto-axial rotatory fixation. J Bone Joint Surg (Am) 1978; 60:1102–1104.
29. Flanders AE, Schaefer DM, Doan HT, et al. Acute cervical spine trauma: Correlation of MR imaging findings with degree of neurologic deficit. Radiology 1990; 177:25–33.
30. Forsyth HF, Alexander E, Davis C Jr. The advantages of early spine fusion in the treatment of fracture-dislocation of the cervical spine. J Bone Joint Surg 1959; 41:17–36.
31. Gehweiler JA, Daffner RH, Roberts L Jr. Malformations of the atlas vertebra simulating the Jefferson fracture. AJNR 1983; 4:187–190, and AJR 1983; 140:1083–1086.
32. Gehweiler JA, Osborne RL, Becker RF. The Radiology of Vertebral Trauma. Philadelphia: W.B. Saunders Co., 1980, p 189.
33. Gehweiler JA, Osborne RL, Becker RF. The Radiology of Vertebral Trauma. Philadelphia: W.B. Saunders Co., 1980, pp 190–191, 194–198.
34. Gehweiler JA, Osborne RL, Becker RF. The Radiology of Vertebral Trauma. Philadelphia: W.B. Saunders Co., 1980, pp 191, 198–200.
35. Gehweiler JA, Osborne RL, Becker RF. The Radiology of Vertebral Trauma. Philadelphia: W.B. Saunders Co., 1980, p 215.
36. Goldberg AL, Baron B, Daffner RH. Atlanto-occipital dislocation: MR demonstration of cord damage. J Comput Assist Tomogr 1991; 15:174–178.

37. Goldberg AL, Rothfus WE, Deeb ZL, et al. The impact of magnetic resonance on the diagnostic evaluation of acute cervicothoracic spinal trauma. Skeletal Radiol 1988; 17:89–95.

38. Greeley PW. Bilateral (ninety degrees) rotary dislocation of the atlas upon the axis. J Bone Joint Surg (Am) 1930; 12:958–962.

39. Green BA, Magana IA. Spinal cord trauma: Clinical aspects. In Davidoff RA (ed). Handbook of the Spinal Cord. Vol 4. New York: Marcel Dekker, Inc., 1987, pp 63–96.

40. Green JD, Harle TS, Harris JH Jr. Anterior subluxation of the cervical spine: Hyperflexion sprain. AJNR 1981; 2:243–250.

41. Grogono BJS. Injuries of the atlas and axis. J Bone Joint Surg 1954; 36:397–410.

42. Hackney DB, Asato R, Joseph PM, et al. Hemorrhage and edema in acute spinal cord compression: Demonstration by MR imaging. Radiology 1986; 161:387–390.

43. Hadley MN, Browner CM, Liu SS, Sonntag VKH. New subtype of acute odontoid fractures (Type IIA). Neurosurgery 1988; 22:67–71.

44. Harrington JF, Likavec MJ, Smith AS. Disc herniation in cervical fracture subluxation. Neurosurgery 1991; 29:374–379.

45. Harris JH Jr, Burke JT, Ray RD, et al. Low (Type III) odontoid fracture: A new radiographic sign. Radiology 1984; 153:353–356.

46. Harris JH, Edeiken-Monroe B. The Radiology of Acute Cervical Spine Trauma. 2nd ed. Baltimore: Williams & Wilkins, 1987, pp 83, 189–191, 202, 213.

47. Harris JH, Edeiken-Monroe B. The Radiology of Acute Cervical Spine Trauma. 2nd ed. Baltimore: Williams & Wilkins, 1987, pp 120–123.

48. Harviainen S, Lahti P, Davidsson L. On cervical spine injuries. Acta Chir Scand 1972; 138:349–355.

49. Hay PD Jr. The Neck: A roentgenological study of the soft tissues: Consideration of the normal and pathological. III. Normal necks (adults). Ann Roentgenol 1930; 9:5–21.

50. Hay PD Jr. The Neck: A roentgenological study of the soft tissues: Consideration of the normal and pathological. III. Normal necks (infants and children). Ann Roentgenol Vol 9. New York: Hoeber, 1930, pp 22–28.

51. Hayashi K, Yabuki T. Origin of the uncus and of Luschka's joint in the cervical spine. J Bone Joint Surg (Am) 1985; 68:788–791.

52. Hinck VC, Hopkins CE. Measurement of the atlanto-dental interval in the adult. AJR 1960; 84:945–951.

53. Iannacone WM, DeLong WG Jr, Born CT, et al. Dynamic computerized tomography of the occiput-atlas-axis complex in trauma patients with odontoid lateral mass asymmetry. J Trauma 1990; 30:1501–1505.

54. Ingebrightsen R. On dislocation and fracture-dislocation of the spinal column. Acta Chir Scand 1946; 94:455–468.

55. Jackson H. The diagnosis of minimal atlanto-axial subluxation. Br J Radiol 1950; 23:672–674.

56. Jefferson G. Fracture of the atlas vertebra. Br J Surg 1920; 7:407–422.

57. Johnson JE, Yang PJ, Seeger JF, Iacono RP. Vertical fracture of the odontoid: CT diagnosis. J Comput Assist Tomogr 1986; 10:311–312.

58. Juhl JH, Miller SM, Roberts GW. Roentgenographic variations in the normal cervical spine. Radiology 1962; 78:591–597.

59. Kadoya S, Nakamura T, Kobayashi S, Yamamoto I. Magnetic resonance imaging of acute spinal cord injury. Neuroradiology 1987; 29:252–255.

60. Kalfas I, Wilberger J, Goldberg A, Prostko ER. Magnetic resonance imaging in acute spinal cord trauma. Neurosurgery 1987; 29:252–255.

61. Kerslake RW, Jaspan T, Worthington BS. Magnetic resonance imaging of spinal trauma. Br J Radiol 1991; 64:386–402.

62. Kim KS, Chen HH, Russell EJ, Rogers LF. Flexion teardrop fracture of the cervical spine: Radiographic characteristics. AJNR 1988; 9:1221–1228, and AJR 1989; 152:319–326.

63. Kowalski HM, Cohen WA, Cooper P, Wisoff JH. Pitfalls in the CT diagnosis of atlanto-axial rotary subluxation. AJNR 1987; 8:697–702, and AJR 1987; 149:595–600.

64. Kulkarni M, Bondurant FJ, Rose SL, Narayana PA. 1.5 Tesla magnetic resonance imaging of acute spinal trauma. Radiographics 1988; 8:1059–1082.

65. Kulkarni MV, McArdle CB, Kopanicky D, et al. Acute spinal cord injury: MR imaging at 1.5T. Radiology 1987; 164:837–843.

66. Lee C, Kim KS, Rogers LF. Sagittal fracture of the vertebral body. AJR 1982; 139:55–60.

67. Lee C, Kim KS, Rogers LF. Triangular cervical vertebral body fractures: Diagnostic significance. AJR 1982; 138:1123–1132.

68. Lee C, Woodring JH, Goldstein SJ, et al. Evaluation of traumatic atlanto-occipital dislocations. AJNR 1987; 8:19–26.

69. Levine AM, Edwards CC. The management of traumatic spondylolisthesis of the axis. J Bone Joint Surg (Am) 1985; 67:217–226.

70. Lipson SJ, Mazur J. Anteroposterior spondyloschisis of the atlas revealed by computerized tomography scanning. J Bone Joint Surg (Am) 1978; 60:1104–1105.

71. Locke GR, Gardner JI, Van Epps EF. Atlas-dens interval (ADI) in children: A survey based on 200 normal cervical spines. AJR 1966; 97:135–140.

72. Marar BC. Hyperextension injuries of the cervical spine: The pathogenesis of damage to the spinal cord. J Bone Joint Surg (Am) 1974; 56:1655–1662.

73. Marar BC. The pattern of neurologic damage as an aid to the diagnosis of the mechanism in cervical-spine injuries. J Bone Joint Surg (Am) 1974; 56:1648–1654.

74. McArdle CB, Wright JW, Prevost WJ, et al. MR imaging of the acutely injured patient with cervical traction. Radiology 1986; 159:273–274.

75. Merriam WF, Taylor TKF, Ruff SJ, McPhail MJ. A reappraisal of acute traumatic central cord syndrome. J Bone Joint Surg (Br) 1986; 68:708–713.

76. Mirvis SE, Geisler FH, Jelinek JJ, et al. Acute cervical spine trauma: Evaluation with 1.5-T MR imaging. Radiology 1988; 166:807–816.

77. Oon CL. Some sagittal measurements of the neck in normal adults. Br J Radiol 1964; 37:674–677.

78. Orofino C, Sherman MS, Schechter D. Luschka's joint: A degenerative phenomenon. J Bone Joint Surg (Am) 1960; 42:853–858.

79. Paakkala T. Prevertebral soft tissue changes in cervical spine injury. Crit Rev Diagn Imaging 1985; 24:201–236.

80. Pal JM, Mulder DS, Brown RA, Fleiszer DM. Assessing multiple trauma: Is the cervical spine enough? J Trauma 1988; 28:1282–1284.

81. Pan G, Kulkarni M, MacDougall DJ, Miner ME. Traumatic epidural hematoma of the cervical spine: Diagnosis with magnetic resonance imaging. J Neurosurg 1988; 68:798–801.

82. Pavlov H, Torg JS, Robie B, Jahre C. Cervical spinal stenosis: Determination with vertebral body ratio method. Radiology 1987; 164:771–775.

83. Penning L. Prevertebral hematoma in cervical spine injury: Incidence and etiologic significance. AJR 1981; 136:553–561.

84. Penning L, Wilmink JT. Rotation of the cervical spine: A CT study in normal subjects. Spine 1987; 12:732–738.

85. Powell JN, Waddell JP, Tucker WS, Transfeldt EE. Multiple-level noncontiguous spinal fractures. J Trauma 1989; 29:1146–1151.

86. Powers B, Miller MD, Kramer RS, et al. Traumatic anterior atlanto-occipital dislocation. Neurosurgery 1979; 4:12–17.

87. Pratt ES, Green DA, Spengler DM. Herniated intervertebral discs associated with unstable spinal injuries. Spine 1990; 15:662–666.

88. Quencer RM. The injured spinal cord. Radiol Clin North Am 1988; 26:1025–1045.

89. Raynor RB, Koplik B. Cervical cord trauma: The relationship between clinical syndromes and force of injury. Spine 1985; 10:193–197.

90. Resnick D, Niwayama G. Diagnosis of Bone and Joint Disorders. 2nd ed. Vol 2. Philadelphia: W.B. Saunders Co., 1988, p 684.

91. Rizzolo SJ, Piazza MR, Cotler JM, et al. Intervertebral disc injury complicating cervical spine trauma. Spine 1991; 16:S187–S189.

92. Roaf R. Lateral flexion injuries of the cervical spine. J Bone Joint Surg (Br) 1963; 45:36–38.

93. Ross SE, Schwab W, David ET, et al. Clearing the cervical spine: Initial radiographic evaluation. J Trauma 1987; 27:1055–1060.

94. Schaaf RE, Gehweiler JA Jr, Miller MD, Powers B. Lateral hyperflexion injuries of the cervical spine. Skeletal Radiol 1978; 3:73–78.

95. Schaefer DM, Flanders A, Northrup BE, et al. Magnetic resonance imaging of acute cervical spine trauma: Correlation with severity of neurologic injury. Spine 1989; 14:1090–1095.

96. Scher AT. Anterior cervical subluxation. AJR 1979; 133:275–280.

97. Schneider RC. The syndrome of acute anterior spinal cord injury. J Neurosurg 1955; 12:95–122.

98. Schneider RC, Cherry G, Pantek H. The syndrome of acute central cervical spinal cord injury. J Neurosurg 1954; 11:546–577.

99. Schneider RC, Kahn EA. Chronic neurological sequelae of acute trauma to the spine and spinal cord. I: The significance of the acute-flexion or "tear-drop" fracture-dislocation of the cervical spine. J Bone Joint Surg (Am) 1956; 38:985–997.

100. Schneider RC, Livingston KE, Cave AJE, Hamilton G. "Hangman's fracture" of the cervical spine. J Neurosurg 1965; 22:141–154.

101. Scott EW, Haid RW Jr, Peace D. Type I fractures of the odontoid process: Implications for atlanto-occipital instability. J Neurosurg 1990; 72:488–492.

102. Shapiro R. Myelography. 4th ed. Chicago: Year Book Medical Publishers, Inc., 1984, pp 253–269.

103. Skold G. Sagittal fractures of the cervical spine. Injury 1978; 9:294–296.

104. Spence KF Jr, Decker S, Sell KW. Bursting atlantal fracture associated with rupture of the transverse ligament. J Bone Joint Surg (Am) 1970; 52:543–549.

105. Steele HH. Anatomical and mechanical considerations of the atlanto-axial articulations. J Bone Joint Surg (Am) 1968; 50:1481–1482.

106. Stoltmann HF, Blackwood W. An anatomical study of the role of the dentate ligaments in the cervical spinal canal. J Neurosurg 1966; 24:43–46.

107. Suss RA, Bundy KJ. Unilateral posterior arch fractures of the atlas. AJNR 1984; 5:783–786.

108. Suss RA, Zimmerman RD, Leeds NE. Pseudospread of the atlas: False sign of Jefferson fracture in young children. AJNR 1983; 4:183–186, and AJR 1983; 140:1079–1082.

109. Tarr RW, Drolshagen LF, Kerner TC, et al. MR imaging of recent spinal trauma. J Comput Assist Tomogr 1987; 11:412–417.

110. Templeton PA, Young JWR, Mirvis SE, Buddemeyer EU. The value of retropharyngeal soft tissue measurements in trauma of the adult cervical spine. Skeletal Radiol 1987; 16:98–104.

111. Thomeier WC, Brown DC, Mirvis SE. The laterally tilted dens: A sign of subtle odontoid fracture on plain radiography. AJNR 1990; 11:605–608.

112. Torg JS, Pavlov H, Genuario SE, et al. Neurapraxia of the cervical spinal cord with transient quadriplegia. J Bone Joint Surg (Am) 1986; 68:1354–1370.

113. Uddenberg N. Differential localization in dorsal funiculus of fibers originating from different receptors. Exp Brain Res 1968; 4:367–376.

114. Walsh JW, Stevens DB, Young AB. Traumatic paraplegia in children without contiguous spinal fracture or dislocation. Neurosurgery 1983; 12:439–445.

115. Washington ER. Non-traumatic atlanto-occipital and atlanto-axial dislocation. J Bone Joint Surg 1959; 41:341–344.

116. Weir DC. Roentgenographic signs of cervical injury. Clin Orthop 1975; 109:9–17.

117. Whalen JP, Woodruff CL. The cervical prevertebral fat stripe: A new aid in evaluating the cervical prevertebral soft tissue space. AJR 1970; 109:445–451.

118. White AA III, Johnson RM, Panjabi MM, Southwick WO. Biomechanical analysis of clinical stability in the cervical spine. Clin Orthop 1975; 109:85–96.

119. White AA III, Panjabi MM. Clinical Biomechanics of the Spine. 2nd ed. Philadelphia: J.B. Lippincott Co., 1990, p 643.

120. White AA, Southwick WO, Panjabi MM. Clinical instability in the lower cervical spine: A review of past and current concepts. Spine 1976; 1:15–27.

121. Wholey MH, Bruwer AJ, Baker HL Jr. The lateral roentgenogram of the neck. Radiology 1958; 71:350–356.

122. Wood-Jones F. The ideal lesion produced by judicial hanging. Lancet 1913; 1:53.

123. Yamashita Y, Takahashi M, Matsuno Y, et al. Acute spinal cord injury: Magnetic resonance imaging correlated with myelography. Br J Radiol 1991; 64:201–209.

124. Zupruk GM, Mehta Z. Brown-Séquard syndrome associated with post-traumatic cervical epidural hematoma: Case report and review of the literature. Neurosurgery 1989; 25:278–280.

125. Zwimpfer TJ, Bernstein M. Spinal cord concussion. J Neurosurg 1990; 72:894–900.

CHAPTER 7

The Thoracic and the Lumbar Spine, and the Spinal Cord

DIANNE B. MENDELSOHN, M.D.
GEORGIANA GIBSON, M.D.

The increasing number of motor vehicle accidents has resulted in an inexorable annual increase in the number of spinal column and spinal cord injuries. Since the lumbar and the thoracic spine are both larger and stronger than the cervical spine, greater traumatic forces are usually required to cause thoracolumbar fractures and dislocations. The thoracic spine is also rather rigid and is braced by the ribs, compounding the force needed to fracture a thoracic vertebra. Only rarely are thoracic or lumbar spinal dislocations present without associated fractures. During the evaluation of patients with a spinal injury, both the radiologist and the clinician must recognize that the radiographs depict only the residual dislocation present when the films are taken. This degree of dislocation is not necessarily the same as the actual dislocation that occurred at the time of injury. A very unstable fracture-dislocation of the thoracic or the lumbar spine can reduce spontaneously when the patient is in the supine position, thus obscuring the true severity of the bone and soft tissue injury. In addition, the overall incidence of multiple level but noncontiguous fractures of the spine in patients who have sustained a spinal cord or column injury is sufficiently high to warrant a mandatory search for the commonly associated fractures of the cervical spine and the thoracolumbar junction.[1, 17] Approximately 40% of thoracolumbar junction fractures are associated with neurologic deficits, a frequency exceeded only by that for fractures in the lower cervical region.[2]

RADIOLOGIC EVALUATION USING PLAIN FILMS, COMPUTED TOMOGRAPHY, MAGNETIC RESONANCE IMAGING, TOMOGRAPHY, AND MYELOGRAPHY

Patients with thoracic or lumbar spine trauma can be evaluated with several imaging modalities. Following an injury, spine films should be obtained quickly with the least amount of patient movement

• • • • APPROPRIATE RADIOGRAPHIC STUDIES

I. **Plain Films**
   A. Anteroposterior and lateral spine films should be performed first.
      1. They should include both the region of primary concern and areas of commonly associated injury.
      2. Although these films may not be completely diagnostic, they serve as a localizer for computed tomography (CT) and magnetic resonance (MR) imaging.
      Comment: Films should be obtained with as little patient motion as possible. If hyperflexion has occurred, particularly with seat belt injuries, a full abdominal film may be needed to look for free air or fluid in the abdomen.

II. **Computed Tomography**
   A. Axial images serially using 3-mm sections may be needed to detect subtle, nondisplaced fractures or to perform sagittal or coronal reconstructions.
   B. Thicker sections (5 mm) can be used for survey purposes.
   Comment: CT requires movement of the patient only from the stretcher to the scanner. CT demonstrates soft tissues in addition to bones. CT is preferable to MR imaging for complex fractures and for bone or metallic fragment localization.

III. **Enhanced Computed Tomography**
   A. Requires the instillation of a water-soluble contrast medium either via a lumbar or a C1–2 puncture.
   B. Improves CT delineation of the spinal cord and the nerve roots.
   C. Primarily used to locate dural tears.

IV. **Magnetic Resonance Imaging**
   A. Axial, sagittal, coronal, or oblique images may be obtained as needed. T_1-weighted images are generally of most use for anatomic delineation. T_2-weighted sequences are useful for intrinsic cord and pathologic evaluation.
   B. Far superior to CT even with enhancement for evaluation of the spinal cord. MR imaging should totally replace myelography for this purpose. MR imaging provides excellent soft tissue contrast, including cancellous bone (marrow) evaluation. However, it is not as good as CT for cortical bone evaluation.

V. **Tomography**
   A. Can provide a thorough evaluation of spinal fractures but generally requires patient motion for lateral projections.
   B. Tomography is a time-consuming procedure.

VI. **Myelography**
   A. Unless MR imaging or contrast-enhanced CT are not available, myelography has little place in the evaluation of acute spinal injury.
   B. Can detect dural tears with cerebrospinal fluid leaks.
   Comment: Myelography virtually always requires some patient motion, which may be contraindicated in the presence of an unstable fracture.

possible. At a minimum, anteroposterior and cross-table lateral views must be obtained. These views may not be completely diagnostic, but they do serve as a roadmap and a localizer for further imaging with CT or MR imaging. The plain film radiographic signs of thoracolumbar injury are listed in Table 7–1.

Vertebral injuries with interspinous widening or with evidence of disruption of the vertebral arch complex are clinically unstable, and extreme care must be used in moving patients with such injuries. The integrity of the apophyseal joints is particularly important to evaluate on the plain films because

TABLE 7–1. Radiographic Signs of Thoracolumbar Injury

> **Soft tissue signs**
>   Loss of psoas muscle stripe
>   Widened paraspinal line
> **Spinal abnormalities**
>   Abnormal intervertebral disc
>   Widened apophyseal joint
>   Widened interspinous space
>   Displacement (malalignment) of vertebrae
>   Scoliosis, kyphosis, or both
>   Widened interpedicular distance
>   Fracture of vertebra

these joints are the most sensitive indicator of dislocation or of an unstable spine injury (Fig. 7–1).[6, 7] Stability of the spine depends on the integrity of the posterior osteoligamentous complex. Transverse or oblique fractures through the transverse processes should always alert the radiologist or the clinician to the possibility of a horizontal arch fracture. When associated abdominal trauma is suspected, in particular with seat belt injuries, a full-sized abdominal radiograph should be carefully scrutinized for free air or fluid within the peritoneal cavity.

In order to identify dislocated or locked facets the radiologist must be familiar with the normal appear-

ance of the facets both on plain films and on CT scans. Normally, the superior facet articular surfaces are concave and directed posteromedially, and the inferior articular surfaces are flat or convex and are directed anterolaterally. Visualization of only the superior or the inferior facet should suggest that a subluxation or a dislocation of the facets exists.[13] This radiographic finding is referred to as the "naked facet" sign (see Fig. 7–1C).

CT in particular and MR imaging to a lesser degree are not screening procedures for thoracolumbar trauma, but if used they should be directed at a specific area of known or suspected injury. Tomography and myelography have been gradually decreasing in use owing to the increasing availability and greater diagnostic capabilities of both CT and MR imaging. Another advantage of these latter modalities is that once the patient is placed on the examination table, he or she need not be moved or change position during the study. This is preferable for patient stabilization, airway control, and other life support measures.

CT and MR imaging demonstrate the surrounding soft tissues (information that is not provided by

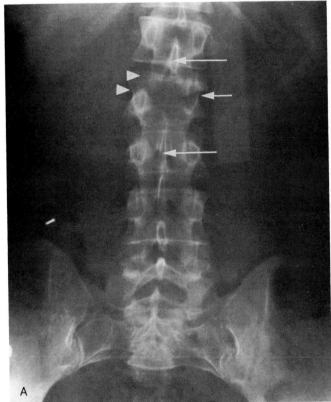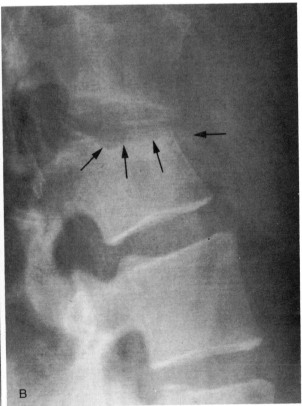

FIGURE 7–1. Unstable Spine Fractures

• • • •

A, This anteroposterior abdominal radiograph shows a flexion distraction injury involving L2. Note the widened L1–2 interspinous distance and the dislocation of the right L1–2 facet joint *(arrowheads).* The left facet joint remains congruous; however, there is a fracture through the left L2 pedicle *(short arrow).* The L1 and L2 spinous processes *(long arrows)* are widely separated. *B,* A lateral radiograph shows the kyphotic deformity related to this L1–2 flexion distraction injury. The anterior column of L2 is compressed *(arrows),* and the middle and posterior columns have failed under tension.

Illustration continued on following page

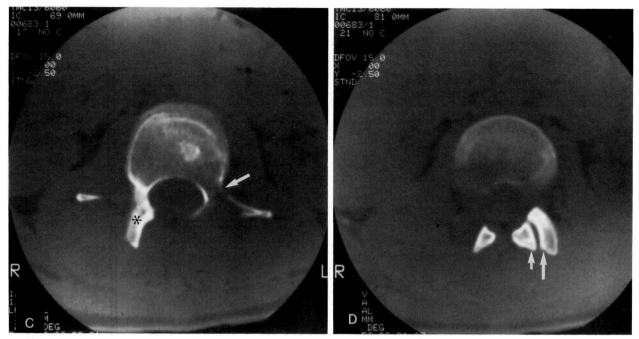

FIGURE 7–1 *Continued* **Unstable Spine Fractures**

• • • •

C, This axial computed tomography scan through the body of L2 shows the "naked facet sign" on the right. The superior articular process of L2 *(asterisk)* is seen without its corresponding inferior articular process of L1. Also notice the fracture through the left pedicle *(arrow).* *D,* The left superior and inferior articular processes of the L1–2 facet joint have a normal relationship as is apparent on this adjacent slice. The superior articular surface of L2 *(long arrow)* faces posteromedially, whereas the inferior of L1 *(short arrow)* faces anterolaterally.

routine radiographs) and visualize the spine and the spinal canal and its contents. Myelography has the disadvantage of necessitating patient manipulation and invasiveness, since a contrast agent must be injected within the spinal subarachnoid space. If for any reason a myelogram is indicated in an unstable patient in whom minimal movement is required, this can be performed using a C1–C2 puncture with the patient lying in the supine position and the head end of the table slightly elevated. The main indication for myelography with or without CT scanning is a suspected dural tear with cerebrospinal fluid (CSF) leak or a known contraindication to MR imaging (Table 7–2 and Figs. 7–2 to 7–4).

CT is superior to MR imaging in the detection and the localization of fractures as well as the demonstra-

TABLE 7–2. Contraindications to Magnetic Resonance Imaging

Pacemakers
Intracranial aneurysm clips not compatible with MR* imaging technology
Suspected metallic foreign body in the globe
Cochlear implants
Uncooperative, agitated, or restless patient
Life support systems not compatible with MR imaging technology
Marked obesity or any other reason that makes it impossible for the patient to be placed in the MR scanner

*Magnetic resonance.

tion of small displaced bone fragments within the spinal canal, the lateral recesses, or the exit foramina (Figs. 7–5 and 7–6). The degree of encroachment on the spinal canal by retropulsed bone or disc material can be demonstrated with CT or MR imaging. CT accurately assesses the degree of congruity of the facet articulations.[16] Seat belt injuries, particularly Chance fractures (see p. 277) with their primary horizontal component, are difficult to detect on axial CT scans and may require sagittal reconstructions for accurate delineation of the fracture and alignment of the fragments.

CT performed after intrathecal contrast medium instillation is often necessary for adequate visualization of the spinal cord and the thecal sac, particularly in the thoracic and the upper lumbar spine where little contrasting epidural fat is present. MR imaging is far superior to CT in evaluating the spinal cord itself and is able to detect contusion or cord compression by a hematoma, a disc herniation, or a large retropulsed bone fragment (Figs. 7–7 to 7–9).[11, 12, 15] The development of post-traumatic spinal cord cysts is a well-recognized complication of spinal cord injury. These are completely and noninvasively shown on MR images (Fig. 7–10). Complex fractures are better seen with CT, but MR imaging should completely replace myelography in the acute setting for spinal cord evaluation when it is technically feasible.

Text continued on page 275

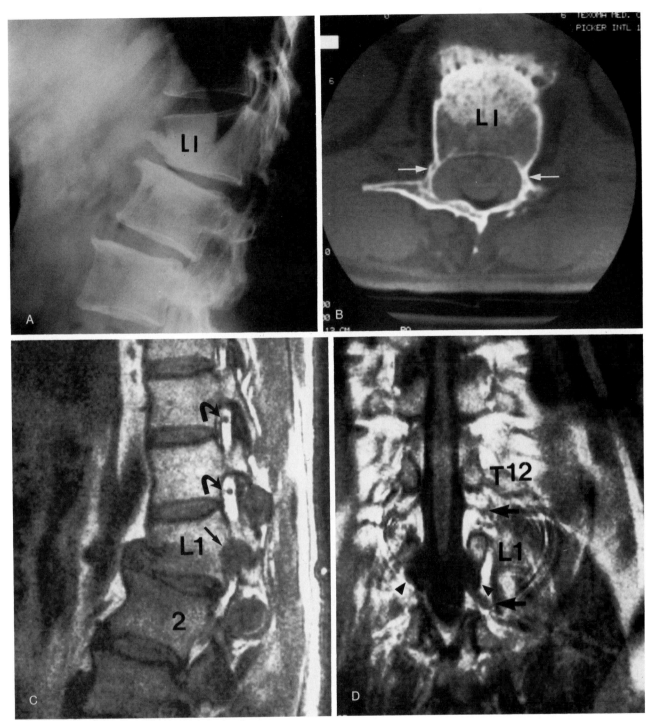

FIGURE 7–2. Post-Traumatic Pseudomeningoceles
• • • •
A, This lateral thoracolumbar radiograph shows an old wedge compression fracture of L1 with anterior L1–2 osteophytes and abnormal kyphosis. *B,* An axial computed tomography scan through L1 after the instillation of intrathecal contrast medium shows the presence of bilateral post-traumatic pseudomeningoceles with resultant thinning of the adjacent pedicles *(arrows). C,* This parasagittal T$_1$-weighted magnetic resonance (MR) image demonstrates the wedge compression fracture of L1 and a decreased signal (pseudomeningocele) extending into the superior aspect of the L1–2 exit foramen with loss of the normal epidural fat in this location *(straight arrow).* Normal fat-filled exit foramina with the centrally located exiting nerves are seen at T11 and T12 *(curved arrows). D,* A T$_1$-weighted coronal MR image at the level of the pedicles shows the bilateral pseudomeningoceles beneath the L1 pedicles *(arrowheads).* The exiting T12 and L1 nerves are delineated *(short black arrows).* The L1 nerve on the left is inferiorly displaced by the pseudomeningocele immediately above it.

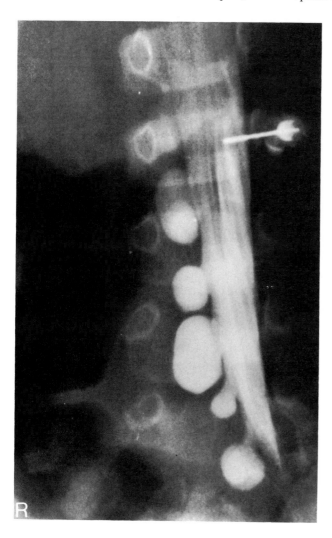

FIGURE 7–3. Post-Traumatic Nerve Root Avulsions

• • • •

Post-traumatic right nerve root avulsions with pseudomeningoceles are shown at five contiguous levels in this lumbar myelogram.

FIGURE 7–4. Traumatic Dural Tears

• • • •

This anteroposterior myelographic view shows frank leakage of contrast medium on the right side at T12–L1 and to a lesser degree at T10 (arrow) through dural tears incurred during a severe motor vehicle accident. The horizontal metal spring and band density are within the underlying mattress.

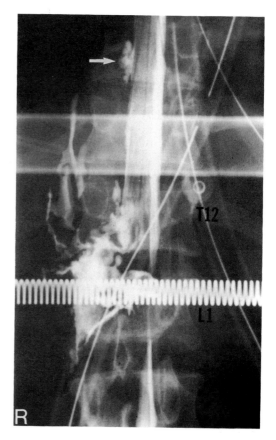

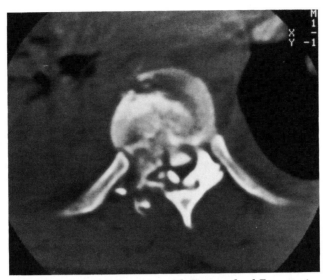

FIGURE 7–5. Burst Fracture with Retropulsed Fragments

• • • •

This axial computed tomography scan through L2 demonstrates an unstable burst fracture with retropulsion that markedly compromises the underlying anteroposterior spinal canal diameter. In addition, several small bone fragments are noted within the spinal canal.

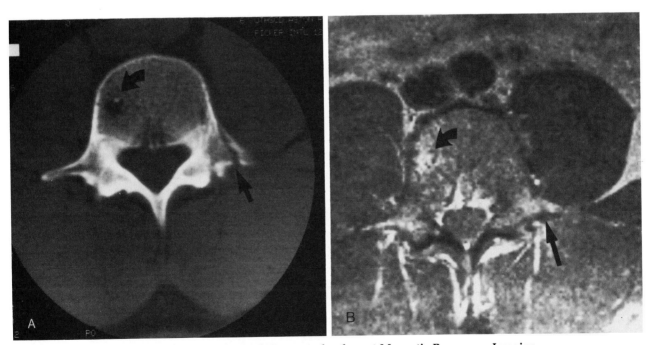

FIGURE 7–6. Fracture Seen Better at Computed Tomography than at Magnetic Resonance Imaging

• • • •

A, This axial computed tomography (CT) scan through L4 shows a fracture of the left transverse process *(straight arrow)*. A vertebral body hemangioma *(curved arrow)* is incidentally noted. *B*, This axial magnetic resonance (MR) image (2000 msec/40 msec) was recorded at the same level. The fracture of the transverse process is seen as a subtle area of decreased signal intensity *(arrow)*. The hemangioma is again seen *(curved arrow)*. Cortical fractures are better evaluated and defined with CT than with MR imaging.

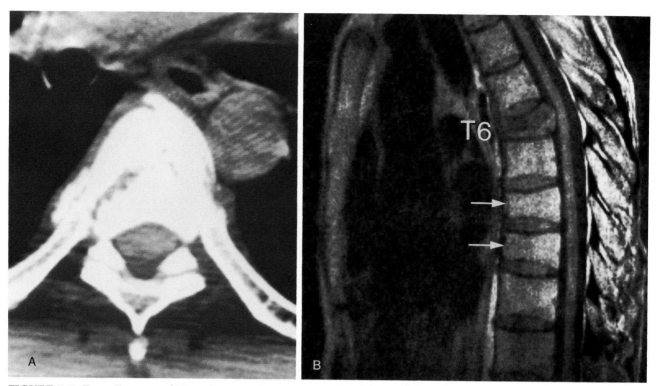

FIGURE 7–7. Burst Fracture of T6 at Computed Tomography and Magnetic Resonance Imaging

• • • •

A, This axial computed tomography scan through the T6 vertebral body confirms the presence of a burst-type compression fracture. The underlying cord and surrounding subarachnoid space cannot be evaluated because these structures are poorly delineated. Intrathecal contrast medium would permit a better evaluation of these structures. *B*, This sagittal T$_1$-weighted magnetic resonance image taken through the thoracic spine demonstrates that the burst fracture of T6 has a retropulsed fragment. This bone fragment effaces the anterior subarachnoid space, indenting the underlying spinal cord. Note also the mild anterior wedge compression fractures involving the anterior aspects of the T8 and T9 vertebral bodies *(arrows)*.

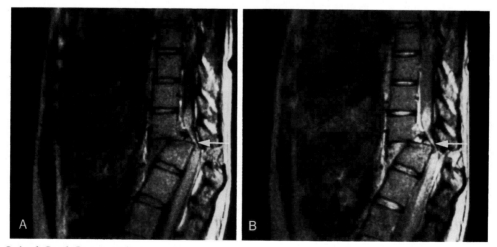

FIGURE 7–8. Spinal Cord Compression

• • • •

A sagittal T$_1$-weighted magnetic resonance (MR) image *(A)*, and a proton density (2000 msec/40 msec) MR image *(B)* taken after a motor vehicle accident show severe cord compression and/or transection *(arrows)* at the T10–11 level caused by posterior translation of the T11 vertebral body. An increased signal in the cord extending from T10 through the conus, consistent with a severe cord contusion, is demonstrated with both techniques but is more easily seen on the proton density scan.

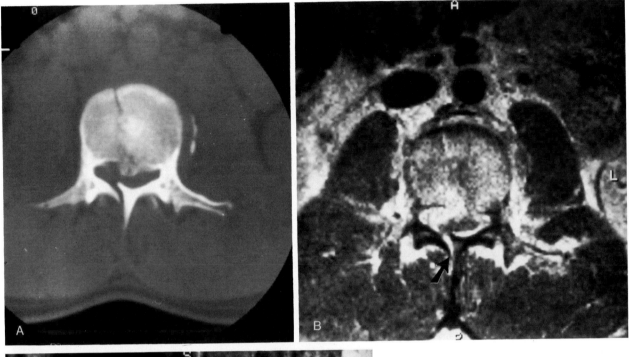

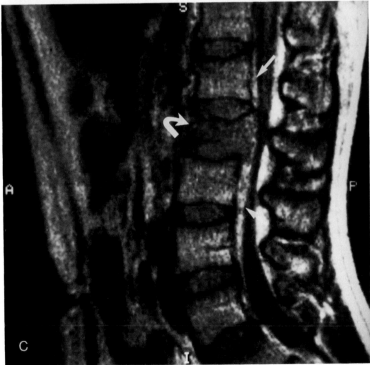

FIGURE 7–9. Compression Fracture with Retropulsion

• • • •

A, A computed tomography scan shows the L2 vertebral body fracture, laminar fracture, and retropulsed fragment to good advantage. *B,* The corresponding axial proton density (1500 msec/40 msec) magnetic resonance (MR) image demonstrates attenuation of the thecal sac and the right laminar fracture *(arrow).* The vertebral body fracture is barely perceptible. *C,* The T_1-weighted sagittal MR image through the lumbar spine shows both the L2 *(curved arrow)* retropulsed fracture compressing the thecal sac and an associated epidural hematoma *(arrows).*

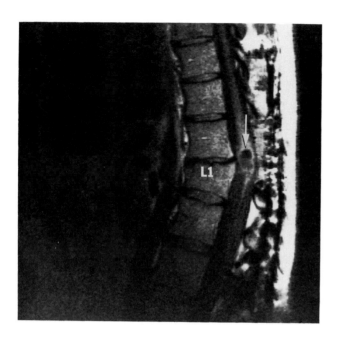

FIGURE 7–10. Post-Traumatic Spinal Cord Cyst

• • • •

A T$_1$-weighted sagittal midline magnetic resonance image through the conus shows the old L1-wedged vertebral body slightly distorting the contour of the spinal canal. In addition, there is a small septated post-traumatic cyst in the conus (*arrow*).

FIGURE 7–11. The Three Column Classification

• • • •

1. Anterior: anterior longitudinal ligament, anterior half vertebral body, anterior half disc; 2. Middle: posterior longitudinal ligament, posterior half vertebral body and disc; 3. Posterior: neural arch, ligamentum flavum, facet joint capsules, and interspinous ligament.

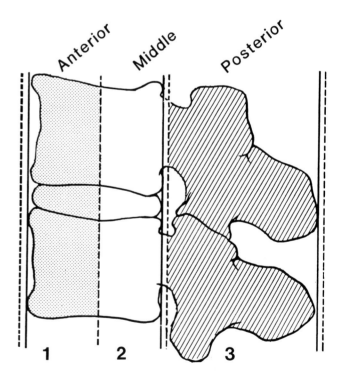

CLASSIFICATION OF THORACOLUMBAR SPINE FRACTURES

Several different classifications of stability in thoracolumbar spine fractures have been developed. The *three longitudinal column concept* is the most practical classification available (Fig. 7–11).[3, 8, 14] The anterior column consists of the anterior half of the vertebral body, the anterior part of the annulus fibrosus, and the anterior longitudinal ligament. The middle column includes the posterior half of the vertebral body, the posterior part of the annulus fibrosus, and the posterior longitudinal ligament. The posterior column consists of the facet joint capsules, the ligamentum flavum, the osseous neural arches, the supraspinous ligament, the interspinous ligament, and the articular processes.

MECHANISMS OF INJURY

There are six basic types of injury in the thoracolumbar spine as well as many complex injuries that are not assignable to one specific group.[14] The six basic injury types include:

1. The wedge compression fracture, which is caused by forward flexion. This injury results in isolated failure of the anterior column. This type of fracture rarely causes a neurologic deficit because it involves only the anterior column (Fig. 7–12).

2. A stable burst fracture, in which the anterior and the middle columns fail, but the posterior elements remain intact (Fig. 7–13). Neurologic symptoms may occur if the fracture fragments impinge on the spinal cord or nerves as they exit the spinal canal.

3. An unstable burst fracture, which involves failure of the anterior and the middle columns and has associated disruption of the posterior column (Fig. 7–14). Neurologic symptoms are frequent with these fractures.

4. Seat belt injuries, which are caused by hyperflexion around a fulcrum anterior to the vertebral body usually where the seat belt contacts the anterior abdominal wall.[7, 10] There are two basic categories. The first is *posterior ligament avulsion without bone fracture*, a type of injury that is more likely to occur in younger patients. The second category is a *posterior distraction fracture*, which has three variants:

a. The Smith fracture, which is a horizontal fracture through the neural arch that includes a small

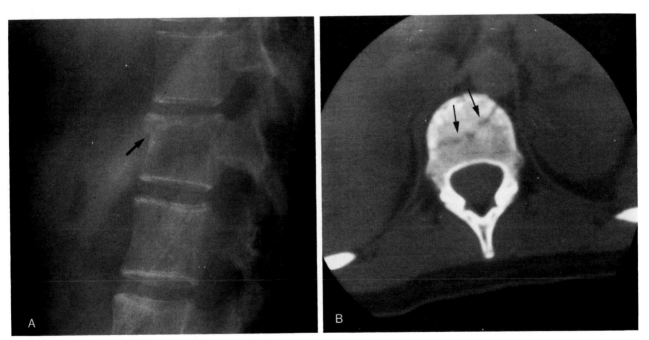

FIGURE 7–12. Anterior Wedge Compression Fracture

A, This lateral spinal radiograph shows the T12 compression fracture *(arrow)*. *B,* An axial computed tomography scan demonstrates the anterior wedge compression fracture of T12 *(arrows)* with an intact posterior vertebral body and ligamentous complex.

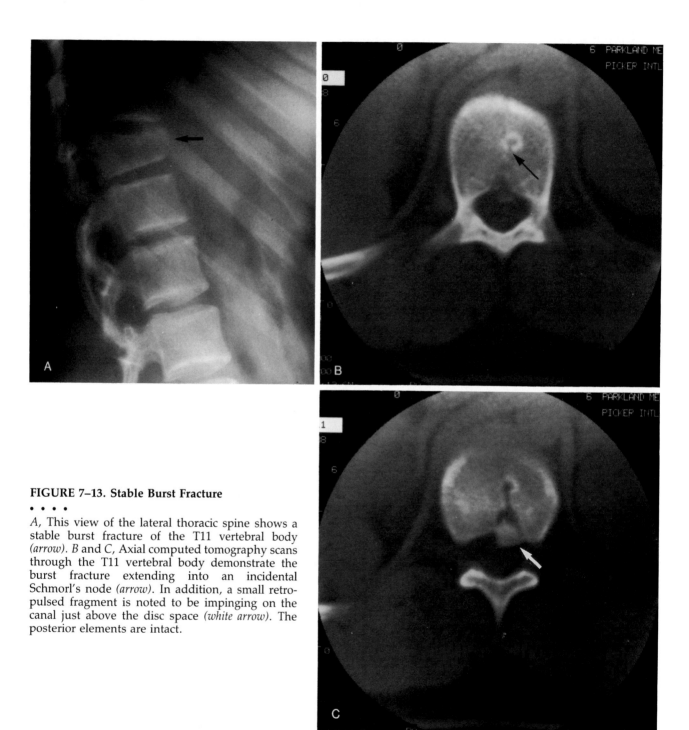

FIGURE 7–13. Stable Burst Fracture

• • • •

A, This view of the lateral thoracic spine shows a stable burst fracture of the T11 vertebral body *(arrow). B* and *C,* Axial computed tomography scans through the T11 vertebral body demonstrate the burst fracture extending into an incidental Schmorl's node *(arrow).* In addition, a small retropulsed fragment is noted to be impinging on the canal just above the disc space *(white arrow).* The posterior elements are intact.

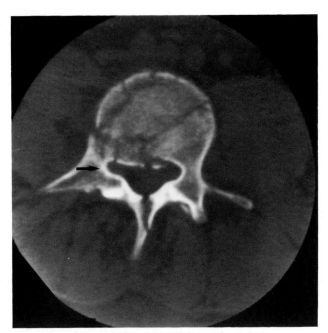

FIGURE 7–14. Unstable Burst Fracture

• • • •

This axial computed tomography section demonstrates an unstable burst fracture with failure of the anterior and middle columns in association with a left laminar fracture. Mild posterior retropulsion is seen centrally and to the right; it narrows the right lateral recess of L4 *(arrow)*.

posterior fragment of the vertebral body and the superior articular process. In this variant the spinous process remains intact (Fig. 7–15).

b. A Chance fracture, in which the horizontal fracture line extends posteriorly through the spinous process. A slight anterior compression fracture of the vertebral body may also be present.[4]

c. The horizontal fissure fracture, which occurs when the horizontal arch fracture extends anteriorly through the vertebral body to produce complete transverse splitting of the vertebral body. It also extends through the posterior bony ring. This variant is more common in older patients with brittle or osteoporotic bones.

Due to the fact that the abdominal organs lie between the spine and the seat belt, the possibility of intra-abdominal injury should always be borne in mind when hyperflexion fractures are encountered. The associated abdominal trauma, such as bowel or splenic rupture, is often more acutely life-threatening than the spinal injury.[7]

5. A flexion distraction injury, which results in failure of the anterior column due to compression. The middle and the posterior columns fail owing to the tension caused by the distraction. This causes a tear of the posterior longitudinal ligament, with or without subluxation, dislocation of the facet joints, or fracture of the facets. These fractures may have a

deceptively normal plain film appearance as spontaneous reduction with good resultant alignment can occur, and only subtle widening of the interspinous distance or slight subluxation of facet joints can be seen. Many of these injuries are potentially unstable (see Fig. 7–1).

6. Translational injuries, in which the alignment of the neural canal is disrupted usually after the failure of all three columns during a shear injury (Fig. 7–16).

This simplified classification of thoracolumbar fractures and fracture dislocations into six groups, based on the type of failure of the middle column, utilizes the mechanism of injury as well as its morphology. The forces causing injury of the middle column can be axial compression, axial distraction, and translation in the transverse plane. If the middle column has not failed, operative fixation is rarely indicated.[14] Stability of thoracolumbar fractures is based primarily on the integrity of the posterior vertebral arch complex because all severe vertebral body injuries with evidence of vertebral arch complex disruption are clinically unstable.[9]

Extension injuries of the thoracolumbar spine are extremely rare because the facet joint complex resists rotational forces. The middle column rarely, if ever, fails in extension or rotation injuries.

Sacral fractures are seen in nearly one half of all fractures of the pelvic ring.[7] These fractures are most commonly vertical or oblique, though transverse sacral fractures do occur.[5] Most sacral fractures are unilateral and may be very difficult to see on a plain film examination owing to superimposed bowel content. Careful evaluation of the neural arches bilaterally, particularly for any break in the fine cortical margins, is required (Fig. 7–17). Associated soft tissue injuries are common and include tears of the bladder and the urethra and avulsion injuries of the upper sacral nerve roots in pelvic and sacral fractures. If sacral fracture is suspected, CT should be performed.

• • • •

CLINICAL FINDINGS

Patients with thoracolumbar spine injuries usually have back pain that is sometimes associated with an inability to move the legs. Neurologic injury occurs in 50–70% of all thoracolumbar dislocations.[7] Physical findings are often few, but local ecchymoses or a palpable gap between the spinous processes are sometimes detected.[7, 10] It is important to remember that the extent of skeletal damage is not necessarily a good indicator of the severity of neurologic injury. Patients may have edema of the spinal cord, an

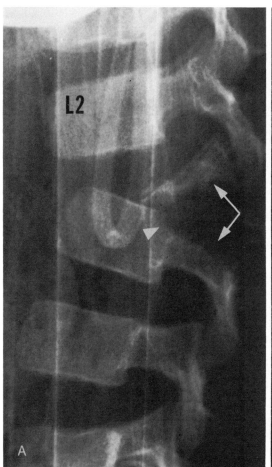

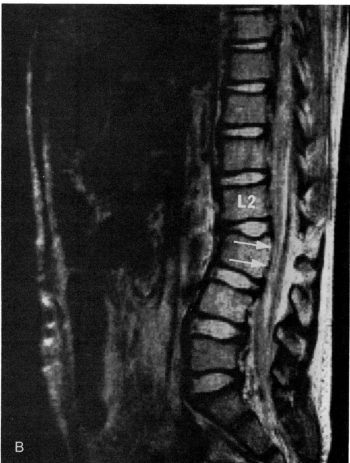

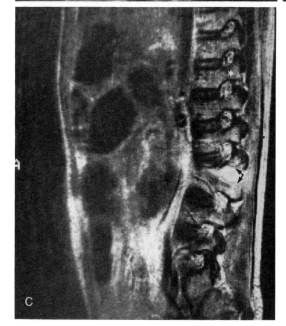

FIGURE 7–15. Posterior Distraction Fracture

• • • •

A, This lateral spinal radiograph shows a posterior distraction fracture at L2–3 associated with an abnormal kyphotic angulation. Note the horizontal shearing fracture *(arrows)* through the pedicle of L3 with extension to involve the posterosuperior corner of the L3 vertebral body *(arrowhead)* (Smith's fracture). The widened interspinous distance implies disruption of the interspinous ligament as well as the posterior longitudinal ligament. The spinous process is intact. *B*, A corresponding midline sagittal (2000 msec/40 msec) magnetic resonance (MR) image taken through the thoracolumbar spine is shown. The kyphotic angulation with normal intact adjacent intervertebral disc spaces is demonstrated. There is mild compromise of the underlying ventral aspect of the thecal sac *(arrows)*. *C*, Parasagittal MR image taken through the left pedicles *(asterisk)* and intervertebral foramina. The diastatic fracture site *(arrows)* and preservation of the adjacent intervertebral exit foramina correlate well with the plain radiograph. The fracture itself, however, is better demonstrated on the plain radiograph.

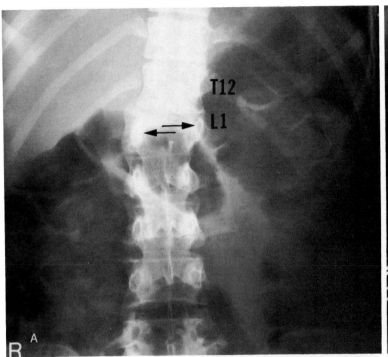

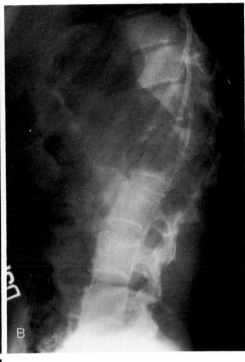

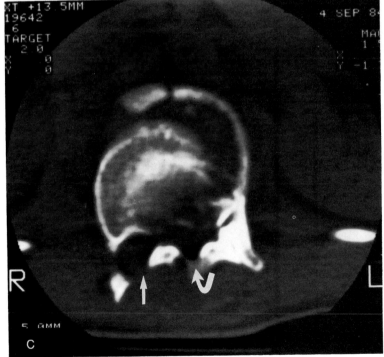

FIGURE 7–16. Translational Injury

• • • •

A, An anteroposterior abdominal radiograph demonstrates lateral subluxation of T12 in relation to the fractured L1 vertebral body. Note the widened interpedicular distance of L1 *(arrows),* implying the interruption of the vertebral body as well as the posterior neural arch—findings indicative of an unstable injury. Loss of the bone cortex of the L1 vertebral body as well as nonvisualization of the normal-sized intervertebral disc spaces are plain film indicators of a vertebral body injury. *B,* This lateral spinal radiograph demonstrates the kyphotic deformity and the severe L1 fracture. A marked T12–L1 subluxation is present. *C,* This axial computed tomography scan recorded at the level of lateral translation shows the lateral subluxation of one spinal canal related to the other. The L1 spinal canal is indicated by the straight arrow, and the canal at T12 is indicated by the curved arrow.

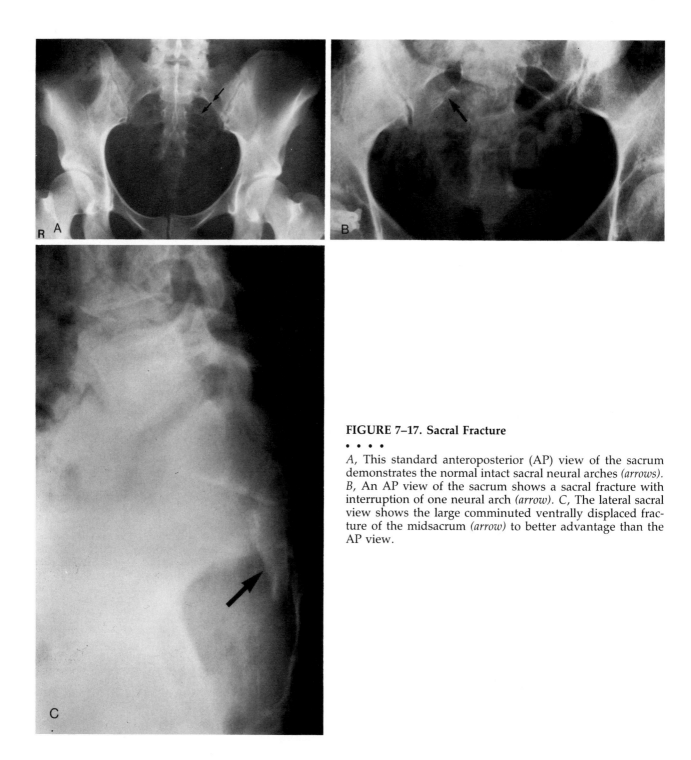

FIGURE 7–17. Sacral Fracture

• • • •

A, This standard anteroposterior (AP) view of the sacrum demonstrates the normal intact sacral neural arches (arrows). B, An AP view of the sacrum shows a sacral fracture with interruption of one neural arch (arrow). C, The lateral sacral view shows the large comminuted ventrally displaced fracture of the midsacrum (arrow) to better advantage than the AP view.

epidural hematoma, or bone or disc fragments compressing the spinal cord. Some impressive fractures of the vertebral body, however, may have no associated neurologic injury.

• • • •
SPINAL CORD AVULSION

An uncommon phenomenon worthy of note is spinal cord avulsion, which occurs in infants and young children (Fig. 7–18). In contrast to adults, in whom spinal cord trauma is extremely rare in the absence of skeletal fracture or dislocation, children can have spinal cord injury without skeletal injury. Cord transection occurs with severe injuries, such as those that are sustained in motor vehicle accidents, and is also a recognized obstetric complication of fetal hyperextension, which occurs during a breech delivery. Whenever a neurologic deficit does not correlate with the known bone or ligamentous level

of injury, further MR imaging is warranted to exclude a remote spinal cord injury. It is important to be aware that spinal cord injury in children that is caused by severe distraction forces often occurs without evidence of underlying skeletal injury or is remote from the site of the skeletal injury.

• • • •
PENETRATING TRAUMA

Penetrating trauma to the spine is a special class of abnormality that presents slightly different imaging problems. CT scans depict both small bone and metallic (bullet) fragments to best advantage, whereas MR images are superior in demonstrating spinal cord compression or contusion and epidural collections. Myelography may be necessary when a dural leak or nerve root injury is suspected.

Of particular interest in penetrating trauma is evaluation of images to define the path of the missile. This allows inferences as to potential neurologic structures that may be involved. Ultimately, however, neurologic involvement is determined clinically.

• • • •
CONCLUSION

Owing to the complex nature of many thoracolumbar injuries, which may include a structural component, a neurologic component, or both, patients often require both CT scans and MR images in addition to routine spine radiographs to evaluate the extent of fracture and to assess the underlying cord, especially prior to surgical reduction and internal fixation.

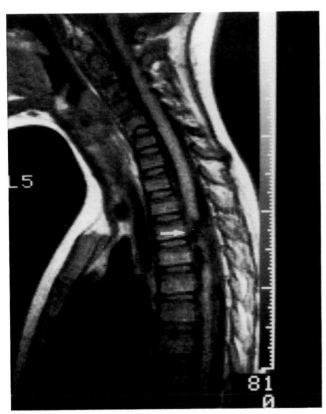

FIGURE 7–18. Spinal Cord Avulsion
• • • •
This T$_1$-weighted sagittal magnetic resonance image taken through a child's cervicothoracic spine shows complete transection of the spinal cord at the level of T3 *(arrow)*. No associated skeletal injury was present. (From Mendelsohn DB, Zollars L, Weatherall PT, Girson M. MR of cord transection. J Comput Assist Tomogr 1990; 14:909–911.)

References

1. Atlas SW, Regenbogen V, Rogus LF, Kim KS. The radiologic characterization of burst fractures of the spine. AJR 1986; 147:575–582.
2. Brant-Zawadzki M, Jeffrey RB Jr, Munagi H, Pitts LH. High resolution CT of thoracolumbar fractures. AJR 1982; 138:699–704.
3. Bucholz RW, Gill K. Classification of injuries to the thoracolumbar spine. Orthop Clin North Am 1986; 17:67–73.
4. Chance GQ. Note on a type of flexion fracture of the spine. Br J Radiol 1948; 21:452–453.
5. Fountain SS, Hamilton RD, Jameson RM. Transverse fractures of the sacrum. J Bone Joint Surg [Am] 1977; 59:486–486.
6. Gehweiler JA Jr, Daffner RH, Osborne RL Jr. Relevant signs of stable and unstable thoracolumbar vertebral column trauma. Skeletal Radiol 1981; 7:179–183.

7. Gehweiler JA Jr, Osborne RL Jr, Becker RF. The Radiology of Vertebral Trauma. Philadelphia: W.B.Saunders Co., 1980, p 261–398.
8. Holdsworth F. Fractures, dislocations, and fracture-dislocations of the spine. J Bone Joint Surg [Am] 1970; 52:1534–1551.
9. Jelsma RK, Kirsch PT, Rice JF, Jelsma LF. The radiologic description of thoracolumbar fractures. Surg Neurol 1982; 18:230–236.
10. Kaufer H, Hayes JT. Lumbar fracture-dislocation. J Bone Joint Surg [Am] 1966; 48:712–730.
11. Kulkarni MV, Bondurant FJ, Rose SL, Narayana PA. 1.5 tesla magnetic resonance imaging of acute spinal trauma. Radiographics 1988; 8:1059–1082.
12. Kulkarni MV, McArdle CB, Kopanicky D, et al. Acute spinal cord injury: MR imaging at 1.5 T. Radiology 1987; 164:837–843.
13. Manaster BJ, Osborn AG. CT patterns of facet fracture dislocations in the thoracolumbar region. AJR 1987; 148:335–340.
14. McAfee PC, Yuan HA, Fredrickson BE, Lubicky JP. The value of computed tomography in thoracolumbar fractures. J Bone Joint Surg 1983; 65:461–473.
15. Mirvis SE, Geisler FH, Jelinek JJ, et al. Acute cervical spine trauma: Evaluation with 1.5 T MR imaging. Radiology 1988; 166:807–816.
16. O'Callaghan JP, Ullrich CG, Yuan HA, Keiffer SA. CT of facet distraction in flexion injuries of the thoracolumbar spine: The "naked" facet. AJNR 1980; 1:97–102.
17. Rogers LF, Thayer C, Weinberg PE, Kim KS. Acute injuries of the upper thoracic spine associated with paraplegia. AJNR 1980; 1:89–95.

SECTION

THREE

Neck
and
Thorax

CHAPTER 8

Soft Tissues
of the Neck

LINDA O'CONNELL JUDGE, M.D.

Injuries to the soft tissues of the neck that require emergency radiologic evaluation are primarily those to the larynx, the trachea, the esophagus, and the carotid and the vertebral arteries. Vascular injuries and the esophagus are addressed in other chapters. This chapter focuses primarily on the larynx.

Detection of acute injury to the larynx and the trachea demands a high level of clinical suspicion. These infrequent and often obscure injuries may worsen insidiously as more obvious injuries are addressed in the emergency room. Attention to the ABCs of advanced trauma life support (Airway, Breathing, and Circulation) should make establishment of a stable and patent airway the first priority in trauma management. Failure or delay in making the diagnosis of laryngeal injury can lead to life-threatening, even catastrophic consequences. If the patient survives, chronic morbidity with impaired breathing, swallowing, or phonation may ensue.

The clinical signs of laryngotracheal injury are many and varied. They include localized tenderness and swelling, subcutaneous emphysema, anterior neck contusion and ecchymosis, loss of palpable landmarks, tracheal deviation, pneumothorax, and hemoptysis. Hoarseness is the primary symptom, followed by cough, dyspnea, dysphagia, and dys-

phonia. Restlessness or inability of the patient to maintain a supine position are important observations and may be the only clues to laryngeal injury when the patient is unable to speak. Subcutaneous emphysema caused by interruption of the larynx, the trachea, or the major bronchi is both a sign and a symptom. It can be massive and readily evident on physical examination. Alternatively, there may be minimal or no physical findings, and the emphysema may be detected as subtle radiolucent streaks on plain films. As so often is the case, accurate diagnosis is predicated on clinical suspicion, and thus a careful, methodic evaluation of the airway and the neck is mandatory in all trauma victims.

The comparatively rare occurrence of laryngeal trauma is well known and has been estimated at 0.04% of all emergency room visits.[3, 4] This means that in even the largest trauma centers no individual physician has much experience in the diagnosis and care of laryngeal injury. As a result, controversy persists with respect to both the diagnostic and the therapeutic approaches to this injury. Published recommendations are frequently based on anecdotal experience or a compilation of data from several centers rather than on extensive individual first-hand experience and follow-up.

• • • • *APPROPRIATE RADIOGRAPHIC STUDIES*

I. Plain Films
   A. Lateral view of the neck using a soft tissue technique
   B. Anteroposterior view of the neck using a soft tissue technique
Comment: Portable views of the neck are often of poor quality and are taken for bone detail of the cervical spine. These films may suffice for the soft tissues, but when laryngeal injury is likely, films taken with a soft tissue technique are mandatory.

II. Laryngography
   A. Rarely indicated or feasible in the acutely injured patient.
   B. May be needed in a patient seen for a collapsing or stenotic airway several weeks or months after injury. Even in such a patient, laryngography is rarely needed as an emergency procedure.
Comment: Requires a cooperative patient and is time-consuming. This procedure is preferably performed with the anticholinergic atropine, and it requires good topical anesthesia.

III. Tomography
   A. Can demonstrate bones and air column in the larynx and the trachea, but it is rarely indicated acutely.
Comment: Has been largely replaced by computed tomography (CT) and magnetic resonance (MR) imaging, which provide more information about soft tissues. Tomography requires a cooperative patient.

IV. Computed Tomography
   A. An axial thin-section technique using 3–5-mm sections is performed.
   B. Does not require intravenous contrast material routinely.
Comment: Demonstrates the submucosal soft tissues and cartilage that cannot be evaluated by direct or indirect laryngoscopy. CT requires that the patient lie flat and motionless and therefore cannot often be performed in the presence of acute injury.

V. Magnetic Resonance Imaging
   A. Axial sections
   B. Sagittal and coronal sections as indicated
Comment: Produces exquisite images. MR imaging isolates a patient who is often unstable and may have acute airway problems. Furthermore, the procedure is not readily available on an emergency basis.

The uncommon occurrence of laryngeal injury is directly related to the small size of the larynx and its inherent elasticity and mobility. Posterior support is provided by the cervical spine, and anterior protection is provided by the mandible when the patient is in the usual flexed-neck, tucked-chin position. These same factors also contribute to the precarious nature of the larynx in trauma. The small caliber of the airway, particularly in children, allows little leeway for edema or cartilaginous fragments. Greenstick-like fractures and buckles of the larynx may occur in children and young adults. The rate of mineralization in adults varies, and the severity of injury is directly related to the loss of elasticity that accompanies calcification. The vertically communicating soft tissue planes of the neck permit easy movement of blood and edema and provide very little tamponade effect. Proportionately, the cross-sectional area of the larynx and the trachea in children is small in comparison to that in adults. The propensity of children to develop widespread edema in response to mild trauma or noxious fumes is well known. The tendency of children to easily obstruct the airway is also well recognized. The redundant soft tissues of the skull base and the retropharynx create a funnel configuration, further narrowing the small diameter of the airway in the child with laryngeal injury.

• • • •
CLASSIFICATION OF LARYNGEAL TRAUMA

Laryngeal trauma may be classified by cause or by anatomy. Etiologic factors include blunt, penetrating, thermal, noxious, and iatrogenic trauma, and foreign body inhalation. The blunt and penetrating trauma categories include the majority of injuries seen in the emergency room, with a shift in recent years from blunt to penetrating causes. The enactment and enforcement of seat belt laws as well as the lowering of speed limits have significantly decreased the incidence of blunt laryngeal trauma caused by motor vehicle accidents in which the victim is thrown forward, with his or her neck extended, against the dashboard or the steering column. Supplemental restraint systems, such as air bags, should further protect against this injury. In most major cities, the rate of trauma from blunt violence, including strangulation, direct blows, and aggressive sports, has not kept pace with that of penetrating trauma resulting from stab wounds and bullets, an unfortunate result of our increasingly violent society.

Anatomic divisions are made on the basis of structures extrinsic or intrinsic to the larynx. Extrinsic injuries are mainly extralaryngeal hematomas and edema, including injury to the recurrent laryngeal nerves that supply sensory innervation to the subglottic region and motor capabilities to the remainder of the intrinsic laryngeal musculature.

Intrinsic trauma has been subdivided by Mancuso and Hanafee and Ogura and associates into the following categories[6, 9]:

1. Injury to soft tissues of the larynx, including the aryepiglottic folds and the false and the true vocal folds.

2. Supraglottic injuries, primarily fractures or avulsions of the epiglottis and the thyroepiglottic ligament.

3. True glottic injuries, usually fractures of the thyroid cartilage.

4. Infraglottic injuries, which may be either cricoarytenoid dislocations or fractures of the cricoid ring.

5. Tracheal fractures, which are rare due to the open-C configuration of the tracheal rings, and complete tracheal transection.

• • • •
RADIOGRAPHIC PROCEDURES

Plain Films

Patients who are suspected of having neck, cervical spine, or laryngeal trauma usually have a cross-table lateral film of the cervical spine performed early during triage. Although the primary plain film findings of laryngeal trauma are often obscure and nonspecific owing to the limited amount of laryngeal calcification, the secondary sign of subcutaneous or retropharyngeal free air must prompt a more aggressive investigation (Fig. 8–1). The lateral cervical spine film also provides an assessment of the alignment and the integrity of the cervical spine in the event that direct or indirect laryngoscopy, intubation, or tracheostomy become necessary. If placement of an airway is needed before the lateral cervical spine film can be obtained, or if there is any question about the integrity of the cervical spine after the film has been taken, all manipulations must be performed without extension of the neck. Occasionally, interruption of the tracheal air column is seen in patients with tracheal transection. Nearly complete obstruction of the airway caused by edema, hematoma, or hemic drowning is also sometimes seen (Fig. 8–2).

Laryngography

Other fluoroscopic or diagnostic radiologic examinations have a limited role in the acute management of laryngeal trauma. Laryngograms are usually not helpful. They are time-consuming, difficult to perform (particularly in uncooperative patients) and are contraindicated in patients with unstable airways. They are of some use in acute penetrating injuries and in following patients with earlier neck trauma. To perform a contrast laryngogram, the patient must fast for several hours. Atropine is administered 1 hour prior to the examination to decrease secretions except in those patients who have glaucoma, obstructive uropathy, or other contraindications to the drug. Local anesthesia is given by spraying the oropharynx and the hypopharynx with 2% lidocaine (Xylocaine); the anesthetic is then painted or dripped onto the pyriform sinuses and the vocal folds. The patient is asked to phonate to expose the vocal folds and then inspire deeply to propel the anesthetic farther into the trachea. When sufficient anesthesia is achieved, an oily contrast agent is instilled, and anteroposterior

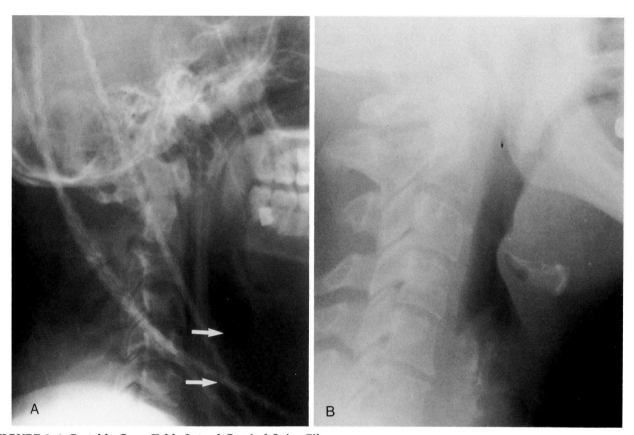

FIGURE 8–1. Portable Cross-Table Lateral Cervical Spine Film

• • • •

A, This cross-table lateral cervical spine film demonstrates both subcutaneous and retropharyngeal air. Note the subglottic edema narrowing of the airway *(arrows).* This lateral film of the neck illustrates the challenge the radiologist faces in evaluating the trachea. The film is portable, the shoulders are not down, a nasogastric tube is in place, and various other lines cross the soft tissues of the neck. The film could have been improved by using a soft tissue technique and by moving all lines that are external to the patient. *B,* A normal cross-table lateral film of the neck performed using the soft tissue technique demonstrates why an appropriate radiographic technique is mandatory when the presence of laryngeal trauma is of concern. Soft tissue air, swelling, and the disruption of calcified laryngeal cartilage can be more easily evaluated on a film of this quality.

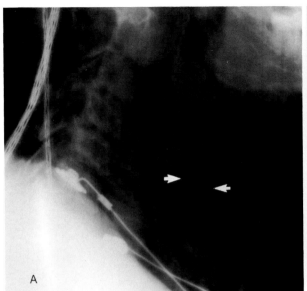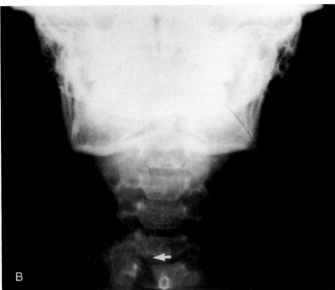

FIGURE 8–2. Airway Obstruction

• • • •

A and *B, respectively,* Lateral and anteroposterior projections of the neck in a patient with severe combined blunt and penetrating trauma that caused fragmentation of the laryngeal frame, severe subcutaneous edema, and obvious obstruction of the larynx *(arrows)* demonstrated by a cut-off of the air column. These films could have been improved by using a soft tissue technique.

and lateral spot films are taken of the patient during quiet respiration, "E" phonation, inspiratory "E" phonation, and the modified and the true Valsalva maneuvers. Oily contrast material coating is superior to that of water-soluble preparations. This examination provides information about the mucosal contour and the capacity of the vallecula, the aryepiglottic folds, the pyriform sinuses, the vocal folds, and sometimes the laryngeal ventricles (Fig. 8–3).

Computed Tomography

As in most head and neck radiology, computed tomography (CT) has significantly improved the ability to identify and pinpoint submucosal abnormalities. CT is a perfect adjunct to laryngoscopy. However, CT generally plays a limited role in the initial diagnosis of laryngeal trauma. Although the patient needs only to lie on the table and breathe quietly, this is precisely what a patient with an acute tracheal or laryngeal trauma is unable to do. If CT is employed in the acute stage, the patient must be closely monitored, and resuscitative equipment and personnel must be available in the immediate vicinity. The scan should be performed using thin sections of 3–5 mm in thickness. Intravenous contrast material is generally not required.

In general, CT is superior to laryngoscopy and plain films in the evaluation of the cartilaginous and

the osseous framework of the larynx as well as the submucosal fat and the fascial planes, whereas indirect or direct visualization is recommended for determining mucosal integrity. Massive and gaping injuries are easily recognized clinically. Patients with such injuries are taken directly to surgery for direct laryngoscopy, primary closure, and diversion of the airway. Otherwise, the initial evaluation is usually indirect laryngoscopy, sometimes performed with a flexible nasopharyngoscope. The decision can then be made as to how to proceed. CT is reserved for instances in which only edema of a mild to moderate degree is encountered in a minimally symptomatic or asymptomatic patient (Fig. 8–4). CT detects isolated submucosal injury, evaluates the alignment of laryngeal fractures, and can confirm the endoscopic observations, thereby allowing conservative management. Thus, CT is generally reserved for those patients in whom the results directly influence treatment (Fig. 8–5).

Magnetic Resonance Imaging

Although magnetic resonance (MR) imaging yields exquisite images of the larynx in axial, sagittal, and coronal planes, this examination is often not available on an emergency basis, is costly, and is more dependent on patient cooperation than CT. It also requires isolation of a potentially unstable patient and is

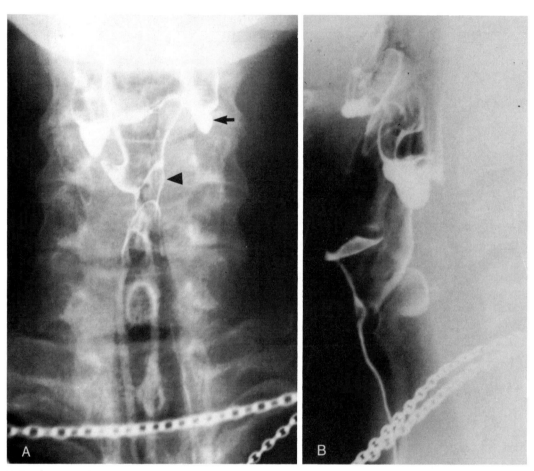

FIGURE 8–3. Laryngography

• • • •

A and *B, respectively,* Anteroposterior and lateral radiographs from a contrast laryngogram demonstrating deformity of the left pyriform sinus *(arrow)* and obliteration of the left laryngeal ventricle *(arrowhead)* due to edema from an acute stab wound. Although there is significant swelling, the airway is not narrowed.

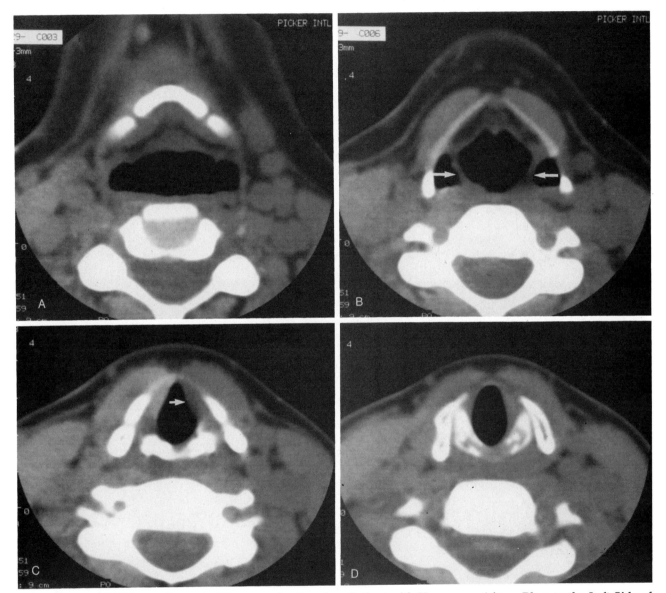

FIGURE 8–4. Mild Edema. Computed Tomography Scan in a Patient with Hoarseness After a Blow to the Left Side of the Neck

• • • •

A, The tripartite hyoid bone is well demonstrated and is normal. *B,* The cephalad aspect of the thyroid alae and aryepiglottic folds *(arrow)* are also normal. *C,* There is very mild focal edema of the left vocal fold *(arrow). D,* The edema is also present in the subglottic area on the left. These minimal abnormalities can be safely treated using conservative methods.

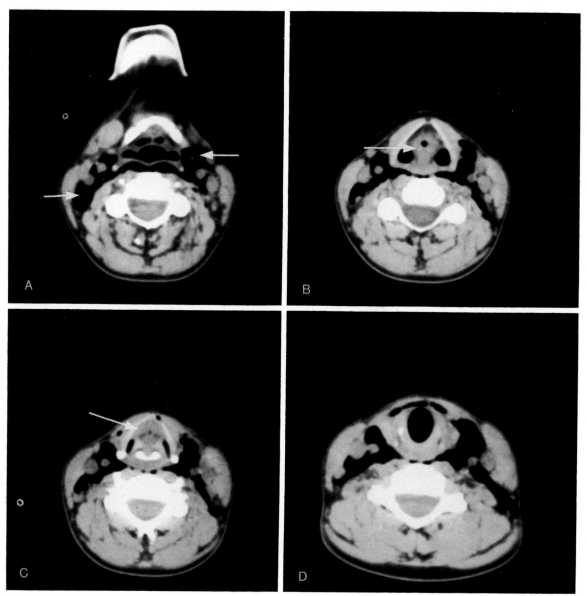

FIGURE 8–5. Computed Tomography Used to Confirm an Isolated Vocal Fold Injury
• • • •
A, There is marked subcutaneous emphysema *(arrows)*, but the hyoid bone is normal. *B*, There is symmetric edema of the aryepiglottic folds *(arrow)* at this level. *C*, The vocal folds are quite edematous *(arrow)*, and the pyriform sinuses are compressed. Subcutaneous air is still seen. *D*, No subglottic edema is seen. Laryngoscopy had demonstrated a right true vocal fold laceration. The computed tomography scan demonstrated no other injury, thereby aiding in planning therapy.

therefore an unsuitable emergency diagnostic technique for most laryngeal and tracheal injury.

Examinations for Associated Injuries

Esophageal injury is the most frequent companion injury when laryngeal soft tissue trauma is present. Barium-based or water-soluble contrast examination of the esophagus is indicated when esophageal integrity is questioned (Fig. 8–6). Other associated injuries of major concern are those to the carotid and the vertebral arteries and to the spine and the spinal cord. Angiography, CT, MR imaging, and myelography are appropriate techniques in specific patients with laryngeal injury. Penetrating trauma, in partic-

ular, may warrant angiography when a laryngeal injury is identified.

• • • •
ANATOMY OF THE LARYNX

The injuries occurring to the larynx (from the hyoid bone to the cricoid ring) are usually the result of an undefended assault on an extended or hyperextended neck. The anatomy of the larynx is complex and should be understood (Fig. 8–7). The thyroid cartilage normally protects the glottis by arching over it like a butterfly and by draping its alae over the lateral reflections. The posterior aspect of the superior cornu is attached to the hyoid bone by the thyrohyoid membrane. Inferiorly, synovial joints ar-

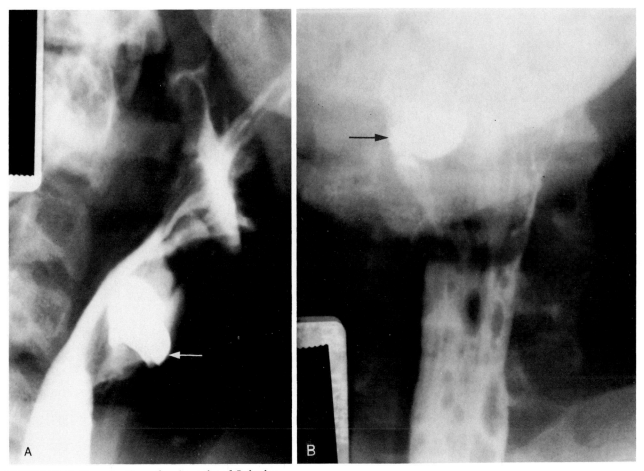

FIGURE 8–6. Examinations for Associated Injuries
• • • •
A–D, A bullet *(arrows)* is lodged in the right pyriform sinus.

A and *B*, Lateral and anteroposterior views of the esophagus performed using a water-soluble contrast material do not demonstrate any injury. Delayed films showed no extravasation.

Illustration continued on following page

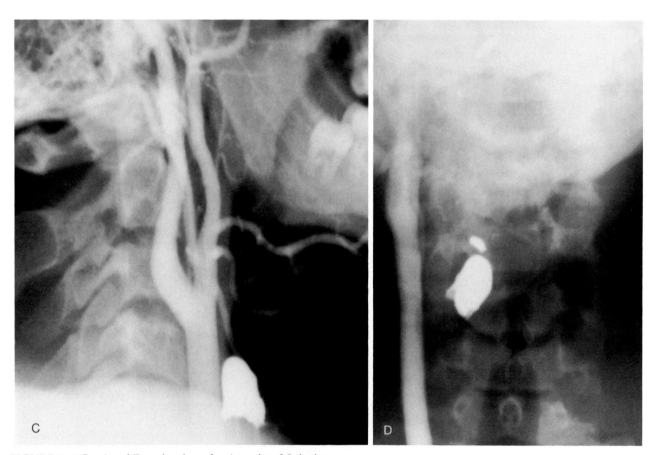

FIGURE 8–6 *Continued* **Examinations for Associated Injuries**
• • • •
C and *D*, The right common carotid angiogram is also normal. Since the entrance site of the bullet was the right lateral side of the neck, the potential for right common carotid artery injury was significant.

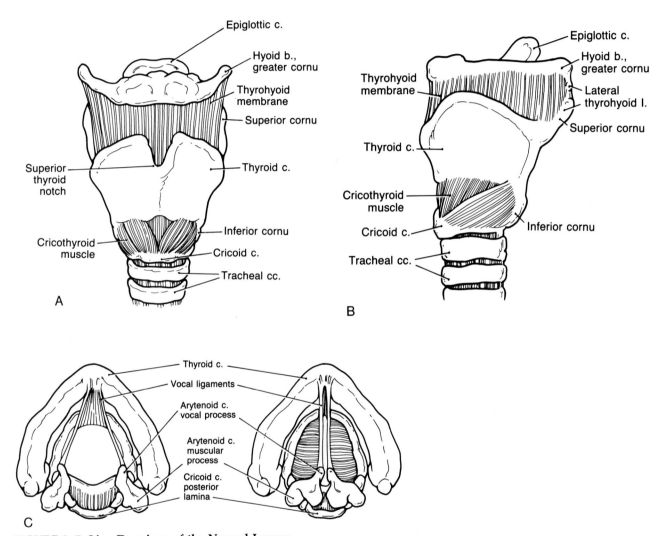

FIGURE 8–7. Line Drawings of the Normal Larynx.

• • • •

A, A frontal view. *B*, A lateral view. *C*, A cross-sectional view showing the vocal folds open and apposed.

ticulate with the cricoid cartilage, and the cricothyroid membrane anchors the anterior thyroid cartilage to the narrower aspect of the signet ring-shaped cricoid cartilage. Injury to the superior laryngeal branch of the vagus nerve inhibits sensory innervation to the supraglottic area and motor stimulation to the cricothyroid muscle. Subglottic sensation and the remainder of intrinsic laryngeal muscular innervation is from the recurrent branch of the vagus nerve. The recurrent laryngeal nerves run posterior to the cricothyroid articulation; and integrity of this joint is vital for stability of the glottic aperture.

The hyoid bone is composed of three parts that frequently remain unfused into adulthood (see Figs. 8–4 and 8–5). The fibrous connections are radiolucent and must not be mistaken for fractures, nor should fractures be considered a lack of fusion (Fig. 8–8). The hyoid is a useful landmark for indicating the transition from the fixed to the free portions of the epiglottis, the upper boundary of the pre-epiglottic space, and the lower margin of the jugulodigastric nodes.

The epiglottis is suspended from the hyoid bone by the hyoepiglottic ligament, which runs from the posterior hyoid to the anterior surface of the free border of the epiglottis. It is attached inferiorly to the thyroid cartilage by the thyroepiglottic ligament at its petriole. It is inverse U-shaped and composed of elastic cartilage. Its role in deterring aspiration by covering the glottis during swallowing has been shown to be secondary to the sphincteric action of the supraglottic laryngeal musculature.

The structures called the *pyriform sinuses* have a disputed anatomic definition. They may be considered lateral recesses or gutters that project from the pharyngoepiglottic folds inferiorly and posteriorly from the hypopharynx to the upper margin of the cricopharyngeus. Here they fuse and join the lumen of the esophagus. Alternatively, a more rigid description details three sections, all triangular, bordered anteriorly, and open posteriorly. The most superior is between the pharyngoepiglottic fold and the mucosal fold over the internal laryngeal nerve. A midsection extends from the aryepiglottic folds through the length of the thyroid cartilage. The lowest region extends between the inferior thyroid cornu and the lateral aspect of the posterior cricoid cartilage.

Pyramidal arytenoid cartilages rest upon and articulate with the superoposterolateral surfaces of the cricoid cartilage on synovial joints. During phonation, both of these arytenoid cartilages rotate and tilt on their bases. The thyroarytenoid ligaments, or

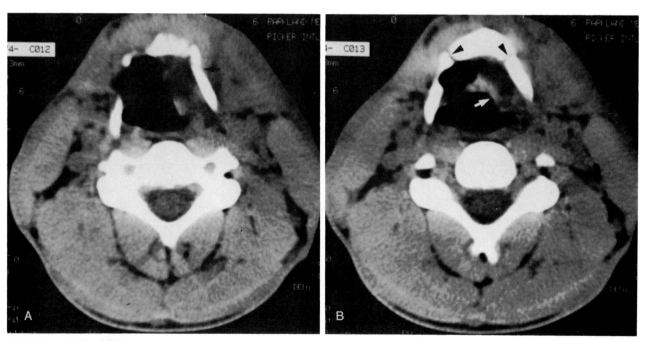

FIGURE 8–8. Hyoid Fracture

• • • •

A, Buckling of the left side of the hyoid bone *(arrow)* is barely perceptible, but the soft tissue edema medial to the bone and the swelling lateral to it are convincing evidence of fracture. *B,* A section done 3 mm caudal to the first again demonstrates the asymmetry of the airway *(arrow)* and lateral soft tissue swelling. There is no hint of hyoid fracture at this level, emphasizing the need for thin section computed tomography studies. The two normal fibrous connections *(arrowheads)* are well demonstrated.

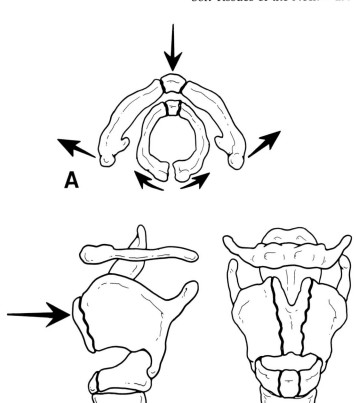

FIGURE 8–9. Diagram of a Blunt Anterior Force Compressing the Thyroid Cartilage Against the Cervical Spine, Causing the Splaying and the Buckling of the Thyroid Alae

• • • •

A, A direct blow to the midline of the thyroid cartilage *(top arrow)* causes at least one paramedian fracture, splaying out the thyroid alae *(lower arrows).* A concomitant cricoid fracture often occurs. *B,* The fracture *(arrow)* as it is seen in lateral view. *C,* The fractures of the thyroid cartilage and cricoid seen face on.

vocal cords, extend from the medial and posterior aspects of the thyroid cartilage to the vocal surface, or process, of each arytenoid cartilage.

• • • •

BLUNT LARYNGEAL TRAUMA

The severity of blunt injuries to the larynx is related to the pliability of the various laryngeal components, particularly that of the thyroid alae, and also to the direction of force exerted on them. The degree of calcification inversely affects the compliance and the resilience of the thyroid cartilage and is directly related to the probability of fracture. When struck in the midline, the larynx is driven posteriorly against the rigid cervical spine, and the thyroid alae splay open (Fig. 8–9). If sufficiently calcified, the thyroid cartilage fractures in at least one paramedian vertical plane or at its symphysis, similar to the cracking of a wishbone (Fig. 8–10). These fractures may be identified by tiny fracture lines, subtle step-offs, unusual contours, buckling of the alae, or by localized hematoma and edema infiltrating the fat plane immediately adjacent to the fracture. The arytenoid cartilages may be torn from their thyroid cartilage

attachments and dislocate. The thyroarytenoid and the cricothyroid ligaments are susceptible to disruption, allowing the thyroid cartilage and cricoid cartilage to telescope upon each other. No thyroid cartilage is normally visible in the CT sections in which the complete ring of the cricoid is seen (Fig. 8–11). The cricoid is inherently more rigid and more calcified and recoils with less ease when it is compressed. Because it is a ring, it usually fractures in at least two places. The displacement of these fractures is determined by the relative stability of the larynx and by the thickening of the posterior cricoid ring, which serves as the cornerstone for the glottis.

When the blow to the thyroid cartilage is off center (Fig. 8–12), the thyroid alae may fracture directly (Fig. 8–13). On the other hand, a pliable ala may deform inward at the point of impact, indenting and even crossing the midline to transmit the force to the contralateral mucosal surface (Fig. 18–14). It then recoils with little ipsilateral mucosal disruption. This mechanism is proposed for the infrequent "contrecoup" injury (Fig. 8–15).

Glottic edema (with or without laryngeal fracture), extrinsic laryngeal soft tissue contusion, hematoma, and subcutaneous emphysema dissect quickly in a craniocaudad direction owing to the loose areolar tissue beneath the mucosa (Fig. 8–16). The loose

Text continued on page 307

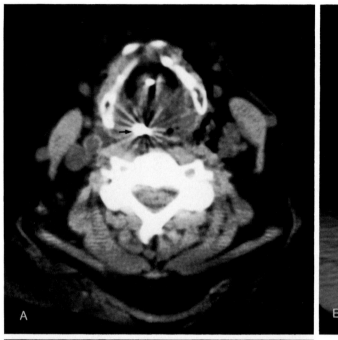

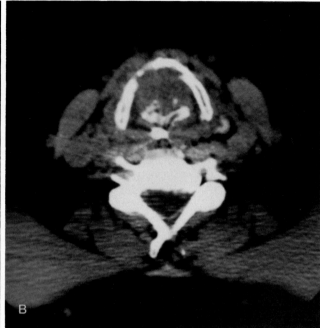

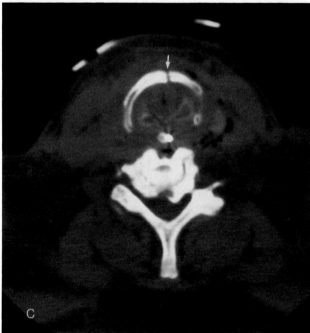

FIGURE 8–10. Fractures of the Thyroid Cartilage and the Cricoid Ring Caused by Blunt Trauma

• • • •

A, The airway is markedly narrowed by edema. A naso-gastric tube is present *(arrow),* causing artifacts to be seen on this computed tomography section. Some subcutaneous emphysema is present. *B,* A section recorded 15 mm caudal to the first demonstrates complete obliteration of the airway by edema. *C,* A 3-mm section done 9 mm caudal to that in *B* displayed with a bone technique. A thyroid cartilage fracture *(arrow)* is present. The airway is a narrow slit.

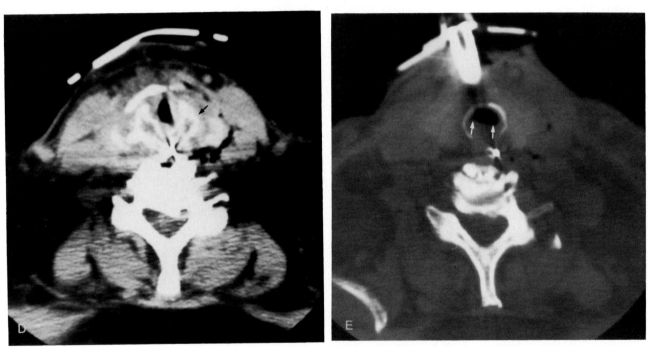

FIGURE 8–10 *Continued* **Fractures of the Thyroid Cartilage and the Cricoid Ring Caused by Blunt Trauma**

• • • •

D, The next section displayed with a narrow window demonstrates the thyroid cartilage fracture again. In addition, the cricoid is fractured *(arrow).* The artifacts from the nasogastric tube interfere with evaluation of the cricoid ring. A wider window would diminish the spray effect and improve visualization of the bone structures. *E,* The final section is 12 mm caudal to that in *D* and is displayed with a wide window. An air fluid level *(arrows)* is seen in the trachea, indicating that this patient is at serious risk of hemic drowning. Part of a tracheostomy tube and very bulky osteophytes are also seen.

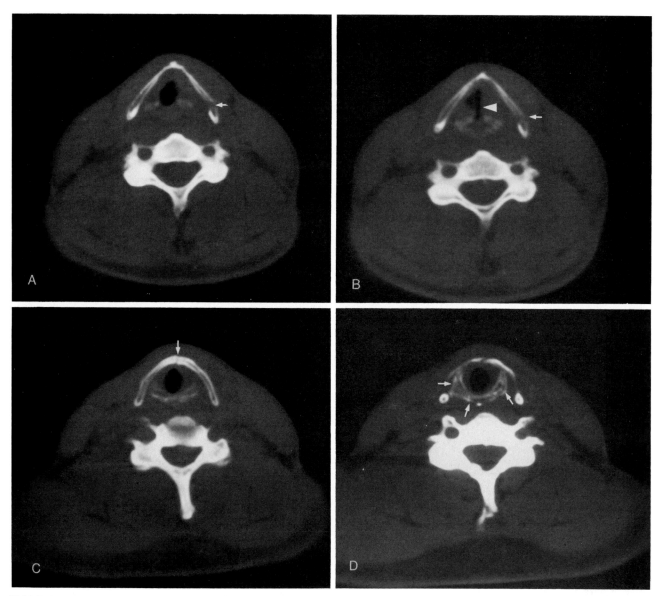

FIGURE 8–11. Injury to the Cricothyroid Ligament Permitting Telescoping of the Thyroid Alae over the Cricoid Ring
• • • •
A, A fracture of the left thyroid ala *(arrow)* is associated with moderate glottic edema. *B*, A computed tomography section taken 3 mm caudal to the first demonstrates the thyroid ala fracture *(arrow)*. In addition, the left vocal fold is in a paramedial position *(arrowhead)*. Clinically, the patient had poor voice quality. *C*, A third section recorded 5 mm below the last demonstrates the midline thyroid cartilage fracture *(arrow)*. On this section the thyroid alae are overlapping the cricoid ring. *D*, The fourth scan is 5 mm more caudal and demonstrates significant overlap of the thyroid and cricoid *(arrows)* cartilages, indicating injury to the cricothyroid ligament that will require surgical repair.

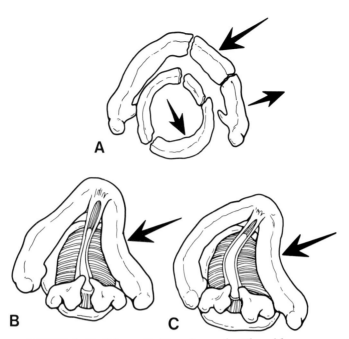

FIGURE 8–12. Schematic Drawings of a Thyroid Cartilage Injury When the Force Is Not Applied to the Midline

• • • •

A, The blow *(top arrow)* can fracture the ala, displacing the comminuted fragments *(lower arrows).* Fractures of the cricoid ring may also occur. *B,* A more pliable, less calcified ala may simply deform inward and then recoil to its original shape. *C,* A pliable ala may be deformed inward forcefully enough to cross the midline and cause contralateral mucosal disruption—a contrecoup type of injury. In such a case there may be minimal ipsilateral injury or edema.

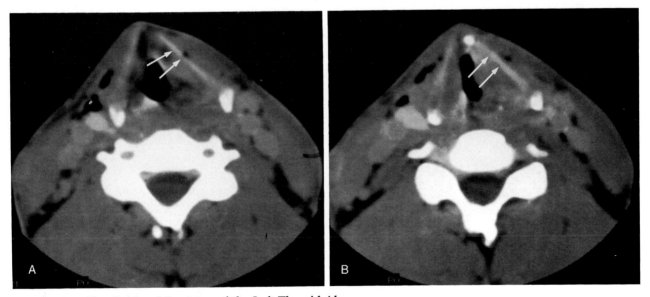

FIGURE 8–13. Nondisplaced Fractures of the Left Thyroid Ala

• • • •

A, The thyroid cartilage is only moderately calcified. The nondisplaced fractures *(arrows)* are difficult to see, but the underlying edema of the false cord on the left is obvious. *B,* The fractures *(arrows)* are slightly more obvious on the second section at the level of the true cords. Again, swelling is present on the left.

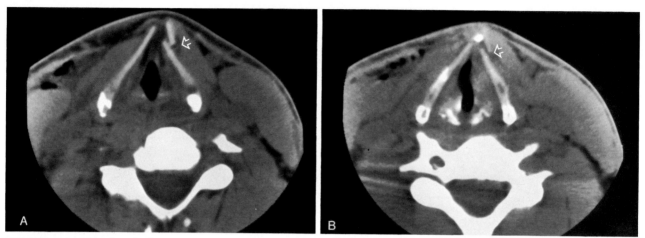

FIGURE 8–14. Displaced Thyroid Ala Fracture

• • • •

A, Displaced fracture of the left thyroid ala *(arrow). B,* Lower computed tomography section demonstrating edema of the left vocal fold in the paramedian position. The thyroid ala fracture is seen more anteriorly at this level *(arrow).* (Courtesy of James Fleckenstein, M.D.)

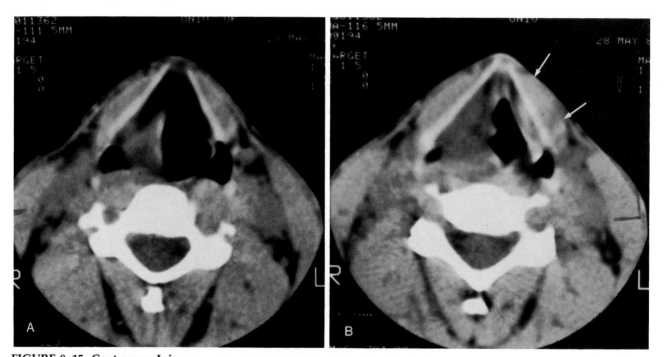

FIGURE 8–15. Contrecoup Injury

• • • •

A, This patient was struck on the left side of the neck. The left thyroid ala is normal, but there is edema of the right aryepiglottic fold and compression of the pyriform sinus on the right. *B,* A lower section demonstrates a superficial hematoma *(arrows)* on the left as well as the edema on the right.

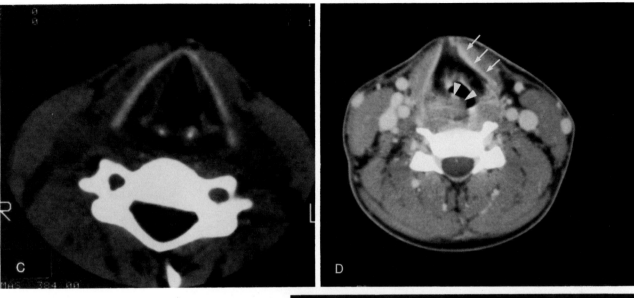

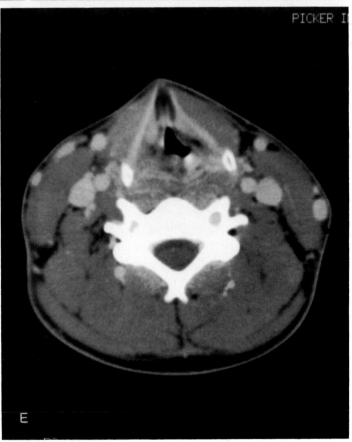

FIGURE 8–15 *Continued* **Contrecoup Injury**

• • • •

C, A third lower section demonstrates mild right vocal fold edema. *D*, A second patient, also struck on the left, demonstrates buckling of the left thyroid ala *(arrows)*, but no fracture could be identified. There is marked soft tissue swelling on the right *(arrowheads)*. *E*, A slightly lower section again demonstrates the buckling and the soft tissue swelling. There is slight left-sided edema at this level.

Illustration continued on following page

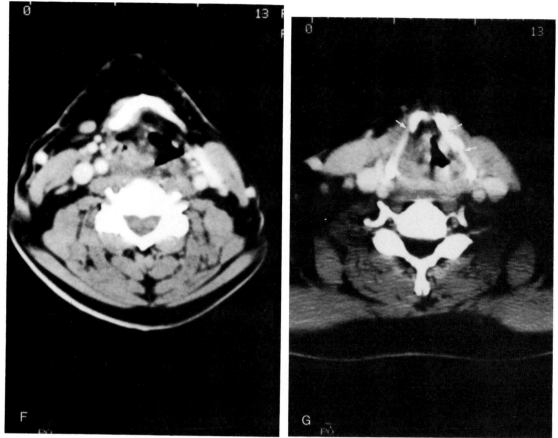

FIGURE 8–15 *Continued* **Contrecoup Injury**
• • • •
F, A third patient with a blow to the left side of the neck has marked, primarily right-sided edema. *G*, A lower section demonstrates bilateral thyroid alar fractures *(arrows)*, but again the edema is primarily right-sided.

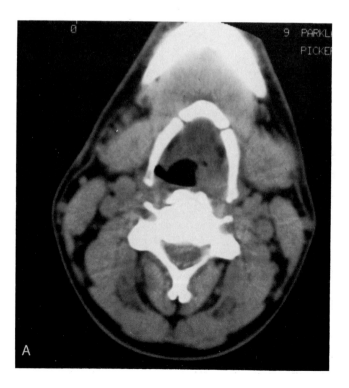

FIGURE 8–16. Marked Edema from a Small Left Mucosal Laceration
• • • •
A, The left pyriform sinus is obliterated.

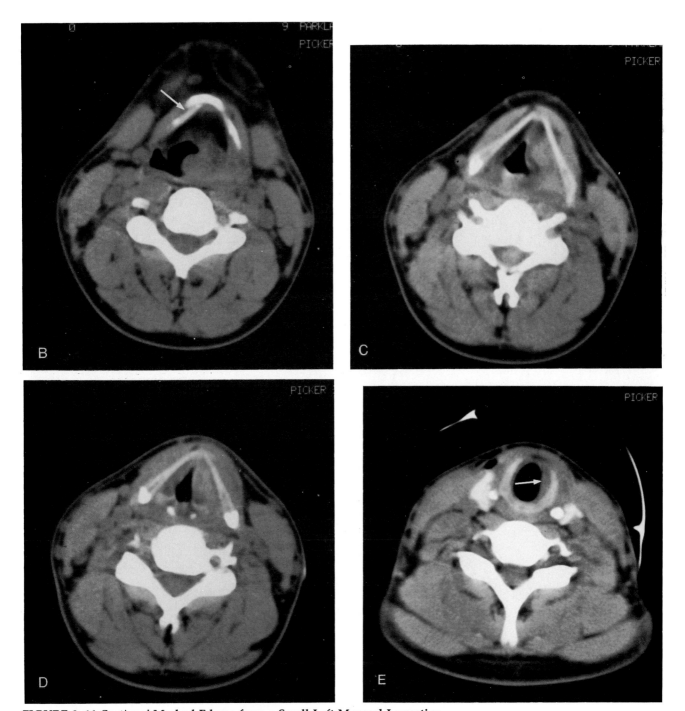

FIGURE 8–16 *Continued* **Marked Edema from a Small Left Mucosal Laceration**

• • • •

B, The left aryepiglottic fold is markedly swollen. Note the overlapping of the right thyroid ala with the hyoid bone *(arrow)* due to incomplete extension of the neck. *C,* The left false cord is markedly swollen. *D,* The left true cord is distorted by edema. *E,* There is even mild subglottic edema *(arrow)*; some right subcutaneous emphysema is also seen.

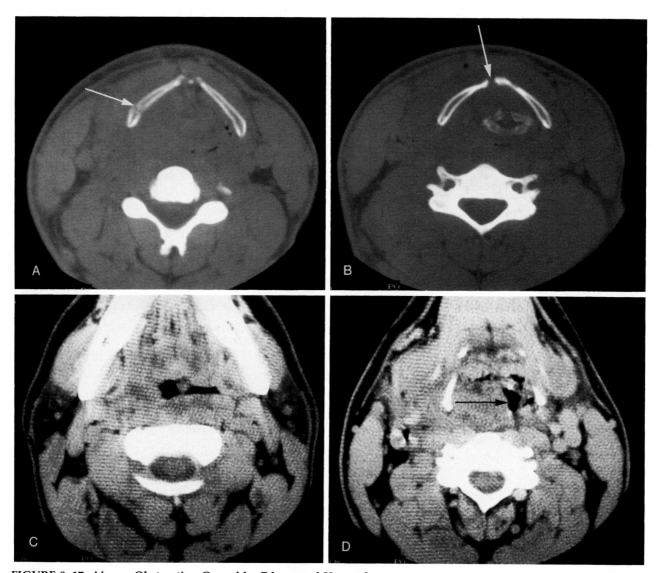

FIGURE 8–17. Airway Obstruction Caused by Edema and Hemorrhage

• • • •

A, The right thyroid lamina is fractured *(arrow)* and slightly displaced. The associated swelling has obliterated the airway. This section is displayed for bone detail. *B,* Another section demonstrates a right paramedian fracture of the thyroid cartilage *(arrow).* Notice the marked soft tissue swelling and obliteration of the airway. *C,* This more cephalad section uses a soft tissue technique. Though the airway is patent at this level, there is significant swelling in the right parapharyngeal space. Notice the asymmetry of the airway. *D,* The right pyriform sinus is obliterated, and the right aryepiglottic fold is edematous. The airway is displaced to the left and is distorted *(arrow).*

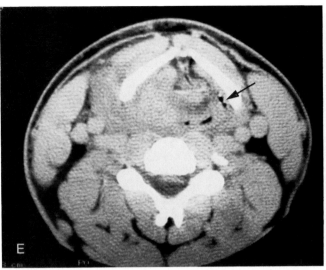 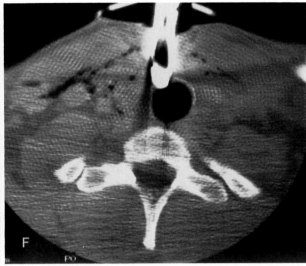

FIGURE 8–17 *Continued* **Airway Obstruction Caused by Edema and Hemorrhage**
• • • •
E, This section is at the same level as that in *A,* but it is displayed for the soft tissues. The airway is virtually obliterated. There is some air in the soft tissues *(arrow). F,* The final computed tomography section demonstrates the low tracheostomy tube and more soft tissue air. The trachea at this level is not edematous.

connective tissue also permits any of these abnormalities to cross the midline with ease. The potential for airway obstruction caused by swelling of any cause is greatest in the supraglottic and the subglottic areas, which do not have the support of the laryngeal framework (Fig. 8–17).

INHALATION INJURY

Massive soft tissue edema may be caused by inhalation of noxious elements, such as smoke, and by thermal irritation, particularly when exposure has been in an enclosed space (Fig. 8–18). The edema from thermal trauma may not occur immediately because patients with such trauma are usually hypovolemic on admission to the hospital. The edema may appear when the patient is rehydrated, so close monitoring is warranted. Edema is unpredictable and highly variable in appearance and location. Laryngeal edema occurs in 2–3% of all burn patients and most commonly in those with a greater than 50% body surface area burn. Normally, the supraglottic mucosa effectively absorbs heat prior to its passage to the trachea. Steam, however, has greater heat-carrying capacity than does dry air and is able to pass into the trachea prior to reflex glottic closure; this causes significant injury. Nuclear medicine xenon scanning is of some use in assessment of smaller airway injury in the lung in the first few days after injury and

before any infection develops. Gas trapping longer than 90 sec in the setting of trauma indicates bronchiolar spasm or edema, though chronic obstructive pulmonary disease, asthma, and retaining blebs can have a similar appearance.

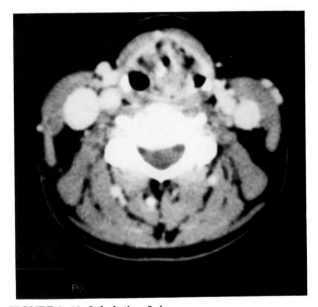

FIGURE 8–18. Inhalation Injury
• • • •
The airway is small. The left aryepiglottic fold in particular is edematous though there is diffuse edema. This computed tomography scan was performed with the use of an intravenous contrast material that enhanced much of the edematous tissue.

• • • •
PENETRATING INJURY

Penetrating injuries, usually lacerations from stab wounds or gunshot wounds, are also unpredictable and are dependent on both the instrument used and the specific structures traversed (Fig. 8–19). They are commonly associated with other soft tissue injuries to vascular, neural, and gastrointestinal structures. Radiologic evaluation of the associated injuries must be planned on an individual basis. Transverse slash wounds of the neck cause readily visualized horizontal disruptions to the cartilaginous structure of the larynx, sometimes permitting respiration through a gaping wound. Stab wounds, on the other hand, cause fewer lacerations in any orientation and may be only puncture wounds.

A penetrating injury with airway obstruction is more likely to cause drowning by aspiration of blood from lacerated carotid arteries or jugular veins than are injuries from blunt trauma. Injuries to the strap muscles and the thyroid gland and mucosal lacerations are also much more common. Symptoms correlate poorly with the severity of penetrating injury. Respiration may be maintained through a traumatically caused aperture without the patient's knowledge. These apertures can be closed acutely by atten-

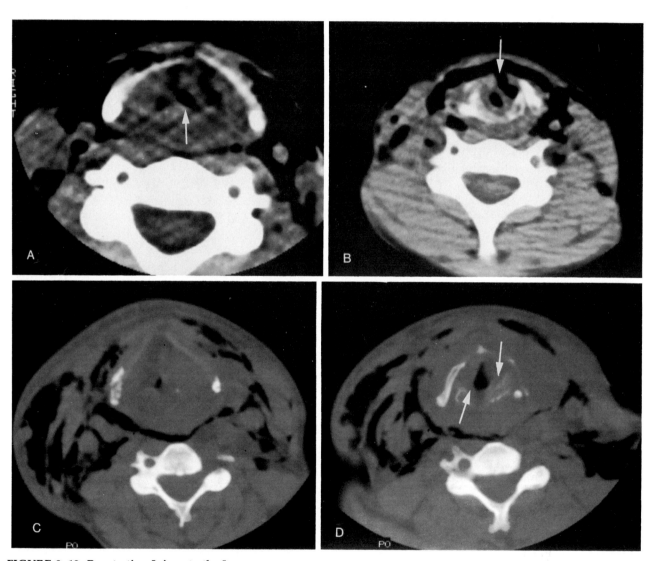

FIGURE 8–19. Penetrating Injury to the Larynx
• • • •
A, A stab wound to the neck has caused massive transglottic edema and extensive subcutaneous emphysema. The airway is quite small (arrow). The quality of this image is poor as a result of respiratory embarrassment and motion. B, A second section on this patient demonstrates the wound entering the anterior aspect of the subglottic space (arrow). C, A second patient was first stabbed and then strangled. There is extensive soft tissue emphysema and marked edema compressing the airway. A thyroid cartilage fracture is seen. D, A lower section also demonstrates cricoid fractures (arrows).

dant edema or clotting blood, or the patient may be seriously compromised when medical personnel close the lacerations. Penetrating injuries of the hypopharynx require treatment with antibiotics and mucosal closure of the exposed fascial spaces with appropriate drainage to avert the development of abscesses. Angiography and barium swallow may be needed following stabilization of the airway.

• • • •
FOREIGN BODIES

Foreign body injury to the larynx is equally common in pediatric and adult populations. Despite the propensity of young children to inhale or swallow inappropriate objects, the majority (85–90%) of these objects that successfully negotiate the oropharynx are small enough to descend into the bronchial tree. Most of the others are retained in the larynx. Adults, however, harbor the peculiar habit of attempting to selectively sort out bones, pits, and other inedible objects mixed with their food after they are placed in the mouth. In order to increase the challenge, these adults frequently imbibe intoxicating bever-

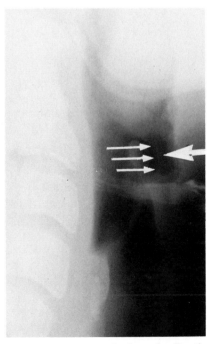

FIGURE 8–20. Soft Tissue Technique for Foreign Bodies
• • • •
This lateral film of the neck shows a very faint linear density (*arrows*) lying in the vallecula. This proved to be a fish bone. The very faint calcification of the fish bone emphasizes the need for an excellent film technique.

ages, impairing their discrimination, reaction time, and common sense. This practice leads to an equal number of adults and children with foreign bodies trapped in the larynx or the trachea.

The symptoms caused by laryngeal foreign bodies are nonspecific and, like other types of laryngeal trauma, include stridor, wheezing, cough, and sternal retractions. The patient may not realize that foreign material has been aspirated. A deft and focused interview about the circumstances at the onset of symptoms is paramount in making the diagnosis. Soft tissue films of the neck are appropriate when a laryngeal foreign body is suspected (Fig. 8–20).

In contrast to a rather innocuous early presentation, a 24-hour delay in diagnosis and treatment leads to a complication rate of 67% in patients with retained laryngeal foreign bodies. Complications include perforation, abscess formation, and glottic and subglottic edema sufficiently severe to require intubation and to cause chronic laryngotracheal stenosis and dysfunction as well as aspiration pneumonia (Fig. 8–21). An initial chest radiograph is usually not helpful, but soft tissue films of the neck are frequently diagnostic. Either the radiopaque foreign material itself is directly visualized or secondary evidence, such as subcutaneous or retropharyngeal gas, is seen. Although improved product design has significantly decreased the incidence of aspiration of pull tabs, the tabs on soda pop cans are made primarily from aluminum and are only faintly radiopaque. On frontal radiographs, a radiopaque foreign material that is planar is seen on its side when it is in the trachea due to the cartilaginous, C-shaped rings that are open posteriorly and distensible only in an anteroposterior plane. Foreign bodies that are seen en face on an anteroposterior film are more likely to be within the esophagus, which is more distensible transversely.

The extraction of these foreign bodies is often difficult. Although they may lend themselves to endoscopic capture, the retrieval can also dislodge the material and move it further into the tracheobronchial tree to more fully obstruct a narrower lumen. If the material rotates or expands to totally occlude the trachea during retraction, the endoscopist often must advance the foreign body into a main stem bronchus to allow ventilation through the contralateral bronchus. These problems have led to the practice of fragmenting the foreign body in situ and removing it in pieces. Simultaneous bronchoscopy and tracheotomy should be considered if the material is larger than a main stem bronchus. When this is done, the foreign bodies are removed through the tracheotomy with the bronchoscope, thus assuring an airway.

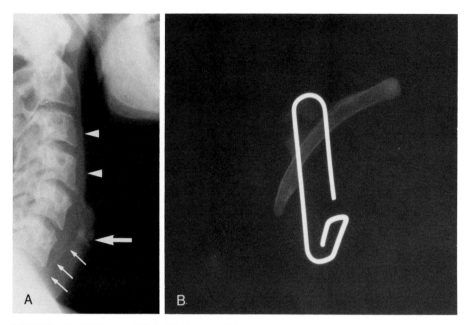

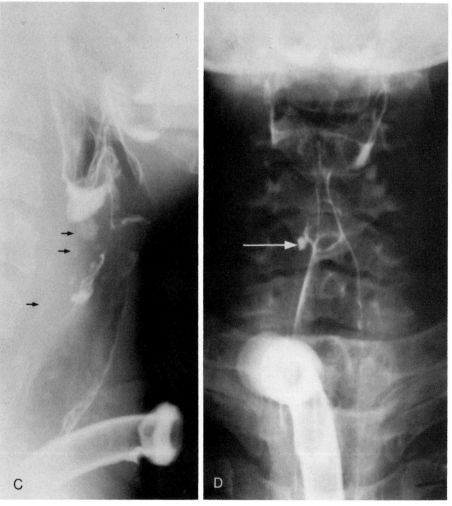

FIGURE 8–21. Delayed Presentation of a Foreign Body

• • • •

A, Initial lateral neck film demonstrates a long, faintly radiopaque foreign body *(arrows)* more or less over the esophagus. In addition, there are other subtle calcifications *(arrowheads)* ventral to C3 and C4. *B,* The surgical specimen, a chicken bone, was removed during surgery. *C,* A lateral film from a laryngogram performed 5 days later demonstrates that a retropharyngeal mass displaced the larynx as well as residual bone fragments *(arrows). D,* An anteroposterior film of the laryngogram demonstrates a pseudodiverticulum *(arrow)* at the site of perforation.

IATROGENIC INJURY

Iatrogenic trauma to the larynx can cause chronic laryngeal and subglottic stenosis. Although injury to the larynx may occur acutely during endotracheal intubation, iatrogenic injury usually occurs after difficult or prolonged intubation. Forceful or blind intubation may cause hematoma, contusion, laceration, perforation, and cord avulsion. Endotracheal tube trauma occurs at two levels: (1) glottic injury usually to the posterior wall that is caused by pressure from the endotracheal tube, which results in mucosal ischemia and breakdown, and (2) tracheal injury due to excessive pressure generated by the cuff or the tip. This latter problem can be avoided by the use of high-volume low-pressure cuffs.[13] Compromised mucosal perfusion leads to pressure necrosis, secondary infection, pseudomembrane formation, and scarring.

Intubation trauma can be minimized in several ways. The most experienced hospital staff member available should perform the intubation. Optimal visualization of the larynx diminishes both immediate and delayed complications. Use of an appropriately sized endotracheal tube is essential. The length of time of endotracheal intubation is critical, since complications increase remarkably after 2½–3 weeks.[12] Decreasing the amount of movement of the endotracheal tube within the larynx diminishes mucosal irritation. Unfortunately, the greatest predictor of endotracheal intubation success is the general health and well-being of the patient in his or her premorbid and acute state. Patients with diabetes mellitus, congestive heart failure, stroke, or tuberculosis tolerate intubation poorly.

The phenomenon of arytenoid dislocation deserves special attention. Recognized as a risk of endotracheal intubation only in the 1980s, arytenoid dislocation causes persistent hoarseness and odynophagia, which can affect patients for more than 48 hours after intubation. The pyramidal arytenoid cartilages, which are perched on the posterolateral aspect of the cricoid cartilage, may dislocate either anteriorly or posteriorly. Anterior dislocation of the arytenoid cartilage is better tolerated by the patient because those that have been dislocated posteriorly protrude into the hypopharynx, rock during swallowing, and cause pain. The left arytenoid cartilage is more often affected than that on the right, which may reflect the general tendency for the endoscopist or the anesthesiologist to handle the laryngoscope with the left hand and to exert more pressure along the left aspect of the larynx.

Arytenoid dislocation and other types of postintubation sequela are not benign, and their importance extends beyond the inconvenience of poor voice quality. These injuries impair the function of the larynx and impede pulmonary toilet both by allowing aspiration and by inhibiting the ability to cough. Pain on swallowing can postpone or limit oral intake and adversely affect postoperative recovery. Gastroesophageal reflux, which occurs asymptomatically in 9% of the normal population and in 40% of intubated patients not receiving antacid therapy, can also delay healing. Although the diagnosis may be made by CT using a high-resolution technique and vocalization maneuvers (prolonged "EEEEE" vocalization), it is readily diagnosed and treated by closed reduction using direct laryngoscopy. This problem should be addressed as soon as possible to avoid fibrosis, cricothyroid joint degenerative change, and recurrent laryngeal nerve dysfunction, all of which make later reduction more difficult and success of the reduction less likely (Fig. 8–22).

DISCUSSION

Mild degrees of edema, with or without the presence of nondisplaced fractures, or mildly ecchymotic cords are generally treated conservatively with voice rest, humidification, antibiotics, possibly steroids, and in-patient observation. It is in this group of patients that CT has a pivotal role in defining unsuspected submucosal abnormalities that require surgical intervention, or conversely, affirming conservative management. Displaced fractures and lacerations require mucosa-to-mucosa apposition for repair, and interposition flaps are needed to separate combined tracheoesophageal injuries, which necessitates surgical closure, temporary tracheostomy, and possibly stenting. Patients initially seen with obvious obstruction are treated with an emergency low tracheostomy at the fourth or the fifth tracheal ring by making a vertical incision upwards from the sternal notch rather than by attempting cricothyrotomy, which is difficult owing to the loss of landmarks and useless in separation of the larynx and the trachea. No attempt is made acutely to search for the recurrent laryngeal nerves, since dissection in these circumstances may actually result in their transection.

Blood in or around the larynx is either absorbed by macrophages or organizes into fibrous tissue. When the collagen contracts, airway stenosis may develop. This process is accelerated when laryngeal cartilage is denuded of its blood-supplying mucosa. The ischemic cartilage acts as a foreign body, inciting further granulation tissue and fibrosis. Cartilage loss also weakens the structural support of the larynx, making it subject to collapse on inspiration and again

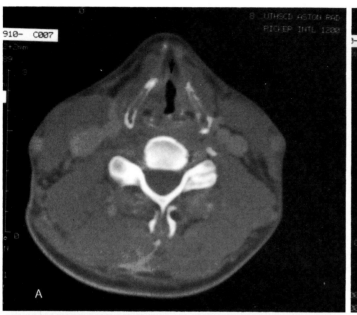

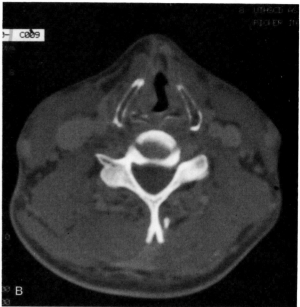

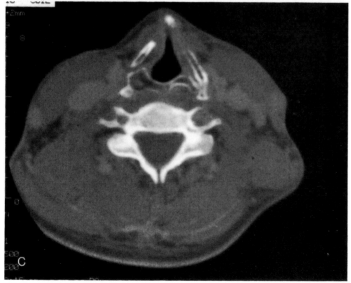

FIGURE 8–22. Post-Traumatic Abnormalities of the Larynx

• • • •

A, There has been resorption of the anterior commisure of the thyroid cartilage *(arrow).* The vocal folds are fixed in a paramedian position. The arytenoids are asymmetric because of the earlier bilateral injury. *B,* A section slightly lower again demonstrates the fixed vocal fold position. The arytenoids are partially resorbed and still asymmetric. *C,* A third lower scan demonstrates that the right arytenoid fragment has coalesced with the cricoid ring. The airway remains deformed.

compromising the narrowed airway. Flow of air drops by the fourth power as the radius of the tube, such as the larynx or trachea, decreases. This is particularly critical at the cricoid or subglottic level, which is the most restricted cross-sectional area of the normal airway. Subglottic stenosis, either in isolation or in combination with other sites, has poor long-term results. When chronic laryngeal stenosis occurs, the surgical goals are to excise scar tissue, return skeletal support, and provide mucosal covering of exposed cartilaginous surfaces without inciting further fibrosis. The role of an intraluminal stent after these goals have been addressed remains controversial.

Paralysis of either the true or the false vocal folds, acutely or chronically, does not preclude reconstitution of the airway and voice. Just as a set of objectively defined measurements has been developed to evaluate respiration and oxygen exchange, the maximum phonation time, the mean airflow rate, the fundamental frequency range, and the electromyography of the intrinsic muscles of phonation have been shown to have a high predictive value for recovery. Speech therapy greatly assists these patients in regaining laryngeal control in the months following their trauma.

The greatest advance in the management of chronic laryngeal stenosis has been in its prevention. The choices made in the acute management of laryngeal trauma have a profound effect on the post-traumatic consequences. The goal is to apply the basic tenets of life support and stable airway establishment while rapidly gathering as much information as possible with which to make prudent therapeutic decisions, some of which become irrevocable as the narrow window of interventional opportunity closes. This explains the limited role of CT in the acutely injured patient, since this study places the patient at some risk and may or may not provide useful clinical information. The time and energy are often better spent in indirect or direct visualization of the larynx. A satisfactory goal is one in which a functional airway provides adequate ventilation and protects from aspiration; this airway should also permit vocalization in a socially acceptable mode for communication.

References

1. Dudley JP, Mancuso AA, Fonkalsrud EW. Arytenoid dislocation and computed tomography. Arch Otolaryngol 1984; 110:483.
2. Edwards WH Jr, Morris JA, DeLozier JB 3rd, Adkins RB. Airway injuries: The first priority in trauma. Am Surg 1987; 53:192.
3. Fuhrman GM, Steig FH 3rd, Buerk CA. Blunt laryngeal trauma: Classification and management protocol. J Trauma 1990; 30:87.
4. Gussack GS, Jurkovich GJ, Luterman A. Laryngotracheal trauma: A protocol approach to a rare injury. Laryngoscope 1986; 96:660.
5. Handler SD. Trauma to the larynx and upper trachea. Int Anesthesiol Clin 1988; 26:39.
6. Mancuso AA, Hanafee WN. Computed tomography of the injured larynx. Radiology 1979; 133:139.
7. Myer CM 3rd, Orobello P, Cotton RT, Bratcher GO. Blunt laryngeal trauma in children. Laryngoscope 1987; 97:1043.
8. Myers EM, Iko BO. The management of acute laryngeal trauma. J Trauma 1987; 27:448.
9. Ogura JH, Henneman TT, Spector GJ. Laryngo-tracheal trauma: Diagnosis and treatment. Can J Otolaryngol 1973; 2:112.
10. Schaefer SD, Close LG. Acute management of laryngeal trauma. Ann Otol Rhinol Laryngol 1989; 98:98.
11. Stanley RB, Colman MF. Unilateral degloving injuries of the arytenoid cartilage. Arch Otolaryngol Head Neck Surg 1986; 112:516.
12. Weymuller, EA Jr. Laryngeal injury from prolonged endotracheal intubation. Laryngoscope 1988; 98:1.

CHAPTER 9

Injuries of the Chest: The Lungs, the Pleura, the Tracheobronchial Tree, the Diaphragm, and the Chest Wall

ANN R. MOOTZ, M.D.

Injury to the thorax may be produced by blunt or penetrating trauma. Some injury to the thorax is seen in at least one half of all patients with multisystem trauma. Automobile and motorcycle accidents are the most common causes of blunt injury to the thorax. Injuries are also incurred when patients fall from a height or are involved in an aggravated assault. Peacetime blast injury, another form of blunt trauma, generally occurs during industrial accidents. Penetrating trauma is most frequently caused by shooting or stabbing, although any sharp object may penetrate the chest and cause injury. Both blunt and penetrating trauma can cause injuries of the chest wall, the lungs, the pleura, the bronchi, the diaphragm, and the solid organs.

Penetrating chest trauma is usually evident clinically. In blunt thoracic trauma, clinically obvious

external signs of significant internal injury are frequently absent. This is particularly true in patients who have suffered severe multisystem trauma that includes the thorax. The emergency room physician often becomes involved in evaluating other organ systems where the injury is more readily apparent. Severe intrathoracic injury may remain unrecognized if the clinician is not aware of its likelihood. Often it is the radiographic findings on a chest film that lead to the diagnosis of an intrathoracic injury that may be life-threatening.

The portable chest film obtained in the emergency room remains the cornerstone of the radiographic evaluation of chest trauma. Often the patient is unable to be moved to the radiology department for upright posteroanterior and lateral chest films. Portable radiographs, often obtained with the patient in

---

•••• *APPROACH RADIOGRAPHIC STUDIES*

I. **The Lung**
   A. Posteroanterior (PA) and lateral chest films.
   Comment: Often not possible in the injured patient.
   B. Anteroposterior (AP) upright and supine chest films.
   Comment: May be more difficult to evaluate, especially when the patient is in a supine position.
   C. Decubitus chest films.
   Comment: Useful for evaluating fluid collections and some pneumothoraces.
   D. Expiratory chest films
   Comment: Help detect small apical pneumothoraces.
   E. Computed tomography
   Comment: Useful in selected patients for studying chest tube position, pneumothorax, and fluid collections.

II. **The Pleura**
   A. PA and lateral chest films
   B. AP chest films
   C. Expiratory chest films
   D. Decubitus chest films
   E. Computed tomography

III. **The Tracheobronchial Tree**
   A. Chest films
   Comment: The radiographic findings are nonspecific. Bronchoscopy is the primary diagnostic technique employed.

IV. **The Diaphragm**
   A. Chest films
   B. Abdominal films
   C. Barium studies of the bowel
   D. Radionuclide liver scanning

V. **Chest Wall Injuries**
   A. Rib films
   B. Thoracic spine films
   C. Sternal films

---

a supine position, must suffice for radiographic diagnosis in many severely injured patients. The classic radiographic findings of thoracic injury present on an upright radiograph may be much more difficult to detect on a supine film. Recognition of significant radiographic findings on a supine chest radiograph is of the utmost importance in proper patient management and is the focus of this chapter. Proper use of ancillary radiographs, computed tomography (CT), and other imaging modalities are also discussed.

••••
THE LUNG

Pulmonary Contusion

Pulmonary contusion is the single most common manifestation of blunt thoracic trauma. Even rib fractures are less common. Although broken ribs may penetrate the lung and cause contusion, rib fractures are frequently absent in patients with pulmonary contusion. Other forms of penetrating trauma also cause pulmonary contusion. Pulmonary contusion results from the rupture of alveolar capillaries and associated intra-alveolar hemorrhage, which produces the classic radiographic appearance of an alveolar infiltrate.[35] This infiltrate does not conform to a segment or lobe of the lung, an important diagnostic hallmark of pulmonary contusion. The infiltrate may be very extensive, may be bilateral, and can even be in a contrecoup location. The infil-

trate of pulmonary contusion is usually present within 6 hours of the time of injury and is most often seen on the first chest x-ray obtained in the emergency room (Fig. 9–1). Pulmonary contusion may worsen in appearance during the first 24 hours, but worsening after 48 hours rarely occurs. In fact, improvement is generally seen within 48–72 hours of injury, and complete resolution usually occurs within 1 week (Fig. 9–2). Worsening of the infiltration after 48–72 hours should suggest a superimposed prob-

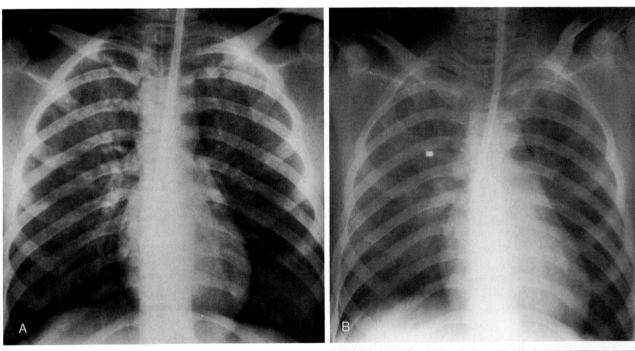

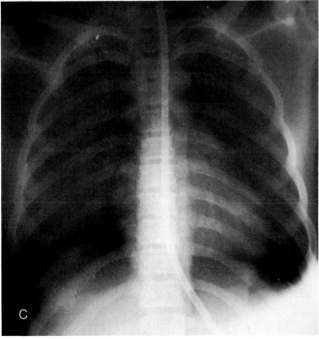

FIGURE 9–1. Bilateral Pulmonary Contusions

• • • •

A, A portable supine chest radiograph obtained shortly after a motor vehicle accident demonstrates bilateral, predominantly upper lobe infiltrates that are pulmonary contusions. There is some involvement of the lower lobes as well. Pulmonary contusion is usually evident on the first film obtained in the emergency room. *B*, Two days later some improvement in the infiltrates is seen. *C*, The pulmonary contusions are completely resolved 5 days after the initial injury.

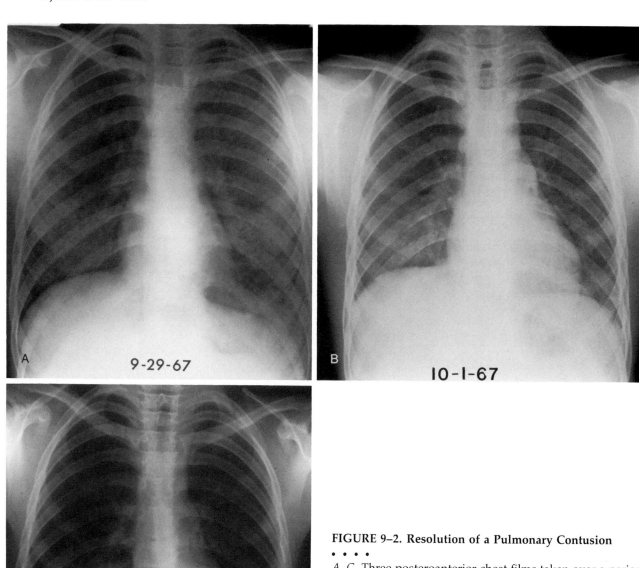

FIGURE 9–2. Resolution of a Pulmonary Contusion

• • • •

A–C, Three posteroanterior chest films taken over a period of 5 days demonstrate the improvement and the resolution of extensive bilateral infiltrates in this patient run over by a car. Complete rapid resolution of uncomplicated pulmonary contusions is to be expected.

lem. Pneumonia, pulmonary infarction, and fat embolism are the most common complications of pulmonary contusion. The diagnosis of pulmonary contusion does not require any special techniques. Chest films are sufficient to make the appropriate diagnosis when the clinical history is appropriate.

Pulmonary Laceration and Hematoma

Penetrating injuries, such as gunshot and stab wounds, are common causes of pulmonary lacerations. Blunt trauma may also have enough force to disrupt or tear the lung and cause a pulmonary laceration. Adjacent pulmonary contusion is almost always present as well. The entities of pulmonary laceration, pulmonary hematoma, and traumatic lung cyst are a radiographic spectrum that is seen when lung parenchyma is actually torn. The radiographic appearance of a pulmonary laceration is determined primarily by the degree of associated contusion and the severity of hemorrhage into the laceration. Pulmonary lacerations are often obscured initially by the adjacent pulmonary contusion. As the contusion begins to clear, a rounded or oval area of radiolucency may be seen in the lung (Fig. 9–3). Further clearing of the contusion may reveal a discrete cavity in the lung (Fig. 9–4). An air-fluid level, caused by hemorrhage into the laceration, may be present within the cavity.

Pulmonary lacerations may be single (Fig. 9–5) or multiple (Fig. 9–6). They can vary in size from as small as 1–2 cm to as large as 10–12 cm. They can occur in any segment of lung and may also be contrecoup in location. Pulmonary lacerations gradually contract in size and usually disappear completely after 1 week to 3 months. They are more common in children and young adults than in the elderly because of the greater compressibility of the chest wall in younger patients. Treatment is conservative, and surgery is rarely required acutely.

Although most lacerations caused by penetrating trauma resolve spontaneously, some pulmonary lacerations caused by bullets may cause tissue necrosis, which can become a focus of infection. Surgical resection may be required for persistent or recurrent infection, recurrent pneumothorax, empyema, persistent purulent sputum, or failure of a cavity to close after a prolonged period of observation.[25]

When a pulmonary laceration is completely filled by hemorrhage it is called a *pulmonary hematoma*. A pulmonary hematoma is seen radiographically as a solid, oval, or rounded radiodensity in the lung (Fig. 9–7). Pulmonary hematomas are often obscured initially by pulmonary contusion. As the contusion begins to clear, a more mass-like, solid opacity becomes apparent. Pulmonary hematomas vary in size from 1 to several centimeters in diameter. As healing occurs they gradually contract in size. Considerable reduction in the size of a pulmonary hematoma usually occurs over the first 6–10 weeks until a solitary pulmonary nodule remains (Fig. 9–8). As the hematoma contracts, a small meniscus of air may be seen in the laceration cavity (Fig. 9–9). Some of the first pulmonary hematomas described in the literature were coin lesions whose true nature was discovered only at thoracotomy. It is the slow progressive reduction in the size of a pulmonary hematoma that led to its description as the "vanishing lung tumor."[31]

Text continued on page 324

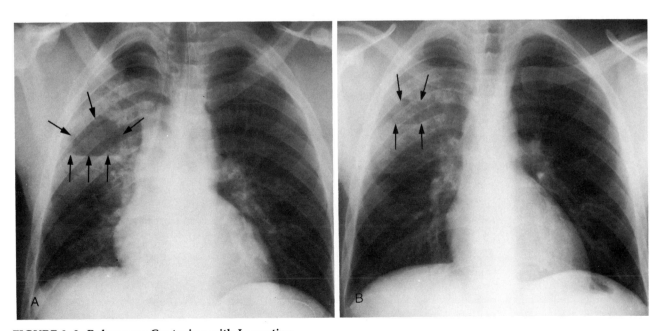

FIGURE 9–3. Pulmonary Contusion with Laceration

• • • •

A, A right upper lobe pulmonary contusion contains a rounded area of radiolucency (*arrows*); this is a pulmonary laceration. The horizontal inferior border is an air-fluid level caused by hemorrhage into the laceration. *B,* Three days later the contusion showed improvement and the pulmonary laceration was decreased in size (*arrows*). The patient had no chest complaints and required no treatment and was therefore discharged.

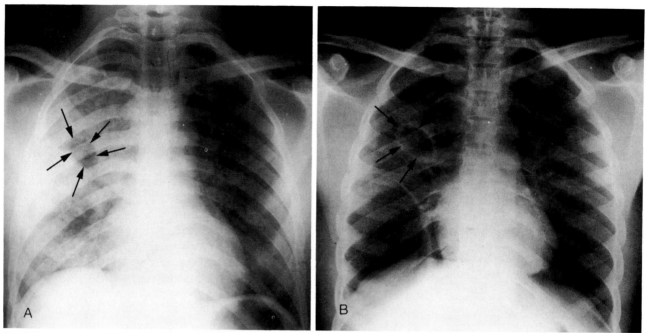

FIGURE 9–4. Pulmonary Contusion with Laceration

• • • •

A, A 3-cm rounded radiolucency (*arrows*) is demonstrated within a large pulmonary contusion that was incurred during a motor vehicle accident. *B*, A posteroanterior film taken after resolution of the pulmonary contusion demonstrates a simple cavity (*arrows*); this is the residual pulmonary laceration.

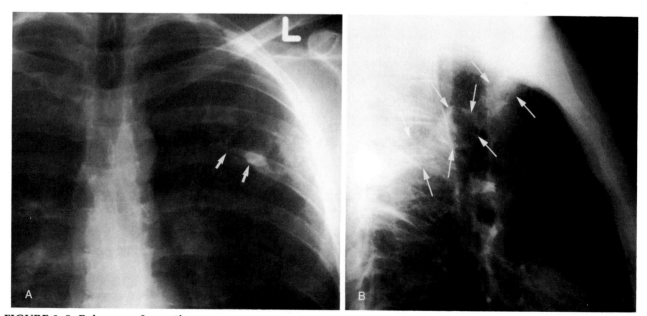

FIGURE 9–5. Pulmonary Laceration

• • • •

A pulmonary laceration was produced by a bullet as it passed obliquely through the left side of the chest. *A*, The posteroanterior film demonstrates both a lucent lesion and a small area of consolidation (*arrows*). *B*, The lateral film demonstrates the tubular nature of the laceration even more clearly (*arrows*).

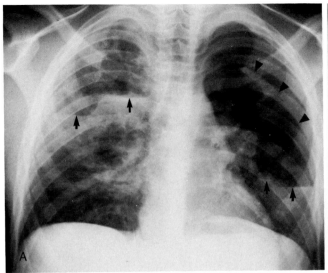
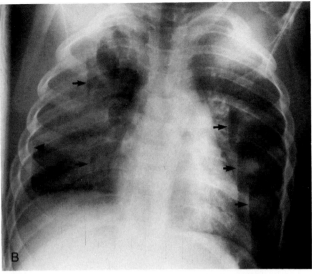

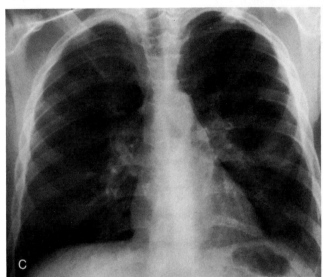

FIGURE 9–6. Extensive Pulmonary Contusion and Laceration

• • • •

A, Extensive bilateral infiltrates with multiple air-fluid levels (*arrows*) are present in this 10-year-old boy following a motor vehicle accident. Note also the large left pneumothorax (*arrowheads*). B, A right lateral decubitus film shows the numerous air-fluid levels to even better advantage (*arrows*). A small right pleural effusion is present (*arrowhead*). C, A follow-up posteroanterior film obtained 3 weeks after injury shows almost complete resolution of the extensive bilateral parenchymal injury.

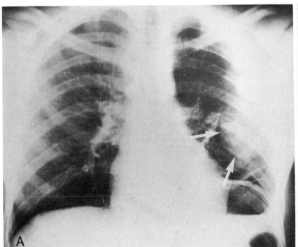
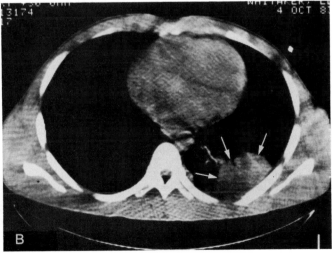

FIGURE 9–7. Post-traumatic Pulmonary Hematoma

• • • •

A, This posteroanterior film obtained 3 days following a motor vehicle accident demonstrates a large mass laterally near the base of the left lung (*arrows*). B, The mass is also well seen on this computed tomography (CT) scan (*arrows*). The rounded appearance at CT is typical of a hematoma that resolved completely after a few months.

321

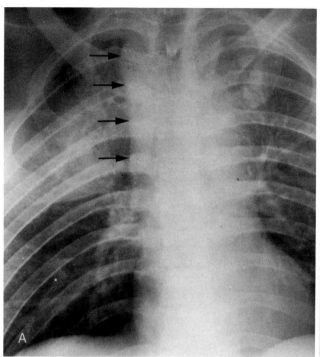

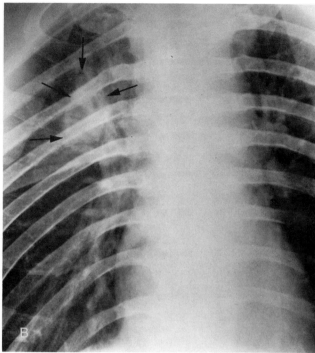

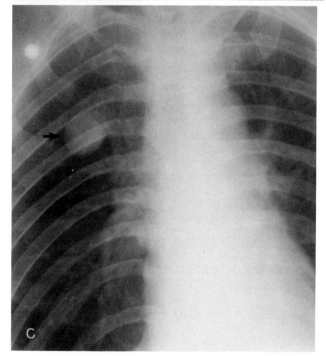

FIGURE 9–8. Pulmonary Contusion with Hematoma

• • • •

A, A supine portable radiograph obtained within hours of an automobile accident demonstrates extensive pulmonary contusion involving the right upper lobe. The mediastinum is widened (*arrows*). A thoracic aortogram showed no evidence of an aortic injury. *B*, When the pulmonary contusion resolves, a more rounded, mass-like density (a pulmonary hematoma) begins to appear (*arrows*). *C*, The pulmonary hematoma has contracted into a smooth, rounded, solitary pulmonary nodule (*arrow*). A hematoma such as this may require months to resolve. It is easy to see how such a hematoma could be suspected of being a carcinoma if no old films or any history of trauma were available.

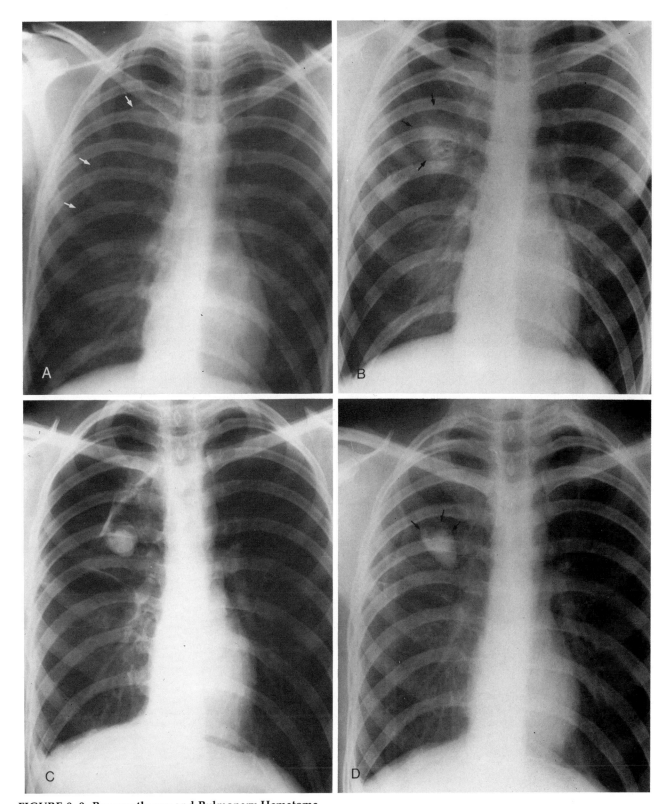

FIGURE 9–9. Pneumothorax and Pulmonary Hematoma

• • • •

A, A large right pneumothorax (*arrows*) is present on the first film obtained after the patient had a screwdriver driven into the upper right side of the chest. *B*, Several hours later, a localized, somewhat poorly defined rounded radiodensity in the upper part of the right lung developed (*arrows*). *C*, Several days later, the pneumothorax is larger. A more discrete mass is now seen; this mass is a pulmonary hematoma. *D*, As the hematoma contracts, a small meniscus of air (*arrows*) is demonstrated at its periphery.

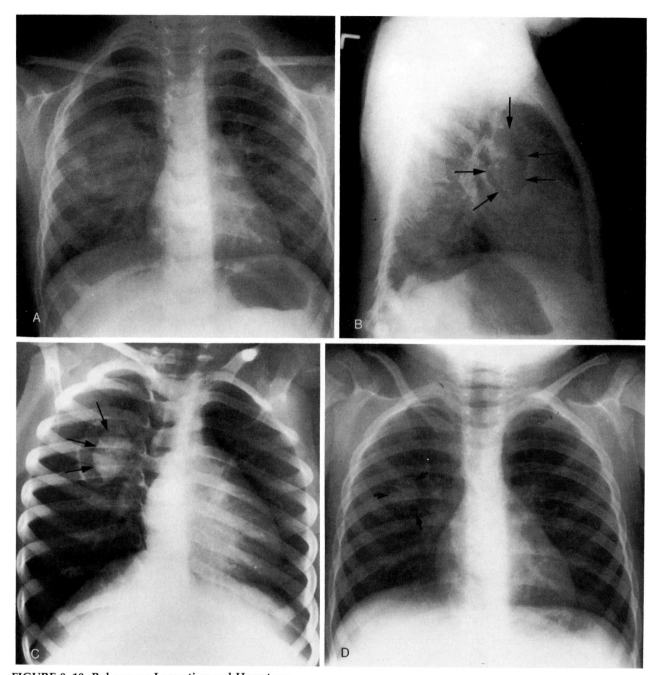

FIGURE 9–10. Pulmonary Laceration and Hematoma
• • • •

A and *B*, Posteroanterior and lateral films obtained on a child shortly after a motor vehicle accident demonstrate a large cavity in the right lung, most easily seen on the lateral film (*arrows, B*). Very little pulmonary contusion surrounds this large laceration. *C*, As the laceration resolves, hemorrhage within the laceration contracts into the hematoma (*arrows*) seen on this decubitus film.

When very little contusion surrounds a pulmonary laceration, a large cystic air collection with or without an air-fluid level is seen (Fig. 9–10). A traumatic lung cyst is a pulmonary laceration into which very little hemorrhage has occurred and around which there is very little pulmonary contusion.[12] Traumatic lung

cysts have been called by a variety of names over the years, including cavitary pulmonary lesions, pneumatoceles, traumatic lung cavities, and traumatic pseudocysts of the lung.

Recently, CT has called into question the basic concepts about pulmonary contusion and laceration.

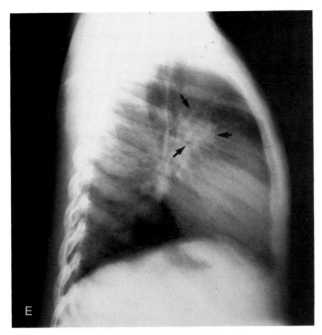

FIGURE 9-10 *Continued* **Pulmonary Laceration and Hematoma**

• • • •

D and *E,* Posteroanterior and lateral chest films obtained several weeks later demonstrate that the laceration has resolved, leaving only the hematoma as a solitary lung mass (*arrows*).

A 1988 report reviewed the CT findings in 85 consecutive patients with chest trauma.[30] Pulmonary contusion was seen on the chest radiographs of 58 of the patients. Only five of these 58 patients had evidence of a pulmonary laceration on the chest radiographs. However, when CT was performed, lung lacerations were seen in 55 of these patients. These data support the belief that pulmonary laceration is the basic component of all parenchymal injuries of the lung and that pulmonary contusion results from spillover of hemorrhage from lacerated lung tissue into adjacent alveoli.

Lung Torsion

Torsion of the lung is rare but can occur in the setting of trauma. However, the majority of cases have been reported in patients following lobar resection or in association with some other underlying pulmonary abnormality such as a lung mass or pneumonia. The most useful radiographic findings include a collapsed or consolidated lobe occupying an unusual position on plain film radiographs, CT scans, angiograms, or bronchograms. Alteration in the normal position and distribution of the pulmonary vasculature has also been described.

• • • •

PLEURA

Injury to the pleura is caused by both blunt and penetrating trauma. In blunt trauma, the sharp ends of fractured ribs may cause tears of the pleura. Blunt trauma may also disrupt the lung directly, causing leakage of air into the pleural space. Rupture of small vessels within the chest wall, the mediastinum, or the diaphragm frequently leads to hemothorax. Penetrating trauma injures the pleura directly. Pneumothorax and hemothorax are the primary injuries seen.

Pneumothorax

A pneumothorax is seen radiographically as a thin pleural line in the apex and the lateral aspect of the lung when the chest film is taken with the patient in the upright position. No lung markings are seen beyond the pleural line (Fig. 9–11). A chest film made during expiration often accentuates a small pneumothorax owing both to the lower pressure and the smaller volume of the lung (Fig. 9–12). Decubitus radiographs are sometimes useful in confirming the presence of a small pneumothorax.

Many chest films obtained in the emergency room are taken with the patient in a supine position out of necessity. This is particularly true in severely injured patients. When the patient is supine, air collects in the most ventral portion of the chest, and the classic apicolateral pneumothorax cannot be seen. Recognition of a pneumothorax in a supine patient is of the utmost importance. In these patients, the most ventral pleural space is anteromedial. Over one third of all pneumothoraces occurring in critically injured or ill patients are located in the anteromedial pleural space. Subpulmonic pneumothorax is seen in about 25% of patients, and the classic apicolateral pneumothorax occurs in another 25% of patients.[79]

An anteromedial pneumothorax is seen radiographically as a paramediastinal lucency, often bordered laterally by a thin, sharp pleural line (the medial visceral pleura). Unlike an apicolateral pneumothorax, lung vessels pass medial to the pleural edge because the lung remains anchored at the hilus more posteriorly (Fig. 9–13). Often a pleural edge is not seen at all. However, mediastinal structures, such as the superior vena cava, aorta and great vessels, the main pulmonary artery, the heart, and the diaphragm, are more sharply delineated than if they interfaced directly with the lung (Fig. 9–14). Differentiation of an anteromedial pneumothorax from pneumomediastinum may be difficult. Upright or

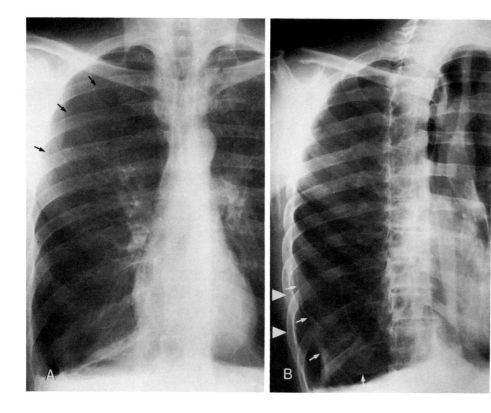

FIGURE 9–11. Pneumothorax

• • • •

A, A typical apicolateral pneumothorax (*arrows*) is seen in this patient following a car crash. A thin pleural line is present, and no lung markings extend beyond this line. *B,* On the oblique radiograph, the subpulmonic component of the pneumothorax is seen to better advantage (*arrows*). Note also the fractures of the eight and ninth ribs (*arrowheads*).

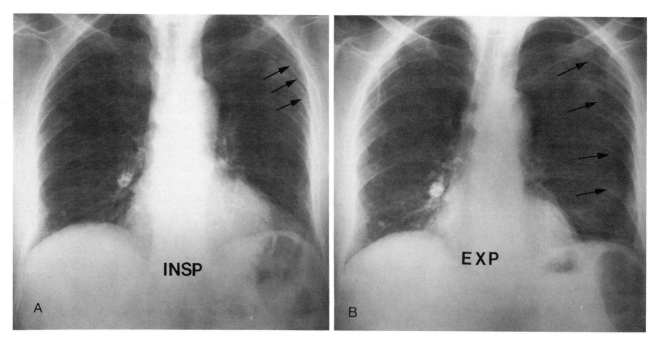

FIGURE 9–12. Pneumothorax with Inspiratory and Expiratory Films

• • • •

A, An inspiratory film demonstrates a small left pneumothorax (*arrows*). *B,* An expiratory radiograph markedly accentuates the pneumothorax (*arrows*).

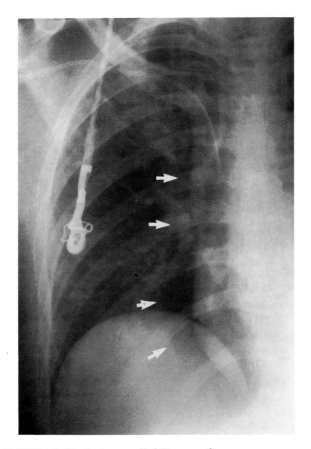

FIGURE 9–13. Anteromedial Pneumothorax
• • • •
An anteromedial pneumothorax is present following the placement of a central line. A very subtle pleural edge is present in a paramediastinal location (*arrows*). Note the unusually sharp delineation of the border of the right side of the heart and the superior vena cava, which are outlined by air. Lung vessels can be seen passing medial to the pleural edge (the lung remains anchored to the right hilus more posteriorly).

decubitus films may differentiate the two when this distinction is important. When an anteromedial pneumothorax is very large, hyperlucency of the involved hemithorax, often accompanied by a mediastinal shift, may be the primary observation. A cross-table lateral or decubitus film is generally helpful in diagnosing these cases, although occasionally such a pneumothorax is so large that the pleural edge is not detectable even with dependent patient positioning (Fig. 9–15).

A variety of radiographic signs have been described to indicate the presence of a subpulmonic pneumothorax. Frequently, the only sign is a subtle increase in the lucency of the lower chest or the upper abdomen. This basilar hyperlucency may cause a double diaphragm sign, which is produced by depression of the anterior diaphragmatic surface (Fig. 9–16). The cardiac apex may be sharply outlined

by air; epicardial fat pads may be seen as rounded or lobulated soft tissue masses that are no longer compressed by adjacent lung tissue (Fig. 9–17). A subpulmonic pneumothorax may extend laterally to produce a deep costophrenic sulcus (see Fig. 9–16). Large pneumothoraces can occupy more than one pleural recess (Fig. 9–18).

Skin folds, which often mimic a pneumothorax, always present diagnostic challenges. Chest tubes have been inserted unnecessarily in patients thought to have a pneumothorax because a skin fold simulated a pleural line. Skin folds produce an edge of radiodensity, often with a thin black line seen just to the outside. This is in contrast to the very thin sharp line produced by the displaced visceral pleura of a pneumothorax. Lung markings extend beyond the edge of a skin fold. The edges produced by skin folds often start and stop abruptly as the skin fold merges with the adjacent chest surface. Skin folds are often multiple, and they may extend across the

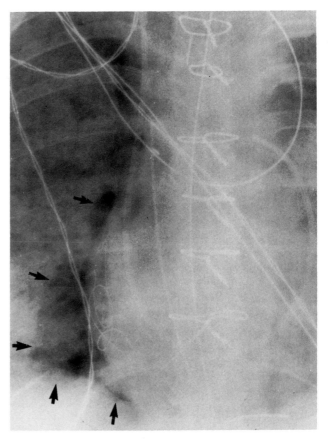

FIGURE 9–14. Anteromedial Pneumothorax
• • • •
An anteromedial pneumothorax is seen as a triangular wedge of hyperlucency adjacent to the border of the right side of the heart (*arrows*). Note the sharp delineation of this border, outlined by the adjacent pneumothorax. This patient developed adult respiratory distress syndrome following cardiac surgery.

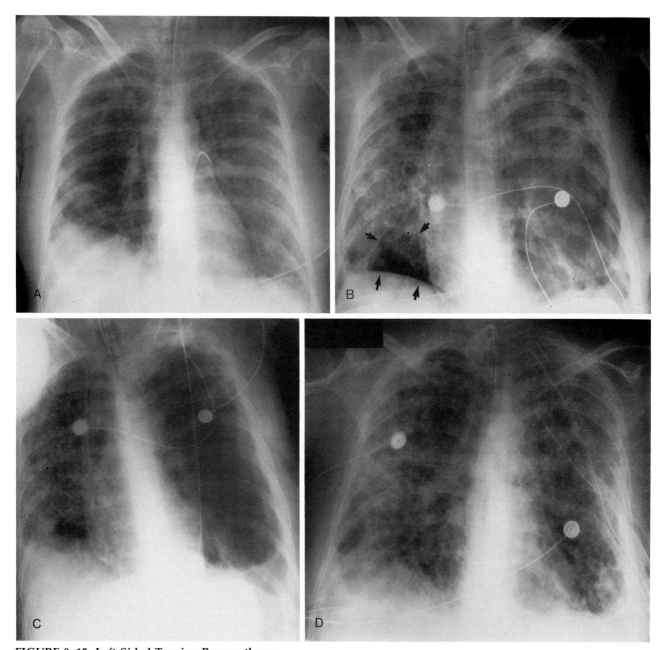

FIGURE 9–15. Left-Sided Tension Pneumothorax

• • • •

A, A supine radiograph in a patient with adult respiratory distress syndrome does not show a pneumothorax. *B,* On a later film the left hemithorax is much more lucent than that on the right, and there is a shift of the cardiomediastinal silhouette to the right. Although a discrete pleural edge could not be seen, a left pneumothorax was suspected. Note the basal pneumothorax on the right (*arrows*). *C,* A right lateral decubitus film was obtained in an attempt to demonstrate a pleural edge, but none is seen. *D,* Because clinical signs of tension were present, chest tubes were placed. Air was successfully evacuated, and the patient's clinical condition improved. The mediastinum returned to a midline position.

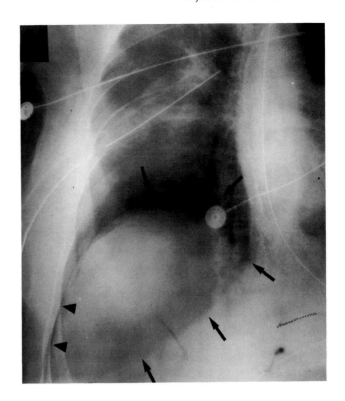

FIGURE 9–16. Subpulmonic Pneumothorax

• • • •

The hyperlucency of the lower chest and the upper abdomen (*arrows*) is caused by a large subpulmonic pneumothorax occurring in spite of the presence of a chest tube. Note also the deep costophrenic sulcus (*arrowheads*). The shift of the cardiomediastinal silhouette to the left is an ancillary sign of a tension pneumothorax.

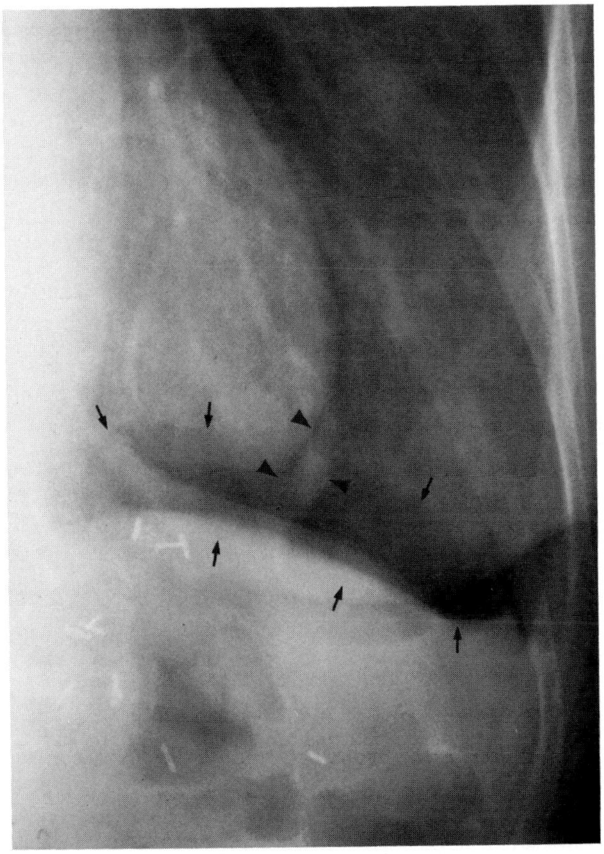

FIGURE 9–17. Subpulmonic Pneumothorax

• • • •

A subpulmonic pneumothorax is present at the base of the left lung (*arrows*). The epicardial fat pad is clearly seen because it is not compressed by the adjacent lung (*arrowheads*).

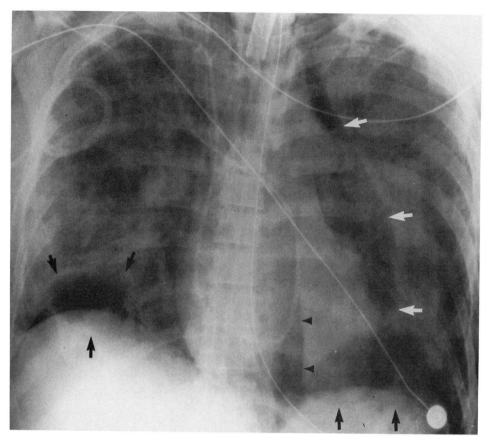

FIGURE 9–18. Pneumothorax Occupying Several Pleural Recesses

• • • •

Bilateral pneumothoraces are present in this patient who developed adult respiratory distress syndrome following a motor vehicle accident. A large anteromedial pneumothorax is present on the left in a paramediastinal location (*white arrows*). Subpulmonic pneumothoraces are present bilaterally as well (*black arrows*). The air outlining the descending aorta (*black arrowheads*) is probably a posterior pneumothorax, which is sometimes seen in patients with lower lobe atelectasis. Air collects in this unusual posterior location due to changes in the elastic recoil of the lung.

midline or outside the rib cage (Fig. 9–19). Repeat chest films often clarify the issue, since skin folds generally disappear or change position recognizably with differences in patient positioning.

Tension Pneumothorax

A pneumothorax is under tension when the intrapleural pressure exceeds atmospheric pressure. A tension pneumothorax is a clinical diagnosis, and is usually manifested by impaired venous return to the heart. Very large pneumothoraces, which often produce radiographic signs of tension, do not necessarily produce clinical signs of tension. In contrast, a very small pneumothorax, which is difficult to detect radiographically, can produce clinical signs of tension. This is particularly true in patients on ventilators or in those with severe chronic obstructive pulmonary disease. In these cases, even a small

pneumothorax may produce devastating clinical results. Radiographic signs of tension include displacement of mediastinal structures away from the pneumothorax, inversion of the diaphragm, atelectasis of adjacent lung tissue, and compression of the superior vena cava, the inferior vena cava, or the border of the heart. Emergency treatment of a tension pneumothorax may be achieved by the insertion of a small catheter.[75]

Hemothorax

Blood enters the pleural space from rupture of small arteries and veins in the chest wall, the pleura, the lung, the mediastinum, and the diaphragm. Hemothorax caused by bleeding from small vessels tends to be moderate in size. A rapidly enlarging hemothorax usually indicates injury to a major systemic or pulmonary artery. If a film showing a

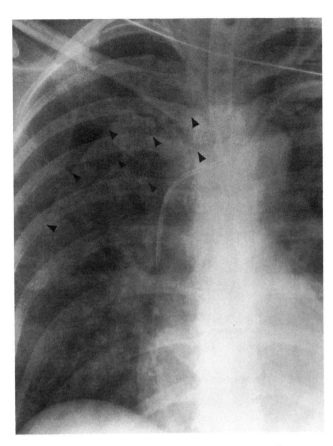

FIGURE 9–19. Skin Folds Mimicking a Pneumothorax

• • • •

A supine chest film demonstrates multiple skin folds. Note that edges bordered laterally by a thin black stripe are present (*arrowheads*). Skin folds often start and stop abruptly, as in this case. The more inferior skin folds also cross the patient's midline, another indication that they are not pneumothoraces.

hemothorax is obtained with the patient in the upright position, the classic meniscus sign with blunting of the lateral costophrenic sulcus can be seen. However, if the film is made with the patient in the supine position, then blood and fluid layer posteriorly, producing only a vague increase in radiodensity located primarily at the base of the lung. No air bronchograms are present, and vascular markings can frequently be seen through the pleural fluid. These observations are in contrast to those of parenchymal disease which obliterates normal vascular markings and often produces air bronchograms. The diaphragm is often silhouetted by the adjacent fluid (Fig. 9–20). Fluid may extend over the apex of the lung to produce an apical pleural cap. Widening of the paraspinous stripe, caused by fluid layering medially, may also be seen in a supine patient. Decubitus radiographs are useful in confirming the presence and the size of pleural fluid collections.

Radiographically a hemothorax cannot be distinguished from pleural fluid of any cause.

Role of Computed Tomography

CT plays a major role in the evaluation of pleural complications of chest trauma because it can detect pleural abnormalities that are not even suspected on chest films. For example, small pneumothoraces are readily apparent on CT scans (Fig. 9–21). Detection of such occult pneumothoraces is especially important in patients receiving ventilation or in those undergoing general anesthesia, since a small pneumothorax may rapidly enlarge to become a tension pneumothorax. CT may demonstrate a large residual pneumothorax unsuspected on chest radiographs in patients who already have a chest tube in place.

CT is used in determining the contribution of parenchymal and pleural disease to an opacity seen on chest radiographs. It can demonstrate a large pleural fluid collection when none is suspected on

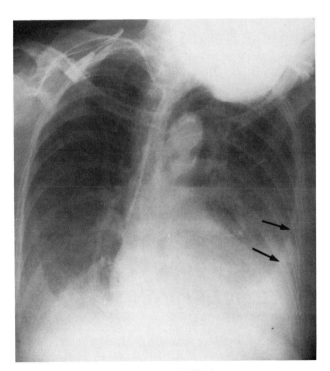

FIGURE 9–20. Bilateral Pleural Effusions

• • • •

An anteroposterior semierect film demonstrates large pleural effusions bilaterally. A haze of increased density extends up both hemithoraces. Note that lung vessels can be seen through the pleural effusion, particularly at the base of the right lung. The left pleural effusion is sufficiently large that a meniscus (*arrows*) is found laterally as well. The diaphragm is silhouetted by the effusions.

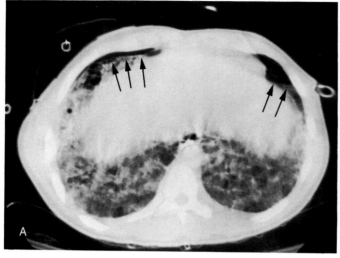

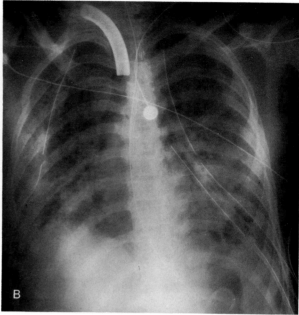

FIGURE 9–21. Computed Tomography Demonstration of Small Pneumothoraces

• • • •

A and B, Computed tomography demonstrates small anterior pneumothoraces bilaterally (*arrows, A*) where none could be seen on chest radiographs. Bilateral chest tubes were already in place in this patient with adult respiratory distress syndrome.

routine radiographs (Fig. 9–22) and detects inadequately drained pleural fluid collections. CT is excellent in detecting malpositioned chest tubes. A single anteroposterior chest film cannot accurately determine the location of a chest tube. CT can demonstrate tubes that have been inadvertently introduced into the substance of the lung or those that lie adjacent to vital mediastinal structures (Fig. 9–23). CT can also provide a guide for accurate placement of chest tubes or drainage catheters into loculated fluid collections (Fig. 9–24). The evaluation of the late complications of thoracic trauma, including the development of lung abscess and empyema, is most appropriately performed by CT (Fig. 9–25).[77]

• • • •

TRACHEOBRONCHIAL INJURIES

Injuries of the tracheobronchial tree are uncommon in closed chest trauma. These injuries are infrequently recognized either clinically or radiographically. Early diagnosis is important in forestalling the late complications of bronchial rupture, especially bronchial stenosis. Complete rupture of a bronchus leads to total atelectasis of the lung or of the lobe involved. If atelectasis is prolonged, marked reduction in lung function occurs, which may not return to baseline even after the injury is surgically cor-

rected. Incomplete rupture of a bronchus often results in a stenotic segment. Infection with resultant bronchiectasis may then occur and often requires a lobectomy for the relief of symptoms.

Penetrating wounds of the trachea usually involve the cervical portion and are most commonly caused by gunshot or stab wounds. Rupture of the cervical trachea is rare in blunt trauma and usually occurs in motor vehicle accidents when the head hits the dashboard; this causes hyperextension of the neck, which tears the trachea (see Chapter 8 for a more complete discussion). Fractures of the thoracic trachea are usually the result of blunt trauma. They usually occur just above the carina. Fractures of the right or the left main stem bronchus constitute 80% of all tracheobronchial injuries. They are usually horizontal and generally occur within 1–2 cm of the carina. Bilateral bronchial injury or injury to lobar bronchi is much less common but can occur. Diagnosis of tracheobronchial injury is difficult and is often delayed. Only about one third of all patients with tracheobronchial rupture are diagnosed in the first 24 hours following injury.[36] Many cases remain undiagnosed for many months or years. Bronchoscopy is used to establish the diagnosis. The preferred method of treatment is primary anastomosis of the ruptured segment.

No single radiographic sign is diagnostic of tracheobronchial rupture. However, several radiographic observations should raise the question of

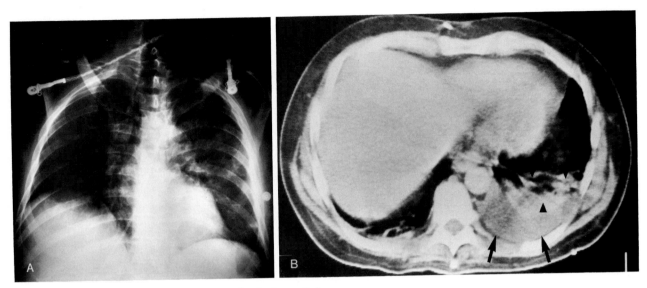

FIGURE 9–22. Use of Computed Tomography in Lung Injury

• • • •

A, An anteroposterior semierect portable radiograph does not demonstrate either parenchymal or pleural disease in this febrile patient who was injured in a boating accident. *B,* A computed tomography scan of the abdomen, performed the same day in order to exclude an abdominal abscess, shows a large left pleural effusion (*arrows*). Left lower lobe consolidation is present as well (*arrowheads*). Note the air bronchograms.

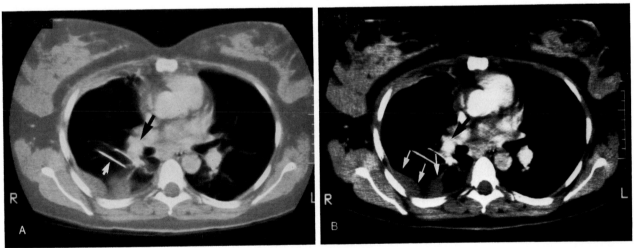

FIGURE 9–23. Computed Tomography Scan of Chest Tube Placement

• • • •

A chest tube has been placed to drain a right pleural effusion in this patient with pneumonia. Because the patient was persistently febrile, a computed tomography (CT) scan was performed. *A,* The chest tube is within the lung parenchyma (*white arrow*), and the tip of the tube abuts the right descending pulmonary artery (*black arrow*). *B,* A small amount of pleural fluid is present posterior to the chest tube (*white arrows*). Because of its position the chest tube was removed. CT clearly demonstrates the precise location of the chest tube in this patient.

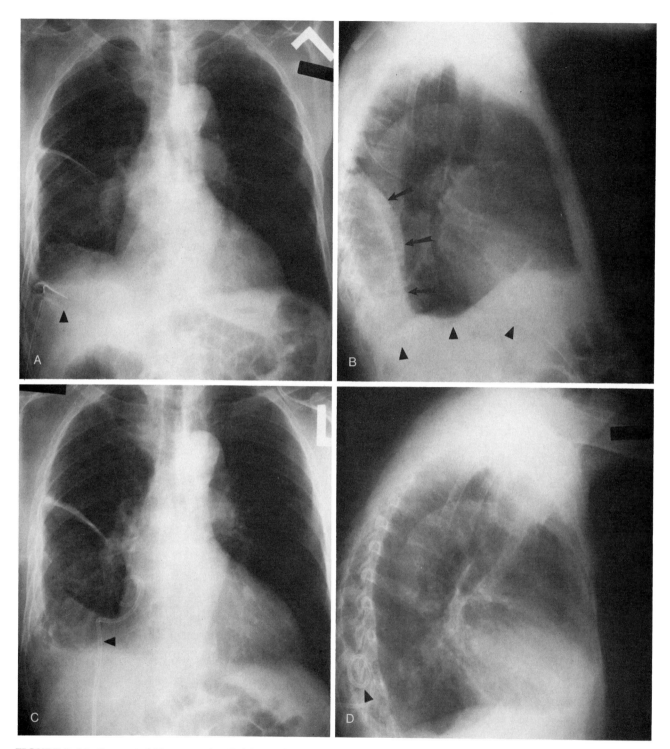

FIGURE 9–24. Computed Tomography Guidance for a Percutaneous Procedure
• • • •

A and *B*, A chest tube was placed surgically to drain this loculated posterior fluid collection (*arrowhead, A*) 5 days after a motor vehicle accident. The tube (*arrowhead, B*) is inferior to the collection (*arrows, B*) which is not being satisfactorily drained. *C* and *D*, A percutaneous drainage catheter (*arrows*) was inserted directly into the collection under computed tomography guidance, achieving complete drainage of the collection.

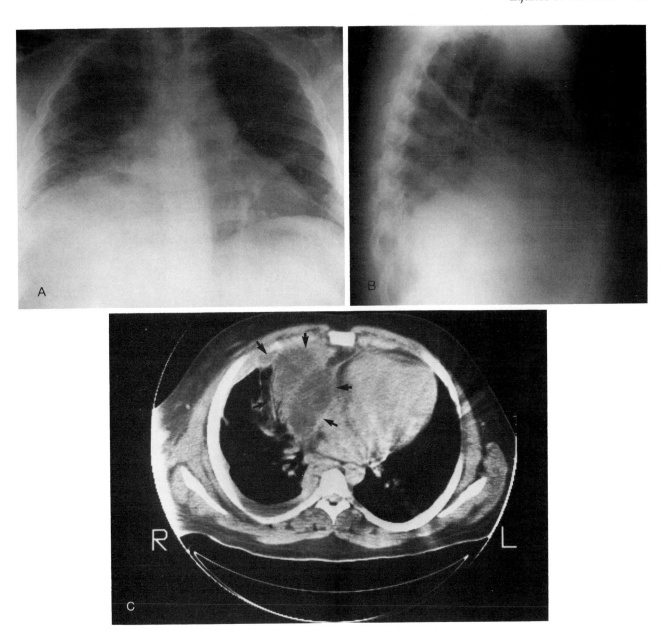

FIGURE 9–25. Empyema

• • • •

This patient had sustained a gunshot wound to the chest and liver 10 days before these films were obtained. *A* and *B*, Posteroanterior and lateral chest films demonstrate elevation of the right hemidiaphragm and an enlarged cardiac silhouette. Because the patient was febrile a computed tomography scan of the lower chest and abdomen was performed. *C*, A large loculated fluid collection is adjacent to the heart (*arrows*). This collection of fluid proved to be an empyema and was surgically drained.

such injury, in a patient who has suffered severe chest trauma. These findings include subcutaneous emphysema; pneumomediastinum, which is seen in over one half of all patients with tracheobronchial tears; pneumothorax, which is also seen in more than one half of these patients; and fractures of the upper thoracic ribs, which occur in about one third of these patients. Clearly these abnormalities are much more commonly associated with other injuries.

However, since early diagnosis of tracheobronchial injuries diminishes the morbidity of the injury, this diagnosis should come to mind when any of these findings are present.

Pneumomediastinum occurs frequently in patients with rupture of the major bronchi. Pneumomediastinum is seen radiographically as thin, linear, vertically oriented streaks of air outlining mediastinal structures. The most common location for mediastinal air in adults is along the left border of the heart. Air may outline the aortic knob, the great vessels, the aortic pulmonic window, and the descending aorta. One unusual sign of pneumomediastinum is the continuous diaphragm sign produced by air outlining the central portion of the diaphragm, which is usually silhouetted by the heart (Fig. 9–26).

Air may extend from the mediastinum into the peritoneal cavity or the retroperitoneum. Air can also dissect along the fascial planes into the neck. Most commonly, such deep cervical emphysema is seen just anterior to the prevertebral fascia and appears as a linear stripe of air just anterior to the cervical spine where its presence in the neck is easier to detect. If pneumomediastinum is suspected on a chest film, a lateral view of the cervical spine may produce convincing, confirmatory proof (Fig. 9–27).

Unfortunately, pneumomediastinum is frequently present in the absence of tracheobronchial injury. The most common cause of pneumomediastinum in the setting of blunt chest trauma is pulmonary interstitial emphysema. A rapid increase in intrathoracic pressure causes the rupture of alveoli. Air escapes

from the alveoli, enters the interstitial network of the lung, and dissects along small vessels in the interstitium to enter the mediastinum. Pneumomediastinum produced in this fashion is a benign and self-limiting process.

Rupture of the esophagus is another, albeit rare, cause of pneumomediastinum. In this instance, pneumomediastinum is often accompanied by basal pleural and parenchymal disease. Traumatic rupture of the esophagus is more thoroughly discussed in Chapter 10.

Pneumothorax was present in just over one half of the patients with tracheobronchial injury reported by Hood and Sloan.[42] A persistent pneumothorax that is unresponsive to chest tube drainage should raise concern for the possibility of tracheobronchial injury (Figs. 9–28 and 9–29). Some patients with tracheobronchial rupture develop a pneumothorax that is initially responsive to chest tube drainage. However, almost all of these patients develop atelectasis within 2–3 weeks as the result of bronchial stenosis. Therefore, delayed radiographs often detect those cases of tracheobronchial rupture that were not recognized initially.

Fractures involving the upper three thoracic ribs have been considered by some to be a reliable sign of tracheobronchial injury. In one series, upper rib fractures occurred in one third of all patients with tracheobronchial injury.[42] However upper rib fractures occur much more often in the absence of any airway injury. Fracture of an upper thoracic rib is an indication that severe trauma has occurred and should alert the clinician and the radiologist that significant intrathoracic and abdominal injuries, including tracheobronchial rupture, may be present.

• • • •

DIAPHRAGM

Traumatic rupture of the diaphragm occurs in both blunt and penetrating trauma. Herniation of some of the abdominal contents into the chest usually results. Diaphragmatic lacerations occur somewhat more commonly on the left side because the liver provides some protection against rupture of the right hemidiaphragm. When laceration occurs on the left side, the most common organs to herniate are the stomach, colon, small bowel, spleen, and omentum. If the laceration occurs on the right side, the liver and the colon are the organs most frequently involved.

Diaphragmatic lacerations tend to be larger in blunt trauma and average 10 cm in diameter in one series. Tears due to penetrating trauma tend to be much smaller, being 2 cm or less in length in 85% of

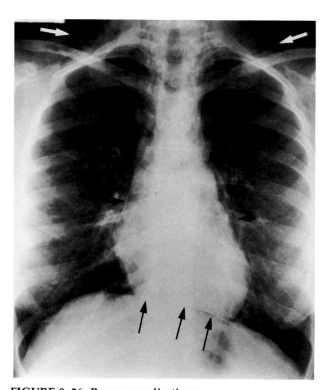

FIGURE 9–26. Pneumomediastinum

• • • •

A pneumomediastinum is seen outlining the right and the left borders of the heart and the upper mediastinum (*small arrows*); it extends into the subcutaneous tissues of the neck (*white arrows*). The central portion of the diaphragm is also outlined by air, producing a continuous diaphragm sign (*large arrows*).

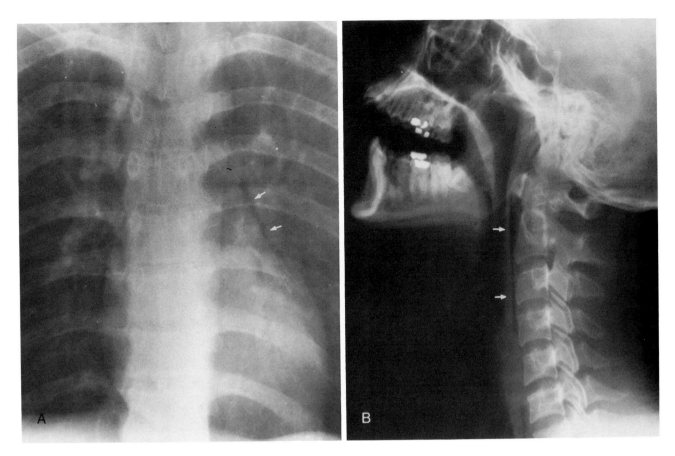

FIGURE 9–27. Pneumomediastinum

• • • •

A, Pneumomediastinum was suspected because of the air outlining the left lower lobe bronchus on the chest radiograph (*arrows*). *B,* Its presence is confirmed by air that can be seen extending from the chest into the neck just anterior to the spine (*arrows*).

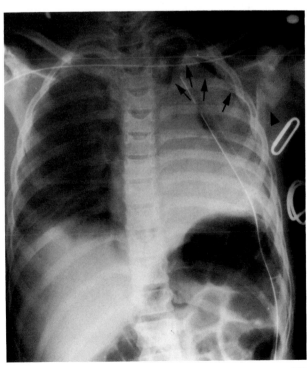

FIGURE 9–28. Laceration of the Left Main Stem Bronchus

• • • •

A portable chest film was obtained several days after insertion of a left chest tube. The persistent pneumothorax (*arrows*) and atelectasis of the left lung were due to a laceration of the left main stem bronchus. Note also the left scapular fracture (*arrowhead*).

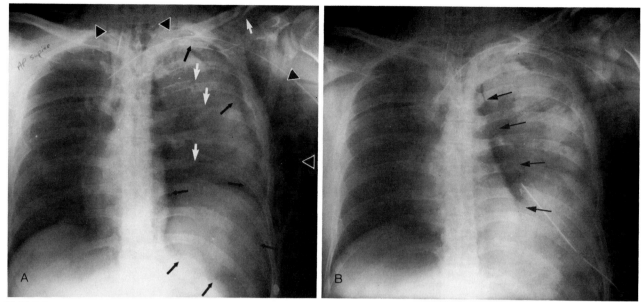

FIGURE 9–29. Laceration of the Left Main Stem Bronchus

• • • •

A, A supine radiograph obtained in a patient involved in a motor vehicle accident demonstrates a very large left subpulmonic pneumothorax with a shift of the cardiomediastinal silhouette to the right (*black arrows*). There is extensive subcutaneous emphysema (*arrowheads*). Note the multiple fractures of the left posterior ribs (*white arrows*) and the left clavicle. *B,* The persistent anteromedial pneumothorax (*arrows*) following chest tube placement was the result of a laceration of the left main stem bronchus. The elevated base of the left lung present on both films was produced by laceration of the left hemidiaphragm.

patients. Strangulation of herniated bowel is more common following penetrating injuries because of the small tear that entraps the herniated bowel.

Associated injuries are present in the majority of patients, reflecting the severity of trauma required to produce diaphragmatic rupture. In patients with blunt trauma, fractured ribs and a ruptured spleen are most commonly reported in association with diaphragmatic rupture. Other injuries include liver lacerations, injury to the bowel, and genitourinary tract injuries. Pelvic fractures are relatively common, as are intracranial injuries. In the setting of penetrating trauma, injuries to the liver or stomach are frequently reported. Death is usually related to the associated injuries rather than to the diaphragmatic injury directly. In the acute phase, injury to other organs is often so severe that the injury to the diaphragm remains undetected. The diagnosis of traumatic rupture of the diaphragm in the acute setting is most likely to be made if the index of suspicion is high. Despite this, fully 50% of traumatic diaphragmatic injuries are diagnosed at the time of laparotomy performed for other injuries. Frequently, the actual herniation of abdominal contents is delayed, which also leads to a delay in diagnosis. Serial films may prove very useful in detecting a diaphragmatic hernia (Fig. 9–30).

If the diagnosis is not made initially, the patient may enter a latent phase lasting several months to many years.[87] Traumatic diaphragmatic hernias are often diagnosed during this period on chest films that were obtained for other reasons. Strangulation of herniated bowel, which may occur many years after the initial injury, is a major concern in unrecognized cases. The presence of a pleural effusion in patients with a chronic diaphragmatic hernia signals strangulation or obstruction.

The chest radiograph is the most valuable tool in the preoperative diagnosis of traumatic diaphragmatic laceration. The radiographic appearance is dependent on the size of the diaphragmatic defect and on the contents of the hernia. Any elevation of the diaphragm in the setting of trauma should raise the possibility that a diaphragmatic laceration exists. If air-filled colon or stomach herniates into the chest, then unusual gas collections are seen at the base of the left lung (Fig. 9–31). The wall of the herniated colon or stomach may simulate the diaphragm itself, causing a misdiagnosis of eventration or elevation of the diaphragm (Fig. 9–32). The pseudodiaphragm produced by the herniated bowel may have a lop-sided appearance, with the dome of the psuedodiaphragm displaced laterally. With elevation of the true diaphragm, the dome maintains its central position within the hemithorax.

If a nasogastric tube is in place, its course may be diagnostic of a diaphragmatic laceration.[96] Because diaphragmatic lacerations usually occur centrally, the

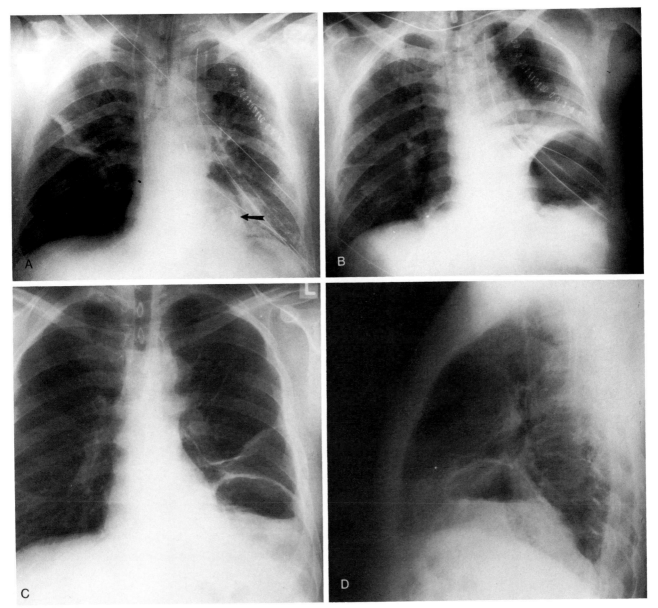

FIGURE 9–30. Diaphragmatic Rupture

• • • •

A, A postoperative radiograph was obtained in this patient who had undergone repair of an aortic laceration following a deceleration injury. The tip of the nasogastric tube (*arrow*) is faintly visible above the level of the left hemidiaphragm. *B,* Following extubation and the removal of the nasogastric tube, a large air collection was seen at the base of the left lung. A diaphragmatic rupture was suggested, but the diaphragm was palpated at the time of the aortic repair and was said to be normal. *C* and *D,* The patient was discharged, and follow-up films again demonstrate what appears to be the stomach in the left hemithorax.

Illustration continued on following page

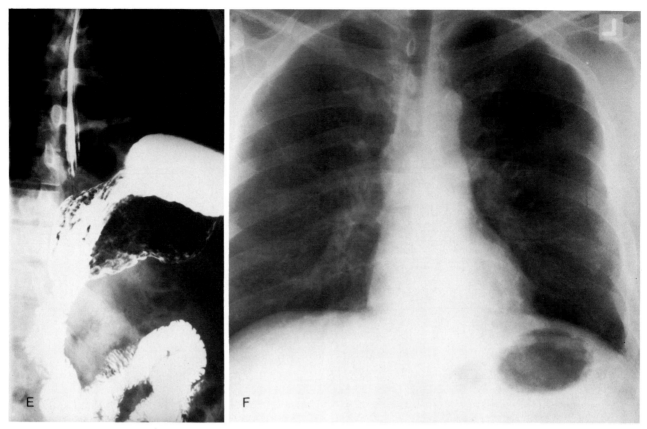

FIGURE 9–30 *Continued* **Diaphragmatic Rupture**

• • • •

E, An upper gastrointestinal study does not demonstrate any constriction of the stomach, though much of the stomach clearly is in the thorax. The diaphragmatic defect was found to be very large at the time of diaphragmatic repair. *F,* A posteroanterior film obtained following the repair of the diaphragmatic laceration shows the stomach in its normal position beneath the left hemidiaphragm.

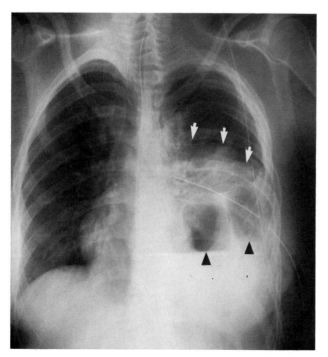

FIGURE 9–31. Diaphragmatic Rupture

• • • •

An anteroposterior semierect film obtained after a car crash demonstrates two unusual air collections at the base of the left lung (*arrowheads*) with a shift of the cardiomediastinal silhouette to the right. A left chest tube has been introduced for the large left pneumothorax (*arrows*). A presumptive diagnosis of a diaphragmatic laceration was made. At laparotomy a large tear in the left hemidiaphragm was found combined with herniation of the stomach and the colon into the chest.

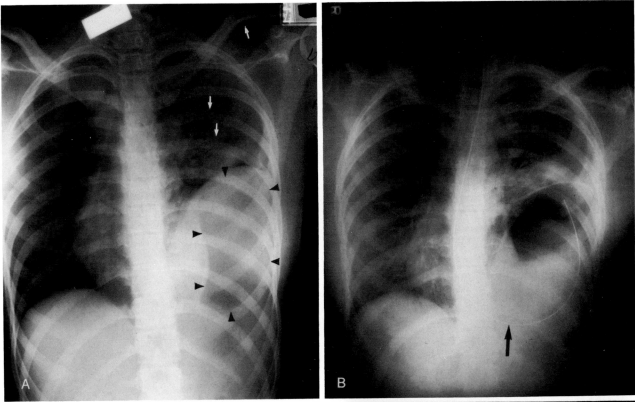

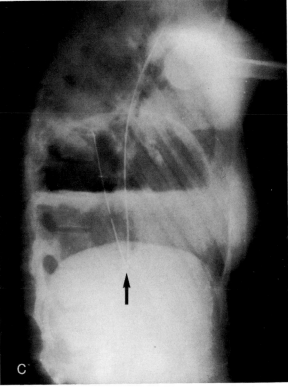

FIGURE 9–32. Diaphragmatic Rupture

• • • •

A, An initial anteroposterior supine radiograph obtained following a motor vehicle accident shows a high position of the left hemidiaphragm with lateral displacement of the "dome." The large air collection at the left base was thought to be the stomach (*arrowheads*). The cardiomediastinal silhouette is shifted to the right. Note the fractures of the left fifth and sixth posterior ribs and the fracture of the left clavicle (*white arrows*). *B* and *C*, Posteroanterior and lateral films obtained following nasogastric tube placement demonstrate the normal position of the gastroesophageal junction beneath the left hemidiaphragm (*arrow*). Entry of the nasogastric tube into the intrathoracic stomach confirms the presence of a diaphragmatic laceration.

gastroesophageal junction remains in the abdomen, whereas the fundus and the body of the stomach herniate through the diaphragmatic rent. Therefore, a nasogastric tube enters the abdomen only to turn cephalad into the chest (Fig. 9–33; see also Fig. 9–32). Indeed, if a nasogastric tube is not already in place, its insertion may be diagnostic. Failure of the nasogastric tube to pass into the fundus or the body of the stomach may also be diagnostic because the stomach may be strangulated or twisted in the diaphragmatic defect (Fig. 9–34).

If a solid organ or fluid-filled bowel herniates into the chest, a mass at the base of the lung is simulated. If the defect in the diaphragm is large and a large hernia is present, shift of the cardiomediastinal silhouette occurs. Atelectasis is frequently present at the base of the lung.

Barium studies may be needed to make the diagnosis. Barium-based contrast material should be administered orally if the stomach is thought to be the herniated organ and rectally if colon herniation is suspected. Constriction of the afferent and the efferent loops of the bowel as they pass through the diaphragmatic rent is usually seen (Fig. 9–35). Barium studies are especially useful in differentiating eventration of the diaphragm from a diaphragmatic laceration. In eventration of the diaphragm, no constriction or waist is seen, and the afferent and the efferent loops retain their normal separation. If the

herniated bowel is completely compressed, then barium-based contrast material can fail to enter the afferent loop of the bowel or exit from the efferent loop (Fig. 9–36). Other procedures, including diagnostic pneumoperitoneum, ultrasound scanning, CT, angiography, and magnetic resonance imaging have been described, but their usefulness in diagnosing diaphragmatic laceration in the acute setting is limited.

Lacerations of the right hemidiaphragm are said to occur less frequently than those of the left hemidiaphragm owing to the protective effect of the liver. However, the difficulty in diagnosis of right-sided injuries is now thought to be responsible for the lower reported incidence.[88] The liver itself, which herniates most commonly in right-sided lacerations, seals the diaphragmatic defect, thereby preventing the herniation of other gas-containing organs, which would increase the likelihood of diagnosis. Instead, the most common radiographic sign of right-sided diaphragmatic rupture is "elevation of the right hemidiaphragm." The presence of a smoothly marginated, mushroom-like mass at the right base of the lung should suggest the diagnosis. The lateral radiograph may be particularly impressive (Fig. 9–37). If herniation of the liver is suspected, the diagnosis can be established by a radionuclide liver-spleen scan. The scan confirms the intrathoracic location of the liver. Often a waist-like constriction around the liver is seen as the liver is pinched in the diaphragmatic rent (Fig. 9–38). If the colon or the small bowel herniates into the chest, unusual gas collections are seen at the right base of the lung that are similar to those seen in left-sided lacerations (see Fig. 9–35).

• • • •

CHEST WALL INJURIES

Rib Fractures

Rib fractures are more common in adults than in children and frequently involve the fourth through the ninth ribs. Multiple rib fractures are more common than solitary ones. Diagnosis of the complications of rib fractures is much more important than the recognition of the fractures themselves. Indeed, nondisplaced rib fractures are often difficult to identify radiographically (see Fig. 9–11). Fractured ribs may cause pulmonary contusion, pulmonary laceration, pneumothorax, or hemothorax, although these same injuries frequently occur in the absence of rib fractures.

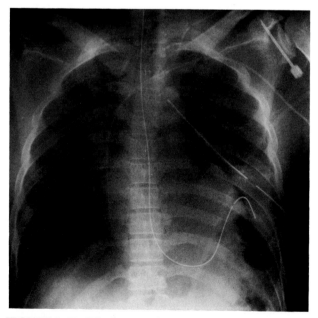

FIGURE 9–33. Diaphragmatic Rupture

• • • •

A portable radiograph obtained after a motorcycle accident demonstrates a high position of the nasogastric tube tip. A diagnosis of rupture of the left hemidiaphragm was made and confirmed at laparotomy.

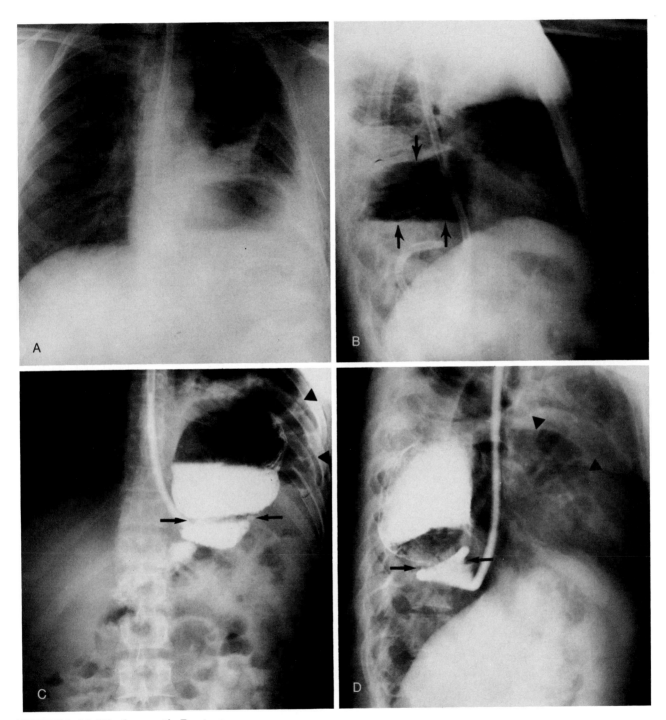

FIGURE 9–34. Diaphragmatic Rupture
• • • •
A and *B*, Posteroanterior (PA) and lateral films were obtained following an automobile accident. A large air collection at the left base posteriorly (*arrows, B*) suggested a diaphragmatic tear combined with herniation of the stomach into the chest, although the nasogastric tube does not enter the fundus of the stomach as might be anticipated. *C* and *D*, PA and lateral films following the introduction of barium through the nasogastric tube demonstrate barium within the intrathoracic stomach. The constricting waist about the stomach (*arrows*) may have prevented the nasogastric tube from entering the fundus of the stomach. Air is also seen in the herniated colon (*arrowheads*).

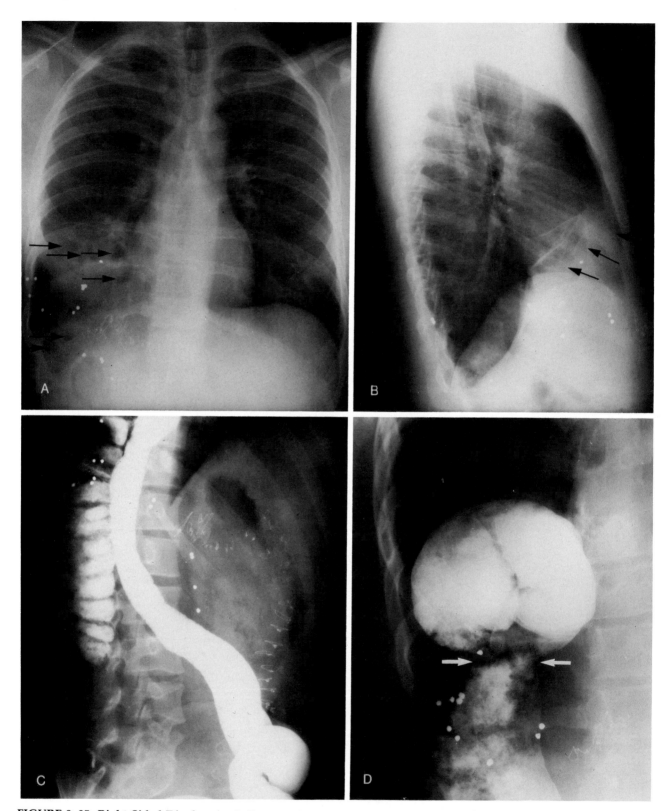

FIGURE 9–35. Right-Sided Diaphragmatic Rupture Combined with Herniated Colon

• • • •

A and *B*, Posteroanterior and lateral chest films of a patient experiencing nausea and vomiting 15 years after a gunshot wound to the abdomen demonstrate multiple air collections (*arrows*) at the base of the right lung. At the time of the initial injury a right hepatic lobectomy was performed. *C*, A barium enema demonstrates herniation of the colon into the chest through a tear in the right hemidiaphragm that had not been repaired at the earlier operation. *D*, Note the constriction on the barium-filled loops as they pass through the diaphragmatic defect (*arrows*).

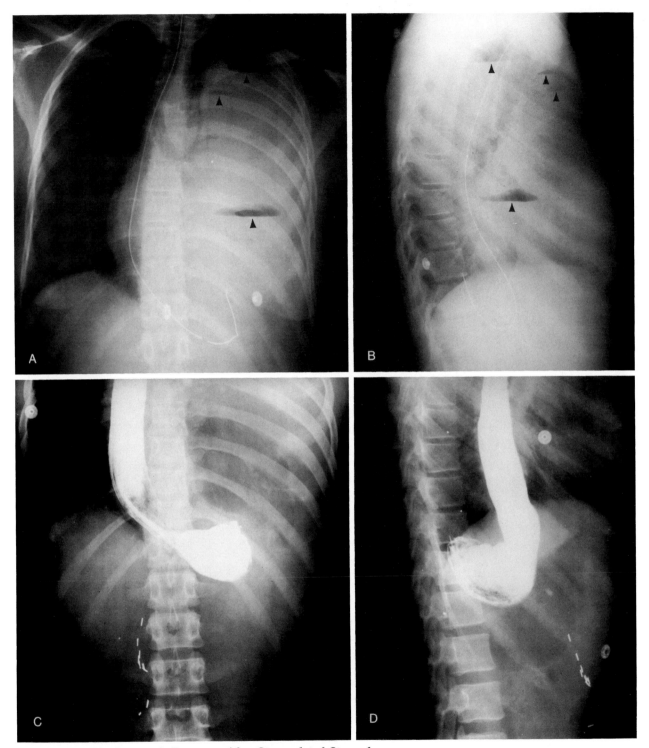

FIGURE 9–36. Diaphragmatic Rupture with a Strangulated Stomach

• • • •

A and *B*, Posteroanterior and lateral chest films were obtained of this patient who was experiencing pain and fever 5 months following a stab wound to the left hemithorax. The left hemithorax is opaque and contains multiple air-fluid levels (*arrowheads*). The cardiomediastinal silhouette and the bronchi are displaced to the right. *C* and *D*, Barium given orally fails to pass into the fundus of the stomach.

Illustration continued on following page

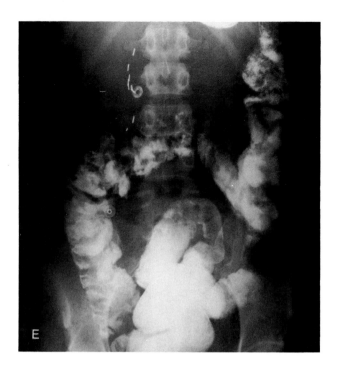

FIGURE 9–36 *Continued* **Diaphragmatic Rupture with a Strangulated Stomach**

• • • •

E, A barium enema demonstrates a normal position of the colon. At surgery, the stomach was intrathoracic and was necrotic secondary to strangulation within a small diaphragmatic defect.

Fractures of the 11th and 12th ribs should raise suspicion for an upper abdominal injury, most notably of the liver, the spleen, or the kidneys. Fractures of the first three ribs have received a considerable amount of attention in the literature because of a suspected association with aortic and bronchial injuries. Fractures of any of the first three ribs is certainly an indication that significant trauma has occurred. However, the presence of an upper rib fracture has a low predictive value for either tracheobronchial or aortic injury. Indeed, the presence of an upper rib fracture alone, in the absence of other clinical or other radiographic signs to suggest aortic injury, is not an indication to perform angiography.

Flail chest occurs when there are either multiple fractures of several ribs, separation of the costochondral cartilages from the sternum, or both. This causes instability of the chest wall with resultant paradoxical respiratory movement. Flail chest is almost always apparent clinically.

Thoracic Spine Fracture or Dislocation

Fractures of the thoracic vertebrae are significant injuries that may remain unrecognized clinically in the presence of severe thoracic injury. On a well-penetrated film on which the spine can be evaluated a fracture or dislocation can be identified. Loss of height of a thoracic vertebral body or a step-off in the normal alignment of the spinous processes indi-

cates a possible fracture or dislocation. However, the thoracic spine is often not well seen on underpenetrated portable radiographs. In such cases, spinal fractures may produce secondary radiographic signs that herald the diagnosis.[107] Spinal fractures often cause mediastinal hemorrhage and widening of the mediastinum identical to that seen with aortic rupture (Fig. 9–39). Other signs of aortic rupture, including widening of the paraspinous stripe, an apical pleural cap, and deviation of the nasogastric tube to the right at the level of T4, may also be produced by fractures of the thoracic spine (Fig. 9–40). If any of these signs are present, both aortic and nonaortic etiologies must be considered. The thoracic and the lower cervical spine should be carefully examined in all patients who have sustained severe thoracic injury. Additionally, well-penetrated, well-collimated views of the thoracic spine may be warranted if any of these findings are present, particularly if an aortogram shows no evidence of aortic injury. Tomography or CT may be necessary in some patients. The thoracic spine is more thoroughly discussed in Chapter 7.

Sternal Fractures

Sternal fractures are usually the result of impact against the steering wheel in motor vehicle accidents. They are difficult to diagnose radiographically even with well-penetrated posteroanterior and lateral

Text continued on page 351

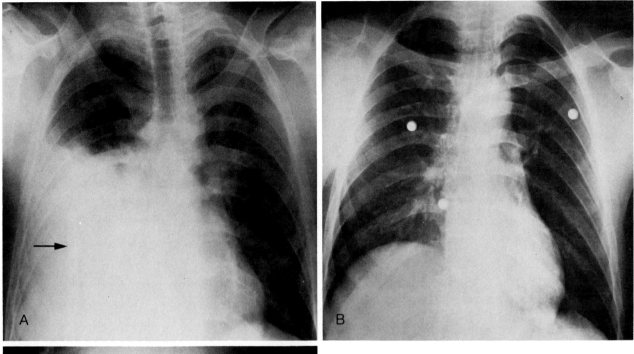

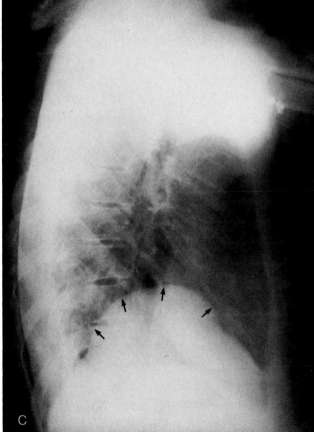

FIGURE 9–37. Right-Sided Diaphragmatic Rupture

• • • •

A, An initial supine radiograph of a patient obtained following an automobile accident. A chest tube (*arrow*) has already been inserted to drain the right hemothorax. *B* and *C*, Delayed radiographs demonstrate the elevation of the right hemidiaphragm on the posteroanterior radiograph. The mushroom-like mass (*arrows, C*) seen on the lateral film is characteristic of liver herniated through an unrecognized diaphragmatic rupture.

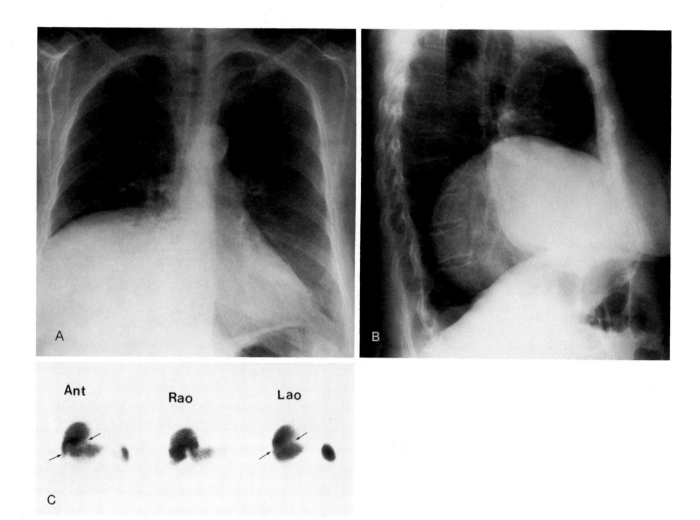

FIGURE 9–38. Right-side Diaphragmatic Rupture

• • • •

A and *B*, Posteroanterior and lateral chest films of a housewife obtained 2 years after a car wreck demonstrate a large mushroom-like mass at the right base. *C*, A nuclear medicine scan of the liver and the spleen confirms the intrathoracic location of the liver. The band of photopenia is produced by the constriction of the liver as it passes through the diaphragmatic defect (*arrows*). (Anterior: Ant; right anterior oblique: Rao; left anterior oblique: Lao)

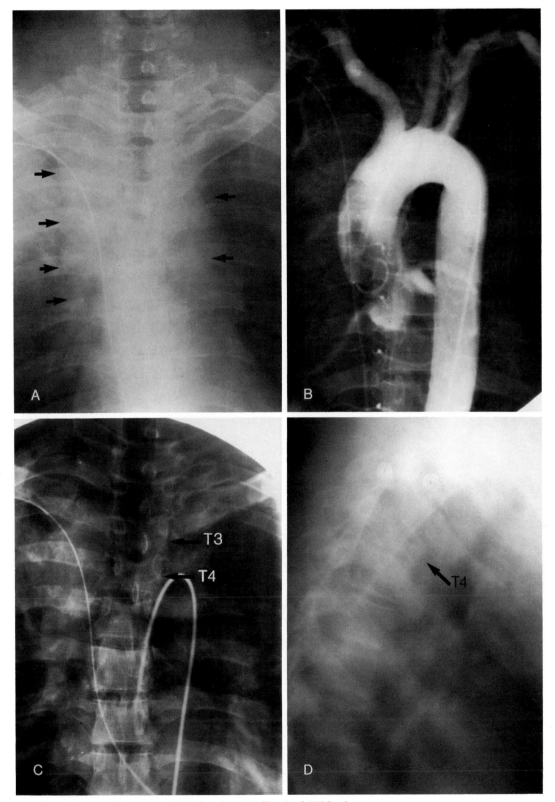

FIGURE 9–39. Compression Fracture of T4 Causing Mediastinal Widening

• • • •

A, A widened mediastinum (*arrows*) is visible on an upright posteroanterior (PA) radiograph taken of a patient following a deceleration injury. *B,* A thoracic aortogram showed no evidence of an aortic injury. *C,* On the scout film for the aortogram, a compression fracture of the T4 vertebral body is present. Note the step-off in alignment of the spinous processes of T3 and T4 (*arrows*). This can be seen in retrospect on the PA chest film and should have raised the suspicion of a fracture-dislocation. *D,* The fractured T4 vertebral body is visible on an underpenetrated lateral view of the thoracic spine (*arrow*).

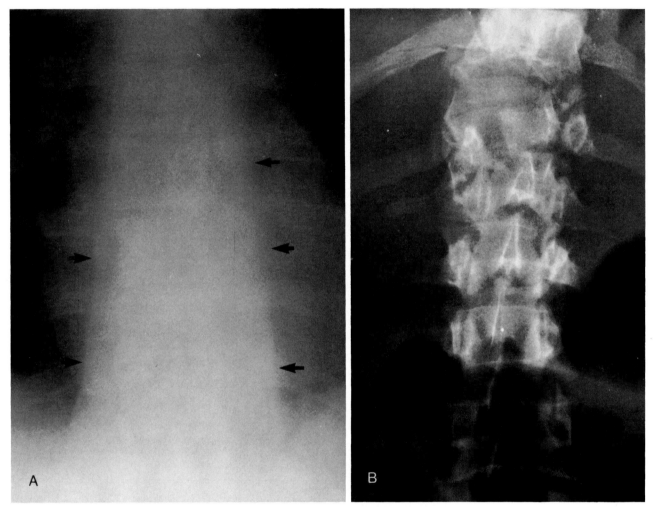

FIGURE 9–40. Thoracolumbar Fracture-Dislocation Causing Mediastinal Widening
• • • •
A, An anteroposterior portable film demonstrates widening of both the right and the left paraspinous stripes (*arrows*) following an automobile accident. Thoracic and abdominal aortograms were performed and showed normal status. *B*, A severe fracture dislocation of the thoracolumbar junction was noted on a follow-up film of the kidney, ureter, and bladder.

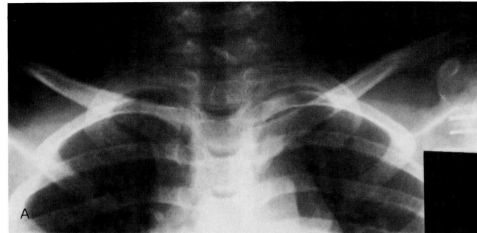

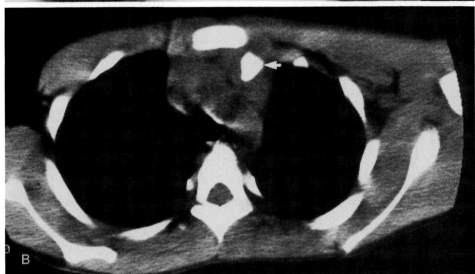

FIGURE 9–41. Clavicular Dislocation

• • • •

A, The medial ends of the clavicles are at different levels in this 9-year-old boy hit by a car while riding his bicycle. *B,* A computed tomography scan confirms a posterior dislocation of the left clavicle (*arrow*).

films. The presence of a convex soft tissue mass adjacent to the sternum, caused by a hematoma, is often the best clue to the presence of sternal fracture. Sternal fractures are important because of their association with injuries to the heart, including myocardial contusion, cardiac rupture, and pericardial tamponade. CT can detect sternal fractures and is also the method of choice for the evaluation of sternoclavicular dislocations. Anterior dislocations of the clavicle are more common than posterior ones. Injury to the aorta and the great vessels may occur with posterior dislocations (Fig. 9–41).

References

General

1. Crawford WO Jr. Pulmonary injury in thoracic and nonthoracic trauma. Radiol Clin North Am 1973; 11:527–542.
2. Goodman LR, Putman CE. The SICU radiograph after massive blunt trauma. Radiol Clin North Am 1981; 19:111–123.
3. Greene R. Lung alterations in thoracic trauma. J Thorac Imaging 1987; 2:1–11.
4. Paredes S, Hipona FA. The radiologic evaluation of patients with chest trauma: Respiratory system. Med Clin North Am 1975; 59:37–63.
5. Reynolds J, Davis JT. Injuries of the chest wall, pleura, pericardium, lungs, bronchi, and esophagus. Radiol Clin North Am 1960; 3:383–401.
6. Tocino I, Armstrong JD. Trauma to the lung. *In* Radiology Diagnosis-Imaging-Intervention. Vol 3. Grand Rapids: J.B. Lippincott Co., 1989, pp 1–15.
7. Williams JR, Bonte FJ. Roentgenological Aspects of Nonpenetrating Chest Injuries. Springfield, IL: Charles C Thomas, Publisher, 1961, pp 1–110.

Pulmonary Contusion, Laceration, and Hematoma

8. Berkmen YM, Yankelenitz D, Davis SD, Zanzonica P. Torsion of the upper lobe in pneumothorax. Radiology 1989; 173:447–449.
9. Bhalla M, Leitman BS, Forcade C. Lung hernia: Radiographic features. AJR 1990; 154:51–53.
10. DeMuth WE, Smith JM. Pulmonary contusion. Am J Surg 1965; 109:819–823.
11. Fagan CJ, Swischuk LE. Traumatic lung and paramediastinal pneumatoceles. Radiology 1976; 120:11–18.

12. Fagan CJ. Traumatic lung cyst. AJR 1966; 97:186–194.
13. Felson B. Lung torsion: radiographic findings in nine cases. Radiology 1987; 162:631–638.
14. Ganske JG, Dennis DL, Vanderveer JB. Traumatic lung cyst: Case report and literature review. J Trauma 1981; 21:493–496.
15. Godwin JD, Webb WR, Savoca CJ, et al. Multiple thin-walled cystic lesions of the lung. AJR 1980; 135:593–604.
16. Greening R, Kynette A, Hodes P. Unusual pulmonary changes secondary to chest trauma. AJR 1959; 77:1059–1065.
17. Hanskins JR, McAslan JC, Shin B, et al. Extensive pulmonary laceration caused by blunt trauma. J Thorac Cardiovasc Surg 1977; 74:519–527.
18. Joynt GHC, Jaffe F. Solitary pulmonary hematoma. J Thorac Cardiovasc Surg 1962; 43:291–302.
19. Milne E, Dick A. Circumscribed intrapulmonary haematoma. Br J Radiol 1961; 34:587–595.
20. Moghissi K. Laceration of the lung following blunt trauma. Thorax 1971; 26:223–228.
21. Moser ES, Proto AV. Lung torsion: Case report and literature review. Radiology 1987; 162:639–643.
22. Santos GH, Mahendra T. Traumatic pulmonary pseudocysts. Ann Thorac Surg 1979; 27:359–362.
23. Sealy WC. Contusions of the lung from nonpenetrating injuries of the thorax. Arch Surg 1949; 59:882–887.
24. Sohrsdal OA, Powell JW. Cavitary pulmonary lesions following nonpenetrating chest trauma in children. AJR 1965; 95:118–124.
25. Spees EK, Strevey TE, Geiger JP, et al. Persistent traumatic lung cavities resulting from medium- and high-velocity missiles. Ann Thorac Surg 1967; 4:133–142.
26. Stevens E, Templeton AW. Traumatic nonpenetrating lung contusion. Radiology 1965; 85:247–252.
27. Taylor DA, Jacobson HG. Post-traumatic herniation of the lung. AJR 1962; 87:896–899.
28. Ting YM. Pulmonary parenchymal findings in blunt trauma to the chest. AJR 1966; 98:343–349.
29. Tomlovovich MC. Pulmonary parenchymal injuries. Emerg Med Clin North Am 1983; 1:379–392.
30. Wagner RB, Crawford WO, Schimpf PP. Classification of parenchymal injuries of the lung. Radiology 1988; 167:77–82.
31. Williams JR. The vanishing lung tumor: Pulmonary hematoma. AJR 1959; 81:296–301.
32. Williams JR, Bonte FJ. Pulmonary changes in nonpenetrating thoracic trauma. Texas State Med J 1963; 59:27–30.
33. Williams JR, Bonte FJ. Pulmonary damage in nonpenetrating chest injuries. Radiol Clin North Am 1963; 1:439–448.
34. Williams JR, Bonte FJ. Pulmonary hematomas secondary to nonpenetrating injury. South Med J 1962; 55:622–625.
35. Williams JR, Stembridge VA. Pulmonary contusion secondary to nonpenetrating chest trauma. AJR 1964; 91:284–290.

Tracheobronchial Fractures

36. Burke JF. Early diagnosis of traumatic rupture of the bronchus. JAMA 1962; 181:682–686.
37. Deslauriers J, Beaulieu M, Archambault G, et al. Diagnosis and long-term follow-up of major bronchial disruptions due to nonpenetrating trauma. Ann Thorac Surg 1982; 33:32–39.
38. Eastridge CE, Hughes FA, Pate JW, et al. Tracheobronchial injury caused by blunt trauma. Am Rev Respir Dis 1970; 101:230–237.
39. Ecker RR, Libertini RV, Rea WJ, et al. Injuries of the trachea and bronchi. Ann Thorac Surg 1971; 11:289–298.
40. Eijgelaar A, Van Der Heide H. A reliable early symptom of bronchial or tracheal rupture. Thorax 1970; 25:116–125.
41. Harvey-Smith W, Bush W, Northrop C. Traumatic bronchial rupture. AJR 1980; 134:1189–1193.
42. Hood RM, Sloan HE. Injuries of the trachea and major bronchi. J Thorac Cardiovasc Surg 1959; 38:458–475.
43. Jones WS, Mavroudis C, Richardson JD, et al. Management of tracheobronchial disruption resulting from blunt trauma. Surgery 1984; 95:319–323.
44. Kirsh MM, Orringer MB, Behrendt DM, Sloan H. Management of tracheobronchial disruption secondary to nonpenetrating trauma. Ann Thorac Surg 1976; 22:93–100.
45. Ramzy AI, Rodriguez A, Turney SZ. Management of major tracheobronchial ruptures in patients with multiple system trauma. J Trauma 1988; 28:1353–1357.
46. Reynolds J, Christensen EE. Early radiologic signs of bronchial rupture. Tex Med 1968; 64:50–60.
47. Rollins RJ, Tocino I. Early radiographic signs of tracheal rupture. AJR 1987; 148:695–698.
48. Silbiger ML, Kushner TN. Tracheobronchial perforation: Its diagnosis and treatment. Radiology 1965; 85:242–246.
49. Wiot JF. Tracheobronchial trauma. Semin Roentgenol 1983; 18:15–22.
50. Unger JM, Schuchmann GG, Grossman JE, Pellett JR. Tears of the trachea and main bronchi caused by blunt trauma: Radiologic findings. AJR 1989; 153:1175–1180.

Pneumomediastinum

51. Cyrlak D, Milne E. Pneumomediastinum: A diagnostic problem. Crit Rev Diagn Imaging 23:75–116.
52. Kleinman PK, Brill PW, Whalen JP. Anterior pathway for transdiaphragmatic extension of pneumomediastinum. AJR 1978; 131:271–275.
53. Levin B. The continuous diaphragm sign: A newly recognized sign of pneumomediastinum. Clin Radiol 1973; 24:337–338.
54. Lillard RL, Allen RP. The extrapleural air sign in pneumomediastinum. Radiology 1965; 85:1093–1097.
55. Lotz AR, Martel W, Rohwedder JJ, et al. Significance of pneumomediastinum in blunt trauma to the thorax. AJR 1979; 132:817–819.
56. Maunder RJ, Pierson DJ, Hudson LD. Subcutaneous and mediastinal emphysema: Pathophysiology, diagnosis and management. Arch Intern Med 1984; 144:1447–1453.
57. Munsell WP. Pneumomediastinum: A report of 28 cases and review of the literature. JAMA 1967; 202:129–133.
58. Naclerico EA. The "V sign" in the diagnosis of spontaneous rupture of the esophagus (an early roentgen clue). Am J Surg 1957; 93:291–298.
59. Rogers LF, Puig W, Dooley BN, et al. Diagnostic considerations in mediastinal emphysema: A pathophysiologic-roentgenologic approach to Boerhaave's syndrome and spontaneous pneumomediastinum. AJR 1972; 115:495–511.

Pleura

60. Casola G, van Sonnenberg E, Keightley A. Pneumothorax: Radiologic treatment with small catheters. Radiology 1988; 166:89–91.
61. Christensen EE, Dietz GW. Subpulmonic pneumothorax in patients with chronic obstructive pulmonary disease. Radiology 1976; 121:33–37.
62. Fleischchner FG. Atypical arrangement of free pleural effusion. Radiol Clin North Am 1963; 1:347–362.
63. Friedman PJ. Adult pulmonary ligament pneumatocele: A loculated pneumothorax. Radiology 1985; 155:575–576.
64. Gordon R. The deep sulcus sign. Radiology 1980; 136:25–27.
65. Heilman RA, Collins VP. Identification of laceration of the thoracic duct by lymphoangiography. AJR 1963; 81:470–472.
66. Hyde I. Traumatic paramediastinal air cysts. Br J Radiol 1971; 44:380–383.
67. Lams PM, Jolles H. The effect of lobar collapse on the distribution of free intrapleural air. Radiology 1982; 142:309–312.
68. Lowman RM, Hoogerhyde J, Waters LL, et al. Traumatic chylothorax: The roentgen aspects of the problem. AJR 1951; 65:529–545.
69. Petersen JA. Recognition of infrapulmonary pleural effusion. AJR 1960; 74:31–41.
70. Raasch B, Carsky EW, Lane EJ, et al. Pleural effusions: Explanation of some typical appearances. AJR 1982; 139:899–904.

71. Rabinowitz JG, Wolf BS. Roentgen significance of the pulmonary ligament. Radiology 1966; 87:1013–1020.
72. Ravin CE, Smith GW, Lester PD, et al. Post-traumatic pneumatocele in the inferior pulmonary ligament. Radiology 1976; 121:39–41.
73. Rhea JT, van Sonnenberg E, McLoud TC. Basilar pneumothorax in the supine adult. Radiology 1979; 133:593–595.
74. Ruskin JA, Gurney JW, Thorsen MR, Goodman LR. Detection of pleural effusions on supine chest radiographs. AJR 1987; 148:681–683.
75. Sargent N, Turner AF. Emergency treatment of pneumothorax: A simple catheter technique for use in the radiology department. AJR 1970; 109:531–535.
76. Stark DD, Federle MP, Goodman PC. CT and radiographic assessment of tube thoracostomy. AJR 1983; 1141:253–258.
77. Stark DD, Federle MP, Goodman PC, et al. Differentiating lung abscess from empyema: Radiography and computed tomography. AJR 1983; 141:163–167.
78. Tocino IM. Pneumothorax in the supine patient: Radiographic anatomy. Radiographics 1985; 5:557–586.
79. Tocino IM, Miller MH, Fairfax WR. Distribution of pneumothorax in the supine and semirecumbent critically ill adult. AJR 1985; 144:901–905.
80. Trackler RT, Brinker RA. Widening of the left paravertebral pleural line on supine chest roentgenograms in free pleural effusions. AJR 1966; 96:1027–1034.
81. Woodring JH. Recognition of pleural effusion on supine radiographs: How much fluid is required? AJR 1984; 142:59–64.
82. Ziter FMH, Westcott JL. Supine subpulmonary pneumothorax. AJR 1981; 137:699–701.

Diaphragm

83. Ammann AM, Bremer WH, Maull KI, et al. Traumatic rupture of the diaphragm: Real-time sonographic diagnosis. AJR 1983; 140:915–916.
83. Andurs CH, Martin JH. Rupture of the diaphragm after blunt trauma. Am J Surg 1970; 119:686–693.
84. Aronhick JM, Epstein DM, Gefter WB, et al. Chronic traumatic diaphragmatic hernia: The significance of pleural effusion. Radiology 1988; 168:675–678.
85. Ball T, McCrory R, Smith JD, et al. Traumatic diaphragmatic hernia: Errors in diagnosis. AJR 1982; 138:633–637.
86. Brown GL, Richardson JD. Traumatic diaphragmatic hernia: A continuing challenge. Ann Thorac Surg 1985; 39:170–173.
87. Carter N, Guiseffi J, Felson B. Traumatic diaphragmatic hernia. AJR 1951; 65:56–72.
88. Estrera AS, Landay MJ, McClelland RN. Blunt traumatic rupture of the right hemidiaphragm: Experience in 12 patients. Ann Thorac Surg 1985; 39:525–530.
89. Fataar S, Rad FF, Schulman A. Diagnosis of diaphragmatic tears. Br J Radiol 1979; 52:375–381.
90. Heiberg E, Wolverson MK, Hurd RN, et al. CT recognition of traumatic rupture of the diaphragm. AJR 1980; 135:369–372.
91. Hoo M. Traumatic diaphragmatic hernia. Ann Thorac Surg 1971; 12:311–324.
92. Jarrett F, Bernhardt TC. Right-sided diaphragmatic injury: Rarity or overlooked diagnosis? Arch Surg 1978; 113:737–739.
93. Mirvis SE, Keramati B, Buckman R, et al. MR imaging of traumatic diaphragmatic rupture. J Comput Assist Tomogr 1988; 12:147–149.
94. Panicek DM, Benson CB, Gottlieb RH, Heitzman ER. The diaphragm: Anatomic, pathologic, and radiologic considerations. Radiographics 1988; 8:385–425.
95. Peck WA. Right-sided diaphragmatic liver hernia following trauma. AJR 1957; 78:99–108.
96. Perlman SJ, Rogers LF, Mintzer RA, et al. Abnormal course of nasogastric tube in traumatic rupture of left hemidiaphragm. AJR 1984; 142:85–88.
97. Schriber M, Brown FE. Traumatic diaphragmatic hernia. Curr Probl Diagn Radiol 1979; 8:1–30.
98. Wise L, Connors J, Hwang YH, et al. Traumatic injuries of the diaphragm. J Trauma 1973; 13:946–950.

Computed Tomography

99. Kerns SR, Gay SB. CT of blunt chest trauma. AJR 1990; 154:55–60.
100. Mirvis SE, Kostrubiak I, Whitley NO. Role of CT in excluding major arterial injury after blunt thoracic trauma. AJR 1987; 149:601–605.
101. Sivit CJ, Taylor GA, Eichelberger MR. Chest injury in children with blunt abdominal trauma: Evaluation with CT. Radiology 1989; 171:815–818.
102. Tocino IM, Miller MH. Computed tomography in blunt chest trauma. J Thorac Imaging 1987; 2:45–59.
103. Tocino IM, Miller MH, Frederich PR, et al. CT detection of occult pneumothorax in head trauma. AJR 1984; 143:987–990.
104. Toombs BD, Lester RG, Ben-Menachem Y, et al. Computed tomography in blunt trauma. Radiol Clin North Amer 1981; 19:17–35.
105. Toombs BD, Sandler CM, Lester RG. Computed tomography of chest trauma. Radiology 1981; 140:733–738.
106. Wall SD, Federle MP, Jeffrey RB, et al. CT diagnosis of unsuspected pneumothorax after blunt abdominal trauma. AJR 1983; 141:919–921.

Chest Wall

107. Dennis LN, Rogers LF. Superior mediastinal widening from spine fractures mimicking aortic rupture on chest radiographs. AJR 1989; 152:27–30.
108. Harris RD, Harris JH. The prevalence and significance of missed scapular fractures in blunt chest trauma. AJR 1988; 151:747–750.
109. Heare MM, Heare TC, Gillespy T. Diagnostic imaging of pelvic and chest wall trauma. Radiol Clin North Am 1989; 27:873–889.
110. Richardson JD, McElvein RB, Trinkle JK. First rib fracture: A hallmark of severe trauma. Ann Surg 1975; 181:251–254.
111. Woodring JH, Fried AM, Hatfield AR, et al. Fractures of first and second ribs: Predictive value for arterial and bronchial injury. AJR 1982; 138:211–215.

CHAPTER 10

•••••••••••••••••••••••••••••••••

The Esophagus

••••••••

LINDA O'CONNELL JUDGE, M.D.

Emergency evaluation of the esophagus and radiographic diagnosis of injury rely on the elicitation of a careful and complete patient history and the communication of this information by the attending physician to the radiologist. In contradistinction to other traumatic insults to the neck and the chest, esophageal injury is usually characterized by a delayed presentation. Protocols for penetrating neck trauma frequently include a contrast medium swallow immediately following angiographic evaluation of the carotid and the vertebral arteries because the risks of overlooking a traumatic esophageal laceration are nearly as great as those leading to angiography. Subtle plain film findings or abnormalities that are unexpected for the injury at hand should alert the acute observer to the possibility of esophageal injury. One example is a unilateral left pleural effusion in a patient with atypical chest pain who is admitted to the hospital for "rule out myocardial infarction," but who is later found to have spontaneous esophageal perforation.

Esophageal injury can be divided into the broad categories of extrinsic, intrinsic, ingestion, and iatrogenic insults, though some overlap in these arbitrary divisions does exist. Extrinsic etiologies are penetrating, blunt, or compressive trauma exerted on the patient's neck or chest. The cause and the time of injury is usually easy to identify. The intrinsic injuries of Mallory-Weiss tears or Boerhaave's syndrome are more insidious in their presentation. Ingestion trauma ranges from inadvertent swallowing of foreign bodies or caustic elements to food impaction, suicide attempts, thermal injury, and direct mucosal irritation from orally administered medications. Iatrogenic injury is the most common cause of esophageal trauma. Medical instrumentation accounts for 75% of all esophageal perforation.

••••

CLASSIFICATION OF ESOPHAGEAL TRAUMA

Extrinsic Trauma

Perforation

Patients with penetrating or blunt esophageal trauma often have other serious major organ injury so that the esophageal signs and symptoms are either overlooked or attributed to the known injuries. Symptoms of esophageal injury include hematemesis, hoarseness, and odynophagia. Chest pain may be unrelenting and often prompts a provisional diagnosis of myocardial infarction, dissecting aneurysm, or perforated peptic ulcer. These complaints should instigate a careful physical examination for

• • • • APPROPRIATE RADIOGRAPHIC STUDIES

  I. **Plain Films**
     A. Lateral view of the neck using a soft tissue technique
     B. Anteroposterior view of the neck using a soft tissue technique
     C. Chest x-ray
        1. Routine posteroanterior and lateral projections are performed.
        2. An expiration view is performed to demonstrate pneumothorax.
  Comment: Excellent quality, detail, and positioning are necessary both to evaluate for foreign bodies, which are often of limited radiopacity, as well as for secondary signs of subcutaneous emphysema, pneumothorax, pneumomediastinum, or mediastinal widening.
 II. **Contrast Studies**
     A. Water-soluble contrast agents
        1. High-osmolality agents
        2. Low-osmolality agents
     B. Barium-based agents
     C. Solid radiopaque tablets
  Comment: Usually the most informative form of acute examination. Contrast study requires some patient compliance and is not appropriate for comatose patients or for those who are unable to drink. The choice of contrast media depends on the anticipated injury. A barium-based agent is preferred if aspiration is likely, but such an agent may cause granulomas and fibrosis if it leaks into the mediastinum. Routine water-soluble contrast is hyperosmolar and has been the preferred agent to demonstrate perforation. It is contraindicated if aspiration or communication with the tracheobronchial tree via a fistula is possible. Early reports indicate that the new low-osmolarity water-soluble compounds may be preferable in *both* situations.
III. **Computed Tomography**
     A. Acutely, computed tomography (CT) may be performed immediately after an oral contrast study to confirm perforation and to evaluate for attendant masses and fluid collections.
     B. Subacutely, CT is excellent for monitoring complications such as abscesses and continued leakage from cervical or thoracic esophageal reanastomoses. The use of an intravenous contrast agent is quite helpful.
 IV. **Nuclear Medicine**
     A. Inflammation localization agents such as gallium or indium are occasionally helpful.
  Comment: Of limited use. Nuclear medicine techniques provide poor spatial resolution. Discrimination of inflammation from infection is generally not possible. These techniques have virtually no acute indication.
  V. **Magnetic Resonance Imaging**
     A. Axial sections
     B. Sagittal and coronal sections as indicated
  Comment: Provides beautiful images in the neck, but cardiac and respiratory motion, even with gating, causes degradation in the chest. Magnetic resonance imaging offers little advantage over CT.

crepitus or the Hamman's sign. Plain films must be scrutinized for subcutaneous or retropharyngeal air (Fig. 10–1), edema, abscess (Fig. 10–2), hematoma, deviated trachea, widened mediastinum (Fig. 10–3), pneumothorax, or pneumomediastinum. Perforations of the distal esophagus usually result in pleural effusion or hydropneumothorax on the left side, whereas perforations of the midesophagus tend to produce a right-sided pleural effusion. Plain chest films are entirely normal in as many as 12–15% of

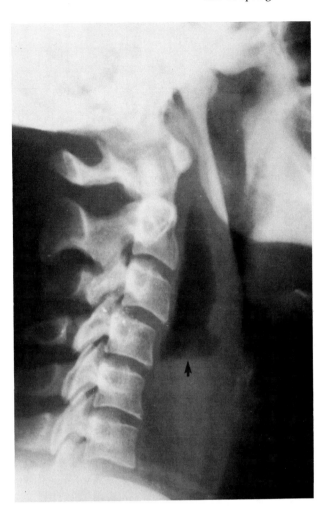

FIGURE 10–2. Retropharyngeal Abscess

• • • •

This patient was treated in an area hospital following a gunshot wound sustained 1 week earlier (note the small metallic fragments). No symptomatology attributable to the esophagus was noted during that admission, and no contrast medium swallow was performed. The patient began to experience dysphagia 5 days later, and at the time of presentation the patient was febrile and unable to eat or control his own secretions. Note the exquisite air-fluid level in the large retropharyngeal abscess in this upright film (*arrow*).

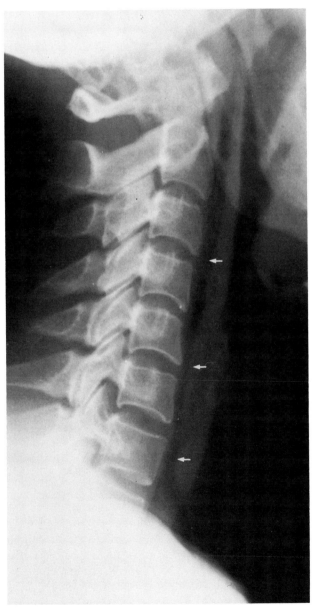

FIGURE 10–1. Retropharyngeal Free Air

• • • •

This cross table lateral view, obtained to evaluate cervical spine integrity, shows retropharyngeal air from esophageal disruption (*arrows*). Although easily identified on this film, a soft tissue technique is often necessary to demonstrate subtle collections.

patients with esophageal injury because the radiographic manifestations are time-dependent.

In penetrating trauma, the path of the bullet or the laceration must be extrapolated by the examiner to determine if esophageal injury is possible. Esophageal perforation carries a high risk of mortality, exceeding a rate of 50% in some series, although most researchers report an approximately 20% mortality rate. The key to successful therapy is early diagnosis, since morbidity and mortality increase significantly when treatment is delayed more than 12 hours after the injury. Although arterial injuries pose the greatest early threat to an injured patient, esophageal injuries are the greatest late threat. Because the consequences of a missed esophageal in-

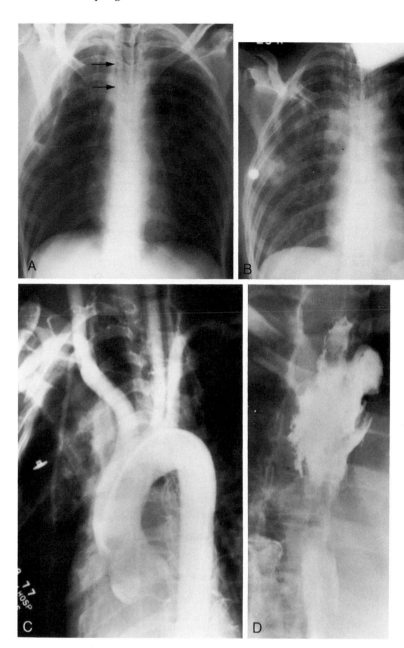

FIGURE 10–3. Ruptured Esophagus After a Motor Vehicle Accident

• • • •

A, This initial portable view of the chest obtained for crush injury demonstrates a right pneumothorax and a minimal right-sided pneumomediastinum (*arrows*). *B,* A film obtained 2 hours later shows continued right pneumothorax and a widened mediastinum. Fractures of the right clavicle and the lateral right ribs are seen. *C,* An aortic arch arteriogram, performed because of the widened mediastinum, is normal. *D,* Subsequent contrast medium swallow shows upper thoracic esophageal disruption with extravasation.

jury are so grave, many trauma centers have a mandatory protocol of barium swallow, regardless of symptomatology, to follow all carotid and vertebral angiography performed for penetrating injury. The even more aggressive approach of surgical exploration of all penetrating injuries through the platysma has been advocated by some. Such a decision should depend upon the institutional track record of sensitivity and specificity in the performance and in the interpretation of the results of esophageal contrast swallows. Consideration should also be given to the relative costs of surgery, angiography, esophagoscopy, and the attendant length of hospitalization.

Blunt or Compressive Injury, Electrical Injury, and Compressed Air Injury

Although stab and gunshot wounds predominate in presentation to the emergency room, blunt or compressive injury to the esophagus resulting from motor vehicle accidents and personal assaults must also be considered (Fig. 10–4). Other less common causes include blunt trauma to the lower esophageal sphincter caused by an improperly positioned seat belt, intraluminal electric burn due to malfunction of an esophageal temperature probe during general

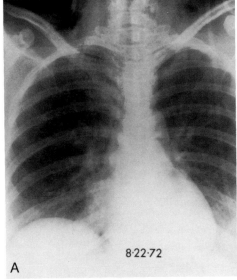

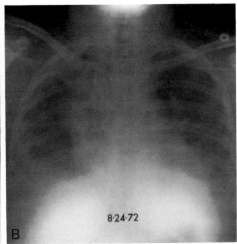

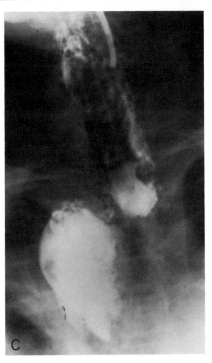

FIGURE 10–4. Ruptured Esophagus Caused by Blunt Trauma

• • • •

This patient arrived at the emergency room 1 hour after her boyfriend jumped and sat on her chest. *A*, Note the right-sided pneumomediastinum above the right hilum and subcutaneous emphysema in the supraclavicular regions. *B*, Two days later there is massive mediastinal widening caused by the development of an abscess and bilateral hydropneumothoraces. Interval fever was clinically attributed to the small right basilar infiltrate seen on the initial film. *C*, The contrast medium swallow demonstrates a perforation of the esophagus at the cervicothoracic junction.

anesthesia, and attempted suicide by swallowing one end of an electric cord while plugging the other end into an outlet. There are reports of midesophageal "blow-outs" from inhaling compressed air from tanks or tires; these injuries usually occur just below the aortic arch. The normal esophagus requires less than 5 lb/in.² of pressure for it to rupture. Lastly, upper mediastinitis has been reported to occur remotely after a whiplash injury, even when a normal swallow was obtained acutely. Tiny tears in the retropharyngeal, perivascular, or pretracheal spaces, which intermittently leak but subsequently close off, are postulated as the cause.

Combined Tracheoesophageal Injury

The esophagus is relatively protected by the spine and the sternum, thus extrinsic injuries to the thoracic esophagus are uncommon and occur in only 0.5% of wartime chest injuries. This infrequent occurrence may also be influenced by its relationship to the heart, since concurrent cardiac injury often results in an immediately fatal outcome. The injuries most commonly associated with extrinsic esophageal trauma, in addition to those of the heart, are to the cervicothoracic spinal cord, the lungs, and the great vessels. A complication rate of 75% is reported in such multiple injuries. Extensive esophageal injuries, even in the cervical region, usually leak after repair (Fig. 10–5). In the neck, interposition of the sterno-cleidomastoid or the strap muscles between the esophagus and the injured trachea or the carotid arteries as well as anterior drainage that does not cross vascular fascial planes is helpful in limiting further complication from anastomotic leakage. Computed tomography (CT) can detect the resultant fluid collections and abscesses.

Intrinsic Trauma

Intrinsic injuries are inadvertently self-induced and are principally Mallory-Weiss tears or spontaneous perforations (i.e., the Boerhaave's syndrome).

Mallory-Weiss Tears

Mallory-Weiss tears are superficial longitudinal mucosal tears of the esophagus. There is a 3:1 predominance of occurrence in the distal hiatal portion of the esophagus in comparison with more proximal

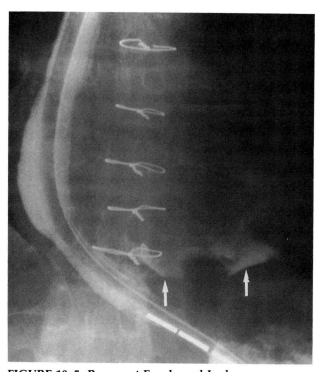

FIGURE 10–5. Recurrent Esophageal Leak

• • • •

Three weeks following the repair of an esophageal tear incurred in a fall from a water tower, this patient's recurrent chest pain and increasing fever resulted in the need to perform a repeat esophagogram. Acute extravasation (*arrows*) of the water-soluble contrast material indicates a recurrence. Both a feeding tube and nasogastric tube are in place.

or multiple locations. The tears are caused by vomiting or blunt chest trauma. Mallory-Weiss tears are generally very shallow, thus they are frequently not seen on contrast esophagograms. Although most heal spontaneously with conservative management, some Mallory-Weiss tears bleed profusely. Angiography is rarely needed to make the diagnosis at the present time because endoscopic evaluation is usually diagnostic. However, angiography may be used therapeutically to embolize a refractory bleeding site. In general, the left gastric artery is occluded during this embolization.

Boerhaave's Syndrome

First described in 1724 by the attending physician to the Dutch admiral Baron von Wasseher, whose reported evening of overindulgence on roast duck and Mozelle wine resulted in his demise and subsequent autopsy, Boerhaave's syndrome of spontaneous esophageal perforation has become synonymous with an episode of forceful vomiting that causes esophageal disruption. This phenomenon is a barogenic rupture due to a precipitous rise in intra-abdominal pressure that is transmitted against a closed glottis. The rapid increase in intraluminal esophageal pressure and the sudden distention of the distal esophagus result in vertical rents, 1–4 cm in length, located in the left lower esophagus 90–95% of the time. This region is generally involved owing to focal thinning of the distal esophageal musculature, segmental defects in the circular muscle layer, and perforating vessels and nerves, which result in transmural weakness. Additional factors are the anterior angulation of the esophagus as it passes through the diaphragm and a lack of discrete supporting structures between the right gastrohepatic ligament and the left gastrophrenic ligament.

Although usually associated with vomiting, any maneuver that causes gastric contents to reflux above the lower esophageal sphincter and increases the intraesophageal pressure by sudden esophageal distention can split the muscularis and allow mucosa to herniate and burst into the mediastinum, resulting in Boerhaave's syndrome. Thus, childbirth, seizure, severe coughing, swallowing, weight lifting, blunt trauma, hyperemesis gravidarum, sneezing, and hiccuping have all been reported as an inciting event. This list is by no means all inclusive, and many additional causes may exist; the important factor to recall is the basic cause of this esophageal injury (Fig. 10–6).

The classic presentation of Boerhaave's syndrome has been termed the *Tetrad of Gott* and consists of (1) lower chest pain with vomiting and hematemesis, (2) subcutaneous emphysema, (3) respiratory distress,

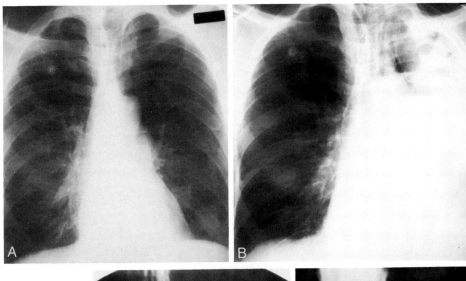

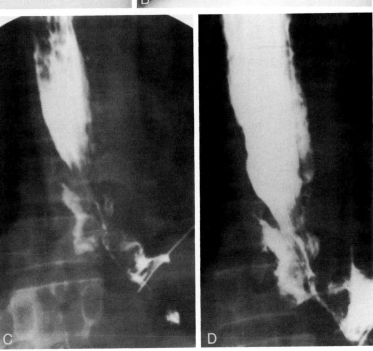

FIGURE 10–6. Boerhaave's Syndrome

• • • •

A, The chest radiograph is normal except for the retrocardiac opacity attributed to underpenetration by the clinician. Note the electrocardiogram leads over the left side of the chest in this patient who complained of relentless substernal pain. *B*, Within 2 days a massive left-sided hydropneumothorax developed. Note the ipsilateral volume loss. *C* and *D*, A contrast medium swallow demonstrates lower esophageal perforation. A left basilar chest tube is in place.

and (4) prostration. This constellation of findings is actually observed in fewer than 50% of patients with spontaneous esophageal perforation. The radiographic findings are both time-dependent and nonspecific. Left-sided effusion or hydropneumothorax is usually not observed until 12–24 hours following the perforation. Pneumomediastinum, mediastinal widening, cervical emphysema, and Niclerio's sign (a V-shaped lucency through the cardiac shadow that is caused by free air in the left lower region of the mediastinum that dissects under the left diaphragmatic crus) may also be seen. Even in a patient with a good history and in whom a concerted effort is made to search for these clues, the correct diagnosis is made within the golden "12-hour window" in only 21% of cases. The average time for diagnosis of

Boerhaave's syndrome is 48 hours. The mortality of Boerhaave's syndrome remained close to 100% until 1947, when Barrett performed the first successful surgery for repair of distal esophageal rupture. Now, the overall survival rate is 70%.

Ingestion of Inappropriate Substances

Ingestion injury covers the broad spectrum of foreign body, caustic, thermal, and drug-induced trauma to the esophagus. These diverse causes have little in common other than the endless litany of items that patients attempt to swallow, which is limited only by the size of their oral cavities. These injuries vary in their intent, mode, sequence, complications, and subsequent prognosis. Ingested objects usually involve other structures in their passage, or lead to aspiration, regurgitation, or perforation.

Foreign Body Ingestion

In the United States 1500 people die annually of foreign body ingestion. It is estimated that 80–90% of ingested foreign material passes spontaneously, 10–20% is removed endoscopically, and less than 1% requires surgical extraction. As has already been stated, the key to diagnosis is an accurate history. The description of ingestion is crucial not only in identifying the nature of the problem, but also in quantifying the volume swallowed. Only 80% of ingestions are correctly diagnosed within the first 24 hours. Symptoms are once again nonspecific. Adults complain of dysphagia, odynophagia, or chest pain similar to that occurring with other types of esophageal injury, whereas children may drool, have respiratory distress or regurgitation, or refuse to eat. Infants may also present with altered consciousness presumed to be from transient hypoxia or vasovagal syncope from an exaggerated vagal response. The physical examination is of little assistance when the foreign material remains within the esophagus or the gastrointestinal tract. Symptomatic localization of dysphagia rarely corresponds with the actual level of impaction.

Foreign bodies lodge at levels of smallest cross-sectional diameter. In the absence of underlying pathology, the majority impact at the level of the cricopharyngeal muscle (C6). Other less common sites are at the thoracic inlet (T1), the aortic arch (T4), the tracheal bifurcation (T6), and the esophageal hiatus (T10/T11). There is a 5–10% recurrence rate even in the absence of stricture or other anatomic abnormality.

Less than 50% of ingested foreign material is sufficiently radiopaque to be identified on plain radiographs. However, the associated complications may be seen and can assist in the diagnosis. When there is concurrent aspiration, a check-valve effect may take place, which causes an overinflation of the affected lung that is exaggerated on expiration views. Alternatively, atelectasis may develop. Other mediastinal changes may suggest perforation, bronchoesophageal fistula, aortoesophageal bleeding, or pericardial injury or tamponade.

The majority of impacted esophageal foreign bodies are foodstuffs. Adults state this fact on arrival in the emergency room, but children often present in a more obtuse fashion even when a choking event has been witnessed by a parent. Peanuts are the most frequently impacted material, but incompletely

chewed hot dogs can also be aspirated into the tracheobronchial tree and are the most common cause of foreign body fatality. Specific, directed questioning of the child's parent may be enlightening.

When children are brought to the emergency room for suspected ingestion, the offending agent is often thought to be a coin. Since coins are clearly radiopaque, radiologic evaluation is warranted in confirming ingestion. In infants or children, films should be obtained from the base of the skull to the anus to document the presence, the size, the number, and the location of the foreign bodies as well as to search for complications of impaction. Coins in the upper esophagus are usually seen en face on frontal radiographs because the esophagus is more distensible transversely, whereas coins within the trachea are seen on edge due to the incomplete posterior cartilage rings comprising the trachea. Dimes are 17 mm in diameter, pennies are 18 mm, and quarters are 23 mm. Greater than 80% of all foreign bodies that successfully maneuver the esophagus to reach the stomach eventually pass through the remainder of the gastrointestinal tract without complication. However, the length of time pennies remain within the stomach is of some concern. The United States Mint switched from the copper penny (containing 95% copper and 5% zinc) to the zinc penny (containing 2.4% copper and 97.6% zinc) in 1982. Zinc is corrosive to the gastric mucosa when it is exposed to gastric acid for prolonged periods. As an incidental note, the American Academy of Pediatrics successfully campaigned against attempts to switch to an aluminum penny in the 1970s because of the limited radiopacity of aluminum and the difficulty of its radiologic identification based on the experience of ingested or aspirated soda pop can pull tabs.

An incompletely chewed bolus of meat is the most frequent impacting agent in the adult patient population (Fig. 10–7), followed closely by the bones of chicken, pork, and fish (Fig. 10–8 and 10–9). Certain other circumstances also deserve mention. Patients with dentures are reported to have a higher incidence of accidental foreign material ingestion because of the diminished tactile sensitivity of the palate. Thus, bones, pits, stems, and other objects usually separated out from food may inadvertently be swallowed.

The explosion of technologic devices available to our population has led to a miniepidemic of button battery ingestions, prompting a National Button Battery Ingestion Study. Its findings show that the majority of these batteries do not exceed 21 mm in diameter and that 89.9% pass out of the gastrointestinal tract without complication in 12–14 days. The most common batteries contain manganese dioxide, silver oxide, mercuric oxide, or lithium and employ a 26–45% mixture of potassium hydroxide or sodium

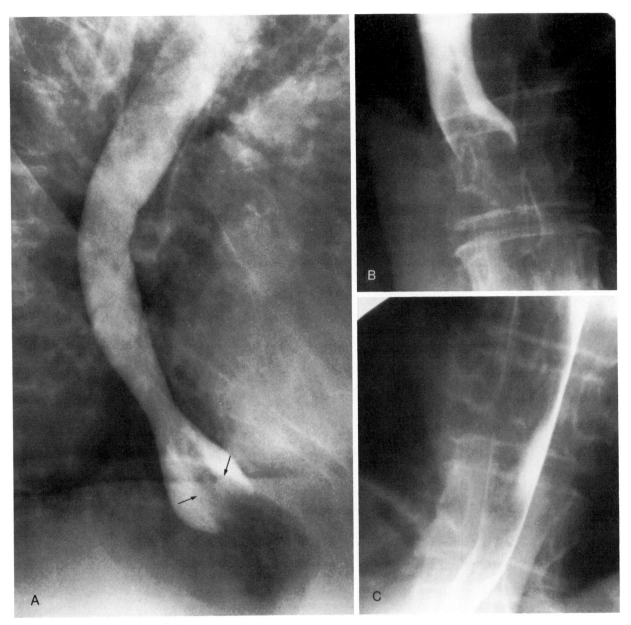

FIGURE 10–7. Impacted Meat Bolus

• • • •

This nursing home resident was brought to the emergency room 3 hours after lunch complaining of chest pain. She had choked on an incompletely chewed bit of pork chop at lunch. *A,* An initial swallow with a diluted water-soluble contrast medium solution shows complete obstruction of the esophageal hiatus by a smoothly marginated intraluminal filling defect (*arrows*). *B,* A spot film of the distal esophagus shows the impacted foreign body very clearly. *C,* The patient immediately underwent endoscopy during which the meat was pushed into the stomach. Re-examination the next morning showed no residual filling defect, no perforation, and no underlying pathology.

hydroxide. The alkaline electrolyte is sufficiently concentrated to produce liquefaction and necrosis if it comes in contact with the gastric mucosa. When damage from these batteries occurs, it is usually caused by direct corrosive action, although low-voltage burns and pressure necrosis have also occurred.

The use of hired agents to transport cocaine has spawned the body packer or body bagger syndrome.

Traffickers volunteer to ingest 30–40 sealed packets each containing 3–5 g of cocaine. These messengers risk far more than legal ramifications should complications develop. In addition to the risk of impaction and gastrointestinal obstruction, the packets are susceptible to leakage and breakage after 12–24 hours, and the ingestion of 1–3 g of cocaine has proved fatal. The packets produce an interesting and pathognomonic "bowel gas pattern." These patients

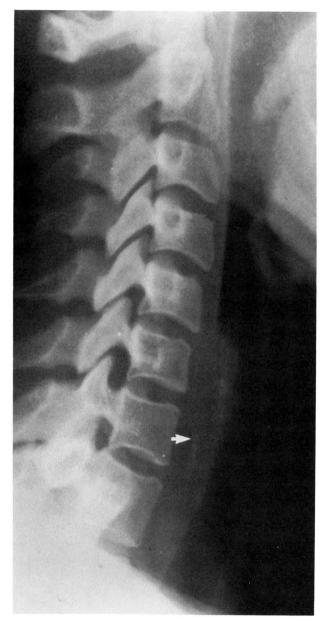

FIGURE 10–8. Chicken Bone Lodged in the Esophagus

• • • •

The patient arrived at the emergency room several hours after choking on a chicken bone. Although the bone can be seen (*arrow*), this examination could have been improved by the use of a soft tissue technique. There is no evidence of perforation.

are commonly fatal, since the direct esophageal access makes tamponade of the rapidly flowing blood virtually impossible. As described by Chiari in 1914,[2] there is first a symptom-free period and then massive hemorrhage into the gastrointestinal tract.

Prior to surgical procedures pioneered in the 20th century, ingestion or impaction of a foreign body

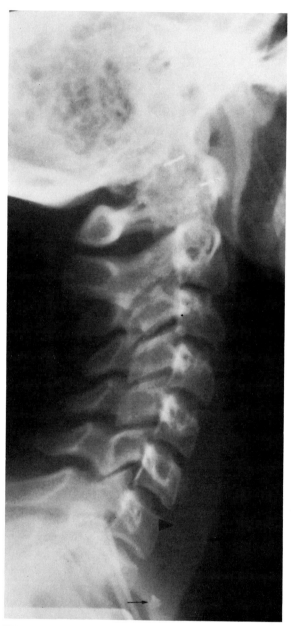

FIGURE 10–9. Lodged Pork Bone

• • • •

This patient presented to the emergency room with the complaint of a sore throat and cervical fullness. No inciting event could be recalled. A cervical spine film nearly excludes a small pork bone (*arrow*), and the bone technique makes the tiny retropharyngeal free air (*arrowhead*) quite subtle. On further questioning, the patient had last eaten meat in a chopped barbecued pork sandwich 3 days earlier.

need stabilization, activated charcoal, and immediate surgery for safest extraction when a packet impacts.

Sharp and pointed foreign bodies should also be removed, usually surgically, as 15–35% perforate somewhere in the gastrointestinal tract, particularly at the ileocecal valve. Aortoesophageal fistulas are usually the result of an aortic aneurysm eroding into the esophagus, but they may also occur from a perforating esophageal foreign body. These fistulas with or without subsequent perforation often led to a prolonged illness and protracted death. Before surgical removal, however, careful reflection is warranted. It must be considered whether the material could pass spontaneously and whether the anticipated therapy poses more threat to the patient than an uninterrupted course of events. The airway must be protected at all times, since dislodging a foreign body impacted in the esophagus into the trachea can have an even more unfortunate outcome. This concern has led to the practice of performing most esophageal manipulations with the assistance of an anesthesiologist. The decision should also be made beforehand whether the goal is to retrieve only, or if either retrieval or advancement into the stomach is acceptable.

Cathartics, stool softeners, and special bulk diets are of no proven benefit in hastening the passage of esophageal foreign material. Postural disimpaction involves inverting a patient, preferably in a myelographic harness on a fluoroscopic table, to 50–60 degrees head down. The patient "drinks" a dilute barium agent through a straw conceivably to force the material to "sink" cephalad. This method has occasional success, requires a high degree of patient compliance, and relies on vomiting, with its inherent risks of perforation and aspiration, to dislodge the material.

Barometric measures have also been tried. Although a number of combinations exist, they all involve administration of a drug to induce smooth muscle relaxation followed by a bolus of gas delivered by nasogastric tube immediately proximal to the impacted material. The tube may also be used to remove pooling fluid cephalad to the obstruction. The gas may be hand-injected from a syringe or formed from 100 ml of a carbonated beverage or the reconstituted contents of a gas-forming agent, such as a cocktail of tartaric acid and sodium bicarbonate. The foreign body is propelled forward into the distal esophagus or the stomach by the expanding gas. The possibilities of re-impaction, barometric rupture, regurgitation, and aspiration exist.

Since the majority of adult foreign body impactions are caused by meat, enzymatic digestion with papain has been attempted without any objective benefit. The enzyme does not discriminate between ingested meat and esophageal muscle and may actually increase esophageal inflammation, causing perforation. It is also hyperosmolar and causes hemorrhagic pulmonary edema on exposure to lung tissue. In addition, some patients have allergic, bronchospastic reactions to the foreign protein.

Interventional methods employed in the radiologic suite, often under fluoroscopic observation, involve basket extraction, magnet retrieval of metallic sub-

stances, and entrapment by a distally positioned Foley catheter with subsequent balloon insufflation and dragging of the impacted material up into the oropharynx. The skill and experience of the interventionalist, a concerted team approach, patient cooperation, the type and the location of the foreign body, and a considerable degree of luck all contribute to the prediction of success of these techniques.

Endoscopic manipulation of foreign bodies has a low complication rate of approximately 0.1%. This reflects both good patient selection and a predetermination that displacement of the object into the stomach by the endoscope is an acceptable outcome. Piecemeal extraction has a lower success rate and a higher complication rate because of complications associated with aspiration.

Caustic Ingestion

Approximately 10,000 visits are made to emergency rooms annually for caustic ingestion. There is a bimodal age distribution in which children 1–5 years of age accidentally ingest these agents, whereas young adults 20–30 years of age drink them in an attempt to commit suicide. As with other forms of esophageal injury, patients present with chest pain and dysphagia; shock, fever, and respiratory distress may be present if the inflammatory process proceeds to perforation and mediastinitis. The extent of injury depends on the material, its concentration, and the volume swallowed. The availability of liquid lye and detergents on the commercial market has significantly increased the potential damage from one swallow of an offending agent, since liquids are able to expose a much greater mucosal surface area than a similar volume of a solid material. This problem has been diminished by prohibition of the sale of high concentrations of these agents in the retail market as well as enactment of the Safe Packaging Act, which legislated the use of child-proof containers for certain cleaners.

As with foreign bodies, the list of possible agents is nearly limitless. In practice, the majority of ingested caustics are alkaline (pH >7), since acids (pH <7) are quite bitter tasting, burn on initial contact with the oral mucosa, and are usually expelled even when the ingestion is intentional. Exposure to acid results in a superficial, coagulation necrosis with gray to white patches progressing to eschar. Toilet bowl cleaners, battery fluid, sulfuric acid, nitric acid, and hydrochloric acid are the most commonly encountered household acids.

Alkaline agents are usually tasteless, but they penetrate rapidly into tissue to cause ulceration, blood vessel thrombosis, liquefactive necrosis, bacterial infiltration, and fatty saponification within 2–3 days. Four to seven days after the injury, the injured mucosa sloughs and fibroblast activity begins. The esophageal wall is weakest at 7–21 days after injury.

First degree burns cause hyperemia and superficial desquamation. These injuries usually do not develop strictures. Second-degree lesions blister and cause shallow transmucosal ulcers with a 15–30% incidence of stenosis. Third-degree or full-thickness burns, or those extending outside the esophagus, result in a clinically significant stricture in more than 90% of patients (Fig. 10–10). These strictures may form as early as 3 weeks after injury or up to several years later. Experimentally, only a few milliliters of a 30% sodium hydroxide solution are needed to cause a full-thickness esophageal injury in 1 second. Typically ingested alkaline agents are lime, Clinitest reagent tablets (40–50% potassium hydroxide or sodium hydroxide), and laundry detergents. Bleaches have a pH in the neutral range, have shown no significant morbidity or mortality, and are considered to be esophageal irritants.

The degree of esophageal injury correlates roughly with increasing pH. Alkaline agents with a pH greater than 12.5 nearly always cause severe injury and stricture, whereas mixtures with a pH of less than 11.4 are rarely associated with anything more severe than a superficial mucosal burn. Experimentally, a better predictor of esophageal injury than pH is the titrable acid/alkaline reserve (TAR). The TAR is defined as the volume of 0.1 M solution of hydrochloric acid (in the case of bases) or sodium hydroxide (in the case of acids) to titrate 100 ml of a 1% solution (or weight/volume in the case of solids) to a pH of 8, which is that of the normal esophageal environment. This is a predictive value only and is not intended for clinical practice. The use of neutralizing agents, such as vinegar for lye ingestion or sodium bicarbonate to neutralize acids, can result in exothermic chemical reactions that further damage the esophagus. Induced vomiting or ipecac syrup administration only repeats the exposure of the agent to the esophageal mucosa and increases the risk of aspiration.

There have been 133 patients who have developed squamous cell carcinoma of the esophagus after lye or caustic ingestion[4, 7, 13]; this is a significantly higher incidence than that occurring in the general population. Although there is a prolonged latent period of more than 20 years, this malignancy still affects a younger age group than usual, that is, those patients who ingested caustics as toddlers. Patients with malignancy following caustic injury demonstrate an unusually equal male-to-female ratio, and 84% of the malignancies occur within 2 cm of the carinal level, regardless of where the most severe injury was noted acutely (Fig. 10–11).

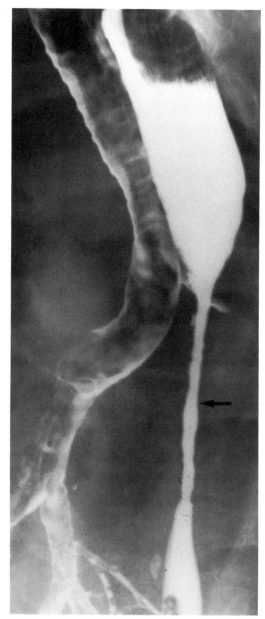

FIGURE 10–10. Esophageal Stricture
• • • •
Esophageal stricture is seen in this patient 2 years following a suicide attempt by drinking Drano. Note the marked midesophageal narrowing (*arrow*), the proximal air-fluid level, and the aspiration. Barium was chosen as the contrast agent because the patient's history strongly suggested the possibility of aspiration during the esophagogram.

Thermal Injury

Thermal burns may occur from the ingestion of dry ice, hot foods, and boiling liquids. They usually produce only superficial lesions because the volume of the offending material is typically small and the exposure time short, since the majority is expelled on initial contact with the oral mucosa.

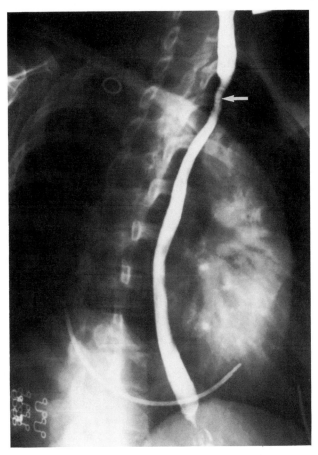

FIGURE 10–11. Squamous Cell Carcinoma Following the Ingestion of a Caustic Material 25 Years Earlier

• • • •

This young woman had ingested a small amount of lye as a toddler. However, she suffered few complications and no stricture until 25 years later. Although the films taken 25 years earlier were not available, the mucosal damage was reported to have been to the distal esophagus. Squamous cell carcinoma was found in this stricture (*arrow*).

Drug-induced Injury

Drug-induced injuries are those in which a medication in proper dosage and intended for oral administration damages the esophageal mucosa by virtue of contact alone. These injuries are dependent on the size and the shape of the capsule or tablet; it should be remembered that anhydrous pills swell on exposure to moisture. The presence of a gelatin or other enteric coating promotes mucosal affinity. Older patients with presbyesophagus and diminished or uncoordinated esophageal contractions can prolong exposure of the drug to the mucosa. The volume of accompanying water plays a critical role. These injuries often present a puzzling diagnostic dilemma, and the drug is usually excluded from consideration because it is often a chronically administered preparation. In patients under 40 years of age, an antibiotic such as tetracycline or doxycycline is often impli-

cated. In patients over 40 years of age, potassium chloride supplements, quinidine, and indomethacin are the more likely culprits. Parenthetically, it has been proposed that this type of injury may be the cause of Plummer-Vinson syndrome, since elderly, iron-deficient, and anemic women with this syndrome are most likely taking an orally administered ferrous sulfate supplement.

Iatrogenic Injury

Injuries Caused by Endoscopy, Instrumentation, and Nasogastric Tubes

Iatrogenic injuries to the esophagus are the most common cause of esophageal trauma. Nearly 75% of all perforations can be attributed to instrumentation. They are discussed last, since they rarely pose a diagnostic dilemma or appear in patients admitted to the emergency room. Rather, the operator usually realizes during the procedure that a complication has occurred; alternatively, the patient becomes symptomatic immediately following the procedure while still under the physician's care.

Any therapeutic procedure occurring in or adjacent to the esophagus carries a risk of injury. As stated before, compilation of various data show a 0.1% incidence of perforation in all endoscopic procedures (Fig. 10–12), approximately 0.06% for fiberoptic endoscopy, and 0.3% for rigid endoscopy. Bougienage procedures carry a 0.55% risk of perforation; mercury dilators have a 0.42% risk, metal olives have a 0.61% risk, and Eder-Puestow autodilators carry a 0.02% risk. Paraesophageal nicks and perforations of the esophagus occur with a 0.55% incidence. Reflecting the markedly increased risk of passing a nasogastric tube when there is underlying pathology, palliative esophageal intubation for carcinoma perforates in 8–9% of attempts. The incidence of routine nasogastric intubation injury is unknown, but it is presumed to be much less than 0.1%.

Radiation Injury

Radiation esophagitis can be caused when the esophagus is exposed to 4500–6000 rads over a 6–8 week period, or at 2000 rads or less if doxyrubicin hydrochloride (Adriamycin) is prescribed concurrently. Once again the symptoms are chest pain, heartburn, and dysphagia. In these patients peristalsis is significantly disrupted. The normal peristaltic wave breaks at the upper margin of the radiation field and again at the lower margin, so that a repetitive and nonproductive contraction pattern is ob-

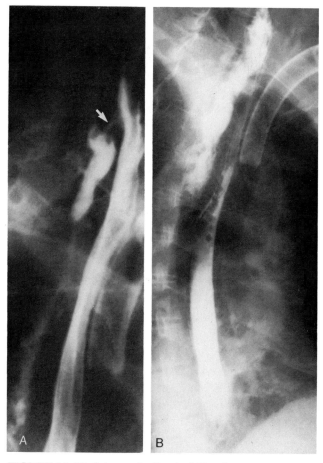

FIGURE 10–12. Iatrogenic Cervical Esophagus Perforation

• • • •

Although perforation was not noted during the procedure, the severity of the patient's complaints afterwards prompted a contrast medium swallow examination. *A,* Discrete perforation at the level of the cricopharyngeal muscle (*arrow*) was identified radiographically and at surgery. *B,* The extravasation extends both cephalad and caudad from the perforation.

served. Occasionally, superficial and diffuse ulceration occurs, resulting in a pattern similar to moniliasis. Delayed fibrosis and stricture are not uncommon.

Injury Caused by Double-contrast Esophagography

Even double-contrast esophagography may rupture an esophagus with a high-grade stenosis or obstruction. The effervescent granules of sodium bicarbonate and citric acid produce 400 cm^3 of carbon dioxide in each 4-g packet within 30 seconds when exposed to liquid. Esophageal rupture may occur at pressures as low as 1.9 lb/in.^{2} (0.13 kg/cm^2) with mean levels at 3.7 lb/in.^{2} (0.26 kg/cm^2). Instances of esophageal perforation during double-contrast

esophagography have been reported, substantiating the time-honored admonition to commence each study with a single swallow of a barium-based agent to exclude high-grade obstruction.

• • • •

EXAMINATION TECHNIQUES

Plain Films

Plain films of the neck and the chest are usually the first films obtained in esophageal injury, even when neither the patient nor the physician suspects injury to the esophagus as the cause. The attendant trauma and the usual presenting complaint of chest pain and dysphagia distract the clinician. This is a reasonable approach, since plain films are easily and quickly obtained and are routinely available. Plain film findings are time-dependent, nonspecific, and may remain entirely within normal limits even 24–28 hours after injury in 10–15% of injuries. Mediastinal emphysema (either "free" pneumomediastinum or the localized Niclerio's sign in the lower left cardiophrenic angle) takes 1 hour or more to develop sufficient volume to be recognized, although nearly 40% of patients manifest this sign before 48 hours. Mediastinal widening from hematoma, the egress of swallowed secretions, or inflammation, or any combination of these are not radiologically apparent until hours after perforation. The integrity of the mediastinum is poor. When intact, the free air remains within the mediastinum, but 77% of hematomas eventually spill over into the pleural space, of which approximately 70% are left-sided, 20% are right-sided, and 10% are bilateral. It is also helpful to remember that the location of the pneumothorax can help to determine the site of the esophageal perforation. The most common location is the left distal region of the esophagus, where perforation causes a left pleural effusion and free air, whereas a mid-esophageal rent is more likely to cause right-sided pleural findings. Also, cervical esophageal injury demonstrates subcutaneous emphysema much earlier than the mediastinal free air of a thoracic esophageal perforation.

Contrast Medium Studies

Once the esophagus has been identified as the source of pathology, a contrast medium swallow is the next evaluation. This recognition, unfortunately, rarely occurs within the "golden 12-hour window" of optimum therapeutic intervention, and spontaneous esophageal perforations require an average of 2 days before diagnosis. The attending physician and the examining radiologist must decide which is the best contrast material to demonstrate the abnormality in each patient. If there is suspicion of perforation alone, a water-soluble contrast material is recommended. Slightly less viscous than even the most dilute barium-based media, these agents are better able to demonstrate small tears. If communication with the tracheobronchial tree is suspected, however, water-soluble hyperosmolar agents are contraindicated and the use of a barium-based agent is advocated. It is anticipated that package labeling on the newer low-osmolarity water-soluble contrast agents will soon include the study of both esophageal perforation and foreign body impaction as an indicated use.

Regardless of the choice of contrast medium, the examination should commence with a single, solid column contrast swallow of small volume observed fluoroscopically without an attempt to obtain spot films. Some centers have found it helpful to videotape the entire examination for review. This initial swallow is useful in excluding total obstruction or complete transection with a small volume of material. If spot films are desired, it is often beneficial to examine the patient in both lateral decubitus positions when the upright swallow shows no abnormalities, since the contrast material may flow too rapidly to demonstrate a small tear. Even if the result of the swallow examination is negative, passage of a nasogastric tube is usually not recommended as long as the possibility of esophageal disruption is entertained. A false-negative rate exceeding 20% on contrast swallows has been found by follow-up endoscopy, observation, or subsequent surgery and autopsy. The addition of a double-contrast examination adds little information in the diagnosis of esophageal trauma, although it may help demonstrate the mucosal irregularities of esophagitis that can explain the patient's chest pain and dysphagia. Similarly, solid agents, such as barium-impregnated foodstuffs or pills of a specific caliber, may assist in showing motility disorders, but they do not enhance the detection of perforation. Contrast swallow is usually not predictive in an acute caustic ingestion, but an examination in the first week may be obtained as a baseline against which subsequent studies can be compared in anticipation of stricture formation.

Computed Tomography

CT evaluation of the neck or the chest is usually not required in the initial diagnostic work-up, but it can prove quite helpful in assessing the complications of esophageal perforation. It is invaluable in documenting the extent of mediastinal infection, which directly determines the type and the approach of surgical intervention (Fig. 10–13). Mediastinal processes that track subdiaphragmatically into the lesser sac can also be followed directly, a feat not possible with other modalities. For maximum information, both intravenously and intraesophageally introduced contrast material should be used to discriminate mature abscesses from other inflammatory collections as well as to search for persistent sites of leakage.

Magnetic Resonance Imaging

Although magnetic resonance imaging can provide exquisite multiplanar images of neck pathology, the unavoidable motion artifacts from respiratory and cardiac motion limit its usefulness in study of the chest. It offers little advantage over CT, is less accessible, and requires a higher level of patient compliance to obtain images of average diagnostic quality. Sonography of the chest may localize and quantitate pleural fluid collections identified on other examinations in anticipation of thoracentesis, but it has only a slight effect on the radiographic diagnosis of disease. Inflammatory localization agents, such as gallium or indium, may ferret out an acute infection against a field of chronic fibrosis and scar, but they do not discriminate well between the massive inflammation accompanying esophageal perforation from focal regions of infection. The poor spatial resolution they provide also limits their usefulness.

• • • •
DISCUSSION

Esophageal trauma frequently masquerades as other more common maladies when presenting spontaneously and is often overlooked when there is associated chest and neck injury. A high level of suspicion must be coupled with an exacting patient history and careful scrutiny of plain films if the diagnosis is to be made in a timely fashion. The ability of the patient to eat and maintain a positive nutritional status profoundly affects his or her prognosis from all injuries. The late complications of abscess, recurrent leak, and sepsis exact a high toll on mortality. Caustic ingestions carry the additional late complications of stricture and a thousandfold increase in the incidence of squamous cell carcinoma of the esophagus. Even seemingly innocent insults, such as foreign body ingestion, may progress to

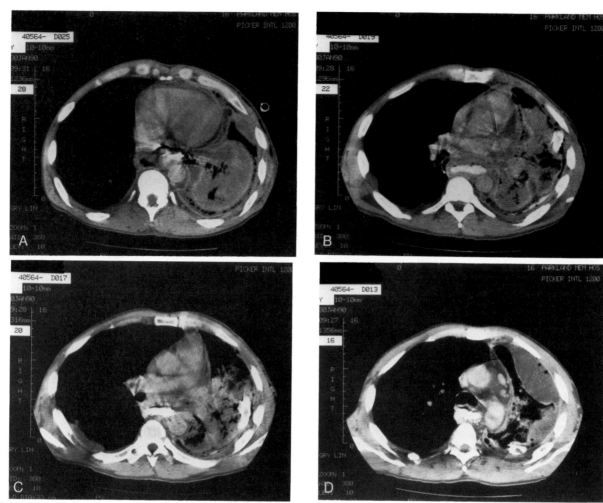

FIGURE 10–13. Computed Tomography Study in a Patient with Boerhaave's Spontaneous Esophageal Perforation
• • • •
Computed tomography study at the levels of the carina (A), the midesophagus (B), the lower esophagus (C), and the hiatus (D) assist in demonstrating mediastinitis, loculated pleural collections, chest tubes, and parenchymal disease. Although free air persists (D), no leakage was identified.

perforation or aspiration if managed inappropriately. Although advances have been made in therapeutic approaches, esophageal injury remains a serious disorder with significant mortality and morbidity, and efforts toward its prevention must remain the primary goal.

References

1. Bloom R, Nakano PH, Gray SW, Skandalakis JE. Foreign bodies of the gastrointestinal tract. Am Surg 1986; 52:618.
2. Chiari H. Über Fremdkörperverletzung des Oesophagus mit Aortaperforation. Berl klin Wschr 1914; 51:7.
3. Endicott N, Molony TB, Campbell G, Bartels LJ. Esophageal perforations: The role of computerized tomography in diagnosis and management decisions. Laryngoscope 1986; 96:751.
4. Friedman EM. Caustic ingestions and foreign bodies in the aerodigestive tract of children. Pediatr Clin North Am 1989; 36:1403.
5. Han SY, McElvein RB, Aldrete JS, Tishler JM. Perforation of the esophagus: Correlation of site and cause with plain film findings. Am J Roentgenol 1985; 145:537.
6. Henderson CT, Engel J, Schlesinger P. Foreign body ingestion: Review and suggested guidelines for management. Endoscopy 1987; 19:68.
7. Howell JM. Alkaline ingestions. Ann Emerg Med 1986; 15:7.
8. Kramer TA, Riding KH, Salkeld LJ. Tracheobronchial and esophageal foreign bodies in the pediatric population. J Otolaryngol 1986; 15:6.
9. Moghissi K. Instrumental perforations of the oesophagus. Br J Hosp Med 1988; 39:231–236.
10. Pass J, LeNarz LA, Schreiber T, Estrera AS. Management of gunshot wounds. Ann Thorac Surg 1987; 44:253.
11. Perry A, Dean BS, Krenzelok EP. Drug-induced esophageal injury. Clin Toxicol 1989; 27:281.
12. Rohrmann CA Jr, Acheson MB. Esophageal perforation during double-contrast esophagram. Am J Roentgenol 1985; 145:283.
13. Rothstein C. Caustic injuries to the esophagus in children. Pediatr Clin North Am 1986; 33:665.
14. Singh GS, Slovis CM. "Occult" Boerhaave's syndrome. J Emerg Med 1988; 6:13.
15. Van der Zee DC, Festen C, Severijnen RSVM, van der Staak FHJ. Management of pediatric esophageal perforation. Thorac Cardiovasc Surg 1988; 95:692.
16. Weigelt JA, Thal ER, Snyder WH, et al. Diagnosis of penetrating cervical esophageal injuries. Am J Surg 1987; 154:619.

CHAPTER 11

Cardiac Trauma

GEORGE MILLER, M.D.

Cardiac injuries occur in up to 20% of patients with significant blunt chest trauma. The spectrum of blunt cardiac injury ranges from arrhythmias, which have no demonstrable cardiac muscle injury, to traumatic rupture of the myocardium, with minor contusions being far more common than more severe injuries. The diagnosis of minor cardiac contusions rests on physical examination, electrocardiography, and serial cardiac enzyme analysis. Although technetium pyrophosphate scanning may be helpful in documenting large areas of myocardial injury and in determining the distribution of injured tissue, this information is not essential to the acute care of these patients, and technetium pyrophosphate imaging has proved to be relatively insensitive in detecting clinical myocardial contusion. Magnetic resonance (MR) imaging may prove to be more sensitive in the detection of injured myocardial tissue, but MR imaging must be considered investigational for the evaluation of cardiac contusions at this time.

Severe cardiac contusions may result in decreased cardiac output and cardiac chamber enlargement and cause the plain film findings of congestive heart failure. The plain film findings are nonspecific, and therefore this diagnosis remains almost entirely in the realm of the clinician.

Severe crushing or deceleration injuries may result in rupture of the myocardium. If the rupture involves the free wall of a heart chamber, then acute cardiac tamponade results. If the rupture involves the atrial or the ventricular septum, then the patient may develop clinical and radiographic signs of an acute left-to-right shunt.

Penetrating injuries of the heart usually result in cardiac tamponade, although rarely a left-to-right shunt can occur in the absence of tamponade (Fig. 11–1). Gunshot wounds to the heart can infrequently result in the lodging of bullet fragments within a cardiac chamber or in the wall of the heart itself. More commonly, intracardiac bullet fragments are the result of a peripheral venous penetration with central embolization of the bullet fragment (Fig. 11–2). Intracardiac fragments can be retrieved using percutaneous catheter techniques (Fig. 11–3).

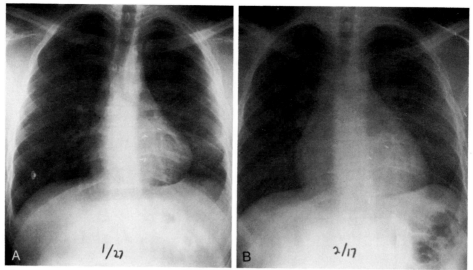

FIGURE 11–1. Left-to-Right Shunt

• • • •

A, This patient was admitted 5 days before this chest x-ray with a stab wound on the left side of the chest. The patient was taken directly to the operating room because of hypotension and a 2500-ml blood output from the left chest tube. A cardiac injury was found and repaired. This film was taken prior to the patient's discharge. *B*, This chest x-ray was obtained 3 weeks later when the patient returned for a clinic visit. He was found to have a holosystolic murmur. Note the interval cardiac enlargement and the development of "shunt" pulmonary vascularity. At repeat thoracotomy the patient was found to have a perforation of Valsalva's sinus which communicated with the right ventricle.

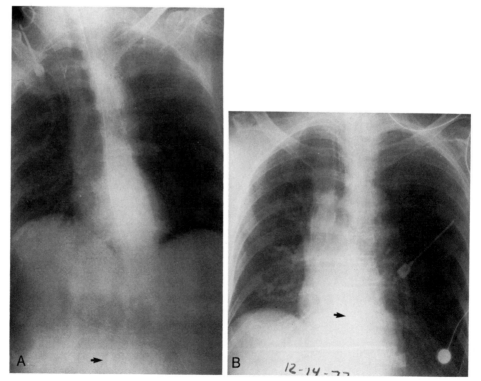

FIGURE 11–2. Peripheral Venous Penetration with Central Embolization of the Bullet Fragments

• • • •

A, This patient sustained a gunshot wound to the abdomen. The paper clip marks the abdominal entrance wound. On this initial film, the bullet is seen in the middle of the abdomen (*arrow*). Surgical repair of the liver, the pancreas, and a tear in the inferior vena cava was performed. *B*, Several days later the bullet had embolized to the right ventricle (*arrow*).

372

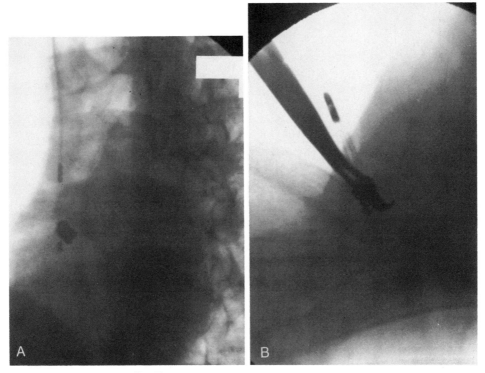

FIGURE 11–3. Retrieval of an Intracardiac Fragment

• • • •

A, This patient was shot in the right groin. Surgical exploration of the groin wound discovered a common femoral arteriovenous fistula (which was repaired). The postoperative chest x-ray showed that the bullet had embolized to the right atrium. A retrieval basket was advanced through a 10 French sheath from the right internal jugular vein to the right atrium. The bullet was trapped in the basket and pulled into the end of the sheath. *B*, Because the bullet was too large to be removed through the sheath, the entire complex was withdrawn into the soft tissues of the neck. The irregularity of the bullet fragment prevented its passage through the soft tissues of the neck, but blunt dissection around the sheath under fluoroscopic guidance allowed successful delivery of the fragment.

Bibliography

Saunders CR, Doty DB. Myocardial contusion. Surg Gynecol Obstet 1977; 144:595–603.

Gay W. Blunt trauma to the heart and great vessels. Surgery 1982; 91:507–509.

Liedke A, Demuth WE. Nonpenetrating cardiac injuries: A collective review. Am Heart J 1973; 86:687–697.

Go RT, Doty DB, Chiu CL, Christie JH. A new method of diagnosing myocardial contusion in man by radionuclide imaging. Radiology 1975; 116:107–110.

SECTION

· ·

FOUR

Abdomen

· · · · · · · · · · ·

CHAPTER 12

The Gastrointestinal System

HELEN C. REDMAN, M.D.

The hollow and the solid organs of the gastrointestinal tract are the major components of the abdomen. There are, however, other aspects of the abdomen that sometimes need radiographic evaluation. These include the abdominal wall itself, the peritoneal space, the pregnant uterus, the adrenal glands, and, of course, the major blood vessels within the abdomen. Evaluation of the blood vessels is considered primarily in Chapter 14 on vascular trauma. As opposed to the genitourinary tract, which has many components that need to be studied by differing radiographic techniques, the procedures applicable to the remainder of the abdomen are relatively similar for most of the involved structures.

RADIOLOGIC STUDIES

Plain Films

Before the development of computed tomography (CT) and ultrasound, evaluation of abdominal plain films was an important primary approach in the evaluation of abdominal trauma. A very fine textbook

on the radiology of abdominal trauma using plain films by James J. McCort was the bible for many radiology residents. However, the plain film, while still useful in the initial evaluation of abdominal trauma, has assumed a markedly decreased significance, primarily because of CT.

The supine film of the abdomen is usually the first radiograph that is obtained. This film should include the diaphragm and extend to the symphysis pubis. It must be of excellent radiographic quality so that subtle differentiation in soft tissues is possible. The second film that is desirable is either an upright or a decubitus film. The primary purpose of these projections is to detect free air within the abdomen. Once again the technique must be meticulous, and the centering of the film must be appropriate for the chosen projection. If a decubitus film is taken, it is helpful to have the patient lie on his side for some minutes prior to taking the film. The delay allows time for small amounts of free air to collect, thus increasing the chance of its detection. The upright abdominal film should be centered to include the dome of the diaphragm at the top of the film. Once again, having the patient in an upright position for a period of time prior to making the exposure is useful.

• • • • APPROPRIATE RADIOGRAPHIC STUDIES

I. **Plain Films**
   A. Supine abdominal (kidney-ureter-bladder) film
      1. May demonstrate fluid in the peritoneal cavity.
      2. May demonstrate free air.
      3. May demonstrate change in organ contour.
      4. May show fractures of the lower ribs, the spine, and the pelvis.
      5. May aid in evaluation of bowel gas pattern.
   B. Decubitus or upright abdominal film
      1. May be used primarily to detect a small amount of free air.
      2. Demonstrates fluid levels in the bowel.
   Comment: Delayed filming increases the chance of detecting free air. Keeping the patient in position for 20 minutes is recommended.

II. **Contrast Studies of the Stomach and the Small and the Large Bowel**
   A. Water-soluble agents should be used if perforation is a concern.
   B. Barium-based agents provide better examination when perforation is not a concern.
   Comment: Both types of contrast media interfere with computed tomography (CT). Barium can interfere with ultrasound imaging. Contrast examinations are rarely performed acutely at this time.

III. **Ultrasound**
   A. Fluid collections and parenchymal disruptions are well demonstrated.
   B. Although used extensively in Europe in the acute evaluation of trauma, this technique is used more often in the United States to follow known injury.
   C. A successful study depends on the skill and experience of the operator.
   D. Bowel contents and patient pain may limit its effectiveness.

IV. **Computed Tomography**
   A. This is the primary radiologic technique to evaluate intra-abdominal injury at the present time.
   B. Evaluation of all solid organs is excellent but is less specific for hollow viscus and mesenteric injuries.
   C. Both oral and intravenous contrast agents should be used whenever possible.
   D. The procedure is very short and requires little patient cooperation.

V. **Angiography**
   A. Indications for use as a primary diagnostic technique at present are rare.
   B. Angiographic interventional techniques may be needed acutely to control hemorrhage.

VI. **Magnetic Resonance Imaging**
   Comment: At present this technique is virtually never indicated for acute gastrointestinal injury. Patient monitoring is cumbersome, units are often not staffed 24 hours daily, and information derived is not more useful than that available with CT. These factors may change over the next few years.

VII. **Scintigraphy**
   A. Demonstrates hepatic and splenic injuries.
   B. Little detail is shown, and no ancillary information is obtained such as is gained from CT or ultrasound.
   C. This procedure is often used to evaluate the course of treatment following injury.

Contrast Studies

Contrast studies of the stomach and of the small and the large bowel can be obtained if there is concern for bowel wall injury. If bowel integrity is of concern, water-soluble contrast agents are preferable to barium-based contrast agents. However, the use of either barium-based or water-soluble contrast agents for evaluation of the bowel interferes seriously with CT; the use of barium-based contrast agents also interferes with ultrasound. Therefore, although at some point in the evaluation of a specific patient these procedures may be required, other studies should be considered and performed first when they are indicated. If a contrast study of the bowel is planned, it should be tailored for the area of concern. As little contrast material as is needed to answer the questions being asked should be used. Seriously injured patients often have a paralytic ileus of the small and the large bowel and sometimes even of the stomach. Barium in these circumstances can inspissate and cause further difficulties for the patient.

Ultrasound

Ultrasound is used extensively in Europe and to some extent in the United States for evaluation of acute injury to the spleen and the liver. Fluid collections and parenchymal disruptions are reliably identified. Ultrasound examinations are not infrequently limited by pain caused by the pressure of the transducer against the bruised abdominal wall or against any broken ribs. Bowel gas can also limit the procedure. In the United States ultrasound has been used more as a follow-up examination than as a primary diagnostic study because of the usefulness of CT scans in detecting injuries throughout the entire abdomen and the pelvis as well as those involving the retroperitoneum and the body wall.

Computed Tomography

CT is the primary radiologic survey technique for abdominal trauma. CT for abdominal trauma is generally performed following the ingestion of dilute contrast medium to opacify the bowel. Whenever feasible, enough time should be allowed between oral administration of the contrast material and performance of the CT scan for the contrast material to fill the small bowel. If needed, dilute contrast material can be instilled directly into the colon. The

procedure is also generally performed following intravenous injection of a bolus of 50–100 ml of 60% contrast material followed by an infusion of 100 ml or more of 30% contrast material during scanning. Scanning for abdominal trauma should start at the diaphragm. In general, 10-mm cuts at 10-mm intervals are performed at least to the lower pole of the kidneys. Depending on the nature of the trauma and the clinical concerns, the study may be continued in the same fashion or 10-mm sections at 20-mm intervals may be used until the symphysis is reached.

Angiography

Diagnostic angiography for abdominal injury is rarely indicated as CT identifies the vast majority of lesions. However, angiographic interventional techniques should be used in specific patients to occlude pseudoaneurysms, anteriovenous fistulas, or bleeding arteries within the abdominal cavity.

• • • •
RADIOGRAPHIC FINDINGS

Plain Films

The plain film findings of trauma are many, but few of these findings are specific (Fig. 12–1). Free air within the abdomen usually indicates a ruptured viscus when the patient has suffered blunt trauma. The absence of free air, however, does not exclude rupture of a hollow viscus. The small bowel, in particular, often does not contain enough air to be detected. Small perforations may not develop any free air at all. When there has been a penetrating injury, free air may be introduced by the actual penetration, but rupture of viscus is also a serious possibility. In fact, most patients with penetrating trauma undergo urgent surgical exploration, thus radiographic studies are generally not indicated. The majority of other observations within the abdomen following serious blunt trauma are caused by abnormal fluid collections and are nonspecific. The paracolic gutter may appear widened, and the properitoneal fat may be obscured. The ground-glass appearance of fluid within the abdomen may be seen. Clearly, ascites has an identical appearance. There may be obscuration of the edge of the liver or the tip of the spleen by fluid. Organomegaly is nonspecific unless a recent previous abdominal film has shown a normal liver or spleen and the current film demonstrates an unequivocal change. The bowel gas

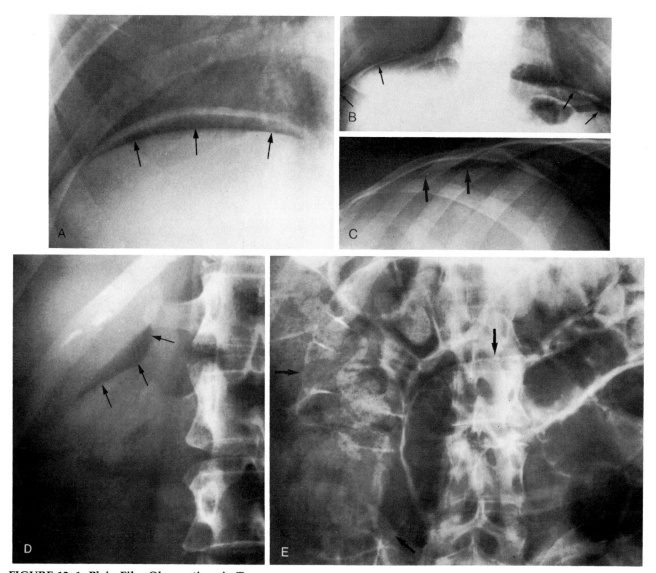

FIGURE 12–1. Plain Film Observations in Trauma

• • • •

A, Free air (*arrows*) is seen beneath the right hemidiaphragm on an upright chest film. *B,* A small collection of free air (*arrows*) is present under each hemidiaphragm. This upright chest film is underpenetrated for the abdomen so that the free air could easily be overlooked. *C,* A lateral decubitus view taken 20 minutes after the patient was placed left side down demonstrates a small collection of free air (*arrows*). *D,* A supine film of the abdomen demonstrates free air (*arrows*) in the subhepatic space. Such collections must be searched for with care since they are easily overlooked in the presence of an ileus. *E,* Massive free air is often difficult to detect on the supine abdominal film in an adult. This patient had a ruptured cecum with a massive pneumoperitoneum. The ability to see both sides of the bowel wall (*arrows*) is the most clear-cut evidence of free air on this film. The ileus makes evaluation of such a patient difficult.

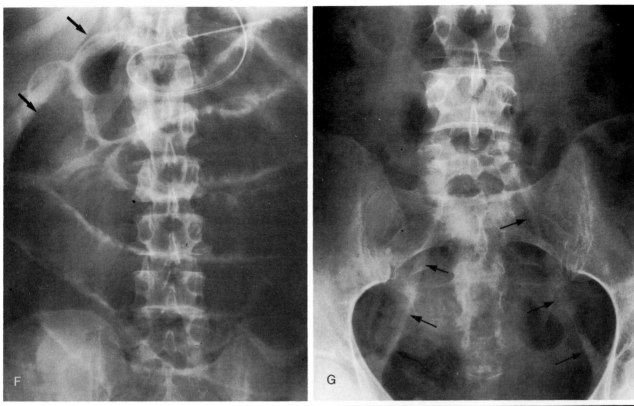

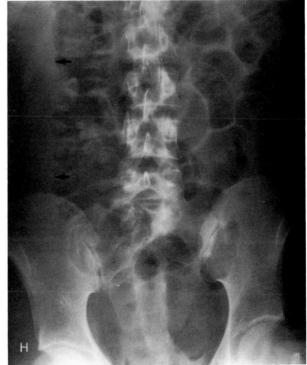

FIGURE 12–1 *Continued* **Plain Film Observations in Trauma**

• • • •

F, The ileus and a massive pneumoperitoneum are most easily identified by the subhepatic air collection (*arrows*). In addition, both sides of the wall can be seen. *G,* A massive pneumoperitoneum outlining the lateral umbilical ligaments (*arrows*) is seen. Little other evidence of pneumoperitoneum is visible on this supine film. *H,* Fluid in the paracolic gutters (*arrows*) is seen displacing the colon medially. The properitoneal fat line appears widened, indicating the presence of fluid (Film courtesy of J. Reynolds, M.D.).

pattern must also be carefully analyzed, since focal dilatation, paucity of gas, or ileus may help in the evaluation of trauma.

Contrast Studies

Probably the most frequent observation on contrast studies of the stomach and of the small and the large bowel is ileus and dilatation. This observation can be made with either barium-based or water-soluble agents, although the progressive dilution of the water-soluble agents in particular often decreases the value of the study. Other observations of importance include mural thickening, such as can be seen with duodenal hematomas and obstruction. Finally, extravasation of contrast material can occur. If bowel perforation is possible and a contrast study must be performed, water-soluble agents are preferable to barium-based ones.

It is critical to remember that all contrast media used for upper and lower gastrointestinal examinations seriously interfere with CT, and that barium-based media also interfere with ultrasound.

Ultrasound

Ultrasound findings of trauma are a shattered or disrupted parenchymal pattern and fluid collections either within or around the organ of interest. In general, ultrasound is more useful for following the treatment course of an injury than for making the original diagnosis, especially since CT is less demanding on the patient. The pressure of the transducer may cause pain or irritate a tender abdomen or a broken rib. CT is also much less dependent on the skill of the operator.

Computed Tomography

The findings of solid organ injury on CT scans are very similar to those described in the kidney (see Chapter 13). Both the liver and the spleen may have a mottled accumulation of contrast material that generally indicates contusion (Fig. 12–2). Actual lacerations cause linear, branching, or rounded areas of decreased CT density (Fig. 12–3). Acute hemorrhage in a noncontrast study is more dense (whiter) than the liver or the spleen. It is less easily recognized as blood following the use of intravenous contrast material, when it generally appears as a collection of fluid (Fig. 12–4). Measurement of the actual atten-

uation identifies blood. Frank hemorrhage at the moment of scanning appears as a higher attenuation focus. Fluid in the area immediately surrounding the liver and the spleen is frequently detected (Fig. 12–5), and, since fluid tends to collect in the most dependent portions of the abdomen, the pelvis should be carefully scrutinized for fluid collections in every patient with abdominal trauma (Fig. 12–6).

Evaluation of the hollow portions of the gastrointestinal tract by CT is less satisfactory. However, thickening of the bowel wall when the lumen is distended certainly suggests injury (Fig. 12–7). Mesenteric thickening also suggests injury. Unfortunately, injuries that involve serosal tears are very hard to detect on CT scans.

Pneumoperitoneum is easily seen on abdominal CT scans (Fig. 12–8). Any pneumoperitoneum that is seen on plain films is easily detected by CT and may even cause degradation of the image with motion. CT detects minute amounts of free air, which do not necessarily indicate bowel perforation. Pneumothorax can lead to pneumoperitoneum. A self-sealing microperforation of the bowel may do the same. In the female patient, air may also enter the peritoneal cavity through the fallopian tubes. In one study,[15] only 22% of patients with CT-detected pneumoperitoneum had significant bowel perforation. It is important, therefore, to evaluate CT-detected free

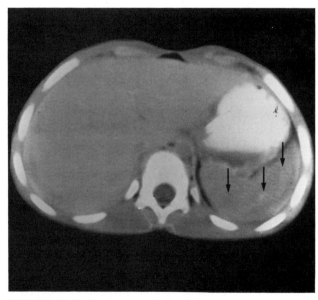

FIGURE 12–2. Contusion of the Spleen

• • • •

The splenic parenchyma has subtle mottled areas of decreased and increased attenuation that are typical of contusion (*arrows*). In addition, curvilinear high attenuation artifacts are seen between the ribs in both the liver and the spleen; they must not be confused with injury. (See also Figs. 12–9 and 12–18.)

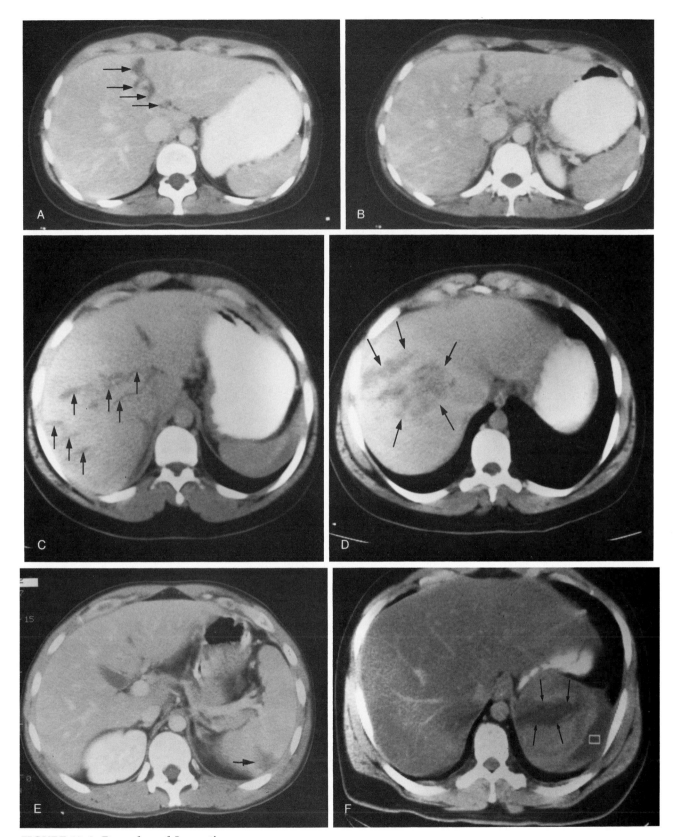

FIGURE 12–3. Parenchymal Lacerations

• • • •

A, This section taken through the liver demonstrates a jagged laceration (*arrows*) in the left lobe. *B,* A slightly lower section of the same injury demonstrates more ramifications of this stellate fracture. *C,* In a second patient, numerous linear fracture lines (*arrows*) in the right lobe of the liver radiate from near the porta to the periphery of the liver. *D,* A slightly higher section demonstrates areas of hemorrhage (*arrows*) within the liver. *E,* The splenic laceration (*arrow*) has jagged edges and is spread apart by hematoma. *F,* This patient with a fatty liver also has a complete transection of the spleen (*arrows*). The laceration is filled with hematoma, and there is blood around the spleen.

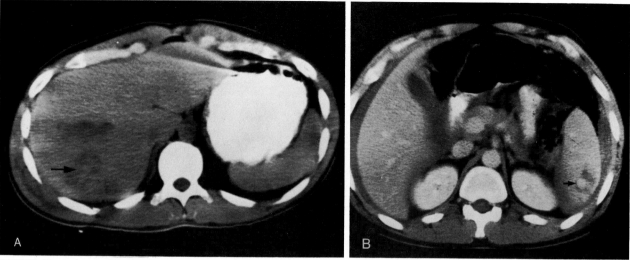

FIGURE 12–4. Acute Hemorrhage Demonstrated with the Use of an Intravenous Contrast Material
• • • •
A, Several hepatic lacerations filled with hematoma have a lower attenuation than the surrounding hepatic parenchyma. One has a central higher attenuation area (*arrow*), probably due to bleeding at the precise time this section was made. *B*, A splenic laceration has a focal high-density area (*arrow*) surrounded by clot; this is again indicative of active hemorrhage. The fluid surrounding the liver and the spleen is also blood that has accumulated in the several hours since the injury.

intraperitoneal air in the context of the specific patient rather than to assume that the free air is synonymous with bowel perforation.

• • • •
LIVER

Plain Films

Evaluation of hepatic injury by plain films is generally unrevealing. The radiographic assessment of liver size is unreliable. Hemorrhage cannot be detected as such on plain films. However, a few observations can sometimes be made. The edge of the liver may be surrounded by fluid; this fluid obscures the fat that normally outlines this edge. If recent abdominal films are available, a marked change in the size or contour of the liver suggests acute hepatic enlargement from hemorrhage either in the subcapsular space or within the liver parenchyma. Air in the parenchyma of the liver, in the bile ducts, or in the portal veins implies serious injury. Portal vein air is most commonly caused by massive infection or devitalization of the bowel and rarely occurs from trauma. Penetrating injuries, especially those caused by high-velocity agents, can introduce air along their track. When there is concomitant right diaphragmatic laceration, the liver may appear to be positioned very high against an elevated hemidiaphragm. Although the liver can herniate through a diaphragmatic laceration, this is an uncommon occurrence. In essence,

the most frequent plain film observation with hepatic injury is that of fluid in the abdomen. This can obscure the edge of the liver or layer in the paracolic gutters lateral to the ascending or the descending colon, obscuring the properitoneal fat. Fluid may also collect in the pelvis, the most dependent portion of the peritoneal cavity. It collects above the bladder, but it is separated from the bladder by perivesical fat. The whimsical "dog's ears" sign is produced by fluid layering in the pelvic recesses lateral to the colon and superior to the bladder. Massive fluid from liver injury can cause the radiographic findings of ascites with the small bowel loops floating toward the midline.

When plain radiographs are obtained to search for trauma, the bones must always be scrutinized. When hepatic injury is of primary concern, right lower rib fractures are an important observation. Rib fragments can cause hepatic laceration. They also clearly show a point of impact. Fractures of the lower thoracic and the lumbar spine also indicate that the injury has been severe, increasing the possibility of hepatic or other soft tissue injury.

Computed Tomography

CT is the technique of choice for the evaluation of acute hepatic trauma. Generally, the scan is performed after both oral and intravenous administration of contrast material, although when necessary a noncontrast examination can be performed. The ab-

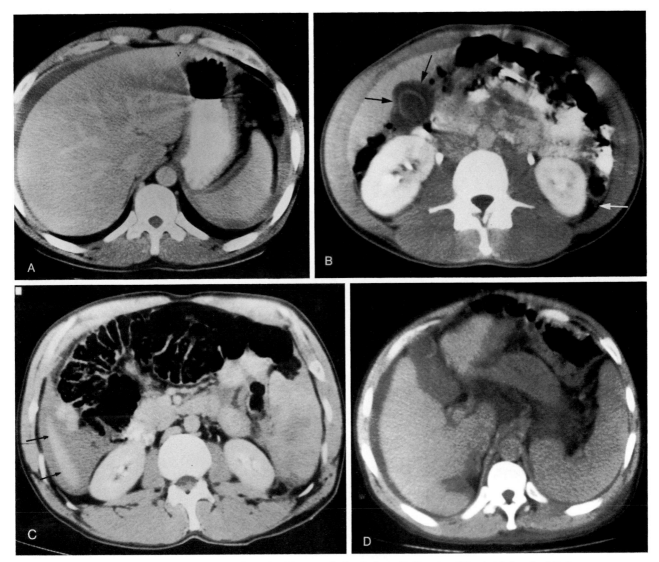

FIGURE 12–5. Hemoperitoneum Surrounding the Liver and the Spleen Following Blunt Abdominal Injury

• • • •

A, Fluid surrounds both the liver and the spleen in this patient. Fluid also surrounds the bowel loops in the left upper quadrant. The collection lateral to the liver had a density measurement of 36 H, which is indicative of blood. *B,* There is a smaller amount of free blood in this patient that has collected primarily around the gallbladder (*black arrows*). A tiny amount of fluid is seen adjacent to the bowel loops (*white arrow*). Lower sections demonstrate a modest hemoperitoneum in the pelvis. *C,* In contrast, this patient with a severe splenic injury had a massive hemoperitoneum. Blood is seen surrounding the tip of the liver (*arrows*). *D,* It is critical to remember that any intraperitoneal fluid can mimic a hemoperitoneum. This patient has extensive fluid and was seen following a high-speed motor vehicle accident in which he was thrown from the car and hit a bridge abutment. The density of this fluid looks like that of the earlier illustrations, but the measurement is 6 H. This patient has ascites, not hemoperitoneum. Fluid attenuation should be measured routinely in such patients.

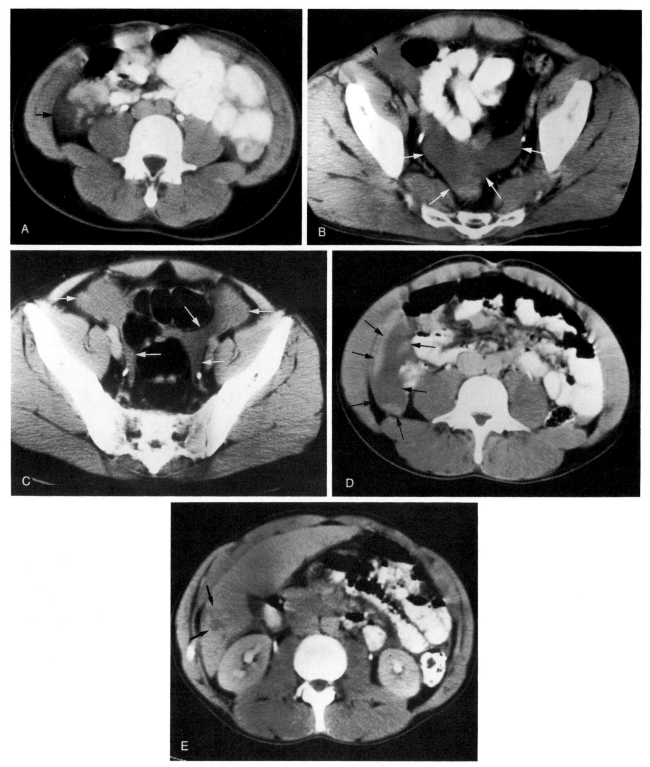

FIGURE 12–6. Hemoperitoneum with Fluid in the Dependent Portions of the Peritoneal Cavity

• • • •

A, This patient had a liver laceration after an aggravated assault. Hemoperitoneum was limited, but there is fluid in the paracolic gutter (*arrow*). *B,* Free fluid (*white arrows*) is present in the pelvis following splenic laceration. There is also hemoperitoneum anteriorly on the right (*black arrow*). *C,* Hemoperitoneum is seen surrounding the bowel loops (*arrows*). *D,* A large paracolic fluid collection (*arrows*) with varying densities is seen in this patient with a liver laceration. *E,* The liver laceration (*arrows*) is easily seen, but there is virtually no fluid around the liver. Dependent areas of the abdomen should be searched for the presence of fluid during computed tomography performed for trauma.

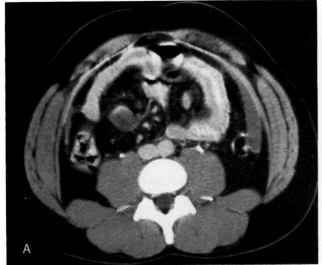

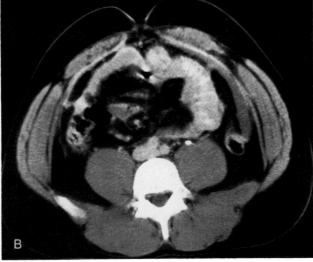

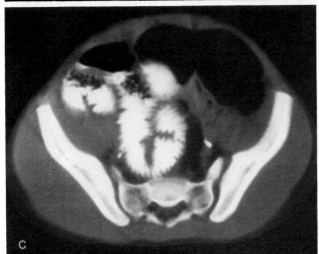

FIGURE 12–7. Bowel Injury

• • • •

This computed tomography scan was performed about 4 hours after blunt abdominal injury. *A,* The striking finding on the first section is an edematous small bowel. There is some cloudiness in the mesentery. The peritoneum is enhanced, an unusual finding in trauma. *B,* A lower section again demonstrates the edematous bowel and the cloudy mesentery. These findings, along with the intraperitoneal free fluid and free air identified on other sections, should raise suspicion for bowel injury. At surgery, two small bowel perforations and several mesenteric tears were found. *C,* This 8-year-old child had mesenteric tears and a single small bowel perforation. The small bowel is edematous, and there is colonic distention. No free air or fluid was identified.

FIGURE 12–8. Pneumoperitoneum

• • • •

A, This section displays a modest amount of intraperitoneal free air (*arrows*). There is also hemoperitoneum. The scan was otherwise unremarkable, but two small bowel perforations were found during surgery. *B,* Very small amounts of intraperitoneal air must be interpreted with caution. This section demonstrates a small collection of free air (*arrow*). The patient is a 5-year-old child who had a pneumomediastinum and no abdominal injury. The sensitivity of computed tomography to air makes it possible to identify air dissecting from the mediastinum and the thoracic cavity.

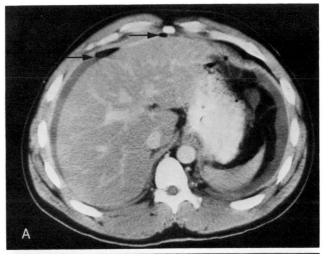

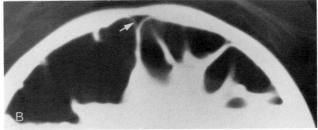

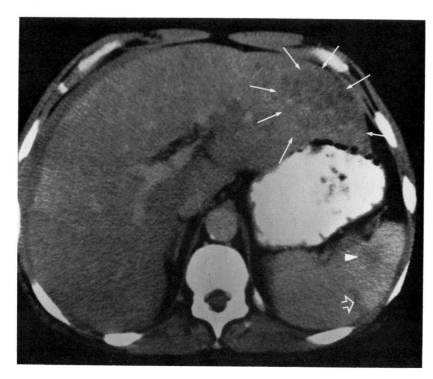

FIGURE 12–9. Hepatic Contusion
• • • •

This computed tomography section demonstrates mottling of the lateral portion of the left lobe of the liver (*arrows*). This appearance is typical of contusion. In addition, there is a splenic laceration (*open arrow*), a small splenic hematoma (*arrowhead*), and hemoperitoneum.

sence of contrast material in the bowel diminishes the accuracy of detection of small amounts of intraperitoneal fluid. Occasional parenchymal lacerations are missed, but larger hematomas generally are detected because they are hyperdense to the unenhanced liver.

Hepatic contusion is seen on a contrast-enhanced CT scan as a poorly defined area of mottled increased density (Fig. 12–9). This observation can be very subtle, and unless other more serious hepatic injuries are present it is very easy to miss. Careful recording of the CT scan at appropriate windows and levels is important in these patients.

Hepatic subcapsular hematomas are seen as low-density crescentic or biconvex collections at the periphery of the liver (Fig. 12–10). Size is highly variable and may be massive. If the patient is actively bleeding at the time of CT, the bleeding point may be seen as extravasated contrast and the subcapsular collection may not be homogeneous. A hepatic subcapsular hematoma may also become nonhomogeneous as it resolves. When CT is performed without contrast enhancement or if the patient is severely anemic or has a fatty liver, the subcapsular hematoma often has increased density relative to the liver.

Hepatic lacerations (Fig. 12–11) can have many configurations and may be multiple. In children, a stellate pattern is often seen. The lacerations are relatively linear and are generally of lower CT density than liver parenchyma on contrast-enhanced scans.

In severe trauma, not only can the liver parenchyma be injured but the bile ducts and the gallbladder may also be avulsed or torn. The CT number of blood is higher than that of bile, so fluid from these two sources can sometimes be distinguished. However, admixture of blood and bile occurs frequently, so that the density difference is not reliable. The

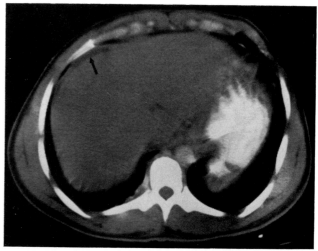

FIGURE 12–10. Hepatic Subcapsular Hematoma
• • • •

A small crescentic collection of blood (*arrow*) that is contained by the hepatic capsule is seen. Subcapsular hematomas may be small, as in this patient, or very large. Early on the configuration is crescentic, but it becomes biconvex with age. Some very large acute collections are also biconvex.

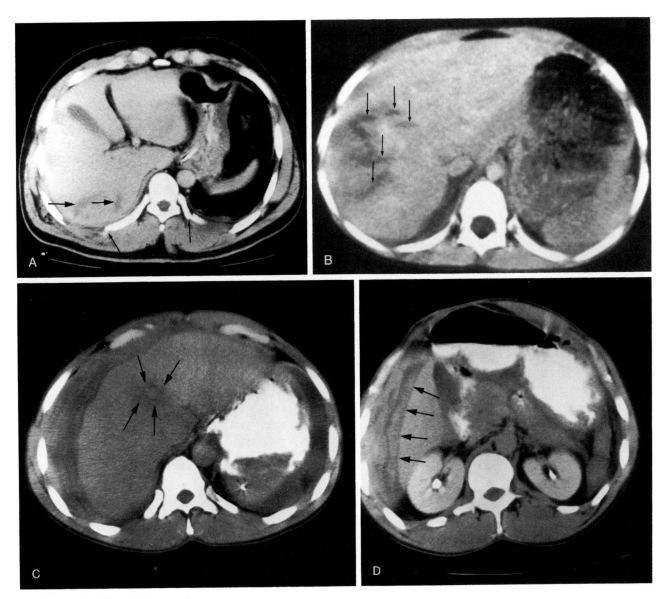

FIGURE 12–11. Hepatic Laceration

• • • •

A, Two lacerations in the dorsal aspect of the right lobe of the liver are demonstrated on this single section (*large arrows*). Though there is hematoma in the lacerations, no associated hemoperitoneum is seen in this patient. Bilateral rib fractures are present (*small arrows*). B, This 8-year-old child has numerous lacerations (*arrows*) associated with diffuse parenchymal disruption, which is seen as mottled high- and lower-density areas. C, This patient has a single laceration that extends from the hepatic capsule centrally. On all sections it was rather poorly defined, as is evident here (*arrows*); a higher density center is demonstrated, which is suggestive of acute bleeding. D, Both this section and the previous one demonstrate laminated blood lateral to the liver. The edge of the liver appears to be straightened in this lower section, suggesting that there is a subcapsular component as well as hemoperitoneum (*arrows*); this finding was confirmed at surgery.

gallbladder should always be identified on CT scans performed for abdominal injury unless it has been surgically removed.

Angiography

Hepatic angiography (Fig. 12–12) was at one time the primary technique for detailed evaluation of

hepatic injury. When properly performed, an angiogram can demonstrate subcapsular hematomas and vascular injuries with regularity. Parenchymal lacerations and contusions are more subtle and are often identified by disruption of the normal hepatic arterial supply or an irregular parenchymal phase. Focal early hepatic vein filling can also be seen.

At present, angiography should not be used as the primary diagnostic technique in hepatic trauma be-

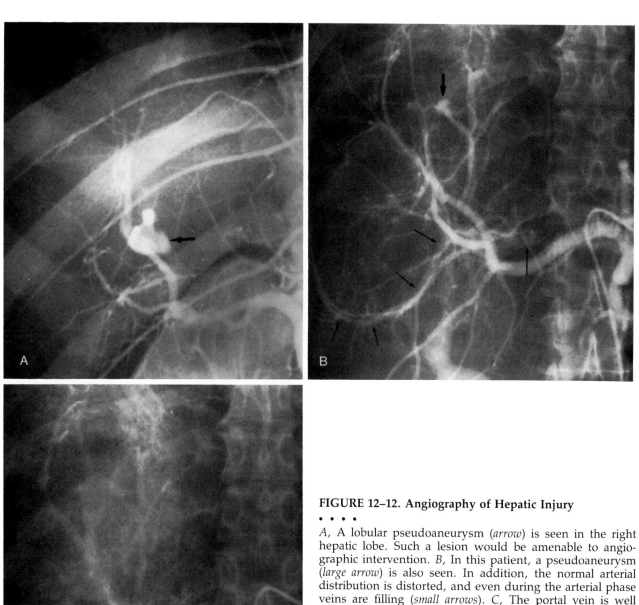

FIGURE 12–12. Angiography of Hepatic Injury

• • • •

A, A lobular pseudoaneurysm (*arrow*) is seen in the right hepatic lobe. Such a lesion would be amenable to angiographic intervention. *B,* In this patient, a pseudoaneurysm (*large arrow*) is also seen. In addition, the normal arterial distribution is distorted, and even during the arterial phase veins are filling (*small arrows*). *C,* The portal vein is well filled on an early parenchymal phase film. The patient had extensive liver lacerations, which caused the arteriovenous shunting, the arterial distortion, and the pseudoaneurysm.

cause CT is far more sensitive, faster, more comprehensive, and less invasive. The role of hepatic angiography is now primarily therapeutic, since pseudoaneurysms, arteriovenous fistulas, and acute bleeding sites can often be definitively treated by angiographic embolization. Such embolization may be performed shortly after the injury or days or weeks later (Fig. 12–13). The embolic material used depends on the precise problem. In general, short-lived embolic material, such as gelatin sponge, controls the bleeding, but delivery of this material may be more difficult than polyvinyl alcohol particles, which can be flow-directed from a site at some distance from the bleeding vessel. Treatment of ar-

teriovenous fistulas may require detachable balloons or coils. The hepatic artery can be occluded without risk only when the portal vein is patent. The liver receives about 70% of its blood supply from the portal vein. When the portal vein is occluded, embolization of the hepatic artery carries a very high risk of hepatic infarction and necrosis.

Hepatic Scintigraphy

Radionuclide studies of hepatic trauma are quite successful in demonstrating the presence of hepatic

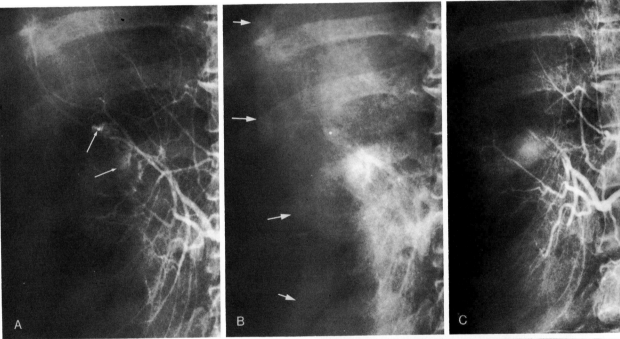

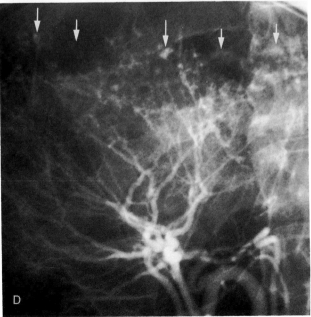

FIGURE 12–13. Embolization of Acute Hepatic Bleeding

• • • •

A, The arterial phase of a common hepatic angiogram demonstrates frank extravasation (*arrows*) from a peripheral right hepatic arterial branch. In addition, the hepatic arterial branches are displaced medially and splayed by a large subcapsular hematoma. *B,* The parenchymal phase demonstrates the displacement of the liver (*arrows*) medially by the large subcapsular hematoma. *C,* The right hepatic artery was embolized with flow-directed small particle polyvinyl alcohol, which occluded the feeding artery but spared most of the hepatic arterial supply. *D,* Another patient with a history of alcohol abuse and several falls was brought to the emergency room in shock after falling down stairs. The angiogram demonstrates an extensive subcapsular hematoma with multiple bleeding sites (*arrows*). In all probability, this is an acute subcapsular hemorrhage superimposed on a chronic one; this assessment is supported by the presence of the increased vascularity at the edge of the liver. It was successfully embolized with gelatin sponge pieces.

injury and can often define the type of injury that has occurred. The spleen can be evaluated at the same time. The drawback of hepatic scintigraphy is its lack of detail. It is very difficult to derive anatomic data or to evaluate the severity of the injury to aid in treatment planning. Therefore, although hepatic scans are sometimes used to follow liver injury, scintigraphy is not a primary diagnostic modality in the emergency setting unless no other technique is available.

Ultrasound

Ultrasound is very accurate in detecting hepatic parenchymal disruption and in finding free fluid and loculated fluid collections. It can also evaluate the gallbladder and larger bile ducts. There are two primary drawbacks to the use of ultrasound during emergency evaluation. First, the pressure of the transducer on the bruised abdominal wall or near broken ribs may cause the patient to be uncooperative, degrading the examination or even making it impossible to complete. At the same time, the adynamic ileus, which often accompanies abdominal trauma, can also limit the ultrasound examination. The second drawback is that ultrasound is very dependent on the skill of the operator. Experienced ultrasonographers are frequently not readily available in an emergency.

Ultrasound is a fine modality for observing the healing of hepatic injury when conservative nonoperative therapy is chosen. It is also useful in detecting delayed complications when the patient is often able to be more cooperative.

• • • •
SPLEEN

The spleen is frequently injured by blunt abdominal trauma that may seem to be minor. Splenic injury in a 10-year-old boy who falls off his bicycle, striking his left side against the curb or the handlebars, is a typical example. Motor vehicle accidents are another frequent source of splenic injury. Following serious trauma, the patient is usually seen in an emergency room shortly after the injury. However, after less obvious injury, the patient may not come to the emergency room for hours or days after the event when left upper quadrant discomfort either does not go away or increases.

Plain Films

Abdominal films cannot make a definitive diagnosis of splenic injury, although there are several observations that may support the clinical suspicion. The normal spleen can be seen on only slightly more than one half of all abdominal films. Therefore, inability to see a spleen cannot be considered abnormal, but visualization of a sharply defined, normal-sized spleen diminishes the chance of injury. In the appropriate clinical setting, visualization of an enlarged and poorly defined spleen increases the chance of injury. When previous abdominal films are available for comparison, change in splenic size or contour also supports the diagnosis. Intraperitoneal fluid is nonspecific but may indicate injury. Oddly, splenic hemorrhage is infrequently retroperitoneal, thus obscuration of the left kidney or other evidence of retroperitoneal hemorrhage suggests injury other than to the spleen. Lower left rib fractures are an important observation and correlate with an increased likelihood of splenic injury.

Chest films may also demonstrate the spleen. Evidence of injury to the left lower lobe of the lung, the left ribs, or the left hemidiaphragm also increases the likelihood of splenic injury.

Computed Tomography

CT is the primary diagnostic modality for splenic trauma. Preferably, CT is performed after the administration of oral contrast material to aid in identification of intraperitoneal fluid and with the use of intravenous contrast material. Generally, 10-mm scans at 10-mm increments provide the diagnosis, but thinner sections may be needed on occasion. Dynamic CT may also increase diagnostic sensitivity. If the patient has a nasogastric tube in place it is important to pull the tube back into the esophagus to avoid artifacts (Fig. 12–14). In general, the spleen is studied during a complete abdominal CT examination rather than in an isolated fashion.

Fluid collections within the spleen, in the subcapsular space, or within the peritoneal cavity should be carefully sought (Fig. 12–15). Although free fluid is often identified in the left upper quadrant in the presence of splenic injury, it may be seen in any dependent portion of the abdomen or pelvis. Since this fluid is blood, it has a moderately high CT density.

The spleen itself may be lacerated (Fig. 12–16). Lacerations are seen as low-density, generally linear

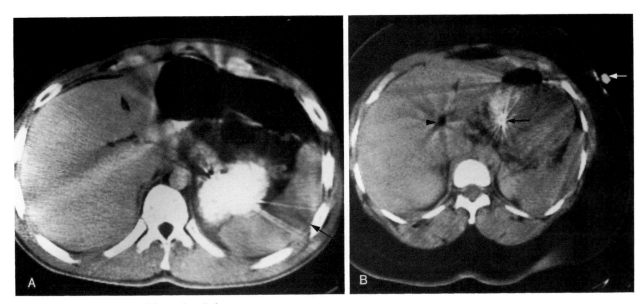

FIGURE 12–14. Artifacts Obscuring Injury

• • • •

A, The dense contrast material in the nondistended stomach and the nasogastric tube produced spray artifacts that obscure the splenic laceration (*arrow*). Less obtrusive artifacts can be seen arising from the distended colon. *B,* In addition to the spray artifact from the nasogastric tube (*black arrow*), this patient has artifacts from a superficial line (*white arrow*) and from air in the bile ducts at the hilum of the liver (*arrowhead*). The first two can be removed, resulting in an improved image.

FIGURE 12–15. Hemo-peritoneum in Splenic Trauma

• • • •

Hemoperitoneum caused by splenic trauma may be minor, but massive hemoperitoneum may also occur as it has in this patient who has blood (*arrows*) filling the pelvis. Free blood may be seen only adjacent to the spleen but often is found around the liver or the surrounding bowel. (See also Fig. 12–5.)

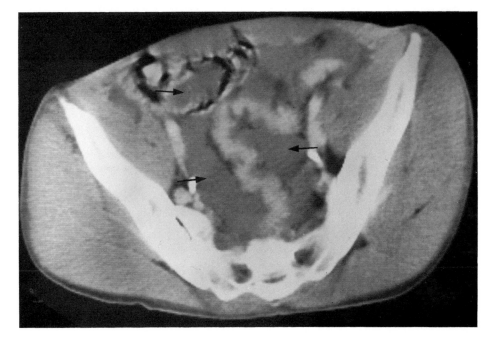

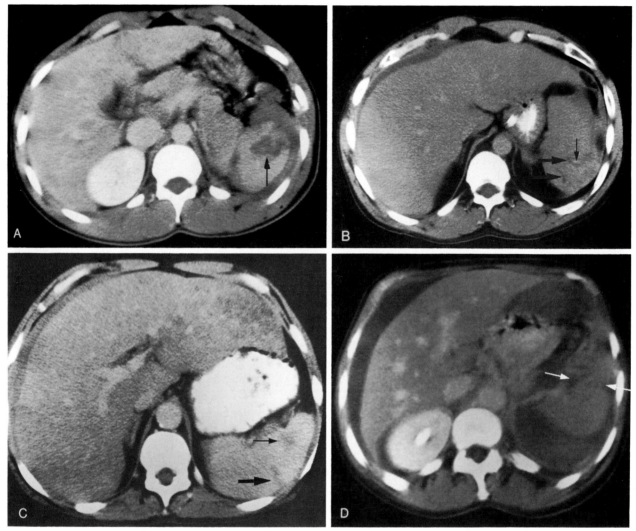

FIGURE 12–16. Splenic Laceration

• • • •

A, A jagged splenic laceration (*arrow*) extends from the capsule toward the splenic hilum. It is filled with lower-density blood or clot. Blood also surrounds the lateral and the ventral aspects of the spleen. *B*, Two fine linear lacerations (*large arrows*) are present in the dorsal aspect of the spleen. The more ventral laceration has an area of increased density within it (*small arrow*), indicative of active bleeding. Free fluid obscures the splenic margin laterally and is also present around the liver. *C*, This patient has both a splenic laceration (*large arrow*) and an area of low density that is probably an intrasplenic hematoma (*small arrow*). Hepatic contusion and fluid around the liver are also seen. (See also Fig. 12–9.) *D*, The splenic laceration in this patient extends completely through the parenchyma (*arrows*). There is a massive hemoperitoneum.

defects in the spleen. Lacerations may be single or multiple, and they may be straight, jagged, or stellate. They may be so numerous that the spleen is fragmented. Lacerations may tear the splenic capsule, in which case peritoneal fluid is generally present, or they may not tear the capsule at all.

Subcapsular hematomas are crescentic or biconvex collections of blood lying between the splenic parenchyma and the capsule (Fig. 12–17). There may be an associated laceration or contusion, but the spleen may appear to be otherwise normal. Dynamic CT with bolus enhancement sometimes reveals an active

bleeding site into a subcapsular hematoma which is seen as a focal high density within the hematoma.

Splenic contusion causes mottling of the splenic parenchyma that is often quite subtle (Fig. 12–18). Contusion may occur as an isolated injury, but it is usually associated with more definitive abnormalities.

The developmental variations of the spleen along its superolateral margin are numerous. They are caused by differing degrees of fusion and are called *fetal lobulations* (Fig. 12–19). These lobulations can simulate lacerations or small fluid collections on CT

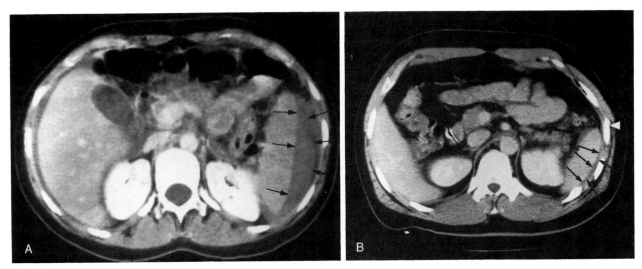

FIGURE 12–17. Splenic Subcapsular Hematoma

• • • •

A, A large subcapsular hematoma (*arrows*) has a crescentic configuration. The splenic parenchyma is displaced medially, and free fluid is also present. *B,* This patient, on the contrary, has a very small subcapsular hematoma (*arrows*), which was the only observation on the entire computed tomography scan except for left rib fractures (*arrowhead*). A small splenic laceration was repaired during surgery.

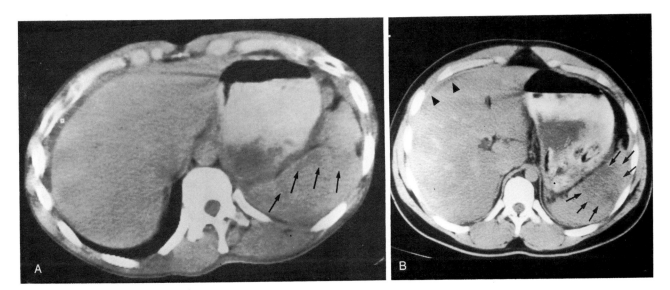

FIGURE 12–18. Splenic Contusion

• • • •

A, This section illustrates the difficulty frequently encountered in detecting splenic contusion. There is a vague higher-density artifact over the anterior and the lateral portion of the spleen caused by the position of the patient in the scanner. In addition, however, there are several poorly defined low-density areas (*arrows*); these are contusions. Hemoperitoneum is present. *B,* Although this patient required a splenectomy, computed tomography findings throughout the spleen are limited to poorly defined areas of decreased attenuation (*arrows*). Hemoperitoneum is also seen (*arrowheads*). The surgeon described complete disruption of the splenic parenchyma.

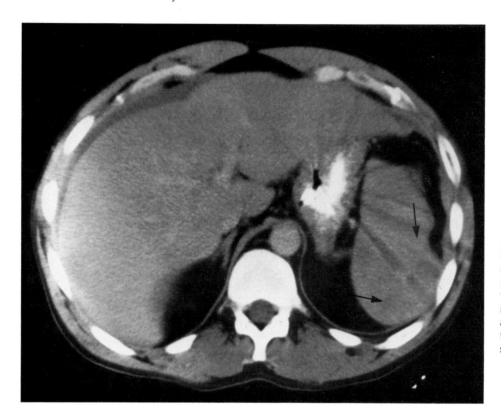

FIGURE 12–19. Splenic Fetal Lobulation

• • • •

The spleen normally fuses into one kidney-bean–shaped organ. However, the process of fusion has many variations, including the complete failure of fusion. These variations are seldom of concern at computed tomography but may cause a wavy anterolateral splenic margin as seen in this patient. Sharp, broad, well-defined clefts may also be encountered. This patient has a splenic contusion (*arrows*) as well as a laceration that was seen on lower sections. Note also the spray artifacts from the air in the nearly collapsed stomach.

scans. They are, however, sharply defined and have a typical location. When care is taken and additional sections are produced as necessary, it is usually possible to determine that these irregularities are fetal lobulations rather than actual laceration or hemorrhage.

Splenic salvage is very important, especially in children. In most trauma centers splenic repair is attempted in both children and adults whenever it appears feasible. Children do very well with conservative therapy and careful observation. Conservative therapy in adults has been less successful. To date, no reliable scheme has been developed to determine which splenic injuries do well with conservative therapy and which require splenorrhaphy or splenectomy. The apparent severity of splenic injury, the presence of associated injuries, and the amount of intraperitoneal blood all do not adequately predict which patients will do well with conservative therapy. Since splenorrhaphy is most successful shortly after the injury, the inability to accurately determine which patients will do well with conservative therapy is a significant problem in patient management. Until there is better understanding of delayed splenic rupture, many trauma centers will continue to handle splenic injury in the adult surgically.

Ultrasound

Ultrasound can demonstrate splenic parenchymal disruption, intrasplenic fluid collections, subcapsular hematomas, and perisplenic fluid very well. In fact, ultrasound is routinely used in Europe for this purpose. The drawbacks of ultrasound are that the study may be limited by pain caused by the transducer pressing on bruised abdominal wall or broken ribs. Ileus may also interfere with the study. Perhaps the greatest drawback is that this technique is very dependent on the skill of the operator, and an experienced ultrasonographer may be less readily available than a skilled interpreter of CT scans.

Ultrasound can be used to follow splenic injury when conservative therapy has been chosen, and it can be used as a guide to evacuate large splenic fluid collections.

Angiography

At one time angiography was the primary nonsurgical technique for the diagnosis of splenic injury. Selective celiac or splenic angiography when performed by an experienced angiographer is both sensitive and specific for this purpose. With the advent of CT, angiography is no longer indicated as a primary diagnostic modality for splenic trauma, although if angiography is being performed for other reasons, such as renal artery injury, the spleen can often be included in the study.

Splenic angiography can be effectively employed for splenic salvage because embolization of the splenic artery can control splenic parenchymal hemorrhage, generally without causing splenic infarction. In some situations, a more selective partial splenic embolization is feasible, again permitting splenic salvage. A current clinical challenge is to learn which splenic injuries benefit from angiographic embolization as opposed to splenorrhaphy or conservative therapy.

Splenic Scintigraphy

Scintigraphy of splenic injury in the acute phase is quite sensitive for injury but less specific than CT. Although the liver may be evaluated at the same time, the remainder of the abdomen and the retroperitoneum are not evaluated. Therefore, although an occasional patient may be better evaluated by scintigraphy because of claustrophobia, agitation, or instability, scintigraphy is rarely indicated as a primary diagnostic technique in splenic trauma. It can be used to follow the course of splenic injuries that are being treated conservatively and demonstrates progressive reconstitution of the spleen when healing progresses satisfactorily.

• • • •
PANCREAS

Injury to the pancreas is relatively rare, occurring in less than 2% of all abdominal trauma patients. The majority of these injuries are caused by penetrating wounds, which are almost universally explored shortly after admission to the emergency room. Blunt injury to the pancreas is more insidious and often accompanies other serious injuries that may divert attention from the pancreas. Severe abdominal pain, an elevated or rising amylase level, and other injuries in the region of the pancreas should all increase clinical concern for pancreatic injury. Pancreatic pseudocysts can become symptomatic days, weeks, or even years after the actual injury. CT is the primary imaging technique for acute pancreatic injury. However, a high index of suspicion

is probably most important in detecting pancreatic injury.

Plain Films

Plain films of the abdomen are virtually useless in diagnosis of pancreatic injury. When present, a dilated duodenum or proximal jejunum, or both, suggests pancreatic injury, but this finding is quite uncommon. Evidence of severe injury, such as fracture of the lumbar spine, increases the possibility of pancreatic injury. Pseudocysts usually take days or weeks to develop so that the presence of a midabdominal mass does not suggest acute pancreatic injury.

Ultrasound

On occasion, ultrasound can demonstrate acute pancreatic injury. Focal or diffuse enlargement of the pancreas is seen. In addition, subtle areas of decreased echogenicity may be present. These are caused either by frank laceration or by areas of fluid or hemorrhage. When seen, such findings are highly suggestive of pancreatic injury. Ultrasound of the pancreas in an acutely injured patient is often limited by abdominal tenderness, ileus, and bowel content. In general, it is more appropriately used in the follow-up evaluation of patients with pancreatic injury than to make the primary diagnosis.

Computed Tomography

CT is the most effective diagnostic procedure for pancreatic injury (Fig. 12–20). However, the CT findings of acute injury are often very subtle. The procedure should be performed after administration of both oral and intravenous contrast material. Good filling of the bowel loops immediately ventral to the pancreas permits an accurate evaluation of subtle pancreatic enlargement. The pancreas is seen on every abdominal CT scan performed for trauma. When there is specific clinical concern for pancreatic injury, added sections at 5-mm intervals should be considered.

The most common CT finding of pancreatic injury is diffuse mild or focal swelling. Retroperitoneal hemorrhage occurs, and the peripancreatic fat may be obscured. Thickening of the left anterior renal fascia should raise the question of pancreatic injury,

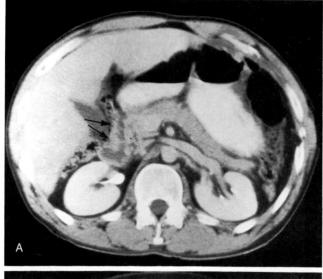

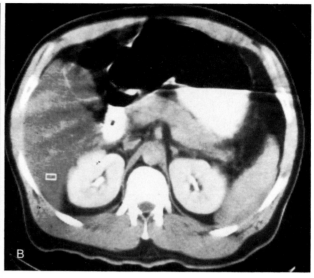

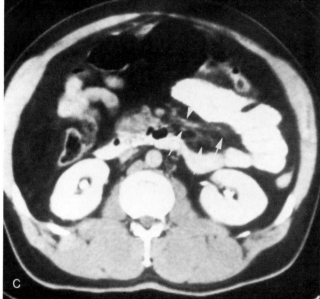

FIGURE 12–20. Pancreatic Injury

• • • •

A, The pancreas often is entirely normal on a computed tomography (CT) scan performed shortly after an injury. This patient developed fulminant acute pancreatitis within hours of this scan. The only questionable abnormality here is possible duodenal wall thickening (*arrows*), but the duodenum is not distended with the contrast medium so no credence can be placed in this finding. *B,* On the contrary, a diffusely and mildly enlarged pancreas with somewhat hazy edges, although seen in trauma, can also have other causes. This patient with a fatty liver had no history of pancreatitis before his trauma but developed clinical pancreatitis in the days immediately following this CT scan. *C,* A section through the pancreatic head on the same patient does demonstrate mild perivascular haziness (*arrows*) in the mesentery immediately caudal to the body and the tail.

as should thickening of the root of the mesentery. These findings can also be caused by injury to the bowel or to other retroperitoneal organs. Fractures of the pancreas are seen as disruptions of the pancreatic contour, but they may not be evident on an initial CT scan. When pancreatic injury is a serious concern but has not been confirmed, a follow-up CT scan at 24 hours or later may demonstrate infiltration of the peripancreatic fat with inflammatory changes or definite pancreatic swelling.

Angiography

Angiography has never been used as a primary diagnostic modality for pancreatic injury. Occasion-

ally, angiography performed for other reasons demonstrates vascular abnormalities in the pancreatic circulation or the parenchymal accumulation in the pancreas may reveal a laceration. A more common use of angiography is for the diagnosis of delayed bleeding days or weeks after the injury. At that time, interventional techniques may be appropriate.

Magnetic Resonance Imaging

At present, there is virtually no use for magnetic resonance (MR) imaging in the immediate acute evaluation of pancreatic injury. Although this may change with advances in both the scanning protocols and MR units, patients with pancreatic injury are currently better evaluated by a CT examination.

• • • •
BOWEL AND MESENTERY

The radiographic detection of significant injury to the stomach, the duodenum, and the small and the large bowel is fraught with hazard. Perforations that cause free air within the abdomen are straightforward. Exploration is mandatory. Unfortunately, perforations of the bowel do not always cause intraperitoneal free air, and not all serious bowel injuries are perforations. Therefore, other radiographic studies are necessary in the attempt to accurately detect bowel injury. The primary radiographic approaches include contrast examinations of the bowel and CT.

It is important to recognize the many possible types of injury that can occur to a hollow viscus. In addition to frank perforation, lacerations that are not transmural can occur. Intramural hematomas, most commonly encountered in the duodenum, can obstruct the bowel lumen. Bowel perforations can be retroperitoneal. The blood supply to a segment of bowel can be disrupted, leading to ischemia or infarction. Mesenteric tears can lead to internal hernias.

Plain Films

The primary observations on plain films include free air in the peritoneal space or air in the soft tissues of the retroperitoneum (Fig. 12–21) (especially in the region of the second portion of the duodenum) bowel gas pattern, and findings of intra-abdominal fluid. Extraluminal air in blunt trauma is almost always due to perforation of some portion of the intestinal tract, although in the very young, pneumomediastinum may dissect into the retroperitoneum and the abdomen. Decubitus and upright films are most appropriate when searching for free air, although free air can also be detected on a supine film (see Fig. 12–1). Visualization of both sides of the bowel wall or of the ligamentum arteriosum indicates free air (Fig. 12–22). Larger amounts of free air may cause an unusual lucency to the abdomen. In infants this is seen as the "football" sign. Distribution of bowel gas may suggest injury if a focal ileus is present, but this is very nonspecific. More important is bowel gas outlining a fixed mural mass or obstruction, such as might be caused by a duodenal hematoma. Free fluid is nonspecific but can be seen in bowel perforation. The absence of all of these obser-

vations in no way excludes serious bowel injury. It also should be remembered that intraperitoneal spill from small bowel injury is less voluminous than that from stomach or even colon injury.

Gastrointestinal Examinations

Water-soluble contrast studies or barium examinations can demonstrate mural abnormalities caused by trauma. If perforation is suspected, water-soluble agents are safer, but otherwise they provide less bowel definition than do the barium-based agents.

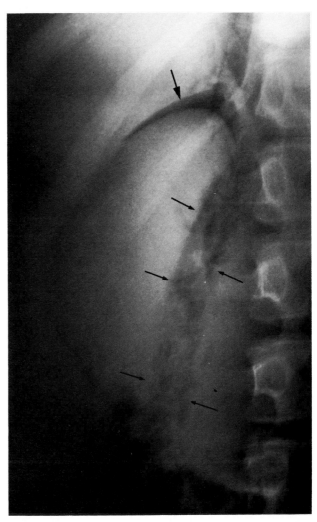

FIGURE 12–21. Retroperitoneal Air Caused by Duodenal Perforation

• • • •

This patient was seen about 6 hours after a blow to the midepigastrium. Air is seen dissecting in the retroperitoneal tissues around the right kidney (*large arrow*) and along the psoas muscle (*small arrows*). While this is unequivocal evidence of injury, all duodenal perforations do not have such easily seen retroperitoneal air.

It is crucial to remember that both types of contrast media designed for overhead filming and fluoroscopy cause severe artifacts on CT scans. Therefore, if CT is planned for the patient, it should be performed first. The barium-based agents can also interfere with ultrasound.

Computed Tomography

CT should be performed using both oral and intravenous contrast agents. Good opacification of the bowel increases the success of CT in bowel injury,

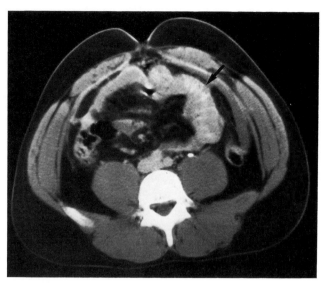

FIGURE 12–23. Thickening of the Mesentery Caused by an Aggravated Assault

• • • •

The mesentery is normally seen as a fat density structure that is traversed by numerous blood vessels. In this young patient, however, the mesentery is hazy. A dilated loop of the bowel is filled with contrast material (*arrow*). Free fluid is also seen but was more readily detected on other sections. At exploration, two small bowel perforations and several mesenteric tears were found.

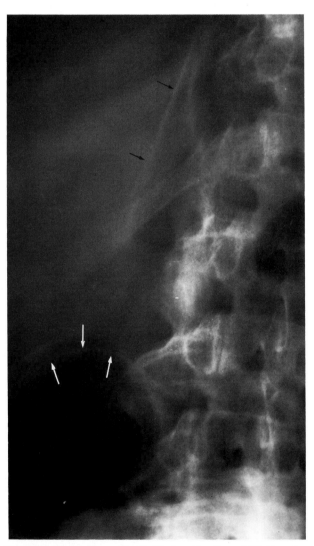

FIGURE 12–22. Free Air Outlining the Bowel Wall and the Ligamentum Arteriosum

• • • •

Both the inner and the outer aspects of a dilated loop of the bowel (*white arrows*) are demonstrated, unequivocally indicating the presence of free air in the peritoneal cavity. In addition, free air outlines the ligamentum arteriosum (*black arrows*).

but detection of bowel injury by CT is not highly reliable overall. Free intraperitoneal fluid is present in most patients but is not specific for hollow viscus injury. Thickening and infiltration of the mesentery is a more specific and also common observation (Fig. 12–23). Bowel wall thickening occurs in over one half of all bowel injuries but is also not specific (Fig. 12–24). Bowel lacerations that are not transmural may have no detectable thickening on CT scans. In general, patients with significant hollow viscus injury have an abnormal CT scan. Unfortunately, the abnormalities are likely to be nonspecific. A high degree of clinical suspicion in addition to meticulous CT technique is mandatory to achieve any level of accuracy in these patients.

Free air within the peritoneal cavity is easily seen on CT scans. It is important to remember that free air seen on the scan is not necessarily indicative of bowel perforation that requires surgical intervention. The sensitivity of CT to air is such that free air from a self-sealing microperforation may be seen. In addition, air may dissect into the peritoneal cavity from a pneumothorax or enter through the fallopian tubes in female patients. Small amounts of free air seen only on CT scans are findings that should be considered in light of the evaluation of the entire patient rather than as indications for immediate exploration.

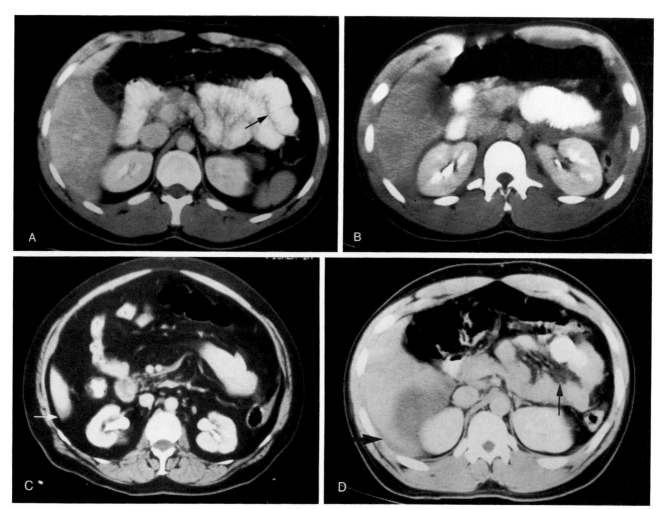

FIGURE 12–24. Bowel Wall Injury

• • • •

A, The small bowel is dilated, the valvulae are swollen, and the bowel wall appears thickened (*arrow*) in this patient with mesenteric hematomas and perforations of the small bowel. The only other abnormality seen on the entire scan was a small amount of free fluid in the pelvis. *B,* This patient, who was stepped on by a horse, has a dilated loop of bowel with some edema of the valvulae. Free fluid was seen primarily in the pelvis. At surgery a jejunal perforation was found. *C,* This patient has a tiny amount of free fluid at the tip of the liver (*arrow*). The entire scan was otherwise normal. At surgery, mesenteric lacerations and colonic deserosalization were found. This scan emphasizes how minimal the computed tomography findings in mesenteric and bowel injuries can be. *D,* This section demonstrates only fluid by the liver (*large arrow*). The bowel is poorly opacified, and thickening of the mesentery could be questioned (*small arrow*). *E,* A lower section on the same patient demonstrates more free fluid that has increased density in its dependent portion (*arrow*), sug-

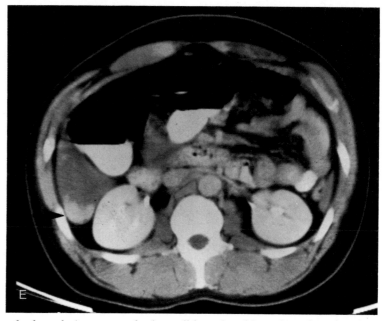

gesting extravasation of the contrast medium from the bowel. At surgery, both small bowel and large bowel perforations were found.

ADRENAL GLAND

Trauma to the adrenal gland is not common and is rarely detected either by clinical examination or radiologic study. The adrenal gland can be injured by both penetrating and blunt trauma. In general, penetrating injuries are explored. CT is often performed in patients in whom surgery is not planned because the injury is believed to be extraperitoneal. CT is also commonly performed in blunt injury to the retroperitoneum. Although ultrasound scans can demonstrate enlarged adrenal glands, CT is by far the simplest way to detect injury. If active hemorrhage is encountered, angiographic therapy is sometimes appropriate.

It should be clear that the discovery of adrenal injury in the adult is usually serendipitous. CT is the most likely source of observation, since the adrenal glands are seen on most abdominal scans performed for trauma. In the unusual circumstance when adrenal injury is of clinical concern, CT is the appropriate diagnostic modality.

ABDOMINAL WALL

The abdominal wall is frequently injured by blunt trauma and is virtually always penetrated when penetrating injury to the peritoneal cavity is present. As a rule there is no role for radiologic studies in the evaluation of these injuries. Most injuries have either no clinical importance or are explored during surgery for a penetrating injury.

In the past, injection of the penetrating injury track was performed in an attempt to determine the depth of penetration. These injections were found to have frequent false-positive and false-negative findings and have been abandoned by trauma centers. CT, on the other hand, includes the entire abdominal wall, and occasionally interesting observations can be made. Rectus sheath hematomas (Fig. 12–25) and other body wall hematomas are easily seen (Fig. 12–26). The track of a penetrating injury is sometimes defined by soft tissue air. Bleeding along the course of penetration also helps to define the track, and the two observations can sometimes accurately determine that the peritoneum has not been violated. Most of these findings have little clinical relevance, but the abdominal wall should always be evaluated during CT for trauma.

PREGNANT UTERUS

The uterus is technically part of the genitourinary tract and is rarely injured in the nonpregnant state. When injury does occur to the nonpregnant uterus, the most appropriate approach is usually surgical exploration. In early pregnancy the uterus remains a pelvic organ and, as such, is protected by the pelvic bones. Again, only very severe trauma injures the uterus. No radiologic study directed at the uterus is

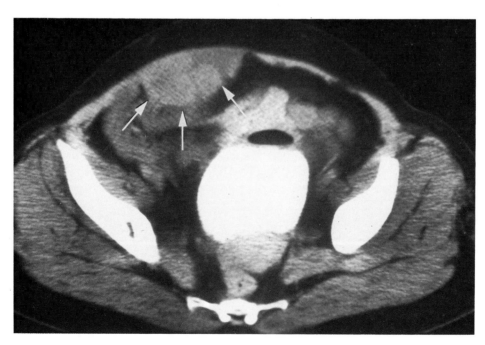

FIGURE 12–25. Rectus Sheath Hematoma
• • • •
A large right rectus sheath hematoma (*arrows*) is seen. This observation explained the tenderness that the patient experienced following an automobile accident.

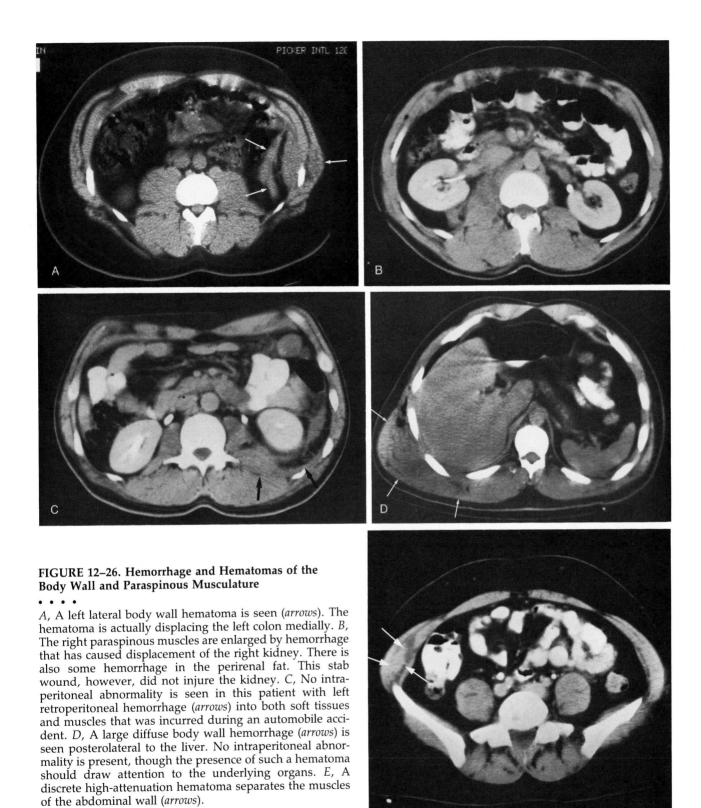

FIGURE 12–26. Hemorrhage and Hematomas of the Body Wall and Paraspinous Musculature

• • • •

A, A left lateral body wall hematoma is seen (*arrows*). The hematoma is actually displacing the left colon medially. *B,* The right paraspinous muscles are enlarged by hemorrhage that has caused displacement of the right kidney. There is also some hemorrhage in the perirenal fat. This stab wound, however, did not injure the kidney. *C,* No intraperitoneal abnormality is seen in this patient with left retroperitoneal hemorrhage (*arrows*) into both soft tissues and muscles that was incurred during an automobile accident. *D,* A large diffuse body wall hemorrhage (*arrows*) is seen posterolateral to the liver. No intraperitoneal abnormality is present, though the presence of such a hematoma should draw attention to the underlying organs. *E,* A discrete high-attenuation hematoma separates the muscles of the abdominal wall (*arrows*).

indicated unless fetal viability becomes an important concern, an issue that ultrasound can resolve. There should be concern about fetal irradiation, and careful records of radiation exposure should be made. Pelvic bone injuries require radiographs that place the fetus directly in the path of the primary beam. Although radiation should be kept to a minimum, the necessary radiographs may lead to a fetal dose in excess of 5–10 cGy at a gestational age when fetal anomalies may occur. The maternal injuries and risks must be balanced against fetal well-being. Maternal well-being is vital to fetal survival. This factor takes precedence in most early pregnancies.

The pregnant uterus becomes an abdominal organ as it enlarges. The pelvis, which protects the uterus until about 12 weeks of gestation, becomes capable of injuring the uterus as it enlarges. There is little role for radiographic evaluation in blunt trauma to the uterus, and it is probably of even less use in penetrating injuries. Direct fetal radiation should be avoided when possible, and careful thought should be given to the real need for maternal radiographic studies. Shielding must be used whenever possible. Careful records of all radiographic studies should be kept so that any fetal radiation dose can be calculated.

The one procedure that has some usefulness in trauma to the pregnant uterus is ultrasound, which can be used to evaluate the status of the pregnancy. Gestational age, fetal cardiac activity, and the volume of amniotic fluid are readily determined. Ultrasound can also be used to check for abruptio placentae. Adverse effects of blunt trauma on the fetus generally manifest themselves quite rapidly. Therefore, fetal evaluation and monitoring as soon as possible after arrival in an emergency room are appropriate. It is important to remember that fetal welfare is directly related to maternal welfare, thus maternal evaluation and stabilization must proceed with efficiency.

References

General

1. Burney RE. Peritoneal lavage and other diagnostic procedures in blunt abdominal trauma. Emerg Med Clin North Am 1986; 4:513–526.
2. Cox EF. Blunt abdominal trauma: A 5-year analysis of 870 patients requiring celiotomy. Ann Surg 1984; 199:467–474.
3. Drysdale WF, Kraus JF, Franti CE, Riggins RS. Injury patterns in motorcycle collisions. J Trauma 1975; 15:99–115.
4. Fabian TC, Mangiante EC, White TJ, et al. A prospective study of 91 patients undergoing both computed tomography and peritoneal lavage following blunt abdominal trauma. J Trauma 1986; 26:602–608.
5. Filiatrault D, Longpré D, Patriguin H, et al. Investigation of childhood blunt abdominal trauma: A practical approach using ultrasound as the initial diagnostic modality. Pediatr Radiol 1987; 17:373–379.
6. Fischer RP, Beverlin BC, Engrav LH, et al. Diagnostic peritoneal lavage: Fourteen years and 2,586 patients later. Am J Surg 1978; 136:701–704.
7. Fletcher TB, Setiawan H, Harrell RS, Redman HC. Posterior abdominal stab wounds: Role of CT evaluation. Radiology 1989; 173:621–625.
8. Foley RW, Harris LS, Pilcher DB. Abdominal injuries in automobile accidents: Review of care of fatally injured patients. J Trauma 1977; 17:611–615.
9. Gelfand MJ. Scintigraphy in upper abdominal trauma. Semin Roentgenol 1984; 19:296–307.
10. Goldstein AS, Sclafani SJA, Kupferstein NH, et al. The diagnostic superiority of computerized tomography. J Trauma 1985; 25:938–946.
11. Hauser CJ, Huprich JE, Bosco P, et al. Triple-contrast computed tomography in the evaluation of penetrating posterior abdominal injuries. Arch Surg 1987; 122:1112–1115.
12. Jeffrey RB Jr, Cardoza JD, Olcott EW. Detection of active intraabdominal arterial hemorrhage: Value of dynamic contrast-enhanced CT. AJR 1991; 156:725–729.
13. Jones TK, Walsh JW, Maull KI. Diagnostic imaging in blunt trauma of the abdomen. Surg Gynecol Obstet 1983; 157:389–398.
14. Kane NM, Dorfman GS, Cronan JJ. Efficacy of CT following peritoneal lavage in abdominal trauma. J Comput Assist Tomogr 1987; 11:998–1002.
15. Kane NM, Francis IR, Burney RE, et al. Traumatic pneumoperitoneum: Implications of computed tomography diagnosis. Invest Radiol 1991; 26:574–578.
16. Kelly J, Raptopoulos V, Davidoff A, et al. The value of noncontrast-enhanced CT in blunt abdominal wall. AJR 1989; 152:41–46.
17. Kurdziel JC, Dondelinger RF, Hemmer M. Radiological management of blunt polytrauma with computed tomography and angiography: An integrated approach. Ann Radiol 1987; 30:121–124.
18. de Lacy AM, Pera M, Garcia-Valdecasas JC, et al. Management of penetrating abdominal stab wounds. Br J Surg 1988; 75:231–233.
19. Levine MS, Scheiner JD, Rubesin SE, et al. Diagnosis of pneumoperitoneum on supine abdominal radiographs. AJR 1991; 156:731–735.
20. MacKenzie EJ, Shapiro S, Siegel JH. The economic impact of traumatic injuries: One year treatment-related expenditures. JAMA 1988; 260:3290–3296.
21. Marx JA, Moore EE, Jorden RC, Eule J Jr. Limitations of computed tomography in the evaluation of acute abdominal trauma: A prospective comparison with diagnostic peritoneal lavage. J Trauma 1985; 25:933–937.
22. McConnell BJ, McConnell RW, Guiberteau MJ. Radionuclide imaging in blunt trauma. Radiol Clin North Am 1981; 19:37–51.
23. McCort J. Caring for the major trauma victim: The role for radiology. Radiology 1987; 163:1–9.
24. Mirvis SE, Fritz SL, Siegel JH, Ramzy A. Radiographic system for use in emergency and intensive care units. AJR 1988; 150:691–692.
25. Orwig D, Federle MP. Localized clotted blood as evidence of visceral trauma on CT: The sentinel clot sign. AJR 1989; 153:747–749.
26. Orwig DS, Jeffrey RB. CT of false-negative peritoneal lavage following blunt abdominal trauma. J Comput Assist Tomogr 1987; 11:1079–1080.
27. Pagliarello G, Hanna SS, Gregory WD, et al. Abdominopelvic computerized tomography and open peritoneal lavage in patients with blunt abdominal trauma: A prospective study. Can J Surg 1987; 30:10–13.
28. Phillips T, Sclafani SJA, Goldstein A, et al. Use of the contrast-enhanced CT enema in the management of penetrating trauma to the flank and back. J Trauma 1986; 26:593–601.
29. Soderstrom CA, DuPriest RW Jr, Cowley RA. Pitfalls of peritoneal lavage in blunt abdominal trauma. Surg Gynecol Obstet 1980; 151:513–518.
30. Wing VW, Federle MP, Morris JA Jr, et al. The clinical impact of CT for blunt abdominal trauma. AJR 1985; 145:1191–1194.

The Liver

31. Abramson SJ, Berdon WE, Kaufman RA, Ruzal-Shapiro C. Hepatic parenchymal and subcapsular gas after hepatic laceration caused by blunt abdominal trauma. AJR 1989; 153:1031–1032.
32. Aldrete JS, Halpern NB, Ward S, Wright JD. Factors determining the mortality and morbidity in hepatic injuries. Ann Surg 1979; 189:466–474.
33. Barclay GR, Crampton JR. ERCP in late post-traumatic biliary fistula. Postgrad Med J 1987; 63:147–149.
34. Brick SH, Taylor GA, Potter BM, Eichelberger MR. Hepatic and splenic injury in children: Role of CT in the decision for laparotomy. Radiology 1987; 165:643–646.
35. Brody AS, Kaufman RA, Kirks DR. Case report: Isolated caudate lobe liver injury in a child: CT demonstration. J Comput Assist Tomogr 1988; 12:524–526.
36. Colletti PM, Barakas JA, Ralls PW, et al. Hepatobiliary scintigraphy and scintiangiography in abdominal trauma. Clin Nucl Med 1987; 12:901–909.
37. Epstein BM, Bocchiola FC, Andrews JC, Bester L. Case report: Traumatic arteriovenous fistula involving the portal venous system. Clin Radiol 1987; 38:91–93.
38. Farnell MB, et al. Nonoperative management of blunt hepatic trauma in adults. Surgery 1988; 104:748–756.
39. Feliciano DV, Mattox KL, Jordan GL Jr, et al. Management of 1000 consecutive cases of hepatic trauma (1979–1984). Ann Surg 1986; 204:438–445.
40. Foley WD, Cates JD, Kellman GM, et al. Treatment of blunt hepatic injuries: Role of CT. Radiology 1987; 164:635–638.
41. Froelich JW, Simeone JF, McKusick KA, et al. Radionuclide imaging and ultrasound in liver/spleen trauma: A prospective comparison. Radiology 1982; 145:457–461.
42. Holdaway CM, Douglas R, Shaw JHF. Conservative treatment of traumatic closed hepatic haematoma. Aust NZ J Surg 1988; 58:123–127.
43. Ivatury RR, Nallathambi M, Lankin DH, et al. Portal vein injuries: Noninvasive follow-up of venorrhaphy. Ann Surg 1987; 206:733–737.
44. Leekam RN, Ilves R, Shankar L. Inversion of gallbladder secondary to traumatic herniation of liver: CT findings. J Comput Assist Tomogr 1987; 11:163–164.
45. MacGillivray DC, Valentine RJ. Nonoperative management of blunt pediatric liver injury: Late complications. Case report. J Trauma 1989; 29:251–254.
46. Meyer AA, Crass RA, Lim RC Jr, et al. Selective nonoperative management of blunt liver injury using computed tomography. Arch Surg 1985; 120:550–554.
47. Mirvis SE, Whitley NO, Vainwright JR, Gens DR. Blunt hepatic trauma in adults: CT-based classification and correlation with prognosis and treatment. Radiology 1989; 171:27–32.
48. Mitchell MJ, Nunnerley B. Radiological investigation of liver trauma. Br J Hosp Med 1986; 36:174–177.
49. Panicek DM, Paquet DJ, Clark KG, et al. Hepatic parenchymal gas after blunt trauma. Radiology 1986; 159:343–344.
50. Petersen SR, Sheldon GE, Lim RC. Management of portal vein injuries. J Trauma 1979; 19:616–620.
51. Rubin BE, Katzen BT. Selective hepatic artery embolization to control massive hepatic hemorrhage after trauma. AJR 1977; 129:253–256.
52. Soderstrom CA, Maekawa K, DuPriest RW Jr, Cowley RA. Gallbladder injuries resulting from blunt abdominal trauma. Ann Surg 1981; 193:60–66.
53. Stalker HP, Kaufman RA, Towbin R. Patterns of liver injury in childhood: CT analysis. AJR 1986; 147:1199–1205.
54. Strodel WE, Eckhauser FE, Lemmer JH, et al. Presentation and perioperative management of arterioportal fistulas. Arch Surg 1987; 122:563–571.
55. Thomas JK, Peters JC. CT in the posttraumatic liver. Comput Radiol 1984; 8:85–89.
56. Wagner WH, Lundell CJ, Donovan AJ. Percutaneous angiographic embolization for hepatic arterial hemorrhage. Arch Surg 1985; 120:1241–1249.
57. Watson DI, Williams JAR. Management of the traumatized liver: An appraisal of 63 cases. Aust N Z J Surg 1989; 59:137–142.

The Spleen

58. Federle MP, Griffiths B, Minagi H, Jeffery RB Jr. Splenic trauma: Evaluation with CT. Radiology 1987; 162:69–71.
59. Howman-Giles R, Gilday DL, Venugopal S, et al. Splenic trauma: Nonoperative management and long-term follow-up by scintiscan. J Pediatr Surg 1979; 13:121–126.
60. Jeffrey RB Jr. CT diagnosis of blunt hepatic and splenic injuries: A look to the future. Radiology 1989; 171:17–18.
61. Kakkaseril JS, Stewart D, Cox JA, Gelfand M. Changing treatment of pediatric splenic trauma. Arch Surg 1982; 117:758–759.
62. Levine E, Wetzel LH. Splenic trauma during colonoscopy. AJR 1987; 149:939–940.
63. Livingston CD, Sirinek KR, Levine BA, Aust JB. Traumatic splenic injury: Its management in a patient population with a high incidence of associated injury. Arch Surg 1982; 117:670–674.
64. Lupien C, Sauerbrei EE. Healing in the traumatized spleen: Sonographic investigation. Radiology 1984; 151:181–185.
65. Lutzker LG, Chun KJ. Radionuclide imaging in the nonsurgical treatment of liver and spleen trauma. J Trauma 1981; 21:382–387.
66. Malagoni MA, Levin AW, Droege EA, et al. Management of injury to the spleen in adults. Ann Surg 1984; 200:702–705.
67. Mirvis SE, Whitley NO, Gens DR. Blunt splenic trauma in adults: CT-based classification and correlation with prognosis and treatment. Radiology 1989; 171:33–39.
68. Mishalany HG, Miller JH, Woolley MM. Radioisotope spleen scan in patients with splenic injury. Arch Surg 1982; 117:1147–1150.
69. Morgenstern L, Uyeda RY. Nonoperative management of injuries of the spleen in adults. Surg Gynecol Obstet 1983; 157:513–518.
70. Nallathambi MN, Ivatory RR, Wapnir I, et al. Nonoperative management versus early operation for blunt splenic trauma in adults. Surg Gynecol Obstet 1988; 166:252–258.
71. Olsen WR, Polley TZ Jr. A second look at delayed splenic rupture. Arch Surg 1977; 112:422–425.
72. Pappas D, Mirvis SE, Crepps JT. Splenic trauma: False-negative CT diagnosis in cases of delayed rupture. AJR 1987; 149:727–728.
73. Resciniti A, Frink MP, Raptopoulos V, et al. Nonoperative treatment of adult splenic trauma: Development of a computed tomographic scoring system that detects appropriate candidates for expectant management. J Trauma 1988; 128:828–831.
74. Scatamacchia SA, Raptopoulos V, Fink MP, Silva WE. Splenic trauma in adults: Impact of CT grading on management. Radiology 1989; 171:725–729.
75. Sortland O, Nerdrum HJ, Solheim K. Computed tomography and scintigraphy in the diagnosis of splenic injury. Acta Chir Scand 1986; 152:453–461.
76. Truab A, Giebink GS, Smith C, et al. Splenic reticuloendothelial function after splenectomy, spleen repair, and splenic autotransplantation. N Engl J Med 1987; 317:1559–1564.
77. Umlas S-L, Cronan JJ. Splenic trauma: Can CT grading systems enable prediction of successful nonsurgical treatment? Radiology 1991; 178:481–487.
78. Wiebke EA, Sarr MG, Fishman EK, Ratych RE. Nonoperative management of splenic injuries in adults: An alternative in selected patients. Am Surg 1987; 53:547–552.

The Pancreas

79. Cook DE, Walsh JW, Vick CW, Brewer WH. Upper abdominal trauma: Pitfalls in CT diagnosis. Radiology 1986; 159:65–69.
80. Federle MP, Crass RA, Jeffrey RB, Trunkey DD. Computed

tomography in blunt abdominal trauma. Arch Surg 1982; 117:645–650.

81. Graham JM, Mattox KL, Jordan GL. Traumatic injuries of the pancreas. Am J Surg 1978; 136:744–748.

82. Hall RL, Lavelle MI, Venables CW. Use of ERCP to identify the site of traumatic injuries of the main pancreatic duct in children. Surgery 1986; 73:411–412.

83. Jeffrey RB, Laing FC, Wing VW. Ultrasound in acute pancreatic trauma. Gastrointest Radiol 1986; 11:44–46.

84. Meredith JW, Trunkey DD. CT scanning in acute abdominal injuries. Surg Clin North Am 1988; 68:255–268.

85. Peitzman AB, Makaroun MS, Slasky BS, Ritter P. Prospective study of computed tomography in initial management of blunt abdominal trauma. J Trauma 1986; 26:585–592.

86. Thomasson B, Linna MI, Viljanto J, Aho AJ. Blunt pancreatic trauma: Report of sixteen cases. Acta Chir Scand 1973; 139:48–54.

87. Van Steenberg W, Samain H, Pouillon M , et al. Transection of the pancreas demonstrated by ultrasound and computed tomography. Gastrointest Radiol 1987; 12:128–130.

88. Wilson RF, Tagett JP, Pucelik JP, Walt AJ. Pancreatic trauma. J Trauma 1967; 7:643–651.

The Bowel and Mesentery

89. Brunsting LA, Morton JH. Gastric rupture from blunt abdominal trauma. J Trauma 1987; 27:887–891.

90. Bulas DI, Taylor GA, Eichelberger MR. The value of CT in detecting bowel perforation in children after blunt abdominal trauma. AJR 1989; 153:561–564.

91. Dauterive AH, Flancbaum L, Cox EF. Blunt intestinal trauma: A modern day review. Ann Surg 1985; 201:198–205.

92. Donohue JH, Federle MP, Griffiths BG, Trunkey DD. Computed tomography in the diagnosis of blunt intestinal and mesenteric injuries. J Trauma 1987; 27:11–17.

93. Fischer RP, Miller-Crotchett P, Reed RL II. Gastrointestinal disruption: The hazard of nonoperative management in adults with blunt abdominal injury. J Trauma 1988; 28:1445–1449.

94. French GWG, Sherlock DJ, Holl-Allen RTJ. Problems with rectal foreign bodies. Br J Surg 1985; 72:243–244.

95. Ginai AZ. Clinical use of Hexabrix for radiological evaluation of leakage from the upper gastrointestinal tract based on experimental study. Br J Radiol 1987; 60:343–346.

96. Hughes JJ, Brogdon BG. Computed tomography of duodenal hematoma. J Comput Tomogr 1986; 10:231–236.

97. Jeffrey RB, Federle MP, Stein SM, Crass RA. Intramural hematoma of the cecum following blunt trauma. J Comput Assist Tomogr 1982; 6:404–405.

98. Rizzo MJ, Federle MP, Griffiths BG. Bowel and mesenteric injury following blunt abdominal trauma: Evaluation with CT. Radiology 1989; 173:143–148.

99. Shuck JM, Lowe RJ. Intestinal disruption due to blunt abdominal trauma. Am J Surg 1978; 136:668–672.

100. Talbot WA, Shuck JM. Retroperitoneal duodenal injury due to blunt abdominal trauma. Am J Surg 1975; 130:659–666.

101. Theuns P, Coenen L, Brouwers J. Gastric rupture from blunt abdominal trauma. Acta Chir Belg 1988; 88:309–311.

102. Thoms CA, Ricketts RR. Intramural duodenal hematoma in children: Reappraisal of current management. South Med J 1988; 81:985–988.

The Adrenal Gland, the Abdominal Wall, and the Pregnant Uterus

103. Drost TF, Rosemurgy AS, Sherman HF, et al. Major trauma in pregnant women: Maternal/fetal outcome. J Trauma 1990; 30:574–578.

104. Pearlman MD, Tintinalli JE, Lorenz RP. Blunt trauma during pregnancy. N Engl J Med 1991; 323:1609–1613.

105. Wagner LK, Archer BR, Zeck OF. Conceptus dose from two state-of-the-art CT scanners. Radiology 1986; 159:787–792.

CHAPTER 13

The Genitourinary System

HELEN C. REDMAN, M.D.

THE KIDNEY

The kidneys are vulnerable to both blunt and penetrating injury. Prompt and accurate evaluation of renal injury is essential in preserving renal function when the vascular pedicle is injured and in determining the appropriate therapy for all other injuries. The diagnostic tests are the same for both blunt and penetrating injury. Although it is not realistic to present a universal algorithm for the radiologic approach to renal trauma, since the appropriate procedures depend on all the injuries in each patient, some ground rules can be established. Virtually all renal injury is associated with hematuria, although the hematuria may be microscopic. Hematuria also makes injury to the lower urinary tract a possibility, thus the type of trauma must be considered before deciding to study only the upper urinary tract. Retrograde urethrography, cystography, and even retrograde pyelography may need to be part of the evaluation in a specific patient. The examinations and the order in which they are performed depend on the history and clinical evaluation.

When injury to the lower urinary tract has been excluded by history, clinical findings, or radiographic examination, attention should be directed to the kidneys as the source of bleeding. Several radiographic studies can be employed, and each has a place in the diagnosis of renal injury. The primary modalities include intravenous urography, computed tomography (CT), and angiography. The backup procedures include ultrasound and nuclear scanning. The challenge is to choose the appropriate initial examination for each patient.

Procedures

Intravenous Urography

TECHNIQUE

Intravenous urography is the simplest procedure to perform, but it provides the least specific information. The volume of contrast material required for the urogram may limit further evaluation with CT or angiography. However, the intravenous urogram

407

The Kidney

I. **Intravenous Urography**
   A. Requires the injection of 1–2 ml/kg of 60% contrast medium.
   B. Films at 1–2 minutes, 5 minutes, and 10 minutes after the start of injection.
   C. Can be performed with portable equipment.
   D. Requires little patient cooperation.

Comment: A normal examination excludes most major renal injury. An abnormal one generally requires further evaluation.

II. **Computed Tomography**
   A. Provides best overall survey of renal injury.
   B. Uses 10-mm sections at 10-mm intervals from the diaphragm to the lower pole of the kidneys and at 20-mm intervals to the symphysis pubis.
   C. Requires intravenous contrast material unless contraindicated.
   D. Requires some patient cooperation unless an ultrafast scanner is available.

Comment: As part of computed tomography of the entire abdomen, information can be obtained about all abdominal structures; computed tomography is a very useful technique for following the course of renal injury.

III. **Renal Angiography**
   A. Diagnostic Study
      1. Reserved for questions of renal artery integrity.
      2. A lumbar aortogram generally must be performed first.
      3. Selective renal angiograms are performed when intrarenal detail is important.
   B. Therapeutic Use
      1. Hemorrhage can be controlled.
      2. The catheter should be as selective as feasible.
      3. Permanent or semipermanent embolic materials can be used.

Comment: A significant proportion of renal parenchyma can often be salvaged.

The Ureter

I. **Intravenous Urography**
Comment: Small or distal injuries may be missed.

II. **Retrograde Pyelography**
Comment: Instrumentation is required, but the procedure should demonstrate virtually all lacerations.

III. **Computed Tomography**
Comment: A urinoma can be defined as well as the level of injury.

The Urinary Bladder

I. **Cystography**
   A. Requires a retention-type catheter.
   B. Uses 25–30% contrast material and 36-in. gravity filling.
   C. Requires a fluoroscope or films at 100 ml. If no extravasation is noted, fill the bladder until the patient's level of discomfort is reached.
   D. Should be done in anteroposterior, lateral, and both oblique views and after drainage.

Comment: When the bladder is adequately distended, most tears are seen.

> • • • • *APPROPRIATE RADIOGRAPHIC STUDIES* Continued
>
> ## II. Computed Tomography
> *Comment:* Extravasation of opacified urine identifies the injury.
> ## III. Intravenous Urography
> *Comment:* This technique is unreliable and should not be used for this purpose for two reasons: (1) bladder distention cannot be ensured, and (2) the urine may not be adequately opacified.
>
> ### The Urethra
>
> #### I. Retrograde Urethrography
>
> ### The Penis
>
> #### I. Radiographic evaluation is generally not required.
> #### II. Retrograde urethrography is performed if the urethra might be injured.
>
> ### The Scrotum and the Testicles
>
> #### I. Ultrasound
> #### II. Radionuclide Scan

may be all that is needed in patients with isolated renal trauma.

An intravenous urogram is performed by injecting contrast material intravenously and taking a series of films at specified intervals. The procedure requires little cooperation from the patient and causes only minor discomfort. When the contrast medium is injected, it produces a warm sensation and a peculiar taste in most patients. Nausea and vomiting may occur; a slow injection decreases the chances of this. A preliminary film should be obtained before any contrast material is injected. The scout film not only serves as a baseline, but it also demonstrates bone injuries, calcifications related to the urinary tract, and bowel gas pattern. Following injection of the contrast material (1–2 ml/kg), a nephrogram film taken at about 1 minute should demonstrate bilateral images of the kidneys. When there is an ileus or distended bowel, nephrotomography may be necessary to see the renal contours. If nephrographic images of both the kidneys are present and are symmetric, a second film at about 5 minutes after injection should demonstrate bilateral function, and the study can then often be terminated. However, if visualization of the kidneys is absent or incomplete, additional films are required. The absence of renal delineation on a nephrogram raises the question of main renal artery injury in the trauma patient.

If, on the contrary, the kidneys are delineated but no excretion is seen at 5 minutes, the patient must be followed with delayed films. The patient should also be checked for hypotension as a result of the trauma or a reaction to the contrast medium. Although a serious renal injury may still be present, especially when function is diminished bilaterally, a nephrogram confirms arterial patency and means that immediate surgery for renal salvage is unlikely to be needed. The absence of a kidney visualization on nephrogram cannot be equated absolutely with arterial occlusion. Rather, this diagnosis must be confirmed by angiography.

RADIOGRAPHIC OBSERVATIONS

The radiographic findings in renal trauma at urography are few; ileus and patient motion may make their detection difficult. The first observation is the presence of bilateral and symmetric nephrographic images (Fig. 13–1). This is best seen on a 1–2-minute film but can generally still be evaluated at 5 minutes. The presence of bilateral nephrographic renal visualization guarantees bilateral renal artery patency, although an arterial injury may still be present. The renal contours should be scrutinized for interruptions of the nephrographic image that may be indicative of laceration (Fig. 13–2). Loss of part or all of the

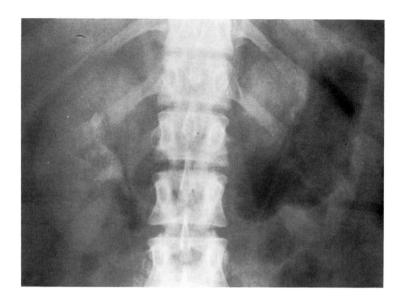

FIGURE 13–1. Normal Nephrograms

• • • •

A film taken approximately 3 minutes after the start of injection of contrast medium demonstrates bilateral nephrograms that are intact and symmetric. Early excretion is also seen.

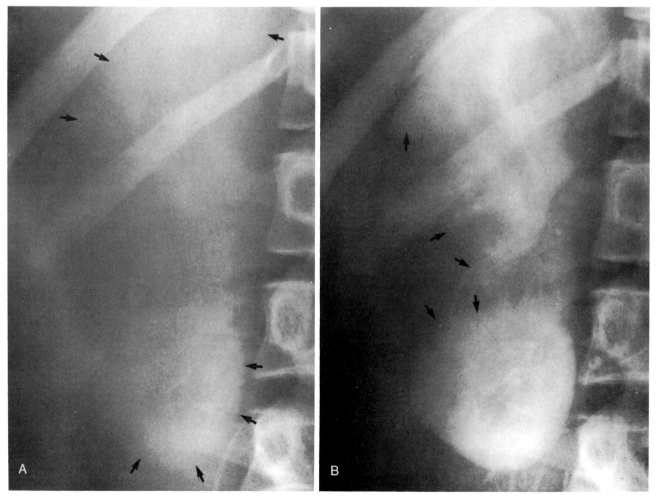

FIGURE 13–2. Nephrogram Demonstrating Renal Laceration

• • • •

A, The nephrogram is faint, but both the upper and the lower poles *(arrows)* can be defined. The lateral aspect of the kidney is indistinct, and contrast medium accumulation is diminished. *B,* The angiographic nephrogram on the same patient more clearly defines the renal laceration *(arrows).*

nephrogram suggests occlusion of the main renal artery, a major branch artery, or an accessory renal artery (Fig. 13–3). Marked asymmetry of the two nephrograms should be noted, as this can indicate renal compression by a subcapsular hematoma or a marked decrease in arterial flow to the side with the diminished nephrographic image (Fig. 13–4). The important caveat is that the kidneys may appear markedly asymmetric or even absent when renal injury is minimal. Therefore, although the observation is an important one, immediate surgical intervention for renal pedicle injury without more specific diagnostic or clinical information is rarely warranted.

The collecting systems normally opacify at about the same time. Asymmetry in excretion may indicate injury, but this finding is difficult to evaluate unless the discrepancy is gross. Differential excretion also has several causes and is a nonspecific observation. Ureteral obstruction, for example, causes delayed function on the obstructed side.

Distortion of the collecting system is often seen in an injured kidney. Extravasation of contrast material, compression of part or all of the collecting system, nonfilling of part of the collecting system, filling defects, and displacement of calyces all may be seen. Aside from filling defects within the collecting system, these observations are either strongly suggestive of renal injury or are unequivocal evidence of injury.

Extravasation of contrast medium from the collecting system is unequivocal evidence of injury. If the extravasation is within the renal parenchyma, the injury is sometimes a relatively minor laceration (Fig. 13–5), but if the extravasation is seen beyond the confines of the kidney, more serious injury, such as

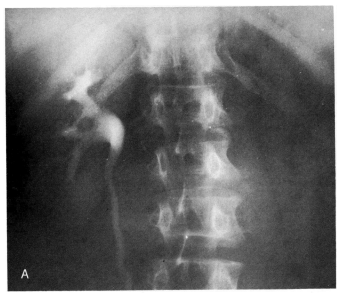
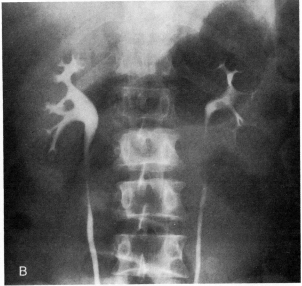
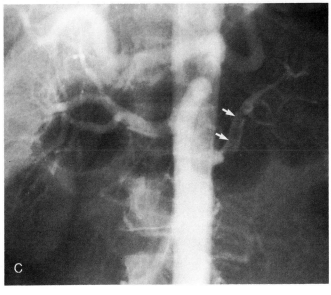

FIGURE 13–3. Absent Nephrogram Caused by Near Complete Occlusion of the Left Renal Artery

• • • •

A, A 10-minute film from an intravenous urogram demonstrates a normal right nephrogram and a normal proximal collecting system. No nephrogram or excretion is seen on the left. *B,* A retrograde pyelogram demonstrates a spidery left-sided collecting system with a possible rounded pelvic filling defect. *C,* Lumbar aortogram demonstrates a large filling defect in the left renal artery *(arrows)* that extends into several primary branch arteries. Very few intrarenal arteries are opacified. At surgery the left renal artery was clotted. Extensive intimal injury was the primary cause.

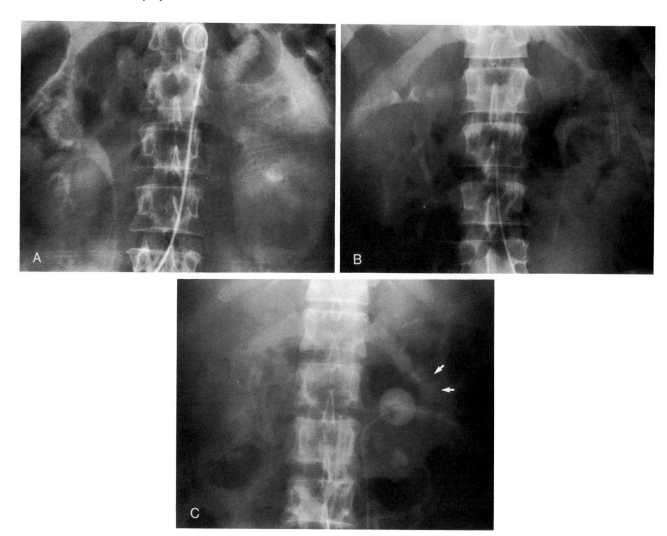

FIGURE 13–4. Abnormal Nephrogram and Collecting System

• • • •

A, A kidney, ureter, and bladder (KUB) image taken after a thoracic aortogram was performed demonstrates asymmetric nephrograms. The right kidney is normal and has a normal collecting system. The left kidney is enlarged, and there is no excretion. The nephrogram was delayed but is now denser than that of the right. While this is a nonspecific sign, in the setting of trauma subcapsular hematoma or other renal injury should be excluded. The opacity is an artifact. *B,* A KUB image taken after a thoracic aortogram was performed in this patient demonstrates a diminished nephrogram in the right lower pole and an unusual configuration of the collecting structures. Angiography demonstrated arterial injury (see Fig. 13–21*A*). *C,* This patient had a percutaneous nephrostomy for stone removal. After the initial percutaneous lithotripsy, the patient became hypotensive. The preliminary film for an aortogram demonstrates a normal right nephrogram and good excretion. The left nephrogram is very faint, and only a few dilated calyces *(arrows)* are demonstrated. There is residual stone in the lower pole. The arteriogram did not identify a specific lesion, but computed tomography demonstrated a large subcapsular hematoma (see Fig. 13–7).

laceration entering the renal pelvis or avulsion of the renal pelvis, is likely (Fig. 13–6). Such injuries are frequently treated surgically, although if adequate drainage can be established by a ureteral catheter or percutaneous nephrostomy, lacerations can heal without surgery.

Compression of part or all of the renal collecting system is seen pyelographically as a splayed out or spidery pelvocalyceal system. The concentration of contrast medium in the collecting system may appear to be less than that on the opposite side. Such compression is generally due to a subcapsular fluid collection, since only fluid in an enclosed space develops sufficient tension to cause visually detectable renal compression. The presence of such a fluid collection is more easily seen on CT scans (Fig. 13–7).

The normal calyceal complement should be present. Avulsion or occlusion of an accessory renal artery or a major arterial branch can cause lack of

FIGURE 13–5. Parenchymal Extravasation of Contrast Medium

• • • •

This intravenous urogram performed after exploratory laparotomy for blunt abdominal trauma demonstrates a normal left kidney. On the right, the renal contour is obscured. Contrast material has extravasated where the right kidney should be *(arrows)*, raising the possibility of a renal injury. Hematuria persisted and a complete renal transection was found at surgery.

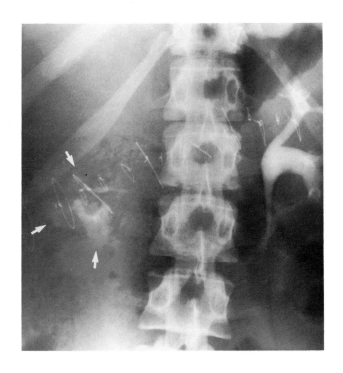

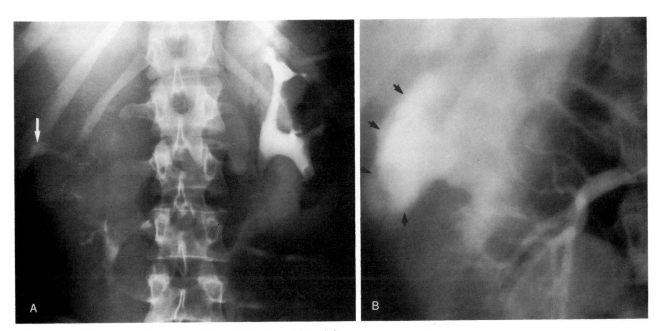

FIGURE 13–6. Extrarenal Extravasation of Contrast Material

• • • •

A, A 10-minute film from an intravenous urogram demonstrates a normal left kidney with sharp definition of the pelvis and calyces. On the right there is some contrast material in the calyces and renal pelvis. In addition, there is extravasation of contrast material beyond the kidney *(arrow)*. *B*, An angiogram performed approximately 1 hour later demonstrates further extravasation *(arrows)*. No arterial injury is seen. At surgery a renal laceration had torn into the renal pelvis.

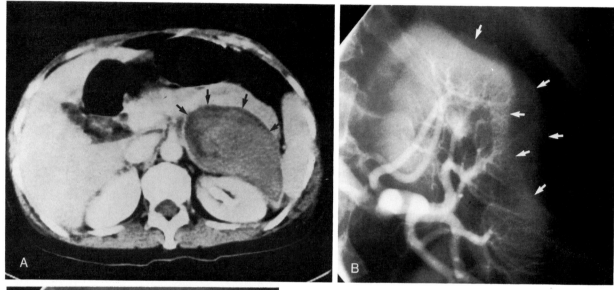

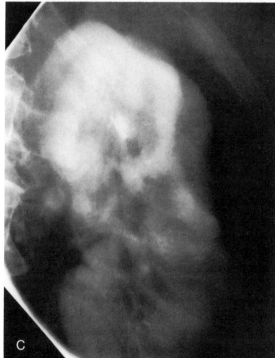

FIGURE 13–7. Subcapsular Hematoma

• • • •

A, A single CT scan demonstrates a large ventral subcapsular hematoma *(arrows)* that compresses the left kidney slightly. It has a nonhomogeneous appearance, suggesting recurrent bleeding. Note: This subcapsular hematoma has ruptured into the perinephric space, accounting for the relatively minor renal compression. When confined by the renal capsule, smaller hematomas may have a more dramatic mass effect on the renal parenchymal contour. *B,* This arterial phase of an angiogram in another patient with a subcapsular hematoma demonstrates an unusual contour *(arrows). C,* The nephrogram emphasizes this unusual "double" contour. The unusual appearance is caused by a subcapsular hematoma, which is frequently very difficult to identify at angiography. Computed tomography makes identification very easy.

the inferior pole of the kidneys to the pubic sym-opacification of some calyces. Another cause of non-filling is a renal parenchymal laceration amputating part of the collecting system (Fig. 13–8). Nonfilling of calyces in these situations is usually accompanied by a nephrographic defect. A focal renal contusion may also lead to compression of some calyces. In this circumstance the nephrogram may not be diminished.

Filling defects within the collecting system are nonspecific for trauma because renal stones are relatively common and may not be calcified enough to be seen on plain films. However, filling defects can also be caused by blood clots in the presence of trauma (see Fig. 13–19F). Generally, such clots are caused by parenchymal lacerations and so a nephrographic defect may also be detected.

Lastly, the calyces may be displaced (Fig. 13–9). Displacement caused by renal trauma is due to either

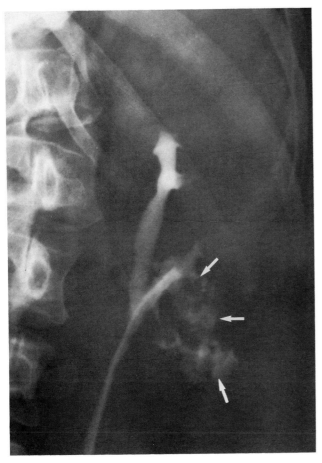

FIGURE 13–8. Renal Laceration Amputating the Lower Pole

• • • •

A retrograde pyelogram performed after an intravenous urogram (which did not demonstrate the lower pole calyces) demonstrates the extravasation of contrast material *(arrows)* into a renal laceration that has amputated the lower pole.

a parenchymal hematoma or a laceration and is usually accompanied by a nephrographic defect. Although calyceal displacement can be caused by simple renal cysts or tumors, the finding suggests renal injury in the presence of an appropriate history. CT displays the cause of the displacement and the extent of injury much more completely than urography.

In summary, although a normal intravenous urogram virtually excludes significant renal injury, an abnormal urogram frequently requires additional procedures to fully evaluate the presence and the extent of injury. The decision to perform an intravenous urogram depends on the degree of suspicion of renal injury and on the other concomitant injuries.

Computed Tomography

CT provides the same information as urography except for fine calyceal detail, which is generally not important in the evaluation of acute renal injury. It also demonstrates the perirenal and the pararenal spaces and gives detailed information about the intraperitoneal organs. It is a short procedure, but the logistics of arranging a CT scan mean that it may take longer to complete than an intravenous urogram. It does require that the patient be able to lie still.

CT can be limited to the kidneys alone, but it is more frequently performed to include the abdomen from the dome of the diaphragm to the symphysis pubis. Generally, the procedure is performed using intravenous contrast material, but when contrast material is contraindicated, CT can still provide useful information about renal injury. The patient must be able to lie quietly, preferably in a supine position, and suspend respiration intermittently for about 15 minutes. The CT scan is degraded by patient motion and also by bullets and other very radiodense objects that cause spray and streak artifacts and can obscure or mimic injury (Fig. 13–10). Nasogastric tubes and intravenous lines should be kept out of the field of view whenever possible. Claustrophobia may be a serious problem when encountered, but fortunately it is rare.

TECHNIQUE

In most institutions, CT for abdominal trauma is performed using an initial bolus injection of 50–100 ml of 60% contrast medium followed by an infusion of 30% contrast medium during the scan to maintain a relatively stable blood level of contrast material. CT sections are taken every 10 mm using 10-mm cuts from the diaphragm to the lower pole of the kidneys, with 10-mm cuts continued at 20-mm intervals from the inferior pole of the kidneys to the pubic sym-

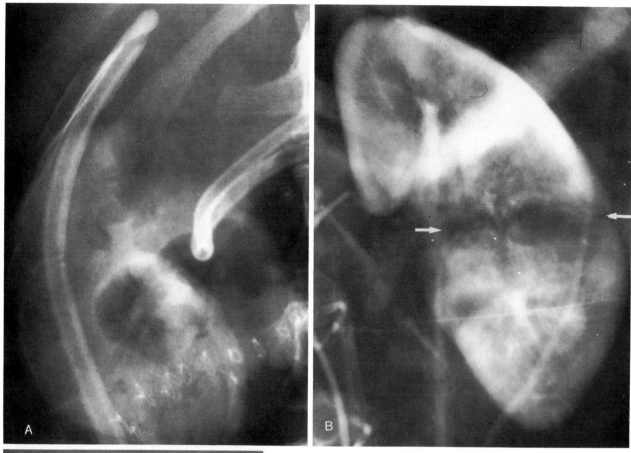

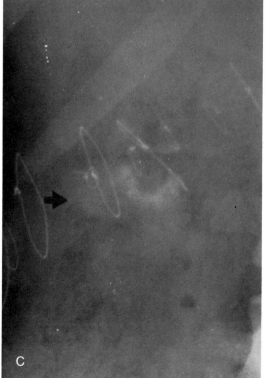

FIGURE 13–9. Displacement of Calyces

• • • •

A, This nephrogram demonstrates that the kidney is rotated and that the upper pole is not opacified. The calyces are displaced down and medially. *B,* The nephrogram in a second patient demonstrates a laceration through the midportion of the kidney. Calyces are displaced by the laceration *(arrows)*. *C,* A urographic nephrogram in a third patient demonstrates a distorted and displaced incomplete complement of calyces *(arrow)*.

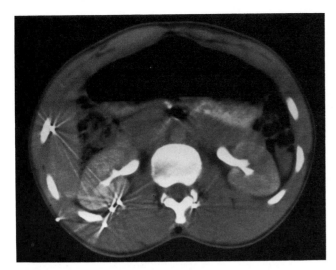

FIGURE 13–10. Streak Artifacts from Shotgun Pellets Degrading Computed Tomography

• • • •

A computed tomography section through the kidneys demonstrates several pellets. Two pellets are immediately adjacent to the right kidney. However, the streak artifacts make it impossible to determine whether the kidney is injured.

physis. Closer sectioning should be used selectively. Dynamic scanning is rarely useful in abdominal trauma.

CT is the most satisfactory current procedure for the definition of renal injury. Intravenous urography is less expensive and can be performed in an emergency room or even in the operating room using portable equipment, but it does not define the injury as completely as CT. Renal angiography is needed only when vascular injury is suspected or therapeutic embolization of a bleeding vessel is planned.

COMPUTED TOMOGRAPHY OBSERVATIONS

The CT examination of the kidneys includes the pararenal and the perirenal spaces in addition to the kidneys. Fluid collections in these spaces are frequent findings in trauma (Fig. 13–11). The fluid may be blood, urine, or a combination of both; as a result, the collections may or may not be homogeneous. These collections of fluid can markedly displace the kidney (Fig. 13–12).

CT for renal injury should be performed with intravenous contrast material unless there is an overwhelming contraindication to its use. The nephrogram can be easily evaluated, and disruptions of the renal parenchyma by lacerations or penetrating injury are readily seen (Fig. 13–13). Care should be taken to section both kidneys entirely, and close interval sections may be needed to evaluate subtle injury. Generally, however, contiguous 10-mm sections demonstrate significant parenchymal injury.

Although the collecting system is not seen with as much detail as is obtained with intravenous urography, the collecting system is seen, the number of calyces can be counted, and contrast medium can be identified as it extravasates through a laceration (Fig. 13–14).

As in urography, absence of a nephrogram and contrast medium excretion generally indicate serious renal disease. In the presence of trauma these findings raise serious concern for renal pedicle injury with arterial occlusion. Although the renal pedicle can be evaluated with CT, angiography is usually necessary to define the presence and the precise nature of the arterial injury. The absence of nephrographic enhancement has causes not related to acute trauma, such as end-stage kidney disease or ureteral obstruction. CT may define these causes of an absent or markedly diminished renal enhancement on the nephrogram. Renal ectopia and congenital absence of a kidney are also well demonstrated by CT.

Lack of excretion of contrast medium also has causes other than trauma. Obstruction, end-stage kidney disease, and renal vein thrombosis, among others, can cause delayed, diminished, or absent excretion. CT may define or suggest these causes but also demonstrates subcapsular hematomas (see Fig. 13–4) and diffuse renal swelling, which can cause slowed, diminished, or absent excretion.

Overall, CT is the most complete diagnostic procedure available for renal injury and should be used as the primary procedure in most patients when renal injury is a primary and serious clinical concern.

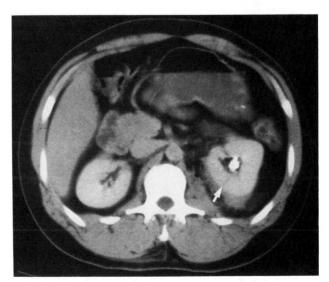

FIGURE 13–11. Fluid Collection Adjacent to the Left Kidney

• • • •

A single computed tomography section demonstrates an irregularly shaped fluid collection at the lower pole of the kidney in a patient who was stabbed. The renal laceration is seen as a subtle line of decreased attenuation *(arrow)*.

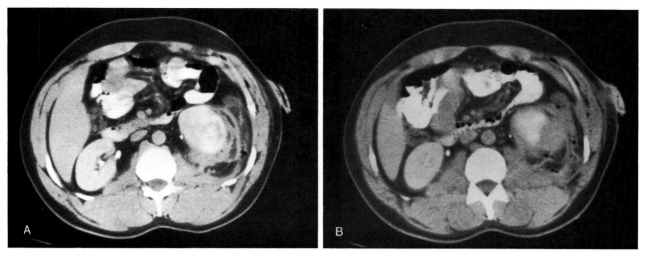

FIGURE 13–12. Displacement of the Left Kidney by a Large Inhomogeneous Fluid Collection After a Gunshot Wound

• • • •

A, This computed tomography section through the lower pole of the left kidney demonstrates that the kidney is displaced anteriorly by an inhomogeneous fluid collection found both dorsal and lateral to the organ. Some air is also seen. The kidney itself has an abnormal shape and shows an inhomogeneous accumulation of contrast material caused by renal laceration and hemorrhage. *B*, A section taken 10 mm caudal demonstrates the extensive fluid collection surrounding the tip of the left lower pole. At surgery it was found that the bullet had passed through the lower pole and that there was a large collection of mixed blood and urine.

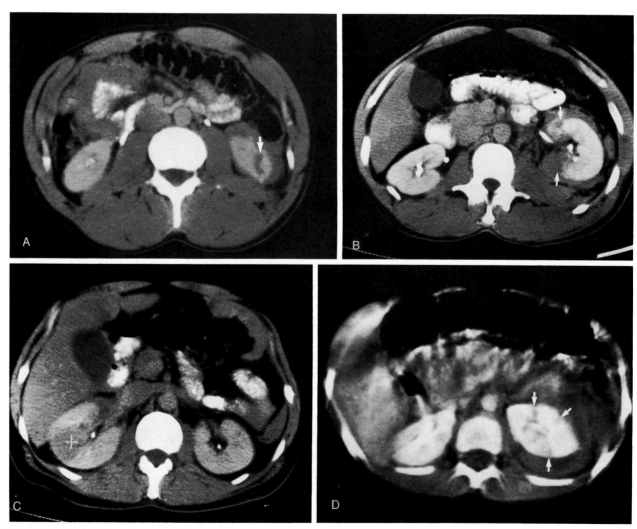

FIGURE 13–13 *See legend on opposite page*

418

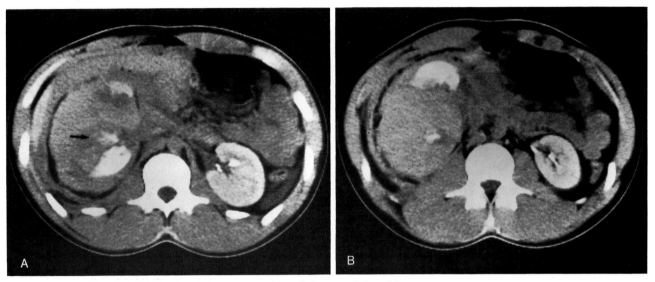

FIGURE 13–14. Renal Laceration with Extravasation of Contrast Material

• • • •

A, The right kidney is transected and surrounded by a large hematoma. The major dorsal component of the kidney is cephalad to this section that demonstrates some extravasation of opacified urine *(arrow)* into the hematoma. The hematoma itself has a higher computed tomography number than usual, probably resulting from the contrast material given earlier during thoracic aortography. *B,* The more ventral portion of the kidney is seen on this section taken 5 cm caudal to the first one. This patient was treated conservatively and had a functioning right kidney 3 months later.

Renal Angiography

INDICATIONS AND TECHNIQUE

Renal angiography should be reserved for patients in whom a vascular pedicle injury is likely or in whom bleeding from a major renal branch artery is suspected. In the latter instance, the angiogram may be performed to stop bleeding by selective embolization. Angiography demonstrates other renal injuries, such as lacerations and subcapsular hematomas, but these lesions are more easily seen on CT scans. Angiography is the most time-consuming of the three modalities and also carries the greatest risk to the patient. If angiography is being performed for other reasons, the kidneys, of course, can be evaluated (within the limitations of total contrast dose).

The need for angiography in renal trauma occurs when injury to the renal arteries is suspected, generally because of the absence of a renal enhancement on the nephrographic phase image at urography or at CT. Angiography must be undertaken expedi-

tiously if the kidney is to be salvaged. Warm ischemia time of much more than 6 hours leads to irreparable renal damage. The patient must be able to lie quietly for about 45 minutes for the procedure and must have an appropriate arterial access available. Generally, a lumbar aortogram is required, and the femoral artery approach is preferable. The left axillary artery can be used if neither femoral artery is accessible because of associated injury or arterial lines. Complications of angiography in a seriously injured patient who may be hypovolemic and hypotensive should occur in less than 1% of cases. The complications include those at the puncture site and those caused by the known renal toxicity of contrast media. This latter problem is minimized in the elective patient by ensuring adequate hydration and the careful monitoring of contrast medium volume. In the emergency situation, aggressive attention to fluid replacement should be employed. Contrast medium volumes should be minimized. The patient should be observed for decreased renal function following

FIGURE 13–13. Renal Laceration

• • • •

A, A computed tomography (CT) section through the lower pole of the left kidney demonstrates a renal laceration *(arrow)* seen as a linear area of decreased attenuation. A fluid collection surrounds the kidney. *B,* A CT scan on another patient demonstrates a laceration *(arrows)* with fluid surrounding the kidney. *C,* This CT section on a third patient reveals a laceration of the right kidney that is filled with a clot. *D,* This CT section in a 9-year-old child demonstrates several lacerations *(arrows)* and fluid surrounding the kidney.

the procedure. Although a serious renal function problem is very uncommon in the typical trauma patient, who is usually young and healthy, acute tubular necrosis may require dialysis for a period of time. Complications at the puncture site are primarily those of arterial occlusion. This problem can be minimized by careful attention to arterial flow distal to the puncture site during and following compression of the artery. If the patient has surgery following angiography, the surgeons and anesthesiologists should be made aware of possible complications at the puncture site with increased or prolonged hypotension.

Angiography may also be used for therapy. Hemorrhage from the kidney following a penetrating injury is often treatable by superselective angiographic embolization to salvage a significant portion of the kidney when a surgical approach is likely to lead to complete resection. Bleeding following blunt trauma can also be treated angiographically in some cases, although such bleeding is often from a torn surface rather than from a point source, decreasing the extent of renal salvage.

Angiography should be reserved for situations in which renal arterial injury is suspected or therapeutic intervention by angiography is planned. Although angiography was a primary diagnostic technique in the past, CT has replaced it in most instances. Unless other indications for angiography are present, it should not be the first diagnostic procedure.

ANGIOGRAPHIC OBSERVATIONS

All the angiographic findings of arterial injury can be seen in renal trauma. Occlusion of the main renal artery or branch arteries occur (Fig. 13–15). Both are associated with an angiographic nephrographic defect. Main renal artery occlusion is generally not flush with the aortic lumen and is seen as a short segment of artery or an irregularity or outpouching of the aorta (Fig. 13–16). When no renal artery is seen, congenital abnormalities such as absent kidney, pelvic kidney, and crossed fused renal ectopia should be excluded by CT. An occluded artery may be the angiographic manifestation of a transected artery or an intimal injury that has thrombosed. Partial transection or even a traumatic dissection is less common.

Extravasation usually occurs from a partially transected major artery or a smaller branch artery (Fig. 13–17). The larger renal arteries go into spasm following complete transection so that extravasation is less common in this situation.

Pseudoaneurysms can be found in the main renal arteries and in their smaller branches (Fig. 13–18). Many pseudoaneurysms heal without therapy, but they can also expand and rupture. Any pseudoaneu-

rysm larger than a few millimeters in size should be considered at risk for rupture. Whereas larger lesions are seen at aortography, smaller ones generally require selective renal angiography in more than one projection to be identified and localized. Pseudoaneurysms can often be treated by selective arterial embolization (Fig. 13–19).

Arteriovenous fistulas are usually caused by penetrating injury (Fig. 13–20). These are characterized by very rapid filling of a renal vein with dense contrast material. Generally, the communicating vein is filled within 1 second of the time the involved artery is opacified with contrast medium. Not infrequently, a pseudoaneurysm lies between the artery and the vein (see Fig. 13–18). Smaller arteriovenous fistulas, such as those caused by percutaneous renal biopsy, often close spontaneously within days of the injury. Larger ones may require treatment that can usually be performed by angiographic embolization (see Fig. 13–19).

Intimal injury to the main renal artery is seen as irregularity of the arterial lumen (Fig. 13–21). Intimal flaps are sometimes identifiable. A traumatic abdominal aortic dissection can extend into a renal artery, and an intimal flap may be present. Intimal injury in the branch renal arteries is rarely encountered, perhaps because smaller arteries with injury usually occlude.

Therapeutic Angiography in Renal Trauma

Bleeding caused by either blunt or penetrating injury may be serious enough to require therapy for the bleeding alone. The surgical approach to the acutely injured bleeding kidney is made difficult by the hematoma surrounding the kidney and often results in a nephrectomy because the renal pedicle must be clamped to control hemorrhage. Angiographic intervention is therefore worth considering in any patient with massive hemorrhage when the renal injury does not inherently require a nephrectomy. Angiography must first define the site and the nature of the hemorrhage. Embolization can then control bleeding in many patients. Important factors include the location of the bleeding artery, its accessibility, whether an arteriovenous fistula is present, and the clinical status of the patient. Ideally, only the bleeding artery is embolized, causing the least renal parenchymal loss. However, if the patient is in shock and bleeding is brisk, occlusion of a more central renal artery may be prudent. If a large arteriovenous fistula is present, occlusion of the actual communication is important. In smaller fistulas, oc-

Text continued on page 428

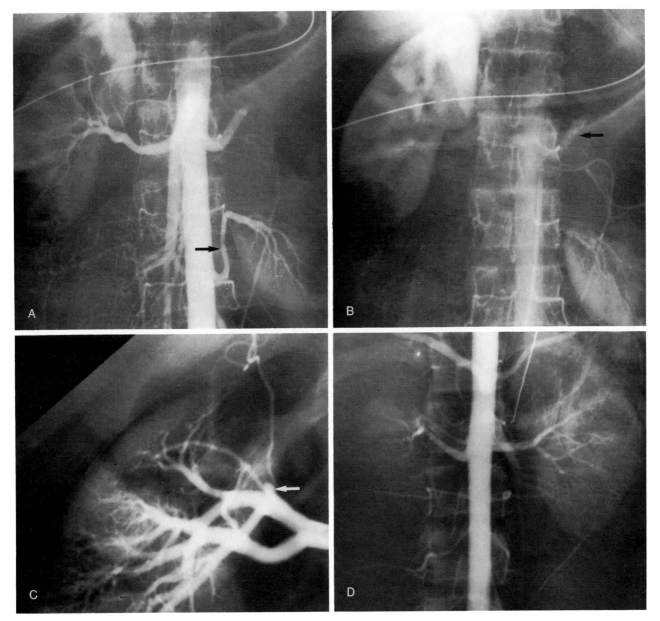

FIGURE 13–15. Renal Artery Occlusion or Injury with a Nephrographic Defect

• • • •

A, The left kidney has two renal arteries. The more cephalad artery is occluded approximately 5 cm distal to its origin. The lower renal artery *(arrow)* feeds a lower pole moiety. *B,* A film taken 2 seconds after completion of the contrast medium injection reveals the holdup of contrast material in the occluded renal artery *(arrow).* No nephrogram is seen in the expected distribution of this artery, but a normal angiographic nephrogram is seen in the renal segment supplied by the lower renal artery. *C,* Selective right renal artery injection in a second patient demonstrates occlusion of an upper pole artery near its origin *(arrow).* Even on this arterial phase film the wedge-shaped upper pole nephrographic defect is suggested. *D,* A lumbar aortogram on another patient demonstrates two right renal arteries. Virtually no intrarenal arterial filling is seen.

Illustration continued on following page

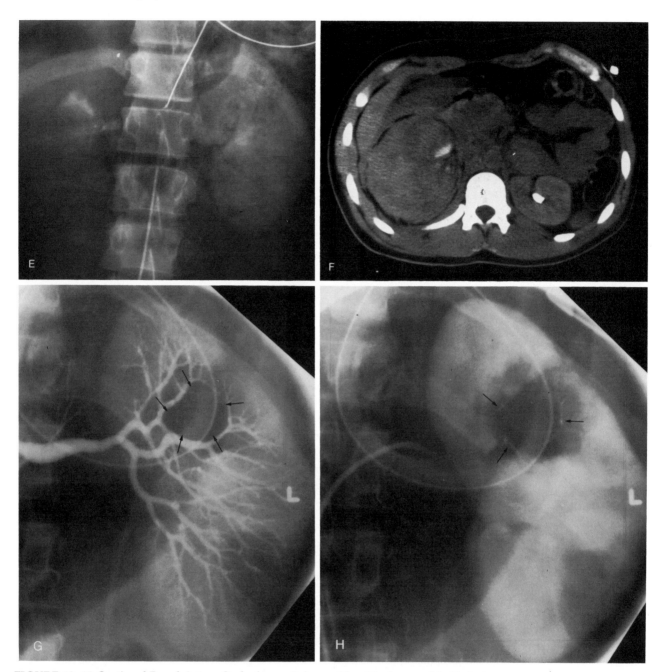

FIGURE 13–15 *Continued* **Renal Artery Occlusion or Injury with a Nephrographic Defect**
• • • •

E, A film taken 7 seconds later demonstrates a very distorted small nephrogram. *F,* Computed tomography performed after angiography reveals a severely injured kidney. Blood is also seen in the pararenal space. *G,* The arterial phase of this angiogram on another patient does not reveal any occluded arteries, but an avascular area should be noted *(arrows).* *H,* The nephrographic phase demonstrates a large defect in the same area with several small damaged arteries *(arrows).* This patient was shot with a small-caliber pistol.

FIGURE 13–17. Extravasation from a Renal Artery Following a Stab Wound
• • • •

A, The extravasation of contrast material *(arrow)* is seen in the arterial phase of this selective right renal angiogram. *B,* The parenchymal phase film demonstrates dense opacification of the renal pelvis and ureter *(arrows).* At surgery there was a communication between the torn artery and the renal pelvis.

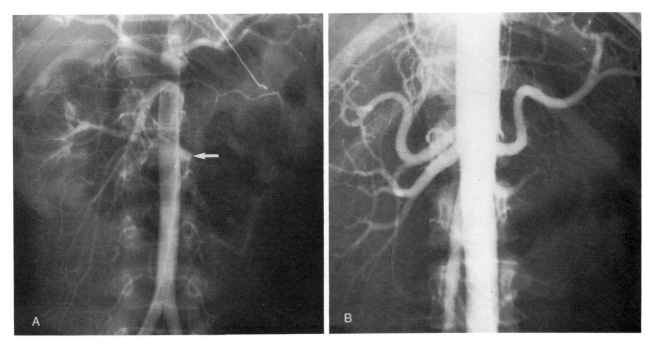

FIGURE 13–16. Renal Artery Occlusion

• • • •

A, The left renal artery is occluded about 1 cm distal to its origin *(arrow)*. B, In a second patient the left renal artery tapers to an occlusion near the bifurcation into the dorsal and the ventral branches. The injury had occurred 3 weeks earlier. The patient developed malignant hypertension during the hospitalization for other injuries.

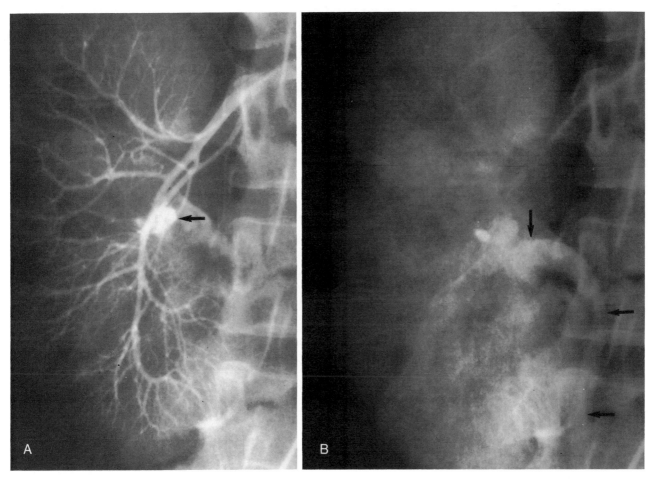

FIGURE 13–17 *See legend on opposite page*

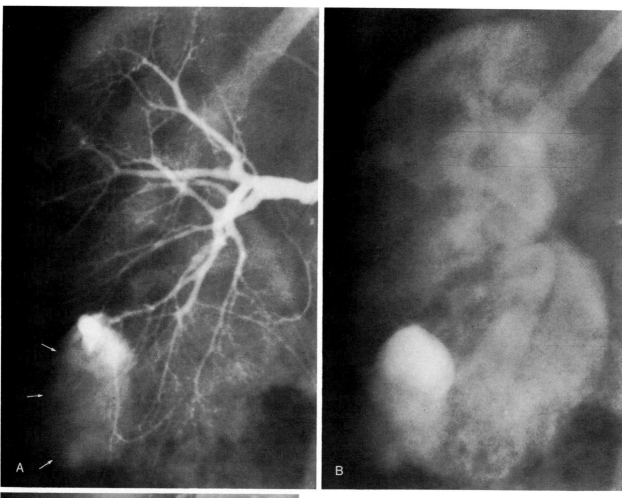

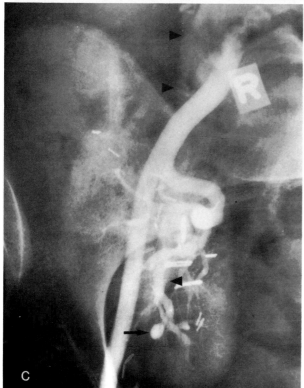

FIGURE 13–18. Pseudoaneurysm

• • • •

A, A very large pseudoaneurysm is seen at the lower pole of the right kidney. The intrarenal arteries are attenuated, and the pseudoaneurysm extends beyond the renal contour *(arrows)*. The patient underwent a renal biopsy approximately 24 hours earlier and was discharged from the hospital. She returned hypotensive and with pain in the right flank. *B*, The parenchymal phase demonstrates the extent of the pseudoaneurysm that ruptured just minutes after this angiogram was taken and before selective embolization could be completed. *C*, A renal biopsy in a transplant kidney caused a small pseudoaneurysm *(arrow)* and an associated arteriovenous fistula *(arrowheads)*. This lesion closed spontaneously.

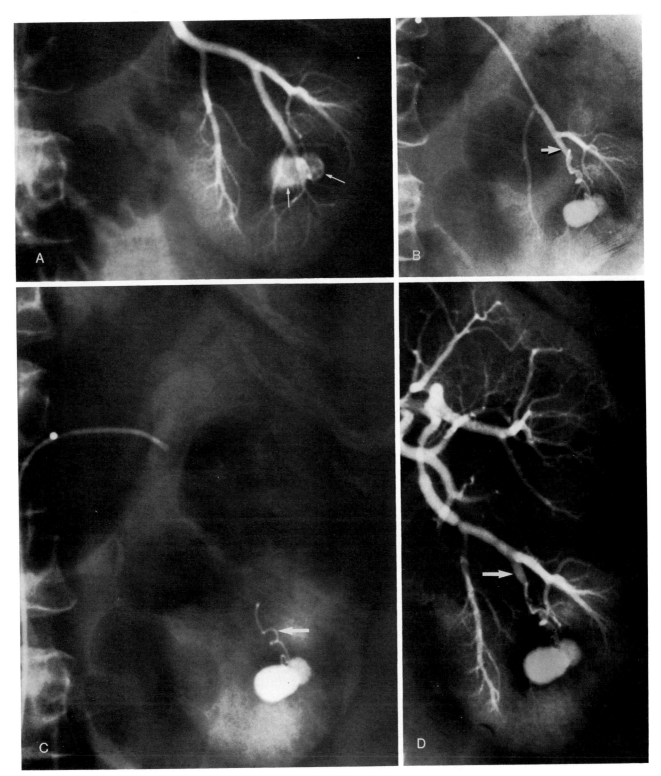

FIGURE 13–19. Embolization for Renal Arterial Injury

• • • •

A, Selective left renal angiogram demonstrates a bilobed pseudoaneurysm in the lower pole of the kidney *(arrows). B,* The arterial branch feeding the pseudoaneurysm has been catheterized selectively *(arrow),* and a single coil has been placed. *C,* This preliminary film of the follow-up angiogram demonstrates residual contrast material in the pseudoaneurysm and also the coil *(arrow). D,* Injection confirms that the coil has successfully occluded the feeding artery *(arrow).*

Illustration continued on following page

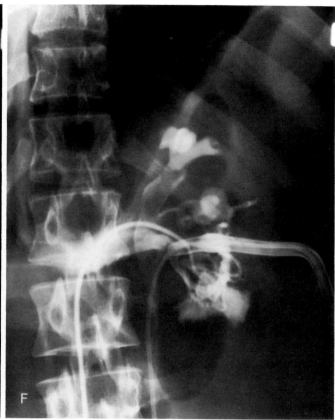

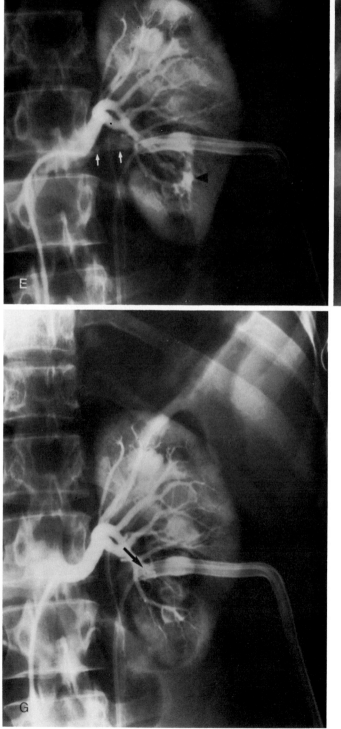

FIGURE 13–19 *Continued* **Embolization for Renal Arterial Injury**

• • • •

E, A second patient developed a small pseudoaneurysm *(arrowhead)* and an arteriovenous fistula *(arrows)* following electrohydraulic lithotripsy. Bleeding occurred into the collecting system. *F*, The catheter has been placed into the feeding artery. *G*, Taken following the placement of two coils *(arrow)*, this angiogram demonstrates the occlusion of the feeding artery.

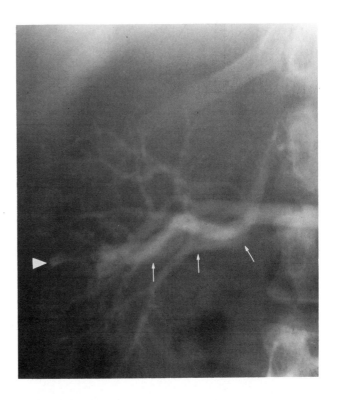

FIGURE 13–20. Arteriovenous Fistula

• • • •

This patient developed hematuria following a stab wound to the kidney. A midarterial film demonstrates filling of the renal vein *(arrows)* from a small arterial branch. A small pseudoaneurysm *(arrowhead)* is interposed between the artery and the vein.

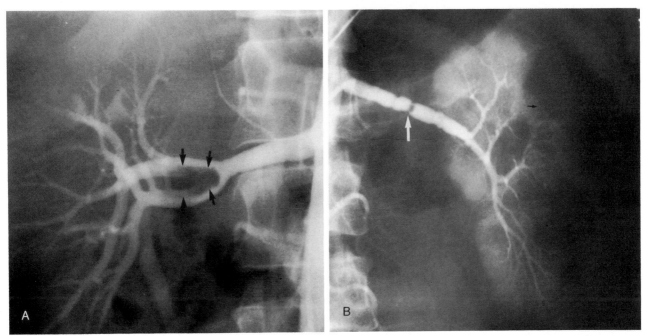

FIGURE 13–21. Intimal Injury

• • • •

A, The right renal artery is normal at its origin, but distal to the origin of the inferior adrenal artery it is slightly irregular in contour and tapers to its bifurcation. Both branches are quite narrow for a centimeter or more and then resume normal caliber. There is an irregular filling defect *(arrows)* causing the narrowing. At exploration intimal injury with clot and some dissection was found. *B,* Selective renal artery injection in a second patient demonstrates marked arterial irregularities caused by intimal tears. Most noticeable is a critical stenosis in its midportion *(arrow).* In addition, there are too few intrarenal arteries and several peripheral nephrographic defects.

Illustration continued on following page

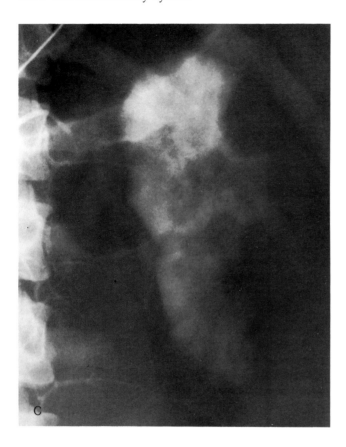

FIGURE 13–21 *Continued* **Intimal Injury**

• • • •

C, This nephrogram phase film more clearly shows the peripheral wedge-shaped nephrographic defects *(arrow)*. The remainder of the nephrogram is patchy and irregular. The entire ventral arterial supply has been occluded.

clusion of the feeding artery suffices. The clinician must weigh these choices while proceeding to control the bleeding artery. Renal hemorrhage can be massive, so speed in performing the procedure is critical.

Occlusion with a resorbable material such as Gelfoam controls many bleeding arteries. Use of a permanent occluder diminishes the possibility of late recurrent bleeding. The decision of what material to use should be made on a case-by-case basis taking into consideration the nature of the lesion, its accessibility, the urgency of the situation, the available materials, and the experience of the operator.

Other Techniques

Nuclear renography and ultrasound scanning can both be used to evaluate renal injury. In general, these examinations are more appropriately used to observe an injury that has already been diagnosed or to evaluate a patient who becomes symptomatic late after an injury rather than as emergency procedures. The renogram can confirm absence of arterial flow, but it does not provide the more specific information available at CT and angiography. However, it is an excellent tool to evaluate patency of an arterial repair. Ultrasound performed at the time of injury can provide detailed information of the injury,

but a technically adequate study is frequently difficult to obtain because of concomitant injuries that make positioning difficult, ileus, and pain on pressure from the probe. When successful, ultrasound can identify intrarenal and extrarenal fluid collection and parenchymal disruptions, and, using Doppler analysis, may identify renal artery occlusion. The procedure is more time-consuming than CT and requires more patient cooperation and operator skill. On the other hand, ultrasound is ideally suited to follow resolution of fluid collections in and around the kidney, and Doppler ultrasound can be used to check patency following renal artery repair.

• • • •

THE URETER

Ironically, the most common cause of ureteric injury is iatrogenic misadventure during pelvic or rectosigmoid surgery. Extensive abdominal vascular surgery and urologic instrumentation can also lead to ureteric injury. Most of these injuries are noticed at the time of the accident; however, unrecognized intraoperative ureteric injury does occur. This possibility should be kept in mind if the postoperative course is not as expected.

Ureteric injury, especially at the ureteropelvic junction, can occur with blunt trauma (Fig. 13–22) but is rarely an isolated abnormality, since severe trauma is necessary to produce the forces needed to disrupt the ureteropelvic junction. Blunt injury to the remainder of the ureter is rare. Penetrating injury may lacerate or transect a ureter (Fig. 13–23) at any point along its course. When the anticipated path of a penetrating injury lies near the course of a ureter, injury should be considered.

Ureteric injury is often asymptomatic, especially initially. Since late recognition of ureteric injury leads to nephrectomy in up to one third of patients, in contrast to less than 5% of patients in whom the injury is recognized early, a high index of suspicion and prompt early evaluation is important. Delayed recognition usually occurs when the patient becomes febrile or develops a flank mass, a fistula, or a renal obstruction, causing pain and hydronephrosis. Delayed recognition of injury also leads to an increased incidence of fibrosis and stricture of the ureter.

Diagnostic Procedures

The diagnosis of ureteral injury can often be made at intravenous urography, although good quality films are mandatory and careful attention must be paid to visualization of the entire ureter. Rupture of the ureteropelvic junction is usually easily seen (see Fig. 13–22). More distal lacerations may be missed if there is a large urinoma that dilutes the extravasating contrast material or if the ureter is not adequately filled. Retrograde and antegrade pyelography also demonstrate lacerations of the ureter (Figs. 13–24 and 13–25). If the retrograde approach is used, fluoroscopic observation is advisable to diminish the amount of contrast medium extravasation from a laceration or transection. CT demonstrates the urinoma and may localize the level of injury when the scan is performed using intravenous contrast material (Fig. 13–26).

If ureteric injury is suspected, the initial radiographic test should either be an intravenous urogram or a retrograde pyelogram. The procedure of choice depends on the nature of the injury. The intravenous

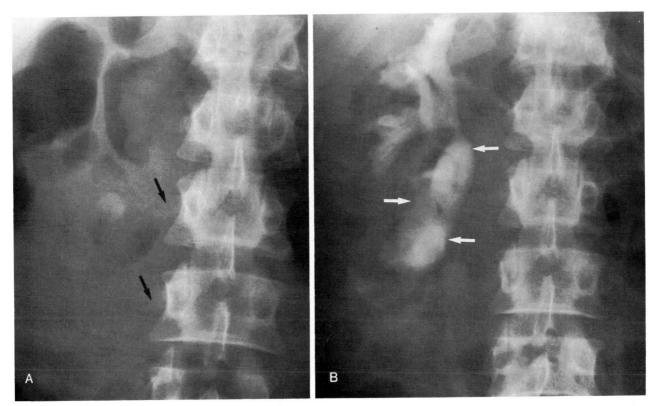

FIGURE 13–22. Avulsion of the Ureteropelvic Junction Caused by Blunt Trauma

• • • •

A, A preliminary film demonstrates fractures *(arrows)* of several transverse processes with displacement of the fracture fragments laterally. *B,* A 10-minute film of an intravenous urogram demonstrates extravasation at the ureteropelvic junction *(arrows);* the extravasation forms a large urinoma.

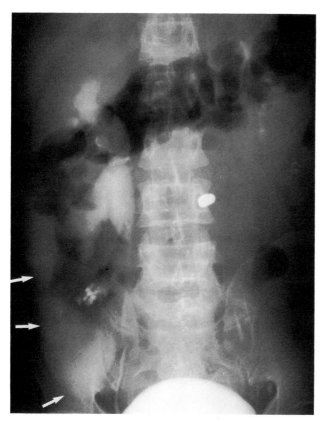

FIGURE 13–23. Penetrating Injury to the Ureter

• • • •

The patient was shot in the abdomen. At exploration the aorta, the inferior vena cava, and the duodenum were found to be perforated. Ascites developed 2 weeks after repair of these injuries. The single film from an intravenous pyelogram demonstrates hydronephrosis on the right side and a large collection of contrast material in the right lower quadrant (arrows). Although the right ureter is seen almost in its entirety, fluoroscopic observation demonstrated leakage from the proximal ureter, which was partially transected.

for prompt intervention. Traditionally this has meant surgical repair, generally by reanastomosis and stenting. When the ureteric injury is extensive or is recognized late, percutaneous or surgical nephrostomy has been employed for decompression until definitive surgical therapy can be undertaken. More

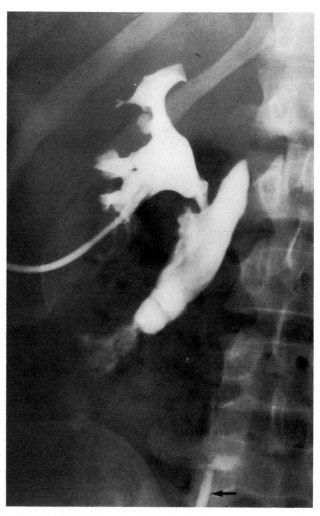

FIGURE 13–24. Antegrade Pyelography Demonstrating a Laceration of the Ureteropelvic Junction

• • • •

A large urinoma is filled by antegrade injection. Note that there is some opacification of the distal ureter (arrow), which was not completely severed.

urogram is simpler and less invasive, but distal ureteric injuries may be missed, especially if the tear is small. Retrograde pyelography that uses standard contrast medium misses few injuries but cannot be performed as readily.

Although the urologic approach to ureteric injury is currently changing, no one argues about the need

FIGURE 13–26. Computed Tomography Demonstration of a Urinoma Caused by a Ureteral Laceration

• • • •

A, This patient was stabbed in the left flank. Computed tomography performed on admission is degraded by patient motion. However, there is extensive extravasation of contrast medium into the left side of the abdomen (arrows). The patient had refused oral contrast media, thus bowel injury could not cause this finding. *B*, A retrograde pyelogram performed after laparotomy, which failed to reveal an injury, demonstrates extravasation from the middle of the ureter (arrow). In this patient, the retrograde injection has been made into the very distal ureter; this is a safer maneuver than more proximal injection.

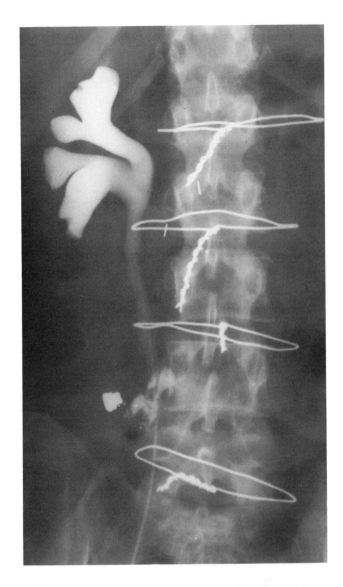

FIGURE 13–25. Retrograde Pyelography Demonstrating a Laceration of the Distal Ureter

• • • •

The retrograde catheter tip is at the ureteropelvic junction. The renal collecting system has been overdistended, and the proximal ureter is well seen. At the level of the bullet there is extravasation of contrast material, and the distal ureter is not filled. The fact that the catheter passed the level of injury indicates the tear is not a complete transection. It is generally safer to inject into the distal ureter rather than to risk further damage to the ureter by instrumentation.

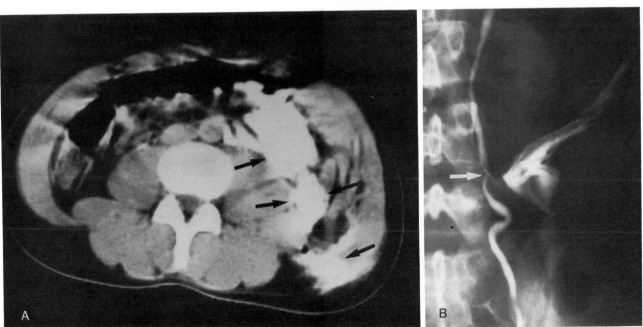

FIGURE 13–26 *See legend on opposite page*

recently, some minor ureteric perforations, such as those occurring during ureteral catheter placement or during percutaneous nephrolithotomy, have been treated successfully by percutaneous nephrostomy with or without stenting. Whether such an approach has any application in noniatrogenic trauma is not yet clear.

• • • •
THE URINARY BLADDER

The urinary bladder is infrequently injured by either blunt or penetrating trauma, probably because of its location deep in the pelvis. In one major trauma center, blunt injury to the bladder requiring laparotomy accounted for less than 2% of all explorations for trauma.[31] Pelvic fractures are strongly associated with blunt trauma to the bladder (Fig. 13–27). Although only 10–20% of patients with pelvic fractures have lower urinary tract injury, pelvic fractures are present in many bladder ruptures. Fractures of the pubic rami and the anterior pelvic ring have the

greatest association with bladder injury. Suspicion of bladder rupture should be high in the presence of such fractures, especially when the patient has hematuria. Penetrating injury of the bladder should be suspected when the course of the projectile has been near the bladder (Fig. 13–28) and also when hematuria is present.

Diagnostic Procedures

Cystography

The first radiographic study to evaluate suspected bladder rupture is the cystogram. This is performed by the retrograde instillation of contrast medium into the bladder, and, therefore, a transurethral catheter must be in place. Urethral injury must always be excluded clinically or by retrograde urethrography before this catheter is placed. Bladder opacification by excreted contrast material following an intravenous urogram, angiogram, or contrast-enhanced CT scan is not reliably dense enough nor can the bladder

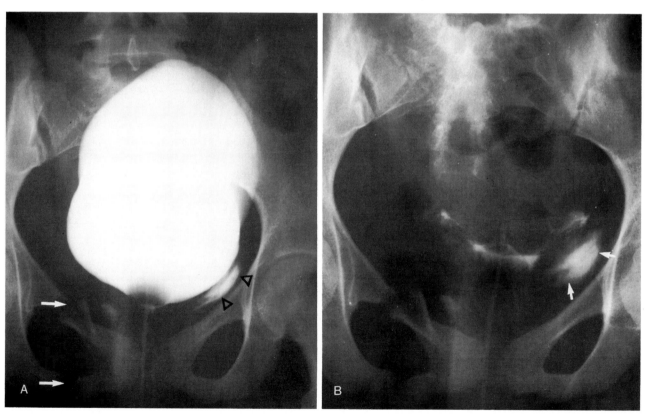

FIGURE 13–27. Pelvic Fractures Associated with Extraperitoneal Rupture of the Bladder
• • • •
A, A filled film of the bladder reveals severe superior and inferior pubic ramus fractures on the right *(arrows).* There is also diastasis of the right sacroiliac joint. The extraperitoneal bladder rupture is seen to the left. *B,* The postdrainage film demonstrates the extravasation *(arrows),* which has the typical hazy contours of extraperitoneal extravasation. The pelvic fractures are again seen.

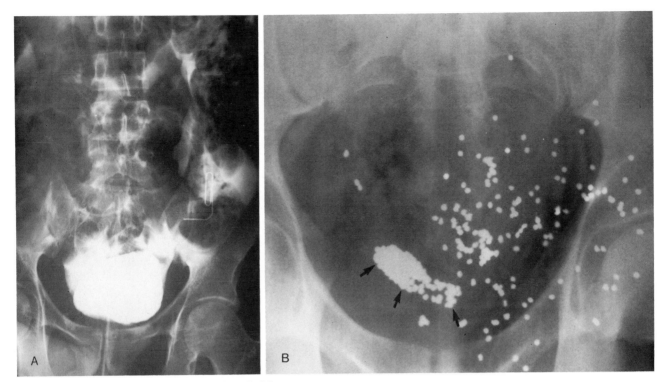

FIGURE 13–28. Penetrating Injury to the Bladder

• • • •

A, The paper clip marks the anterior abdominal wall entry site of a bullet that exited through the right buttock. The cystogram demonstrates an intraperitoneal bladder rupture with contrast material outlining the bowel wall. In such cases two penetrating injuries to the bladder are found unless the bullet has passed tangential to the bladder wall. *B*, A shotgun wound to the pelvis demonstrates innumerable pellets. Those that were clumped together *(arrows)* moved freely with change of position. Many pellets were in the bladder, which had many perforations.

be dependably distended to ensure a diagnostic cystogram.

TECHNIQUE

Following exclusion of urethral injury on clinical or radiologic grounds, a retention-type catheter is positioned in the urinary bladder. A scout film of the bladder is obtained and then dilute (15–25%) contrast medium is instilled into the bladder. About 100 ml of contrast medium should be instilled by gravity with the contrast medium 36 in. above the table top, followed by either fluoroscopy or a film to exclude frank extravasation of the contrast medium. If no extravasation is seen at this point, an additional 200–250 ml should be instilled by gravity. Most patients feel bladder pressure with this volume. After filling, films should be taken of the filled bladder, preferably in anteroposterior, oblique, and lateral projections. At least one postdrainage film should be obtained because the full bladder may obscure subtle extravasation (see Fig. 13–27).

A well-performed cystogram demonstrates the vast majority of bladder tears. Occasionally, a small tear

may be occluded by a clot or the surrounding omentum or bowel, but the usual cause for failure of a cystogram to demonstrate rupture is inadequate bladder distention. Although 300–350 ml distends a normal bladder, a chronically obstructed bladder or one with a capacious diverticulum may require an even larger volume.

RADIOGRAPHIC FINDINGS

The urinary bladder lies in the anterior portion of the pelvis behind the symphysis pubis, from which it is separated by a thin sheet of areolar tissue. The dome of the bladder is covered by peritoneum. Therefore, bladder ruptures can be intraperitoneal, extraperitoneal, or combined (Fig. 13–29). Since the relationship of the dome of the bladder to the peritoneal reflection is highly variable from person to person, both the location of the tear and its relationship to the peritoneal reflection are important in determining the nature of the extravasation. When a rupture occurs near the base of the bladder, the resultant rupture may be complex and extravasation is seen beyond the perivesical space (Fig. 13–30).

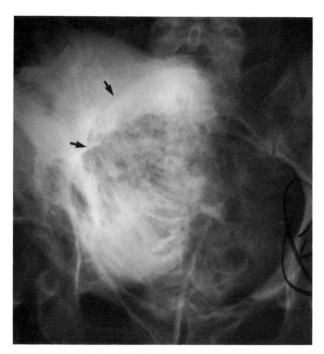

FIGURE 13–29. Combined Intraperitoneal and Extraperitoneal Rupture of the Bladder

• • • •

Contrast material extravasates both in a feathery, ill-defined way and in a better-defined manner indicative of both intraperitoneal and extraperitoneal bladder rupture. The bladder wall *(arrows)* is outlined by contrast material.

Intraperitoneal rupture usually occurs when the bladder is both distended and subjected to an abrupt increase in pressure from a direct blow to the pelvis or lower abdomen. The rupture occurs in the dome of the bladder, which is the weakest point. At cystography, contrast medium generally flows readily through the laceration into the peritoneal space, outlining bowel loops and the paracolic gutters (Fig. 13–31; see also Fig. 13–28A). A small intraperitoneal rupture may be sealed by bowel loops or omentum, but this is uncommon. It should be mentioned that although pelvic fractures may accompany intraperitoneal bladder rupture this is not common. Intraperitoneal ruptures are also more frequent in children than in adults.

Extraperitoneal ruptures are usually associated with pelvic fractures. Laceration by bony spicules has been advocated as the cause of these ruptures, although many ruptures are removed from the pelvic fractures and are more likely bursting injuries. The extravasated contrast material does not flow freely and does not outline bowel loops. It may appear to be contained in a space or may be diffuse or feathery (see Fig. 13–27). Since the pelvic floor is disrupted, complex extraperitoneal ruptures allow the contrast medium to flow beyond the confines of the paravesical space (Fig. 13–32). In these cases, the extrava-

sated contrast material almost always appears feathery and not confined.

Computed Tomography

Bladder rupture with extravasation is readily seen on a CT scan (Fig. 13–33). The ability to discriminate subtle density differences sometimes allows identification of very minor extravasation that could be missed at cystography. Although CT should not be performed as the first diagnostic procedure for bladder rupture, all abdominal CT examinations for blunt trauma should include the bladder and the posterior urethra.

Other Abnormalities

Pelvic fractures that are not accompanied by bladder rupture usually have large pelvic hematomas.

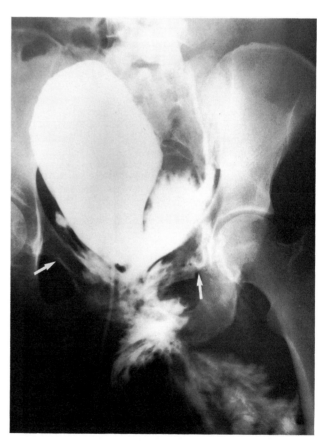

FIGURE 13–30. Extraperitoneal Rupture of the Bladder Near its Base Combined with Injury to the Pelvic Floor

• • • •

The bladder is pear-shaped and displaced to the right. Extraperitoneal extravasation of contrast material is seen to the left of the bladder and tracking down the left thigh and into the scrotum. Bilateral superior pubic rami fractures *(arrows)* are demonstrated. Fractures of the inferior rami are obscured by the contrast material.

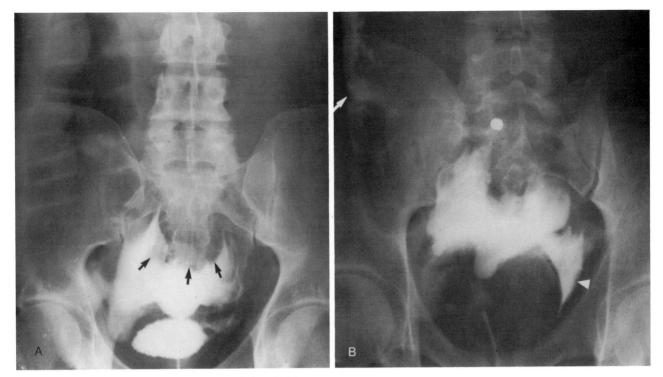

FIGURE 13–31. Intraperitoneal Rupture of the Bladder

• • • •

A, Cystography demonstrates extravasation from the dome of the bladder that outlines bowel loops in the pelvis *(arrows).* The extravasation occurs readily, and the bladder cannot be distended. *B,* Following a gunshot wound, cystography demonstrates the intraperitoneal extravasation of contrast material that has flowed into the right paracolic gutter *(arrow)* and around the dome of the bladder to the left peritoneal reflection *(arrowhead).*

FIGURE 13–32. Extraperitoneal Rupture of the Bladder with Disruption of the Pelvic Floor

• • • •

The bladder base is elevated, and the bladder itself is compressed by surrounding hematoma and urine. The contrast medium extravasation is feathery and ill-defined, which is typical of extraperitoneal extravasation. There is massive bone injury, including fractures of the left acetabulum, the right sacroiliac joint, and the pubic rami.

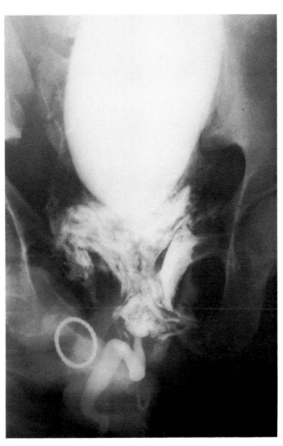

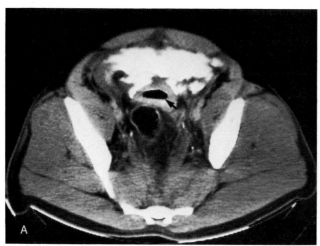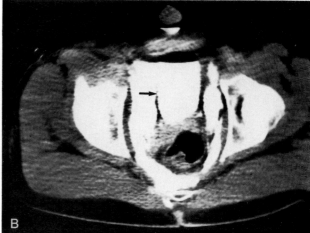

FIGURE 13–33. Rupture of the Bladder at Computed Tomography

• • • •

A, A single section demonstrates the extravasation of contrast material anterior to a small bladder that is filled with air *(arrow).* The intravenous contrast material routinely used for abdominal computed tomography (CT) produced this density in the extravasated urine. *B,* This CT section on a second patient demonstrates the extravasation of contrast material–opacified urine on both sides of the compressed bladder *(arrow).* The very densely opacified urine was also seen surrounding bowel loops in the lower abdomen.

Such hematomas distort and displace the bladder, usually narrowing the transverse dimension of the bladder and increasing the vertical dimension. The deformity has been called "pear-shaped" or "tear-drop-shaped" (Fig. 13–34) and does not indicate bladder injury.

Foreign bodies are sometimes inserted into the bladder through the urethra. The nature of the foreign body determines the likelihood of bladder injury and also the usefulness of any radiographic evaluation (Fig. 13–35).

• • • •

THE URETHRA

Injuries to the urethra can be either blunt or penetrating. The initial radiographic evaluation is usually the same for both and is urgent because the urinary bladder should not be catheterized until the presence or the absence of urethral injury has been established. Blind catheterization of the bladder can exacerbate a urethral injury and is generally impossible to perform when the urethra is lacerated or transected.

The female urethra is short, protected by adjacent bone and soft tissues, and is seldom injured by blunt trauma. The male urethra is longer and less well protected. Although trauma to the male urethra is not common, it can accompany both pelvic straddle injuries and pelvic fractures, especially those of the anterior pelvic arch. Urethral injury must be consid-

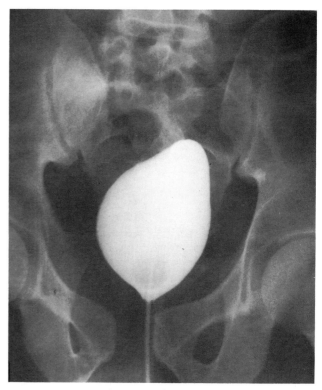

FIGURE 13–34. Pelvic Hematoma Compressing the Bladder

• • • •

Diastasis of the symphysis pubis is demonstrated. The base of the bladder is slightly elevated. The bladder is compressed from both sides by pelvic hematoma, producing a pear-shaped bladder. The bladder is intrinsically normal.

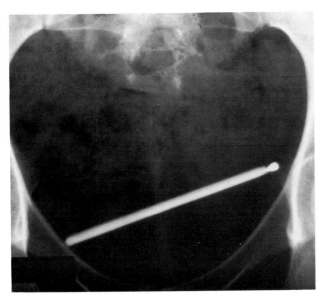

FIGURE 13–35. Thermometer in the Bladder

• • • •

A retarded 24-year-old woman passed a thermometer through her urethra into her bladder. The radiograph was taken to be sure the thermometer was not broken before its removal was attempted.

ered in any male patient who has blood at the urethral meatus, has trouble voiding following pelvic injury even with a full bladder, has anterior pelvic fractures, or has sustained severe perineal or pelvic injury.

Retrograde Urethrography

A retrograde urethrogram should be performed in all patients with urethral injuries, preferably with fluoroscopic control since extravasation can then be minimized. The procedure can be performed using portable filming when the patient is too severely injured to be transported to the radiology department. Several techniques are described for retrograde urethrography, all of which provide satisfactory studies. The simple technique using a Foley catheter is preferable because the equipment needed is available in most emergency rooms and because the hands of the operator are not in the radiographic field.

TECHNIQUE

A 14 or 16 French Foley catheter is filled with 25–30% contrast medium from an attached 50-ml irrigating syringe. Air is cleared from the system. The tip of the catheter is advanced into the urethral meatus for 2–3 cm, and the balloon is inflated with 1–2 ml of fluid so that it is seated in the fossa navicularis of

the penile urethra, permitting gentle traction on the urethra. Filming must be performed during active injection of contrast medium to fully demonstrate all portions of the urethra. If fluoroscopy is available, the injection should be observed to avoid massive extravasation through a laceration or transection. Spot films can be taken during an injection under fluoroscopic control. Otherwise, an overhead film should be obtained during active injection of 15–25 ml of dilute contrast medium (25–30%).

Use of a penile clamp, such as the Brodney clamp, is acceptable if the device is readily available and the operator is familiar with the instrument. Penile clamps obturate the meatus satisfactorily and allow the operator to remove his or her hands from the radiographic field during filming. However, these clamps can be quite daunting if the operator is not familiar with the equipment, which often makes the Foley catheter technique preferable. The use of an irrigating or catheter tip syringe placed in the urethral meatus is unacceptable because the hand of the operator inevitably enters the radiographic field and may even obscure part of the urethra (Fig. 13–36).

Occasionally, a urethrogram is requested on a patient who already has a Foley catheter in the bladder. The very fact that a catheter has been placed correctly into the bladder makes complete transection of the urethra extremely unlikely. However, the catheter should not be removed for urethrography without careful consideration of the management plan for the patient. Urethrography can be performed around the indwelling catheter, but injuries to the posterior urethra may be missed because this portion of the urethra is rarely well visualized when contrast medium is injected around a catheter. A small Foley catheter can be introduced beside the one already in place, or a catheter tip syringe may become necessary.

RADIOGRAPHIC FINDINGS

The male urethra has anterior and posterior components that are divided by the urogenital diaphragm. The anterior urethra consists of the penile (or pendulous) and bulbous portions, and the posterior urethra includes the membranous and prostatic portions. All portions of the urethra must be well distended with contrast medium if subtle injuries are to be detected.

Injuries to the posterior urethra are generally associated with pelvic fractures and are usually caused by shearing or burst forces rather than by perforation caused by a fragment of bone. Colapinto and McCollum[40] have developed a classification of these injuries based on clinical and urethrographic findings. Type I injury is characterized by disruption of

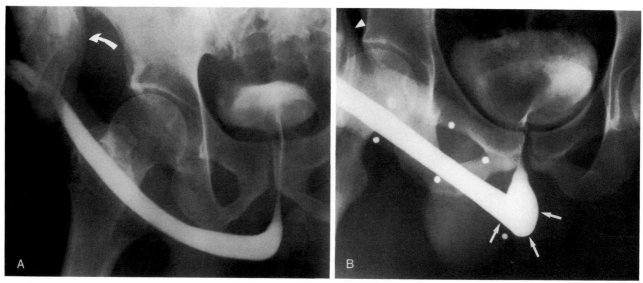

FIGURE 13–36. Normal Urethrogram Using a Catheter Tip Syringe

• • • •

A, The urethra is well distended throughout its entirety. It is also rather well positioned, laying out the entire urethra with no superimposition. However, the hand of the operator *(arrow)* is in the field of view and seen holding the catheter tip syringe in place and also compressing the distal anterior urethra. While no important pathology is obscured in this patient, this is not always the case. *B,* Another normal urethrogram demonstrates both the operator's hand *(arrowhead)* and improper positioning superimposing the bulbous urethra on the penile urethra *(arrows).*

the prostatic attachment to the urogenital diaphragm with an associated hematoma, which causes stretching of the membranous and prostatic portions of the urethra. The urethra is otherwise intact, thus no extravasation of contrast medium is seen at urethrography. Type II injury involves rupture of the membranous part of the urethra above the urogenital diaphragm. Contrast medium extravasates into the fascial planes of the pelvis, but it does not extend beyond the intact urogenital diaphragm. The urethral tear may be partial or complete. Some contrast medium may be seen in the bladder in a partial tear; none enters the bladder if the rupture is complete. Type III injury is the most common form of injury. The urogenital diaphragm is ruptured, and the bulbous and membranous portions of the urethra are torn. At urethrography, contrast medium freely enters the perineal tissues in addition to the pelvic fascial planes (Fig. 13–37). The urethral tear may be partial or complete. Contrast medium in the bladder again indicates an incomplete transection.

The severity of pelvic bone injury does not correlate with the incidence of posterior urethral injury, although the incidence of urethral injury does increase with the severity of the trauma. Even in the presence of anterior pelvic arch fractures, injury is found in only about 10% of male patients. Combined posterior urethral and bladder tears occur in only a slightly greater number (10–15%) of patients.

The anterior urethra is typically injured by direct blows to the perineum, such as the straddle-type injury. Medical instrumentation (Fig. 13–38) and foreign body insertion (Fig. 13–39) are other causes of injury. Blunt pelvic trauma is an uncommon cause of a tear of the anterior urethra.

The radiographic findings in anterior urethral tears depend on whether Buck's fascia is also injured. When this fascia is torn, contrast medium can readily extravasate into the scrotum, the perineum, or the anterior abdominal wall as it is contained only by Colles' fascia (Fig. 13–40). When Buck's fascia is intact, contrast medium extravasates only into the space between that fascia and the tunica albuginea (Fig. 13–41). Blunt injury to the anterior urethra is rather uncommon, even with straddle injury. A more common source of injury to the anterior urethra is iatrogenic, occurring during placement of a Foley catheter (see Fig. 13–38) and during cystoscopy. Such injuries may not be recognized acutely. All these injuries can lead to stricture or other abnormality when therapy is delayed or not instituted (Fig. 13–42).

• • • •

THE PENIS

Fracture of the erect penis is a rare injury that ruptures the tunica albuginea and may disrupt the urethra. Therefore, retrograde urethrography should

Text continued on page 445

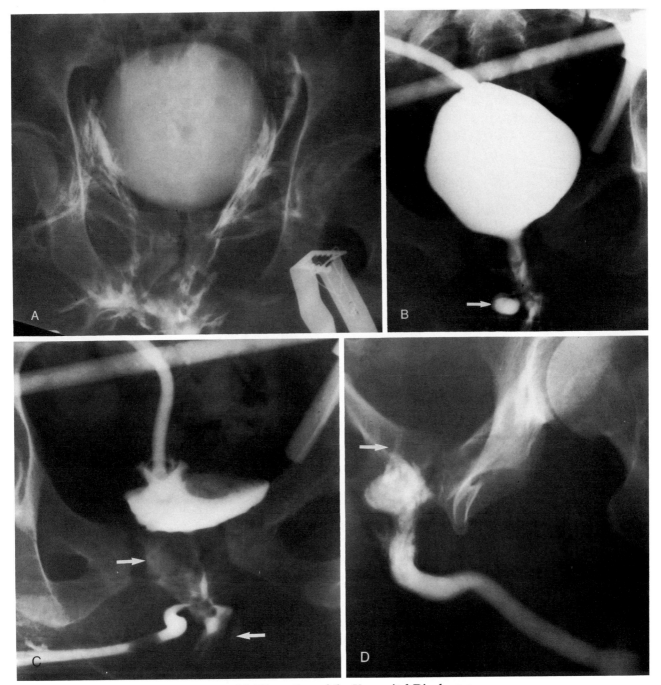

FIGURE 13–37. Posterior Urethral Tear with Disruption of the Urogenital Diaphragm

• • • •

A, At urethrography contrast material extravasates freely into pelvic and perineal tissues, indicating disruption of the urogenital diaphragm in addition to transection of the posterior urethra. The contrast material in the bladder is from an intravenous urogram. *B,* A somewhat less dramatic disruption of the posterior urethra is demonstrated by injection of the suprapubic tube. Focal extravasation is seen at the distal membranous urethra *(arrow)*. At first glance, this is a Type II injury. *C,* This urethrogram in the same patient, however, demonstrates contrast material extravasating into the perineum *(arrows)*, indicating disruption of the urogenital diaphragm. *D,* A urethrogram on a third patient demonstrates frank extravasation at the tear of the prostatic urethra and a small amount of contrast material tracking toward the perineum *(arrow)*.

Illustration continued on following page

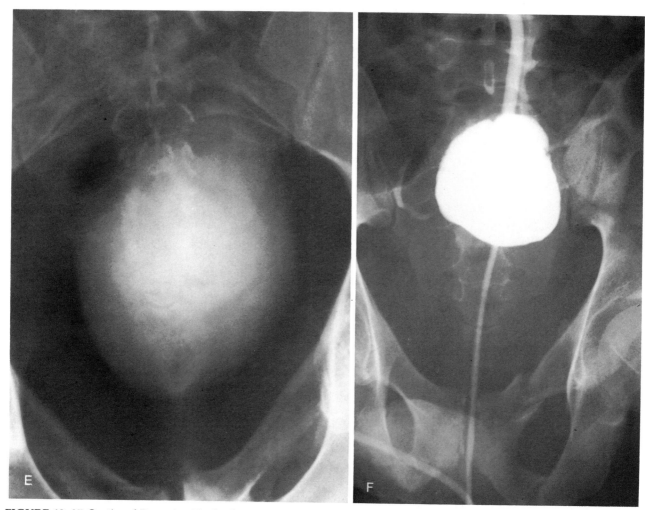

FIGURE 13–37 *Continued* **Posterior Urethral Tear with Disruption of the Urogenital Diaphragm**
• • • •
E, The prostate in this patient was elevated on physical examination. An intravenous urogram demonstrates elevation of the bladder by hematoma from both bone and soft tissue injury. *F,* A cystogram performed through a suprapubic tube demonstrates massive elevation of the bladder. The patient had pelvic fractures and disruption of the prostatic urethra.

FIGURE 13–38. Anterior Urethral Injury

• • • •

Malposition of an indwelling catheter with a 30-ml retention balloon caused a large erosion of the penile urethra in an elderly nursing home patient. The injection has caused some venous intravasation *(arrows)*. The posterior urethra is markedly narrowed by an enlarged prostate, which is the reason for the catheter insertion.

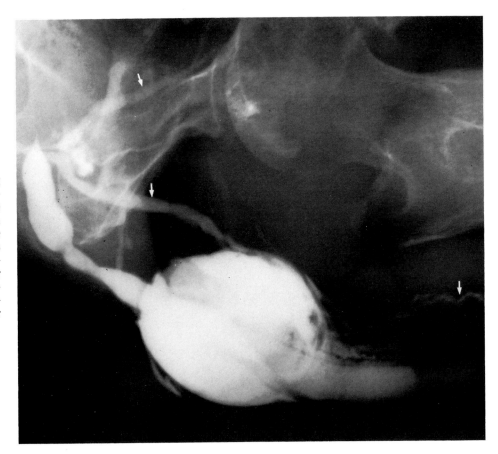

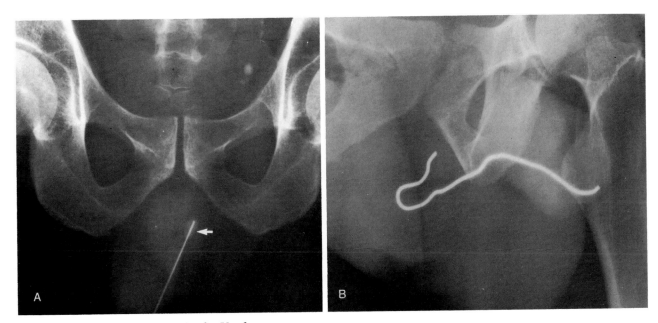

FIGURE 13–39. Foreign Bodies in the Urethra

• • • •

A, A hat pin was inserted into the anterior urethra with its blunt end first *(arrow)*. This type of injury often occurs in mentally disturbed individuals. *B,* Part of a coat hanger in the urethra of a man who had already been treated seven times previously for foreign bodies in the urethra.

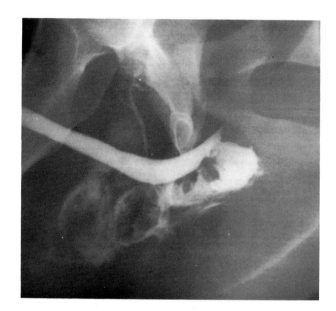

FIGURE 13–40. Anterior Urethral Injury with Disruption of Buck's Fascia

• • • •

A urethrogram demonstrates the extravasation of contrast material into the perineum and the scrotum. Vascular intravasation is also seen.

FIGURE 13–41. Anterior Urethral Injury with Intact Buck's Fascia

• • • •

A urethrogram of a patient with a straddle injury demonstrates extravasation from the bulbous urethra that is confined to the corpus spongiosum. This finding indicates the integrity of Buck's fascia. The venous intravasation is caused by a firm injection and should not be construed as injury.

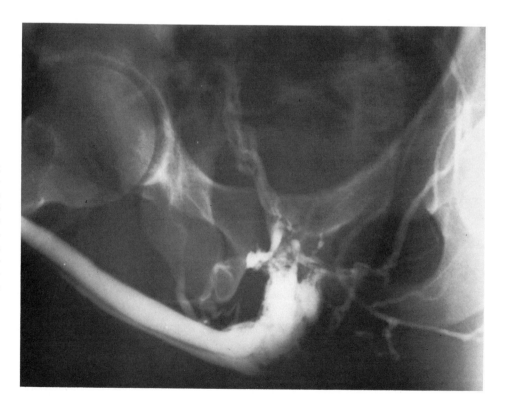

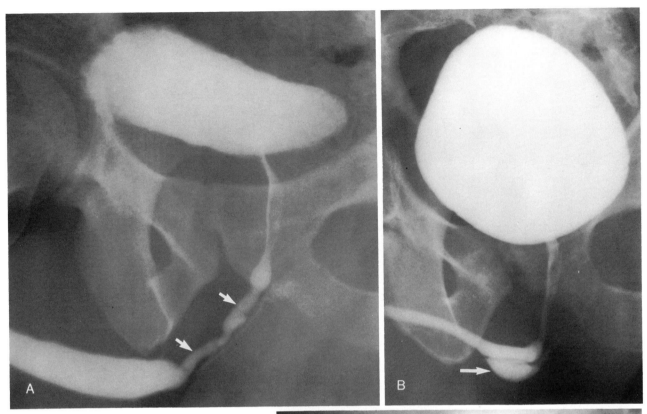

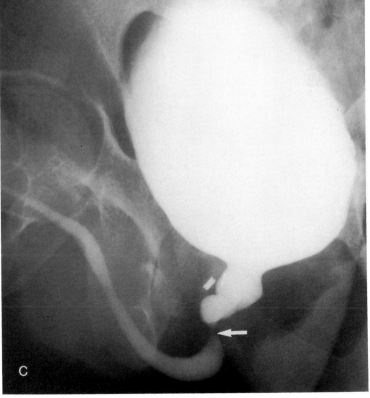

FIGURE 13–42. Complications Following Missed Urethral Injuries

• • • •

A, The patient underwent cystoscopy at 12 years of age. Strictures were identified about 1 year later. This urethrogram performed at 18 years of age demonstrates a long, moderately severe stricture *(arrows)* involving both the anterior and the posterior urethra. *B,* This patient had a straddle injury at 15 years of age but did not see a physician until age 18 years of age, when a urethrogram demonstrating a urethral diverticulum *(arrow),* most likely due to urethral tear, was performed. *C,* A third patient was run over by a tractor. He had a suprapubic tube placed during the repair of a bladder rupture, and his urethral fracture was not recognized for almost 2 weeks. Four years later there is a tight stricture *(arrow)* at the level of the urogenital diaphragm.

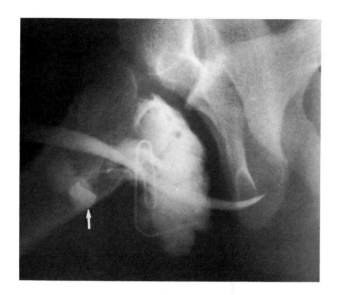

FIGURE 13–43. Penetrating Penile Injury

• • • •

The paper clip marks the bullet entry site. The bullet (*arrow*) is also seen. There is frank extravasation of contrast material at urethrography. Buck's fascia is never intact in this situation, and the extravasation of contrast material can track to the scrotum, the abdominal wall, the perineum, or along the track of the penetrating projectile.

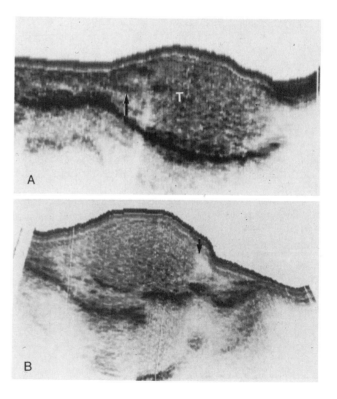

FIGURE 13–44. Normal Ultrasound Image of the Testes

• • • •

A, This sagittal ultrasound of a normal testis demonstrates the fine, even echo pattern of the testes (*T*). The epididymis is more echogenic (*arrow*). A small amount of fluid is often seen between the skin and the testis, though none is seen in this individual. B, A sagittal section of another patient again demonstrates the fine homogeneous testicular echo pattern. A small amount of fluid is seen (*arrow*).

be performed in these patients to evaluate the urethra. Ultrasound has also been used to locate hematomas and tears in the tunica albuginea, which may aid in planning the surgical approach.

Penetrating injuries of the penis usually need no radiologic evaluation unless penetration of the urethra is possible. A retrograde urethrogram should be performed in this situation (Fig. 13–43). Soft tissue films may help to locate foreign bodies but are often not necessary.

• • • •
THE SCROTUM AND THE TESTICLES

Significant blunt injury to the scrotum and the testicles is relatively uncommon. Injury usually results from a direct blow, such as a kick or a blow occurring during football or other contact sport. Straddle injuries can also cause testicular rupture.

Physical examination generally reveals some swelling. Ecchymosis of the scrotum is frequent, and hematocele is commonly present when testicular rupture has occurred. In fact, the presence of a hematocele unfortunately sometimes leads to conservative treatment. Delay in repair of testicular rupture

results in decreased surgical success. For this reason, ultrasound and radionuclide scanning have a role in evaluation of possible testicular rupture.

Ultrasound scans of the normal testicle show a fine, even echo pattern, whereas the epididymis has a coarser pattern (Fig. 13–44). The surrounding capsule is often quite echogenic. Occasionally there is a small amount of fluid between the visceral and the parietal layers of the capsule. In the presence of testicular rupture there is bleeding into the tunica vaginalis; this bleeding is seen as a fluid collection that usually contains numerous echoes (Fig. 13–45). It is this hematoma that makes physical examination of the testicle difficult. Ultrasound may show anechoic areas within an otherwise normal testicle, patchy or geographic abnormalities within the testicles, or lack of differentiation of scrotal contents (Fig. 13–46). Hematomas of the scrotum itself generally appear only as wall thickening, although with age, areas of liquefaction within the clot become hypoechoic.

Testicular radionuclide scanning has been used to differentiate torsion from epididymitis. With the same scanning technique, hematomas are shown as photopenic areas. This may assist in making the decision to explore the testicle for possible rupture.

Many urologists prefer to proceed directly to exploration when confronted by a swollen ecchymotic

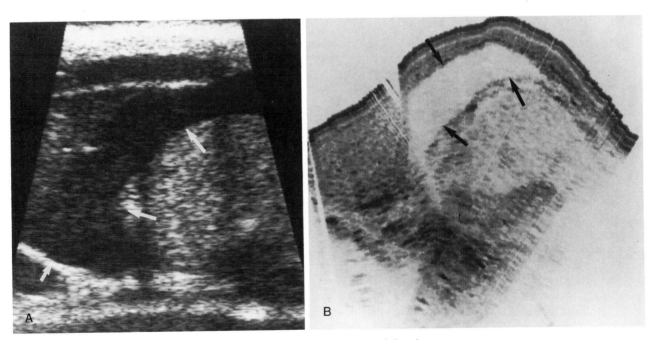

FIGURE 13–45. Hematoma Caused by Testicular Laceration (a Sagittal Scan)
• • • •
A, The testis *(T)* is surrounded by a large fluid collection *(arrows)* that contains many fine echoes; this is the typical ultrasound observation of hematoma surrounding the testicle. *B,* A second patient demonstrates a large fluid collection *(arrows)* with a very fine echo pattern on this sagittal scan.

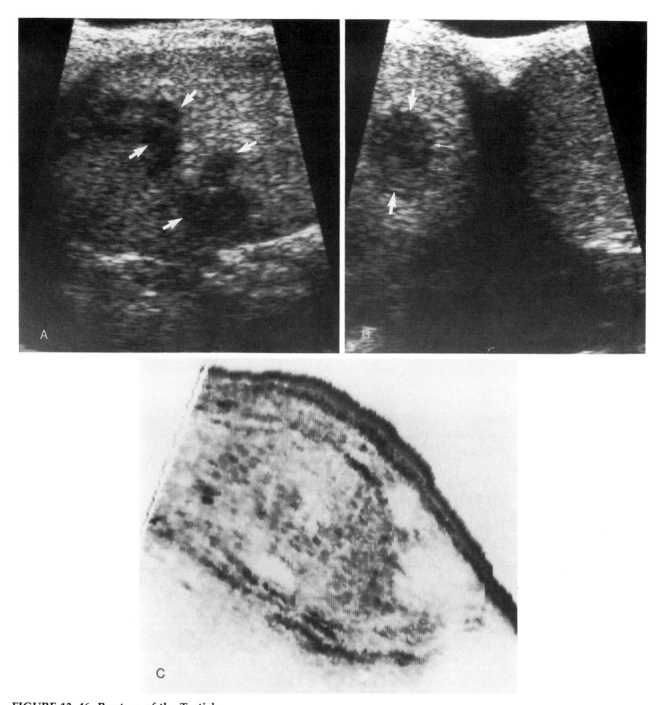

FIGURE 13–46. Rupture of the Testicle

• • • •

A, Patchy hypoechoic areas *(arrows)* are present within the right testicle on this sagittal scan. There is minimal hematoma. *B,* A transverse section on the same patient well demonstrates a hypoechoic area *(arrows). C,* A sagittal scan on another patient with testicular rupture demonstrates a complete lack of differentiation of the scrotal contents and small fluid collections.

scrotum with a hematocele, rather than to perform further tests to confirm testicular rupture. However, both ultrasound and radionuclide scanning have some use in selected patients.

References

The Kidney

1. Bergquist D, Grenabo L, Hedelin H, et al. Long-time follow-up of patients with conservatively treated blunt renal injuries. Acta Chir Scand 1980; 146:291–294.
2. Bergren CT, Chan FN, Bodzin JH. Intravenous pyelogram results in association with renal pathology and therapy in trauma patients. J Trauma 1987; 27:515–518.
3. Bernath AS, Schutte H, Fernandez RRD, Addonizio JC. Stab wounds of the kidney: Conservative management in flank penetration. J Urol 1983; 129:468–470.
4. Carroll PR, McAninch JW. Operative indications in penetrating renal trauma. J Trauma 1985; 25:587–593.
5. Carroll PR, McAninch JW. Major bladder trauma: Mechanisms of injury and a unified method of diagnosis and repair. J Urol 1984; 130:254–257.
6. Cass AS, Cass BP. Immediate surgical management of severe renal injuries in multiple-injured patients. Urology 1983; 21:140–145.
7. Chopp RT, Hekmat-Ravan H, Mendez R. Technetium-99m glucoheptonate renal scan in the diagnosis of acute renal injury. Urology 1980; 15:201–205.
8. Fanney DR, Casillas J, Murphy BJ. CT in the diagnosis of renal trauma. Radiographics 1990; 10:29–40.
9. Fisher RG, Ben-Menachem Y, Whigham C. Stab wounds of the renal artery branches: Angiographic diagnosis and treatment by embolization. AJR 1989; 152:1231–1235.
10. Fletcher TB, Setiawan H, Harrell RS, Redman HC. Posterior abdominal stab wounds: Role of CT evaluation. Radiology 1989; 173:621–625.
11. Furtschegger A, Egender G, Jakse G. The value of sonography in the diagnosis and followup of patients with blunt renal trauma. Br J Urol 1988; 62:110–116.
12. Gelfand MJ. Scintigraphy in upper abdominal trauma. Semin Roentgenol 1984; 19:296–307.
13. Guerriero WG. Trauma to the kidneys, ureters, bladder, and urethra. Surg Clin North Am 1982; 62:1047–1074.
14. Guice K, Oldham K, Eide B, Johansen K. Hematuria after blunt trauma: When is pyelography useful? J Trauma 1983: 23:305–311.
15. Jakse G, Furtschegger A, Egender G. Ultrasound in patients with blunt renal trauma managed by surgery. J Urol 1987; 138:21–23.
16. Kisa E, Schenk WG III. Indications for emergency intravenous pyelography (IVP) in blunt abdominal trauma: A reappraisal. J Trauma 1986; 26:1086–1089.
17. Lang EK, Sullivan J, Frentz G. Renal trauma: Radiological studies: Comparison of urography, computed tomography, angiography, and radionuclide studies. Radiology 1985; 154:1–6.
18. Lupetin AR, Mainwaring BL, Daffner RH. CT diagnosis of renal artery injury caused by blunt abdominal trauma. AJR 1989; 153:1065–1068.
19. McConnell BJ, McConnell RW, Guiberteau MJ. Radionuclide imaging in blunt trauma. Radiol Clin North Am 1981; 19:37–51.
20. Oakland CDH, Britton JM, Charlton CAC. Renal trauma and the intravenous urogram. J R Soc Med 1987; 80:21–22.
21. Peterson NE, Schulze KA. Selective diagnostic uroradiography for trauma. J Urol 1987; 137:449–451.
22. Phillips T, Sclafani SJA, Goldstein A, et al. Use of the contrast-enhanced CT enema in the management of penetrating trauma to the flank and back. J Trauma 1986; 26:593–601.
23. Pollack HM, Wein AJ. Imaging in renal trauma. Radiology 1989; 172:297–308.
24. Rhyner P, Federle MP, Jeffrey RB. CT of trauma to the abnormal kidney. AJR 1984; 142:747–750.
25. Siegel MJ, Balfe DM. Blunt renal and ureteral trauma in childhood: CT patterns of fluid collections. AJR 1989; 152:1043–1047.
26. Stables DP. Unilateral absence of excretion at urography after abdominal trauma. Radiology 1976; 121:609–615.
27. Yale-Loehr AJ, Kramer SS, Quinlan DM, et al. CT of severe renal trauma in children: Evaluation and course of healing with conservative therapy. AJR 1989; 152:109–113.

The Ureter

28. Guerriero WG. Trauma to the kidneys, ureters, bladder and urethra. Surg Clin North Am 1982; 62:1047–1074.
29. Mendez R. Renal trauma. J Urol 1977; 118:698–703.
30. Siegel MJ, Balfe DM. Blunt renal and ureteral trauma in childhood: CT patterns of fluid collections. AJR 1989; 152:1043–1047.

The Urinary Bladder

31. Carroll PR, McAninch JW. Major bladder trauma: The accuracy of cystography. J Urol 1983; 130:287–288.
32. Corriere JN Jr, Sandler CM. Mechanisms of injury, patterns of extravasation, and management of extraperitoneal bladder rupture due to blunt trauma. J Urol 1988; 139:43–44.
33. Hayes EE, Sandler CM, Corriere JN. Management of the ruptured bladder secondary to blunt abdominal trauma. J Urol 1983; 129:946–948.
34. Lieberman AH, et al. Negative cystography with bladder rupture: Presentation of 2 cases and review of the literature. J Urol 1980; 123:428–430.
35. McConnell JD, Wilkerson MD, Peters PC. Rupture of the bladder. Urol Clin North Am 1982; 9:293–296.
36. Oesterling JE, Goldman SM, Lowe FC. Intravesical herniation of small bowel after bladder perforation. J Urol 1987; 138:1236–1238.
37. Sandler CM, Hall JT, Rodriguez MB, Corriere JN Jr. Bladder injury in blunt pelvic trauma. Radiology 1986; 158:633–638.
38. Sandler CM, Phillips JM, Harris JD, Toombs BD. Radiology of the bladder and urethra in blunt pelvic trauma. Radiol Clin North Am 1981; 19:195–211.
39. Wan Y-L, Hsieh H, Lee T-Y, Tsai C-C. Wall defect as a sign of urinary bladder rupture in sonography. J Ultrasound Med 1988; 7:511–513.

The Urethra, the Penis, the Scrotum and the Testicles

40. Colapinto V, McCallum RW. Injury to the male posterior urethra in fractured pelvis: A new classification. J Urol 1977; 118:575–580.
41. Devine PC, Devine CJ Jr. Posterior urethral injuries associated with pelvic fractures. Urology 1982; 20:467–470.
42. Forman HP, Rosenberg HK, Snyder HC III. Fractured penis: Sonographic aid to diagnosis. AJR 1989; 153:1009–1010.
43. Guerriero WJ. Trauma to the kidneys, ureters, bladder, and urethra. Surg Clin North Am 1982; 62:1047–1074.
44. Hricak H, Filly RA. Sonography of the scrotum. Invest Radiol 1983; 18:112–121.
45. Kane NM, Francis IR, Ellis JH. The value of CT in the detection of bladder and posterior urethral injuries. AJR 1989; 153:1243–1246.
46. McAninch JW. Traumatic injuries to the urethra. J Trauma 1981; 21:291–297.
47. McConnell JD, Peters PC, Lewis SE. Testicular rupture in blunt scrotal trauma: Review of 5 cases with recent application of testicular scanning. J Urol 1982; 128:309–311.
48. Morehouse DD. Emergency management of urethral trauma. Urol Clin North Am 1982; 9:251–254.
49. Nymark J, Kristensen JK. Fracture of the penis with urethral rupture. J Urol 1983; 129:147–148.
50. Schuster G. Traumatic rupture of the testicle and a review of the literature. J Urol 1982; 127:1194–1196.

SECTION FIVE

Vascular Injuries

CHAPTER 14

Emergency Evaluation of Vascular Injuries

GEORGE L. MILLER, M.D.
MARGARET E. HANSEN, M.D.

PERIPHERAL ARTERIAL INJURIES

The evaluation of patients for suspected or potential arterial injury has traditionally been performed using catheter angiography. Although new imaging modalities such as magnetic resonance (MR) imaging and color flow Doppler ultrasound scanning have great potential for the demonstration of arteries, their accuracy and precision in the evaluation of acute injury have not yet been proved, and angiography remains the gold standard for the diagnosis of arterial injury. The need for angiographic evaluation of a specific patient must be weighed on an individual basis. The clinical suspicion for arterial injury, the consequences of a suspected arterial injury, the potential complications of angiography or exploratory surgery, and the expertise of the angiographer and surgeon involved in the care of the patient must all be factored into the decision to proceed with angiography or with surgical exploration. The timing of angiography must also be individualized based on the resources and personnel available, the patient's

associated injuries, and the need for other surgical and imaging procedures.

The mechanism of injury should be kept in mind when evaluating a patient for arterial injury. Penetrating injuries are of two types. High-velocity penetrating injuries occur only with high-velocity projectiles such as large-caliber rifle shells. Low-velocity injuries may be caused by handguns or stab wounds. The major difference between these types of injuries is that there must be direct contact between a low-velocity projectile and a vessel for injury to occur, whereas high-velocity projectiles are associated with a surrounding "blast effect" or shock wave that can cause injury to vessels several centimeters away from the direct path of the bullet. Another factor that should be borne in mind is that bullet paths in tissues are not necessarily straight lines. Bullets tumble and ricochet off internal structures and tissue planes and may change course many times between the entrance wound and the final position of the slug or exit wound.

Arterial injuries can also result from direct or blunt trauma such as crush injury, injury by a fracture fragment, or injury from traction on the vessel transmitted from a distant site.

451

• • • • APPROPRIATE RADIOGRAPHIC STUDIES

Peripheral Arterial Injuries

    I. Angiography
Comment: Each study should be tailored to the clinical situation.
    II. Doppler Ultrasound
Comment: May have some use in the future.
    III. Magnetic Resonance Imaging
Comment: May have use in the future.

Venous Injury

    I. Ascending Contrast Venography
Comment: Rarely indicated except for popliteal and femoral veins.
    II. Doppler Ultrasound
Comment: May be useful to evaluate the patency of veins.

Deceleration Injuries of the Aorta

    I. Chest Radiography
        A. Posteroanterior and lateral upright views should be obtained if possible.
        B. Supine anteroposterior views may be helpful.
Comment: Injury is exceedingly unlikely (although it is reported) in a patient with a normal chest film. Further evaluation may be necessary in patients with an abnormal chest radiograph or "mechanism of injury."
    II. Angiography
Comment: A left anterior oblique or lateral view with an additional anteroposterior or right anterior oblique view should be obtained as needed to exclude injury. Caution should be used when negotiating the aortic isthmus.
    III. Computed Tomography
Comment: Can be used to detect mediastinal hematoma, but its true sensitivity and specificity are unknown.
    IV. Magnetic Resonance Imaging
Comment: Can be used to detect mediastinal hematoma, but its true sensitivity and specificity are unknown.

Angiographic Signs of Injury

Regardless of the mechanism of injury, the angiographic appearance of arterial injuries is the same. There are five cardinal signs of arterial injury that may be seen angiographically (Table 14–1). The presence of an arteriovenous fistula, arterial extravasation, intimal flap, pseudoaneurysm, or occlusion is always indicative of arterial injury. Rarely, severe spasm may result in arterial occlusion without arterial injury; however, when an arterial occlusion is seen angiographically, an injury should be presumed to be present until proved otherwise.

Arteriovenous fistulas are abnormal communications between arteries and veins that are caused by partial transection of an adjacent artery and vein (Figs. 14–1 to 14–3). Small arteriovenous fistulas usually close spontaneously, but if they remain patent they can enlarge over time and become symp-

TABLE 14–1. Cardinal Signs of Vascular Injury

Arteriovenous fistula
Extravasation
Intimal flap
Occlusion
Pseudoaneurysm

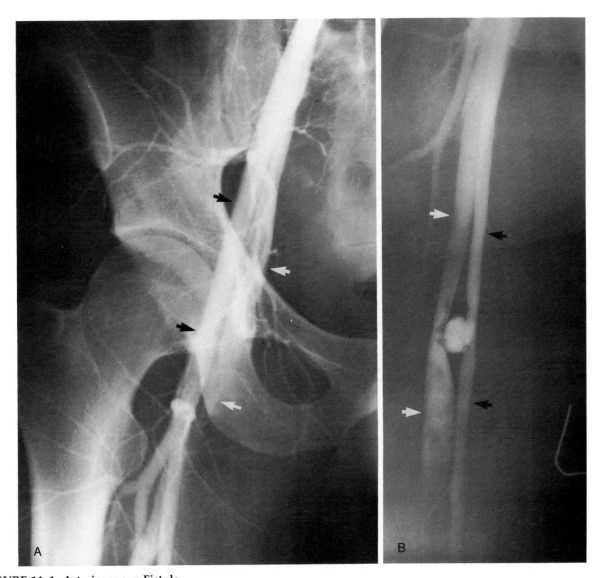

FIGURE 14–1. Arteriovenous Fistula

• • • •

A, Early and dense opacification of the femoral vein *(white arrows)* during the arterial phase *(black arrows)* of an arteriogram indicates a peripheral arteriovenous (AV) fistula. *B,* An AV fistula between the superficial femoral artery *(black arrows)* and the vein *(white arrows)* is demonstrated following a stab wound. AV fistulas are often associated with a pseudoaneurysm, as in this patient.

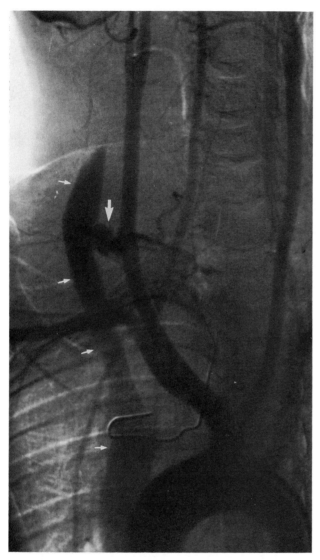

FIGURE 14–2. Arteriovenous Fistula and Pseudoaneurysm

• • • •

An arteriovenous fistula and a small pseudoaneurysm *(white arrow)* between the right common carotid artery and the internal jugular vein *(small white arrows)* is visible. The bent paper clip marks the stab wound entrance.

tomatic. If the actual fistula is not readily apparent on an angiogram, the presence of a fistula should be suspected when an unusually dense vein is seen to opacify early during the arterial phase of an angiogram (see Fig. 14–3). Large fistulas are usually easily seen.

Arteriovenous fistulas, particularly if not identified and treated early, become symptomatic in one of several ways. The presence of a low-resistance communication between an artery and a vein may lead to high-output cardiac failure. If the resistance through the fistula is lower than the peripheral

resistance in the artery, then distal ischemia can occur. As the efferent veins become arterialized, the patient may notice localized venous engorgement or may feel or hear a thrill or bruit (Fig. 14–4).

Extravasation is seen angiographically as extraluminal contrast that appears during the early arterial phase, increases in volume during the arterial phase of the injection, and is not confined to a definable space (Figs. 14–5 to 14–8). This contrasts to a pseu-

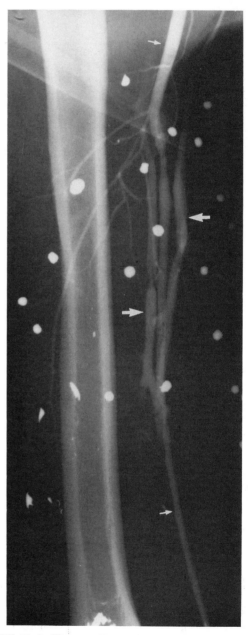

FIGURE 14–3. Shotgun Wound with Multiple Injuries of the Brachial Artery

• • • •

The arteriovenous (AV) fistula is not visible in this projection, but filling of the venae comitantes of the brachial artery *(arrows)* during the early arterial phase of the arteriogram indicates that one or more AV fistulas are present.

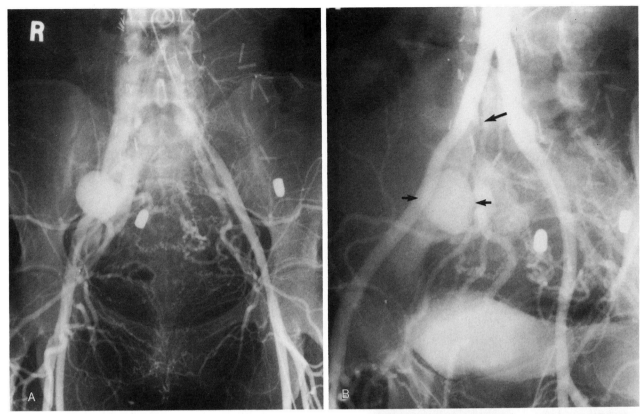

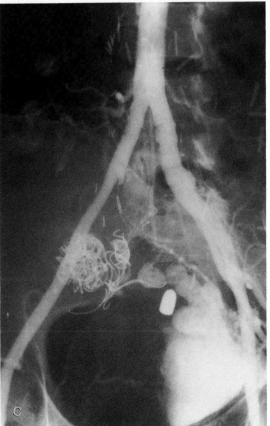

FIGURE 14–4. Chronic Arteriovenous Fistula Associated with a Large Chronic Pseudoaneurysm

• • • •

A and *B,* Anteroposterior and right posterior oblique pelvic arteriographic views in a young woman who had two pelvic gunshot wounds 8 years prior to this study are presented. She developed progressive symptoms of high-output cardiac failure and venous hypertension in the right leg. She has a chronic arteriovenous fistula between the right internal iliac artery and the right external iliac vein associated with a large chronic pseudoaneurysm *(small black arrows, B).* A surgeon had previously attempted to cure this lesion by ligating the right internal iliac artery *(large black arrow, B).* Notice the myriad collaterals reconstituting the proximally occluded internal iliac artery. *C,* This lesion was cured with a combination of transarterial and transvenous embolization.

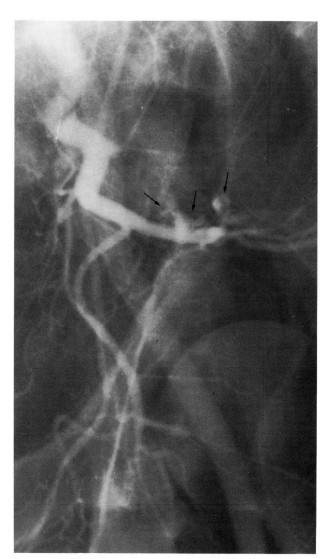

FIGURE 14–6. Extravasation from Branches of the Superior Gluteal Artery

• • • •

This view demonstrates extravasation from branches of the superior gluteal artery *(arrows)* associated with a pelvic fracture sustained in a high-speed motor vehicle accident. This patient's bleeding stopped after selective Gelfoam embolization.

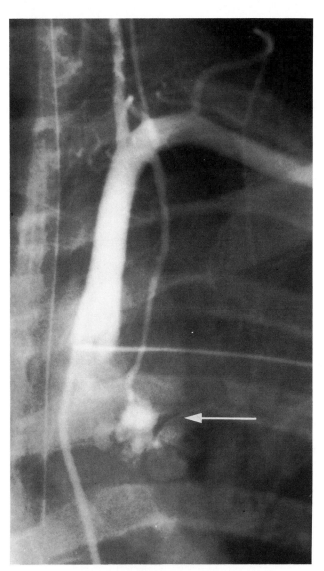

FIGURE 14–5. Contrast Extravasation from a Transected Left Internal Mammary Artery

• • • •

Selective injection of the left subclavian artery demonstrates contrast extravasation from a transected left internal mammary artery *(arrow)* following a stab wound to the left side of the chest. Occlusion with a Gelfoam pledget stopped this patient's bleeding; in general, however, the extensive collaterals to the internal mammary artery make proximal occlusion successful in only about half of all patients.

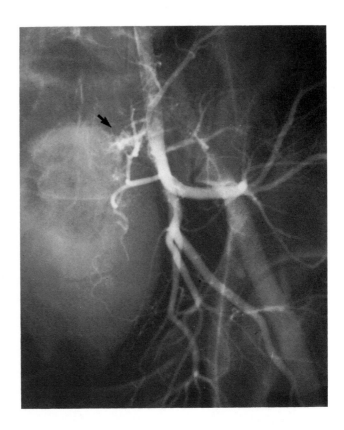

FIGURE 14–7. Extravasation from Medial Sacral Branches of the Internal Iliac Artery

• • • •

Extravasation from medial sacral branches of the internal iliac artery *(arrow)* associated with pelvic fractures sustained in a high-speed motor vehicle accident can be seen. Note the abnormal shape of the bladder due to displacement by a large pelvic hematoma. The proximal origin of these vessels from the internal iliac artery makes transcatheter therapy more difficult. This patient was treated by coil occlusion of the internal iliac artery distal to the origin of the bleeding vessels. This was followed by Gelfoam embolization and proximal coil occlusion.

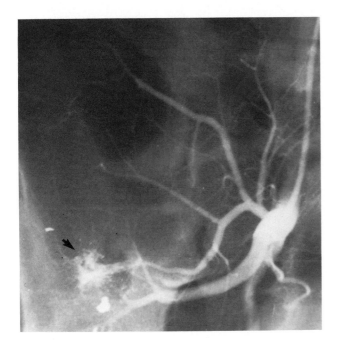

FIGURE 14–8. Extravasation from the Gluteal Branches of the Internal Iliac Artery

• • • •

Extravasation *(arrow)* from the gluteal branches of the internal iliac artery caused by a bullet wound was treated with selective Gelfoam embolization.

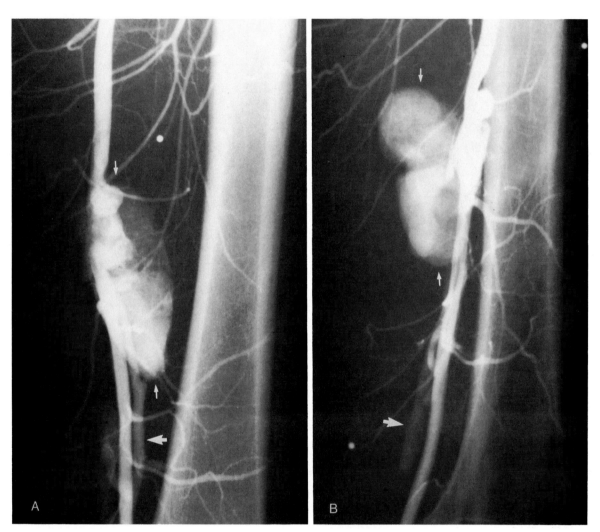

FIGURE 14–9. Pseudoaneurysm Associated with Arterial Wall Irregularity
• • • •

A and *B,* Shown is a large lobulated pseudoaneurysm *(small white arrows)* associated with arterial wall irregularity and a small arteriovenous fistula. The fistula is not seen directly but is inferred from the dense early filling of the popliteal vein *(large white arrow).*

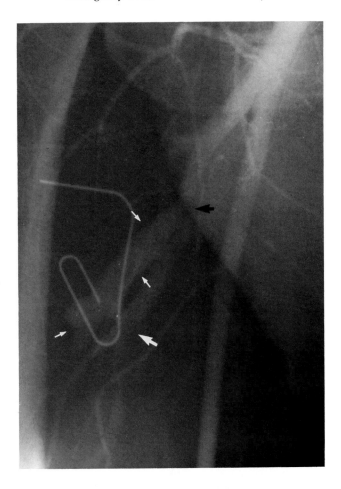

FIGURE 14–10. Short Segment Occlusion with Pseudoaneurysm

• • • •

Short segment occlusion of the deep femoral artery *(large black arrow)* with a pseudoaneurysm *(small white arrows)* arising from the proximal stump is demonstrated in this view. The profunda femoris artery distal to the occlusion is reconstituted *(large white arrow)*.

doaneurysm, which is simply extravasation that is confined (Figs. 14–9 to 14–18). It is sometimes difficult or impossible to determine the difference angiographically between a large pseudoaneurysm and extravasation, but fortunately the distinction is usually of little clinical significance.

Intimal flaps appear angiographically as persistent linear or spiral filling defects within the contrast column (Figs. 14–19 and 14–20). Unopacified collateral inflow defects can simulate intimal flaps, but these tend to be "flame shaped" and vary slightly in size and shape from one film to another. An intimal flap may serve as a nidus for thrombus formation, which may lead to distal embolization or occlusion in situ. Experience with angioplasty-induced intimal flaps would suggest that intimal injuries should usually heal. However, because one cannot differentiate angiographically between an isolated intimal injury and a transmural injury associated with an intimal flap, it is generally considered prudent to surgically explore arteries in which intimal injuries are demonstrated.

Arterial occlusion is easily recognized and may be due to injury with in situ thrombosis or transection with spastic or thrombotic occlusion (Figs. 14–21 to 14–27). Angiographic occlusion of an artery must be considered evidence of injury, but one should bear in mind that occlusive spasm may rarely occur in the absence of arterial injury (Fig. 14–28).

Vasospasm occurs in response to arterial injury and also in association with soft tissue injury without arterial injury. Vasospasm without a concomitant cardinal sign of arterial injury is one of the most difficult areas of angiographic interpretation in trauma. Basically, the angiographic appearance of the vasospastic segment must be considered with the mechanism and the location of injury in order to estimate the likelihood that a particular appearance is due to arterial injury or to simple vasospasm in any individual case. In general, vasospasm not associated with arterial injury involves long segments of vessel, has smoothly tapered proximal and distal margins, and involves the circumference of the artery

Text continued on page 470

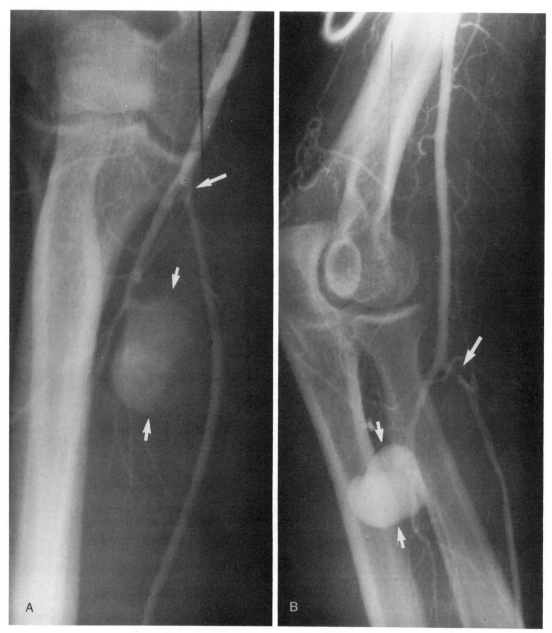

FIGURE 14–11. Pseudoaneurysm of the Ulnar Artery

• • • •

A and *B*, Pseudoaneurysm of the ulnar artery *(small white arrows)* is demonstrated. Note also the intimal injury of the proximal radial artery seen best in *B (large white arrow).*

FIGURE 14–12. Pseudoaneurysm of the Popliteal Artery

• • • •

A small pseudoaneurysm *(arrows)* of the popliteal artery resulting from a stab wound can be seen. A paper clip marks the entrance wound.

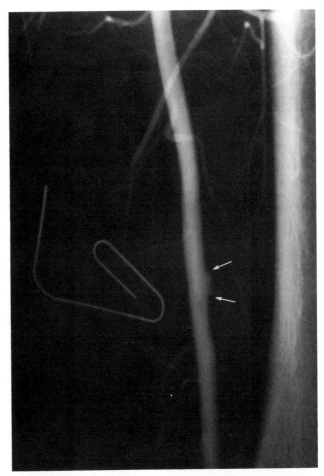

FIGURE 14–13. Shotgun Wound with a Single Pellet in the Neck

• • • •

A and *B, bottom,* There is a pseudoaneurysm of the internal carotid artery *(black arrows)* associated with arterial narrowing *(white arrow).*

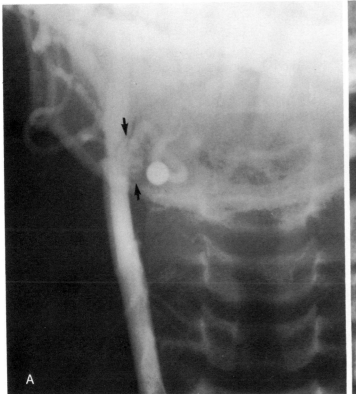

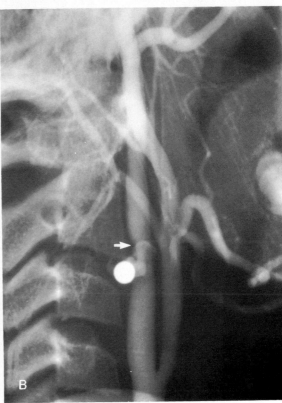

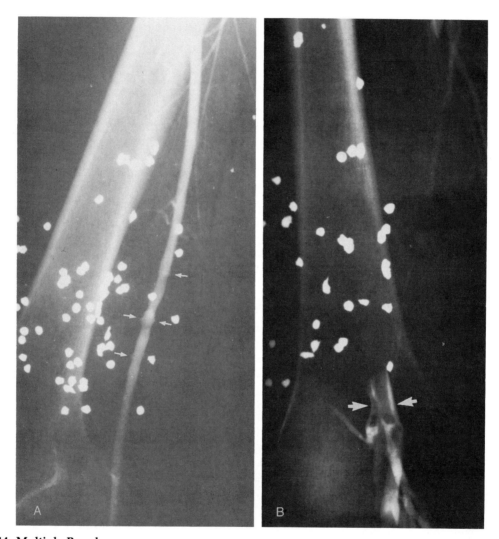

FIGURE 14–14. Multiple Pseudoaneurysms
• • • •
A, Multiple tiny pseudoaneurysms *(arrows)* of the popliteal artery are typical of injuries associated with shotgun wounds. B, An ascending venogram in the same patient shows occlusion of the popliteal vein in the area of injury with some thrombus outlined peripheral to the occlusion *(arrows)*.

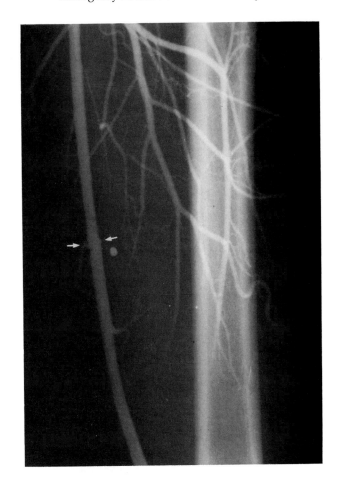

FIGURE 14–15. Tiny Pseudoaneurysms Caused by a Gunshot Wound

• • • •

This view demonstrates tiny pseudoaneurysms *(arrows)* caused by a penetrating injury from a single shotgun pellet.

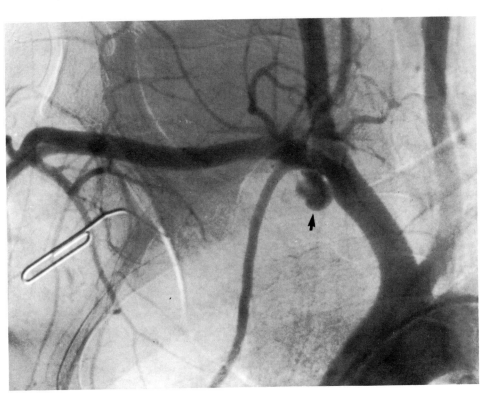

FIGURE 14–16. Pseudoaneurysm of the Proximal Right Subclavian Artery

• • • •

This pseudoaneurysm *(arrow)* was caused by a stab wound. The entrance wound is marked by the paper clip.

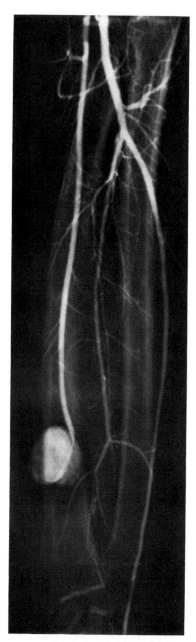

FIGURE 14–17. Large Pseudoaneurysm of the Radial Artery with Occlusion of the Artery Distal to the Injury

• • • •

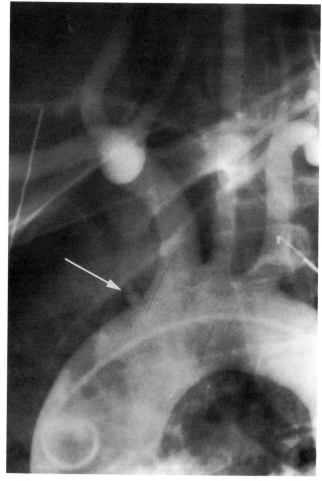

FIGURE 14–18. Small Pseudoaneurysm of the Ascending Aorta

• • • •

This view demonstrates a pseudoaneurysm in a patient with a stab wound in the lower neck. The entrance wound is marked by the paper clip.

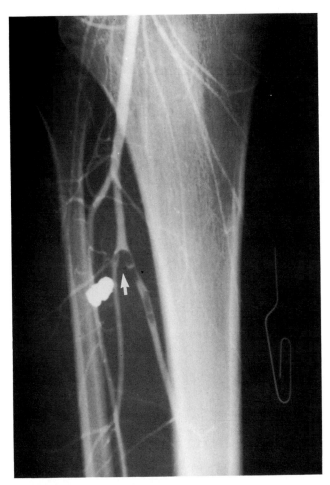

FIGURE 14–19. Intimal Flap

• • • •

This view demonstrates an intimal flap at the bifurcation of the peroneal and the posterior tibial arteries *(arrow)* secondary to a small-caliber gunshot wound. The paper clip marks the entrance wound.

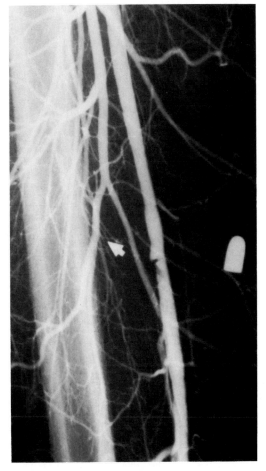

FIGURE 14–20. Intimal Irregularity

• • • •

Intimal irregularity is the only angiographic sign of injury in this gunshot wound. The arrow marks the entrance wound. Partial arterial transection was found at surgical exploration.

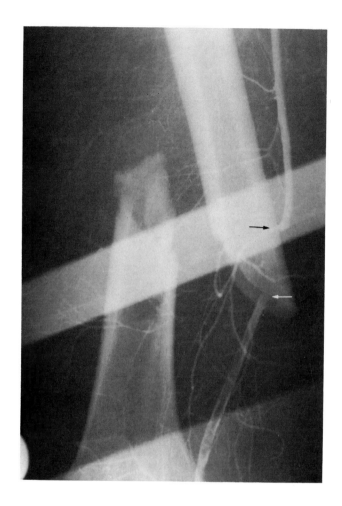

FIGURE 14–21. Arterial Occlusion Caused by Fracture Fragments

• • • •

Note the long intraluminal filling defect in the reconstituted popliteal artery *(white arrow)* caused by an acute nonocclusive thrombus. (Proximal end of occluded segment: *black arrow.*)

FIGURE 14–22. Traumatic Occlusion of an Artery

• • • •

Traumatic occlusion of the axillary artery is demonstrated in a patient who experienced inferior dislocation of the shoulder joint.

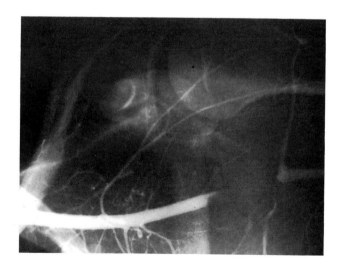

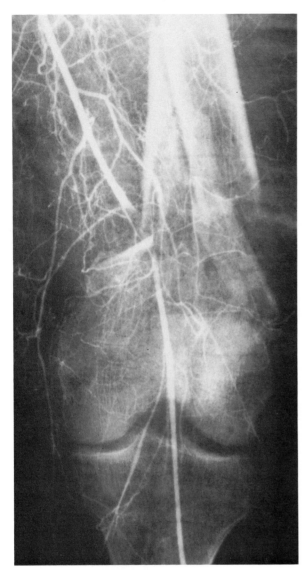

FIGURE 14–23. Popliteal Artery Occlusion Associated with a Distal Femur Fracture

• • • •

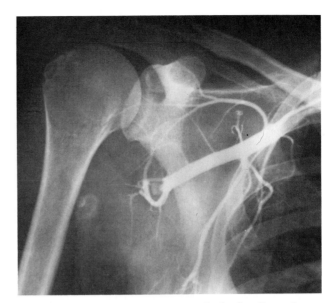

FIGURE 14–24. Subclavian Artery Occlusion Secondary to a Gunshot Wound

• • • •

A complete transection was found at surgical exploration.

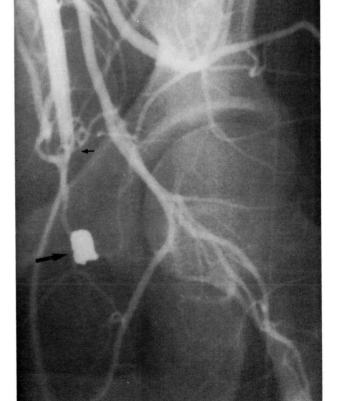

FIGURE 14–25. Embolic Occlusion

• • • •

Embolic occlusion of the left common femoral artery *(arrow)* following a gunshot wound to the chest is demonstrated. Note the bullet lodged in the common femoral artery *(large arrow)*. The bullet entered the pulmonary vein in the lung parenchyma and embolized through the left side of the heart to the systemic circulation.

467

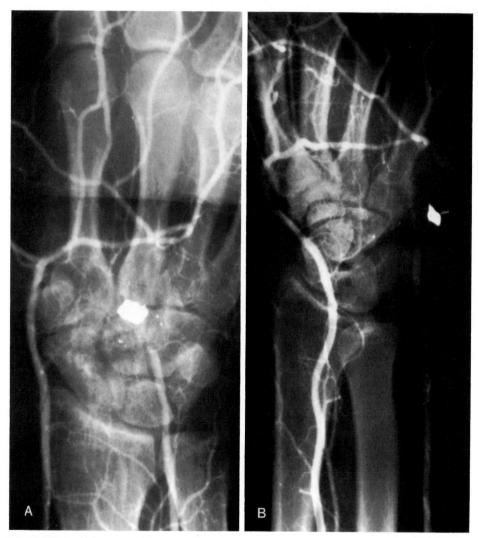

FIGURE 14–26. Distal Ulnar Artery Occlusion

• • • •

A and *B*, These views show distal ulnar artery occlusions associated with gunshot wounds to the hand.

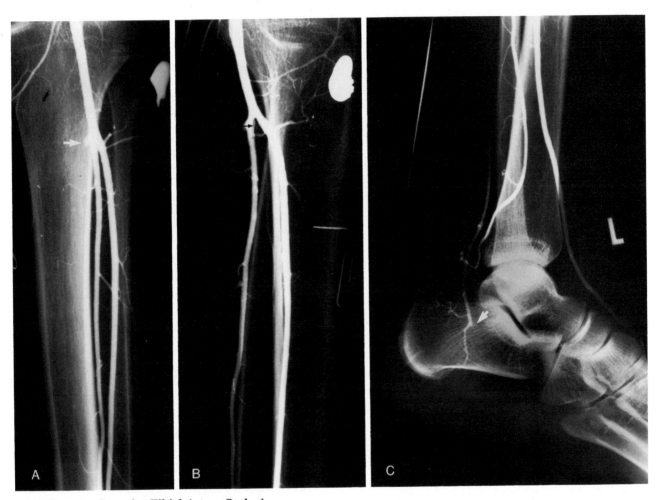

FIGURE 14–27. Posterior Tibial Artery Occlusion

· · · ·

A and *B*, Anteroposterior and lateral views of the lower leg show occlusion of the posterior tibial artery at its origin *(arrow, A)* and a serpiginous filling defect (intimal flap) *(arrow, B)* extending into the proximal peroneal artery. *C*, Lateral view of the foot in the same patient shows abrupt embolic occlusion of the distal posterior tibial artery *(arrow)*.

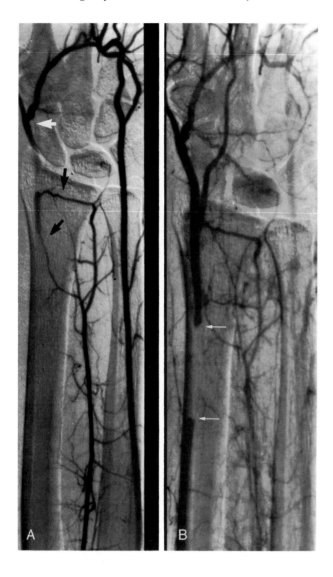

FIGURE 14–28. Occlusive Spasm

· · · ·

A, An early arterial phase film shows delayed flow in the radial artery with distal reconstitution through the palmar arch *(white arrow)* and from the distal interosseous arteries *(black arrows). B,* This late arterial phase film shows segmental occlusion *(arrows).* The artery was found to be normal when it was explored surgically.

symmetrically and concentrically (Fig. 14–29). When vasospasm is associated with an arterial injury, the appearance is often more angular, involves shorter segments of vessel, and has a more eccentric contour (Table 14–2). In the absence of a cardinal sign of injury, however, the angiographic interpretation is an educated guess at best, and therefore the consequences of a missed injury must be weighed against the possible complications of surgical exploration of a normal but spastic artery.

Vasospasm can sometimes be reversed by the intra-arterial administration of a vasodilating agent such as tolazoline (Priscoline), papaverine, or nitroglycerin. If an abnormal artery reverts to a *normal* appearance after the administration of a vasodilator, then the abnormality can be confidently ascribed to vasospasm (Fig. 14–30). If any residual abnormality remains after vasodilator administration, then the previously mentioned considerations still apply. In addition to vasospasm, pre-existing disease must

always be considered when evaluating vascular abnormalities in the trauma patient. Atherosclerosis (Fig. 14–31) is the most commonly encountered problem, and it often mimics intimal injury.

Evaluation Technique

Although every case should be considered and evaluated individually, a few general concepts are applicable to all arteriograms performed on injured extremities.

The area of suspected injury should be studied in at least two projections. Orthogonal projections perpendicular to the long axis of the arteries of interest are ideal. Frequently, however, the local anatomy prevents obtaining views both at right angles to each other and perpendicular to the long axis of the arteries of interest. For example, an ipsilateral pos-

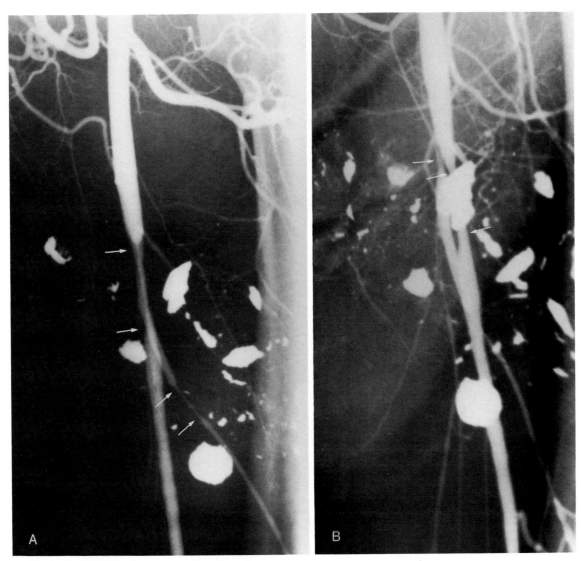

FIGURE 14–29. Vasospasm Not Associated with Arterial Injury
• • • •
A and *B,* Long segments of concentric narrowing of the arteries *(arrows)* are visible in proximity to a large-caliber bullet wound. No large vessel injury was present at surgical exploration. This appearance is typical of spasm.

TABLE 14–2. Angiographic Appearance of Vasospasm

Vasospasm	Injury
Long segment	Short segment
Concentric	Eccentric
Tapered margins	Angular margins

terior oblique view of the femoral bifurcation usually superimposes the superficial femoral artery on the deep femoral artery. The subclavian artery is difficult to study in orthogonal views because the patient's torso prevents positioning perpendicular to the long axis of the artery, and left and right posterior oblique views simply provide foreshortened projections of

the same arterial profile. Angled views of the forearm make identification of the arterial anatomy difficult. A compromise of positioning must be reached that displays the arteries of interest optimally in two projections with the widest separation of angles possible between views. When foreign bodies such as metallic fixation devices or bullet fragments obscure the arteries in orthogonal planes, the views should be modified to clear the foreign bodies from the vessels of interest.

The catheter should be positioned as close as possible to the area of suspected injury to allow good angiographic opacification and to minimize the contrast load administered to the patient, but catheter or guidewire manipulations in the immediate area of

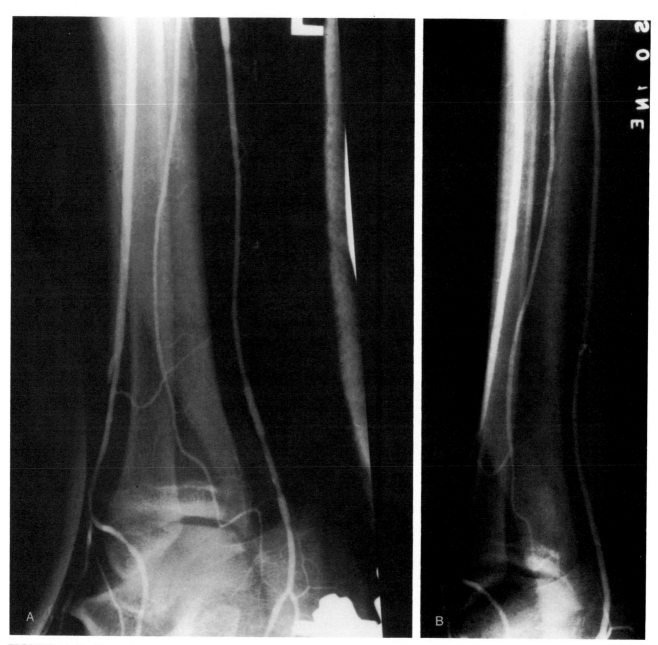

FIGURE 14–30. Normal Appearance of an Artery After Administration of a Vasodilator
• • • •
A, This view demonstrates long segments of concentric narrowing in the posterior tibial artery and the dorsalis pedis artery. The narrowing was caused by spasm. *B,* Arteries are normal after administration of an intra-arterial vasodilator (tolazoline).

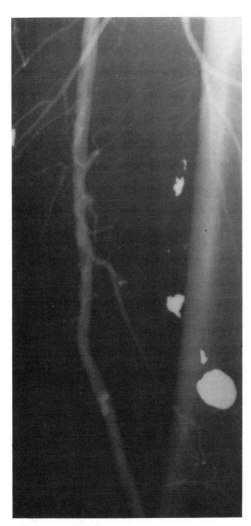

FIGURE 14–31. Atherosclerosis

• • • •

A segment of intimal irregularity is present in the distal superficial femoral artery in proximity to the path of a large-caliber bullet. No injury was found on surgical exploration. This was a focal area of premature atherosclerosis.

suspected injury should be avoided. Catheter or guidewire trauma to the vessel walls can cause spasm or intimal injuries that are indistinguishable angiographically from transmural arterial injuries. Spasm can occur anywhere that a catheter or guidewire has been manipulated and rarely can be seen peripheral to an area of catheter manipulation or a puncture site (see Fig. 14–30).

Careful attention must be given to technical details such as exposure time, collimation, and film markers. As in all vascular contrast studies, a high mA, low kVP technique is preferable, and exposure times must be kept below 0.1 second to minimize physiologic motion artifacts. Careful collimation to the area of interest minimizes scatter radiation fogging of the area of interest and improves image resolution. Ap-

propriate documentation of the patient's name, the hospital number, the date of the procedure, and the side being studied should be *permanently* visible on each film.

Cut film angiograms are the gold standard for the evaluation of arterial injuries, but high-resolution selective arterial digital angiograms (IADSAs) are adequate in some cases. The lower spatial resolution of IADSA compared with film and screen angiography is the limiting factor. If small intimal irregularities are to be treated nonsurgically, then high-resolution IADSA is generally quite acceptable. In some circumstances it may be necessary to use IADSA technique to limit the contrast load when multiple areas must be studied.

Transcatheter Interventions in Vascular Trauma

The vast majority of traumatic arterial injuries must be treated surgically, but there are a few situations in which one should consider transcatheter intervention.

Patients with persistent bleeding associated with pelvic fractures, especially when bleeding persists after emergency stabilization of the fracture fragments, should be studied as quickly as possible with arteriography (see Figs. 14–5 to 14–8). If arterial extravasation or a potential site of extravasation such as a pseudoaneurysm or large vessel occlusion is seen, then transcatheter embolization is the treatment of choice. Surgical intervention in these patients has poor results for several reasons. First, surgical exposure of the internal iliac arteries requires extensive dissection after the retroperitoneal hematoma has been incised and decompressed. These patients often exsanguinate before control of the internal iliac arteries can be obtained. Second, there is extensive collateral supply between the internal iliac arteries across the pelvis and to the internal iliac distribution from the profunda femoris distribution and the body wall. Without angiography, the site of bleeding cannot readily be determined at the time of surgery, and bilateral proximal ligation of the internal iliac arteries is often not effective in stopping hemorrhage because of the extensive collateral blood supply to this area. Therefore, angiographic demonstration of an arterial bleeding site and transcatheter embolization is preferable to surgical intervention in these patients.

Embolotherapy of patients with pelvic arterial bleeding must be aimed at preventing bleeding through collateral channels while attempting to maintain peripheral perfusion to prevent end organ necrosis. This can be accomplished by occluding the large peripheral branches of the internal iliac artery with large particles of gelatin sponge and then occluding the proximal internal iliac artery with a metal coil if necessary (Fig. 14–32).

Acute extremity arterial injuries are rarely amenable to percutaneous embolization because in most cases surgical repair of the injured vessel is necessary for revascularization of an occluded end artery. Extravasation, pseudoaneurysms, and arteriovenous fistulas are amenable to embolotherapy if they arise from branch vessels that can be occluded without jeopardizing the blood supply to an extremity. One must bear in mind that there are extensive collaterals present in the extremities and that it is often essential to occlude vessels both distal and proximal to an injury to prevent collateral reconstitution (Figs. 14–33 to 14–36).

Embolotherapy is often useful in the treatment of renal bleeding from penetrating or blunt injury. Subselective transcatheter embolization allows renal ar-

teriovenous malformations, arteriovenous fistulas, and extravasation to be treated while preserving as much renal parenchyma as possible. Patients with significant injuries of the liver and the spleen are usually treated surgically, but as the surgical treatment of these injuries becomes more conservative there may be an increasing role for transcatheter embolotherapy to control bleeding acutely in these patients (Fig. 14–37).

• • • •
VENOUS INJURIES

Venous injuries are usually inconsequential and seldom require specific diagnostic evaluation. Arteriovenous fistulas are usually diagnosed on arteriography and are significant because of their low resistance, high arterial flow, and consequent poten-

Text continued on page 478

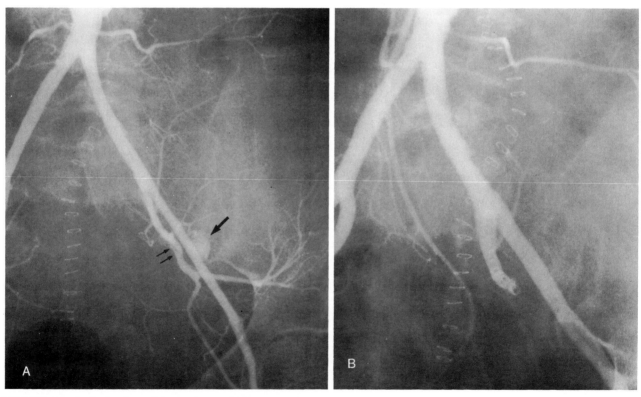

FIGURE 14–32. Occlusion of Large Internal Iliac Artery Branches
• • • •
This elderly patient was involved in a motor vehicle accident and was found to have a large pelvic hematoma at celiotomy. When intra-abdominal injuries were excluded, the abdomen was closed and the patient was sent for immediate pelvic angiography. *A,* This anteroposterior pelvic arteriogram shows a pseudoaneurysm *(large arrow)* arising from a proximal branch of the internal iliac artery. There is also an intimal flap in the internal iliac artery *(small arrows).* Note the severe atherosclerosis of the distal aorta. *B,* After selective catheterization, 2–3-mm gelatin sponge particles were used to occlude the distal branches of the internal iliac artery in order to prevent bleeding from collateral reconstitution. The proximal internal iliac artery was occluded with metal coils 5 mm in diameter.

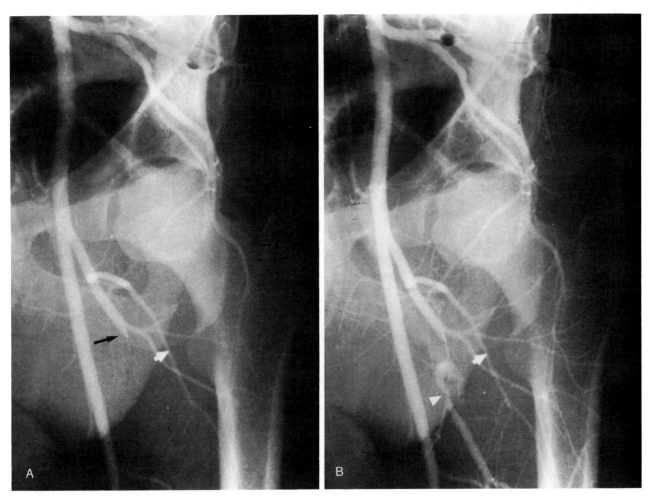

FIGURE 14–33. Pseudoaneurysm of the Deep Femoral Artery

• • • •

The white radiopaque arrow marks the entrance wound in this patient with a stab wound to the groin. *A,* There is occlusion of the proximal deep femoral artery *(black arrow)* with later reconstitution of the distal deep femoral artery (seen in B). *B,* A pseudoaneurysm is seen being filled from the stump of the distal reconstituted artery *(white arrowhead).* This could not be treated with transcatheter occlusion because of the proximal occlusion.

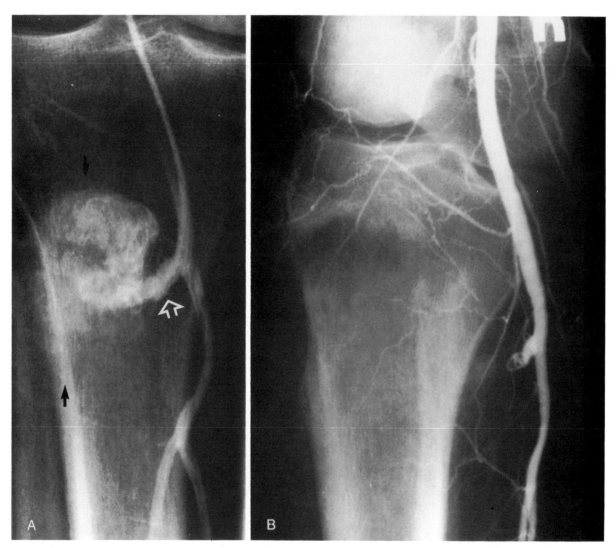

FIGURE 14–34. Pseudoaneurysm of the Anterior Tibial Artery Treated with Transcatheter Occlusion
• • • •

A, This patient has a pseudoaneurysm *(black arrows)* arising from the stump of the anterior tibial artery *(open white arrow).*
B, Because there is no communication between the pseudoaneurysm and the distally reconstituted anterior tibial artery, occlusion of the anterior tibial artery stump with a metal coil is curative.

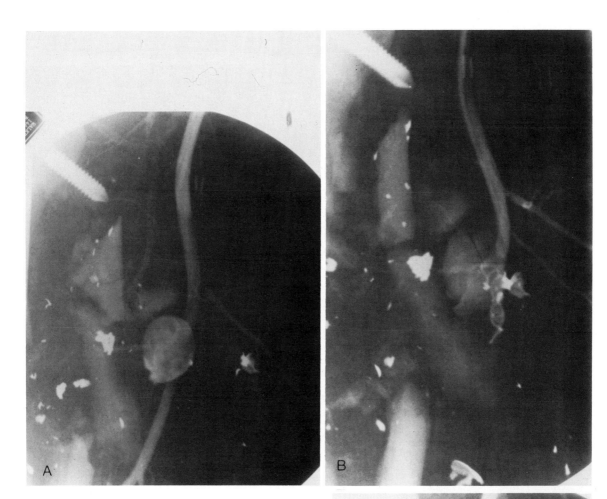

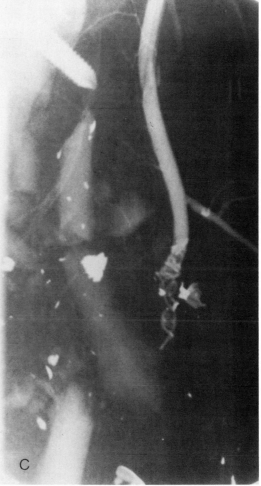

FIGURE 14–35. Treatment of a Pseudoaneurysm of the Deep Femoral Artery with Proximal and Distal Transcatheter Occlusion

• • • •

A, This patient has a comminuted fracture of the femur caused by a gunshot wound associated with a pseudoaneurysm of the main trunk of the deep femoral artery, which is being selectively injected here. He had a massive expanding hematoma in the thigh that progressed over several days. *B,* Following coil occlusion of the deep femoral artery distal to the aneurysm "neck," there is still filling of the aneurysm. *C,* Several more coils are placed and occlude the deep femoral artery proximal to the neck of the pseudoaneurysm. The patient's hematoma stabilized and he had an uneventful recovery following this embolization.

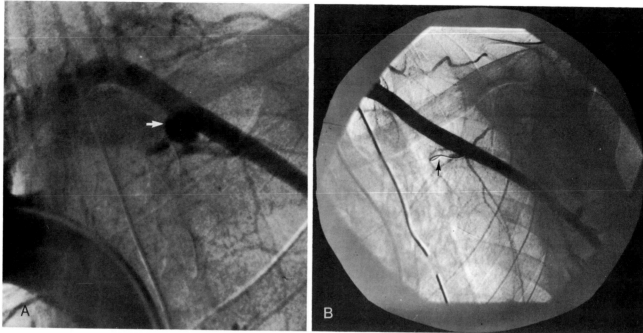

FIGURE 14–36. Pseudoaneurysm of the Distal Subclavian Artery

• • • •

A, This patient has a pseudoaneurysm *(arrow)* arising from a small branch of the distal subclavian artery. *B,* A small platinum coil *(arrow)* occludes the feeding artery with no filling of the pseudoaneurysm. The patient recuperated uneventfully.

tial for enlargement. Venous injuries not associated with arterial lesions are seldom of clinical importance. The exception to this general rule is found in the popliteal and the common femoral veins, which may require surgical repair (see Fig. 14–14). Venous injury is usually manifested by occlusion, but it should be remembered that veins are easily occluded by extrinsic compression from hematoma, bone fragments, or compression dressings. Ascending contrast venography has been the procedure traditionally used to evaluate the popliteal and the femoral veins for injury; however, Doppler ultrasound should be as effective in detecting venous occlusion (Fig. 14–38).

• • • •

DECELERATION INJURIES OF THE AORTA

Deceleration injuries of the thoracic aorta have been recognized for many years but have dramatically increased in frequency with the advent of high-speed motor vehicle travel. Whether traumatic tran-section of the thoracic aorta occurs from deceleration alone or from some combination of deceleration forces and physical compression of the chest has been debated without definitive solution. However, it is well documented that thoracic aortic transection can occur without associated chest wall bone injuries. Traumatic rupture of the thoracic aorta (TRA) has a high mortality rate. Of these patients, 80–90% die before reaching the hospital. Of patients with traumatic rupture of the aorta who reach the hospital alive, approximately 30% die within the first 6 hours, 50% die within the first 24 hours, and 90% are dead within 4 months after hospitalization if the injury is not repaired. Approximately 5% of patients with traumatic rupture of the aorta go on to form "chronic pseudoaneurysms" (Fig. 14–39). Early surgical intervention leads to a dramatically reduced mortality rate for TRA, and therefore it is essential that this diagnosis be considered and made early in the evaluation of patients with deceleration injuries such as those incurred in high-speed motor vehicle accidents and falls from heights greater than 25–30 feet.

There is much debate in the literature regarding the appropriate selection of patients for angiographic

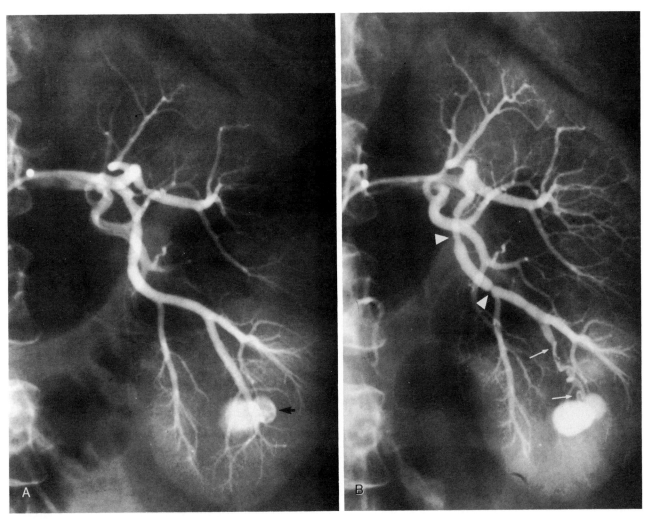

FIGURE 14–37. Transcatheter Embolotherapy

• • • •

A, A selective right renal arteriogram demonstrates a pseudoaneurysm *(arrow)* arising from a lower pole subsegmental branch artery. *B,* A single coil *(small arrows)* occludes the feeding artery. The contrast medium seen in the pseudoaneurysm is static and residual from preocclusion injections. Notice the spasm in the renal artery *(arrowheads)* secondary to manipulation of the catheter.

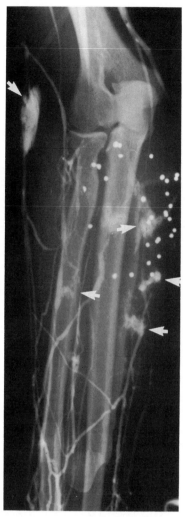

FIGURE 14–38. Contrast Venography

• • • •

This contrast venogram shows multiple areas of venous extravasation *(arrows)* in the forearm of this patient with a shotgun wound.

evaluation of suspected aortic injury. Although some clinical signs such as decreased lower extremity pulses or harsh holosystolic or "machinery" type murmurs suggest aortic injury, the vast majority of patients with TRA have no specific clinical sign suggesting the disorder. Clearly some screening test beyond physical examination is therefore required in patients at risk for this injury. The spectrum of opinions ranges from those who think that any patient who has undergone a significant deceleration force should have an aortic arteriogram, a selection based on "mechanism of injury," to those who believe that a chest film, if normal, is a sufficient screening tool to eliminate the need for further evaluation. The role of computed tomography (CT) and MR imaging, although particularly promising for the detection of mediastinal hematomas that are usually associated with aortic injury, has not yet been scientifically established. It is clear that transmural aortic injuries can occur in the absence of mediastinal hemorrhage; therefore, any screening test such as CT that relies on the detection of mediastinal hematoma fails to identify some patients with TRA.

The most rational approach to evaluation of potential aortic injury would seem to be to first have a high clinical index of suspicion in patients with deceleration injuries. A high-quality chest film should be performed, optimally including both upright posteroanterior and lateral views. When these cannot be obtained because of associated injuries, upright or supine portable chest films may be substituted. Numerous articles have appeared in the radiology literature since the early 1960s that have attempted to correlate isolated plain film findings with the presence of aortic injury. No single plain film finding or constellation of findings has been found to be diagnostic or to meet requirements for a screening test for aortic transection. The abnormalities on the chest film may be quite subtle, but some abnormalities are almost invariably present when TRA has occurred. The clinician must bear in mind that no screening test is perfect; therefore, aortography may be indicated despite negative screening tests (even negative chest x-ray and CT) if there is a strong clinical suspicion and an appropriate mechanism of injury.

Plain film radiographic abnormalities can be divided into three basic categories (Table 14–3). The first are findings that are directly associated with aortic transection and the associated pseudoaneurysm, usually in the region of the aortic isthmus. The second are findings that indicate the presence of mediastinal hematoma. Finally, the third category comprises nonspecific findings that are due to chest wall or pulmonary parenchymal trauma unrelated to aortic injury; these abnormalities are indicative of significant chest wall trauma, deceleration forces, or both.

FIGURE 14–39. Chronic Pseudoaneurysm

• • • •

A and *B*, Posteroanterior and lateral chest x-rays obtained for a routine insurance physical examination show a calcified mass adjacent to the aortic isthmus *(arrows)*. The patient had been involved in a motor vehicle accident 20 years earlier. *C* and *D*, Anteroposterior and lateral aortograms show the chronic pseudoaneurysm.

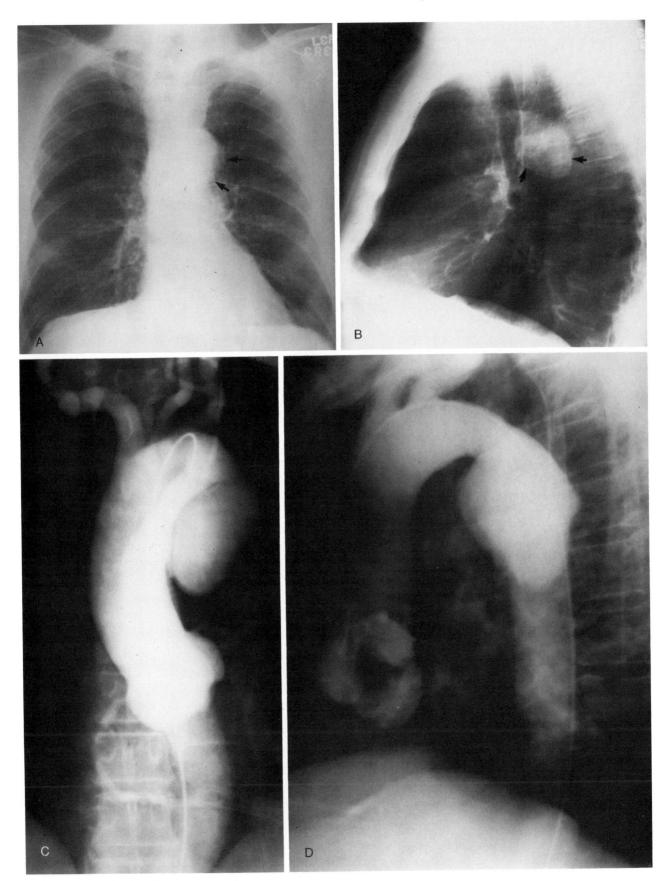

FIGURE 14–39 *See legend on opposite page*

TABLE 14–3. Plain Film Findings in Traumatic Rupture of the Thoracic Aorta

Specific Findings
Trachea displaced to the right at the level of the arch
Esophagus (nasogastric tube) displaced to the right at the level of the arch
Indistinct aortic "knob"
Depressed left main stem bronchus

Mediastinal Hematoma
Widened mediastinum
Widened paraspinous stripe
"Apical cap"
Increased density of the mediastinum
Obliteration of normal mediastinal edges and contours

Nonspecific Findings of Severe Trauma
Pulmonary contusion
Rib fractures
Sternoclavicular dislocation
Hemothorax
Pneumothorax
Diaphragmatic rupture

Clinical Indicators of "Significant Deceleration"
Broken steering wheel
Chest wall bruises/contusions
Cardiac contusion
Major long bone fractures
Spine or pelvic fractures

Plain film radiographic findings related directly to the aortic pseudoaneurysm in the region of the aortic isthmus include irregularity or abnormal contour of the aortic arch, obscuration of the aortic knob, displacement of the trachea to the right at the level of the aortic arch, displacement of the esophagus (usually visualized as a nasogastric tube on the radiograph) to the right at the level of the aortic arch, displacement of the left main stem bronchus, and the obliteration of the aortopulmonic window (see Figs. 14–31 to 14–36).

Plain film findings suggesting the presence of a nonspecific mediastinal hematoma include generalized widening of the mediastinum (8 cm at the level of the aortic arch is a reasonable threshold measurement; however, an experienced radiologic assessment based on degree of inspiration, supine versus upright technique, and so on, is probably as valid). Other findings of mediastinal hematoma include widening of the right or left paraspinous stripes, apical caps, diffuse increased density of the mediastinum, and obliteration of normal mediastinal edges and contours.

Nonspecific plain film findings associated with significant chest trauma include pulmonary contusion, rib fractures (particularly of the first three ribs), clavicle fracture, sternoclavicular dislocation, hemothorax, and pneumohemothorax. Associated clinical information, such as broken steering wheel or steering column, chest wall bruises and contusions, and cardiac contusion, also indicates significant chest trauma. The presence of multiple long bone fractures,

spinal fractures, and pelvic fractures confirms that a rapid deceleration occurred and should raise the clinical index of suspicion for aortic injury.

Findings in the first category are generally associated with a very high incidence of traumatic rupture of the aorta. Findings in the second category are less specific and therefore less often associated with TRA, whereas findings in the third category are completely nonspecific and very poorly correlated with TRA when not found in association with the more specific mediastinal findings.

Evaluation Technique

When a clinical suspicion for TRA exists and the screening chest film is not normal, further evaluation may be obtained with CT, MR imaging, or aortography. The patient's clinical status, the level of suspicion for aortic injury, and resource availability all come into play in deciding the most appropriate next step in evaluation. Thoracic aortography via the transfemoral route has been the traditional mode of evaluation. Studies to assess the accuracy of CT and MR imaging in this setting are ongoing.

After access is obtained through the femoral artery, a soft-tipped guide wire (a 15-mm J-wire or a Bentson wire) is advanced carefully under fluoroscopic observation around the aortic arch and into the ascending aorta. A high-flow pigtail catheter capable of flow rates of at least 35 ml/sec is then advanced over the guide wire and positioned in the ascending aorta approximately midway between the aortic valve leaflets and the origin of the brachiocephalic trunk. Contrast medium is injected to opacify the aorta (usually a flow rate of 35 ml/sec or more is required) for a 2-second injection with rapid sequence imaging (at least three films/sec) in a steep right posterior oblique or lateral projection. The films should include the thoracic aorta from the aortic valve cusps to the diaphragm. The proximal brachiocephalic vessels to the origin of the vertebral arteries can usually be included on this view as well. If an abnormality is seen on this projection, further views may be unnecessary, but an additional anteroposterior or shallow right anterior oblique view is usually performed, particularly if the first view is normal.

Interpretation of Aortograms

Partial or complete transection of the thoracic aorta with pseudoaneurysm formation almost always involves the isthmus of the aorta just distal to the left subclavian artery. The typical radiographic appearance of a complete traumatic transection of the aorta consists of a circumferential, fusiform pseudoaneurysm at the level of the isthmus with jagged intraluminal filling defects caused by the torn edges of the aorta at the pseudoaneurysm margins (Figs. 14–40 to 14–51). Partial or incomplete aortic transection may cause a more subtle abnormality (see Fig. 14–47 and Figs. 14–52 to 14–57), and these more subtle injuries may be mimicked by normal anatomic variations or seen in other diseases such as Marfan's syndrome. Other developmental variants, such as aberrant right subclavian artery (Fig. 14–58) or origin of the left vertebral artery (Fig. 14–59) directly from the aortic arch, may be confusing if they are not recognized.

The ductus bump, located just distal to the aortic isthmus on the anteromedial contour of the aortic arch, is a normal anatomic variant. It may be more or less prominent and may be involved with atherosclerosis even in relatively young patients (Figs. 14–60 to 14–64). Asymmetry or atherosclerosis of the ductus bump may simulate a partial aortic tear (Fig. 14–65). Bronchial or intercostal arteries may arise

Text continued on page 504

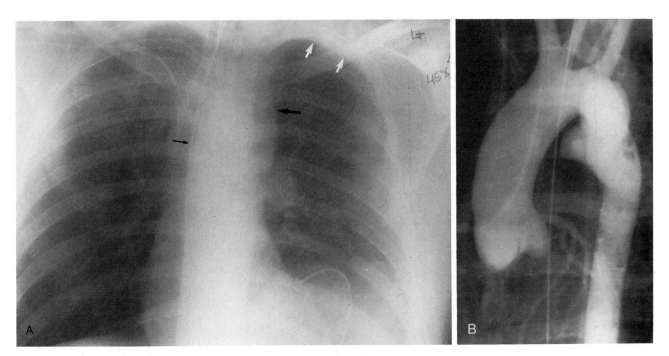

FIGURE 14–40. Traumatic Rupture of the Aorta at the Aortic Isthmus

• • • •

A, This anteroposterior portable chest x-ray in a patient involved in a high-speed motor vehicle accident shows several signs of aortic injury. The nasogastric tube and the tracheal air shadow are displaced to the right at the level of the aortic arch *(small black arrow).* The aortic "knob" has an abnormally straight contour *(large black arrow)* with abnormal density in the "aortopulmonic window" region. There is also elevation of the left hemidiaphragm, and a thin left "apical cap" is present *(white arrows). B,* A right posterior oblique aortogram shows an angular lobulated pseudoaneurysm at the aortic isthmus, the most common site of angiographically identified traumatic rupture of the aorta.

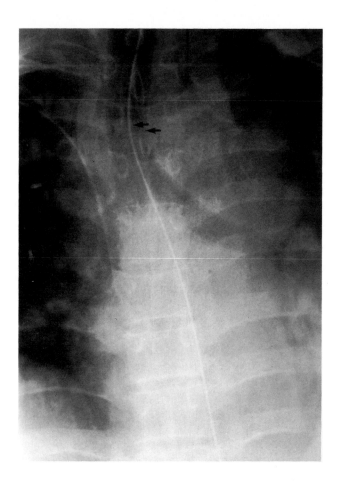

FIGURE 14–41. Tracheal Displacement at the Level of the Aortic Arch in a Patient with Traumatic Rupture of the Aorta

• • • •

An anteroposterior portable chest x-ray shows focal displacement of the nasogastric tube and the trachea to the right at the level of the aortic arch *(arrows)* in a patient with traumatic rupture of the aorta.

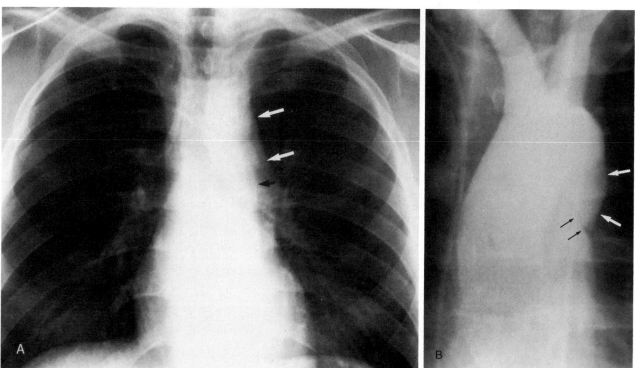

FIGURE 14–42. Intimal Flap and a Small Pseudoaneurysm in Traumatic Rupture of the Aorta

• • • •

A, On this anteroposterior portable chest x-ray, relatively subtle findings suggest traumatic rupture of the aorta. There is abnormal straightening of the left mediastinal contour obscuring the aortic knob and obliterating the normal aortopulmonic window *(white arrows)*. There is also an abnormal edge within the mediastinum *(black arrow)*. *B,* The anteroposterior view of this patient's aortogram shows an intimal flap *(small black arrows)* and a small pseudoaneurysm *(white arrows)*.

484

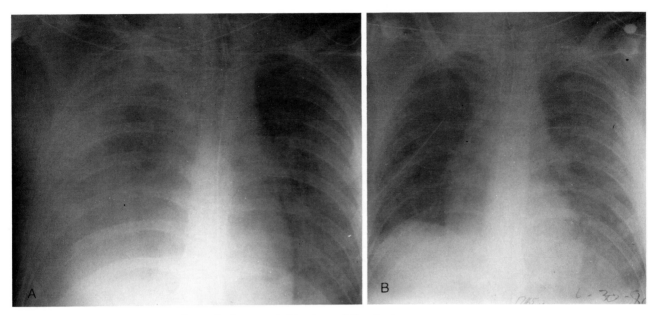

FIGURE 14–43. Bilateral Hemothorax in Traumatic Rupture of the Aorta

• • • •

A, An anteroposterior supine chest x-ray shows a right hemothorax and the normal position of the nasogastric tube and the trachea. *B,* After placement of the right chest tube the patient developed a left hemothorax. The course of the nasogastric tube moves to the patient's right. The aortic knob is not distinct. Traumatic rupture of the aorta was found on the aortic angiogram.

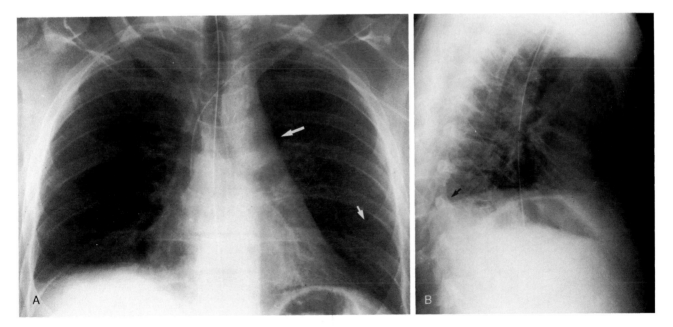

FIGURE 14–44. Pseudoaneurysm in Traumatic Rupture of the Aorta

• • • •

A and *B,* Posteroanterior and lateral chest x-rays show the normal position of the trachea and the nasogastric tube. There is slight straightening of the left mediastinal border *(large arrow, A)* with no distinct aortic knob visible. A fracture of the fourth rib on the left side is present *(small arrow, A)*. The lateral view shows a small pleural effusion *(small arrow, B)*.

Illustration continued on following page

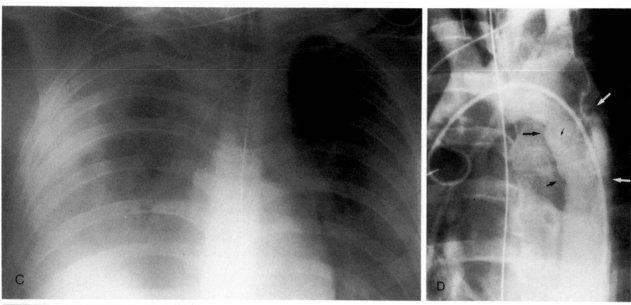

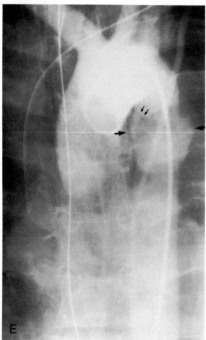

FIGURE 14–44 *Continued* **Pseudoaneurysm in Traumatic Rupture of the Aorta**

• • • •

C, An anteroposterior portable chest x-ray taken 2 hours later, when the patient had sudden hemodynamic decompensation, shows a large right-sided hemothorax. D and E, Right posterior oblique and anteroposterior views from this patient's arch aortogram show a concentric pseudoaneurysm at the level of the isthmus *(large arrows)*. Notice the linear filling defects at the margins of the pseudoaneurysm *(small arrows)* caused by the torn edges of the aorta.

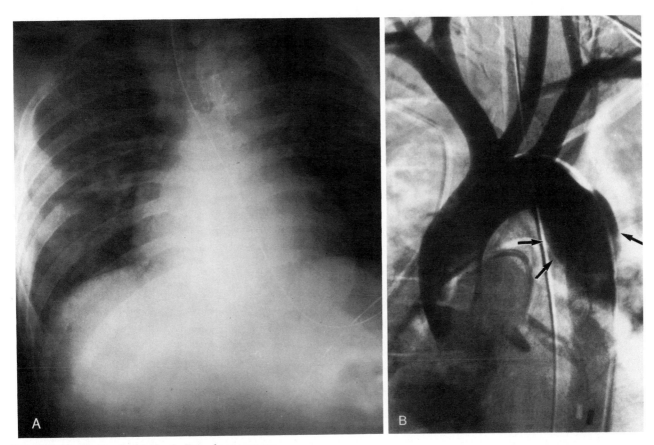

FIGURE 14–45. Typical Isthmic Pseudoaneurysm

• • • •

A, This anteroposterior chest x-ray shows nasogastric tube deviation and right pulmonary contusion associated with a wide superior mediastinum and an abnormal left mediastinal contour. *B,* Film subtraction of a right posterior oblique aortogram shows a typical isthmic pseudoaneurysm *(arrows).*

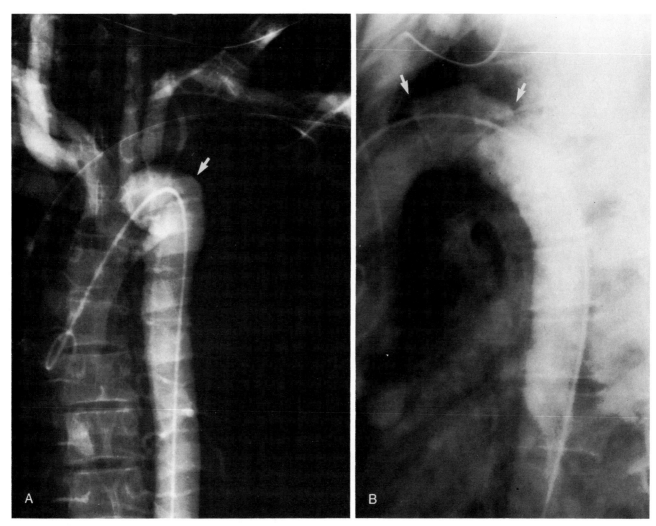

FIGURE 14–46. Transection-Pseudoaneurysm

• • • •

A and *B*, Anteroposterior and lateral views from an aortogram show an unusually proximal-appearing transection-pseudoaneurysm *(white arrows);* it is, however, distal to the left subclavian artery.

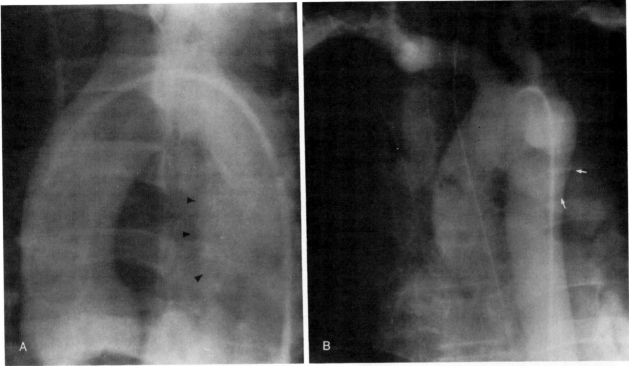

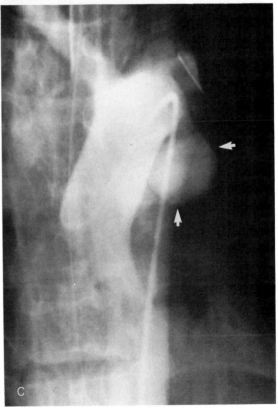

FIGURE 14–47. Pseudoaneurysm in Incomplete Aortic Transection

• • • •

A and *B,* Right posterior oblique and anteroposterior aortograms show a typical isthmic pseudoaneurysm in a patient with an incomplete transection *(arrowheads). C,* This anteroposterior aortogram shows focal pseudoaneurysm *(arrows)* in another patient with partial transection.

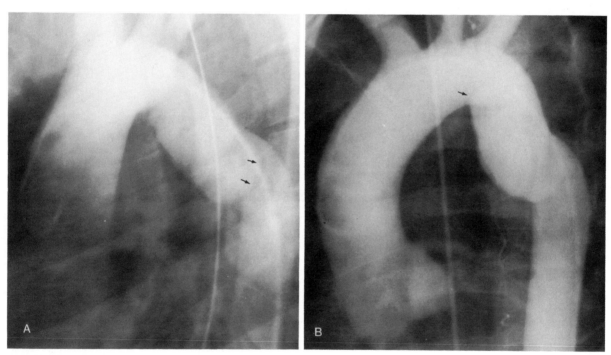

FIGURE 14–48. Pseudoaneurysm in Complete Transection of the Aorta

• • • •

A and *B,* These lateral and right posterior oblique views on an aortogram show elongation and tortuosity of the aortic isthmus with a long pseudoaneurysm in this patient who fell 30 ft. The aorta was completely transected, and the ends of the aorta were 4 cm apart at the time of surgical repair. Again notice the linear lucencies at the margins of the pseudoaneurysm *(arrows)* caused by the torn edges of the aorta.

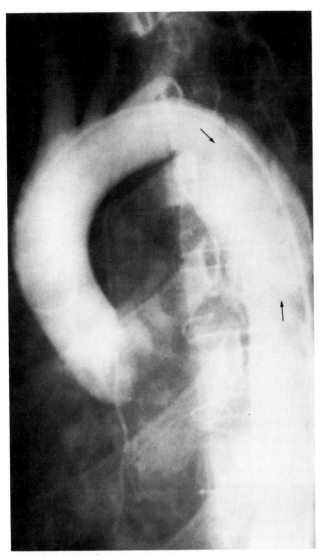

FIGURE 14–49. Pseudoaneurysm and Separation of the Torn Ends of the Aorta

• • • •

This right posterior oblique aortogram shows a long pseudoaneurysm *(arrows)* in a patient with a complete transection and the separation of the torn ends of the aorta.

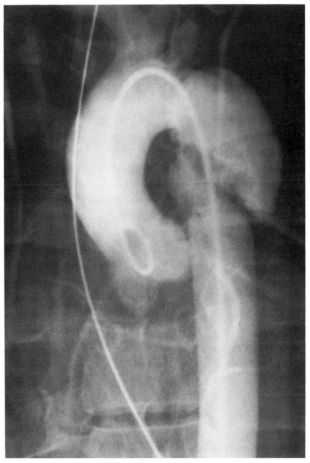

FIGURE 14–50. Irregular Isthmic Pseudoaneurysm in a Complete Transection

• • • •

An anteroposterior aortogram shows a lobulated irregular isthmic pseudoaneurysm in a complete transection.

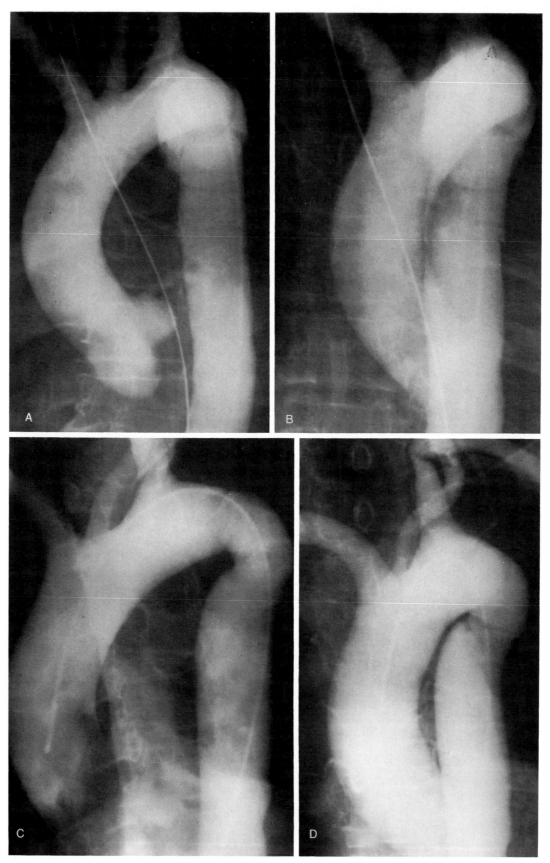

FIGURE 14–51. Typical Isthmic Traumatic Rupture of the Aorta

• • • •

A and *B*, These right posterior oblique and anteroposterior views show typical isthmic traumatic rupture of the aorta. *C* and *D*, This is the same patient after repair with a Dacron tube graft. (The patient had another motor vehicle accident several months after his discharge from the hospital, necessitating this second study.)

492

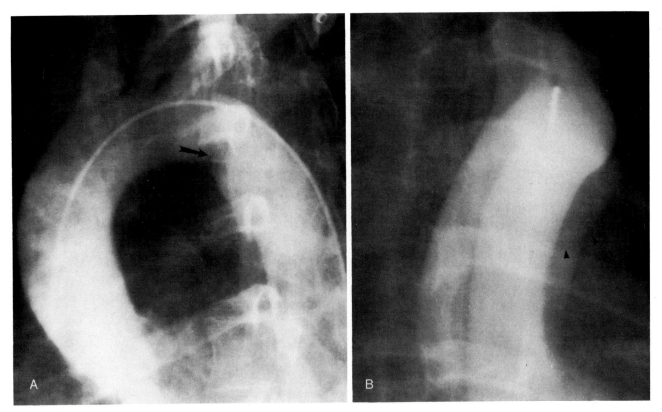

FIGURE 14–52. Subtle Findings of Aortic Transection

• • • •

A, This right posterior oblique aortogram demonstrates a minimal bulge along the anteromedial aorta. This could be a normal "ductus bump." Notice the linear lucency at the cephalad margin *(arrow)*. *B*, A left posterior oblique aortogram shows a pseudoaneurysm *(arrowheads)* extending lateral to the wall of the aorta. This patient had a two-thirds transection.

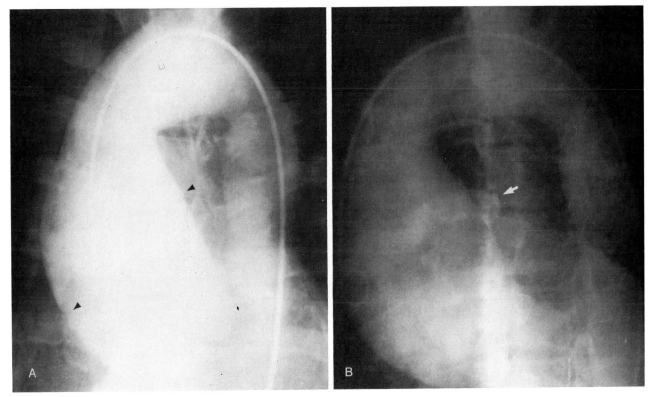

FIGURE 14–53. Annuloaortic Ectasia in a Patient with Marfan's Syndrome

• • • •

The patient had acute chest pain that was found to be caused by a spontaneous rupture of the ascending aorta. *A*, The anteroposterior aortogram shows the dilated ascending aorta and a circumferential tear *(arrowheads)*. *B*, This right posterior oblique view shows a focal pseudoaneurysm adjacent to the posterior wall of the ascending aorta *(arrow)*.

493

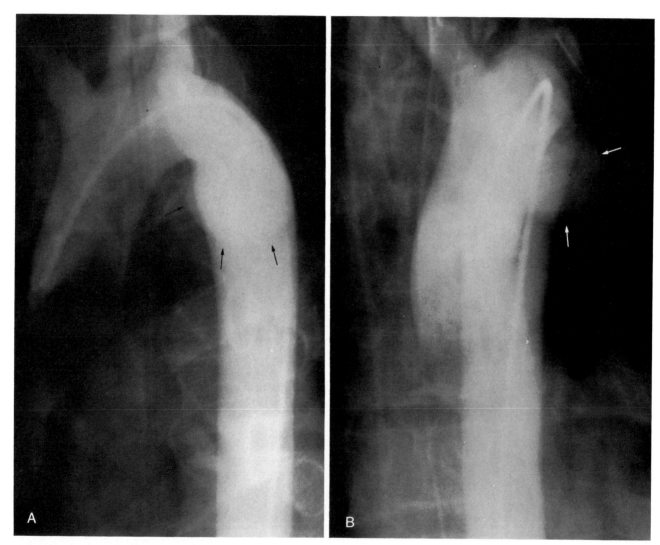

FIGURE 14–54. Focal Pseudoaneurysm in Partial Aortic Transection

• • • •

A and *B,* These anteroposterior and right posterior oblique views on an aortogram show a focal pseudoaneurysm projecting from the lateral aorta *(arrows)* in this patient with a partial transection.

FIGURE 14–55. Pseudoaneurysm in Partial Transection of the Aorta in the Descending Thoracic Aorta
• • • •
A lateral view shows partial transection of the descending aorta with an associated eccentric pseudoaneurysm. The lesion is unusually distal in the descending aorta.

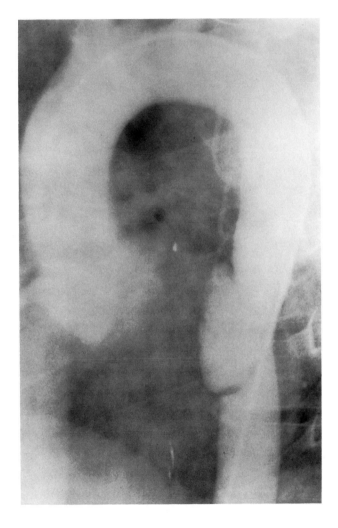

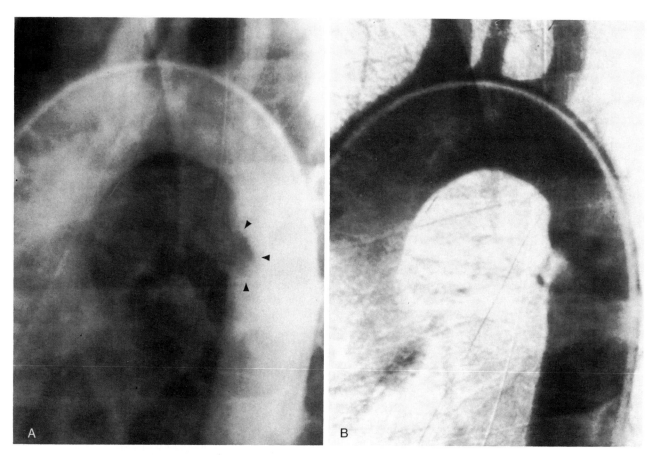

FIGURE 14–56. Small Partial Tear in the Isthmus of the Aorta

• • • •

A and *B*, Right posterior oblique views (film angiogram and film subtraction) show a patient with a small partial isthmic tear. The filling defect seen in the lumen of the aorta *(arrowheads, A)* was caused by an intimal flap with adherent clot.

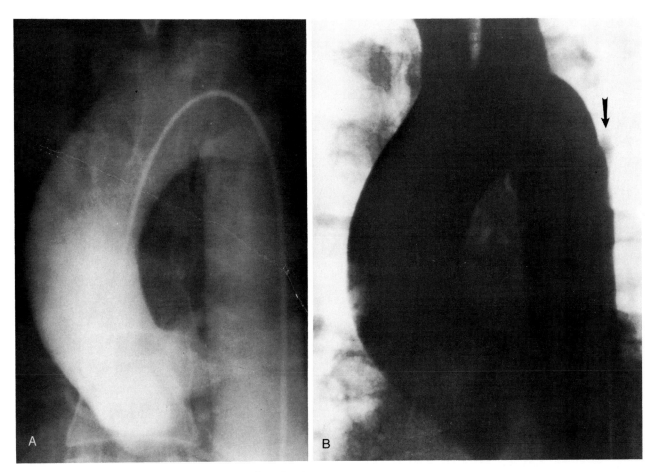

FIGURE 14–57. Small Pseudoaneurysm Lateral to the Aorta

• • • •

A, This anteroposterior view of an aortogram could be misinterpreted as normal. Careful hot lighting shows a small pseudoaneurysm lateral to the aorta. *B,* A subtraction view demonstrates the tear to better advantage *(arrow).*

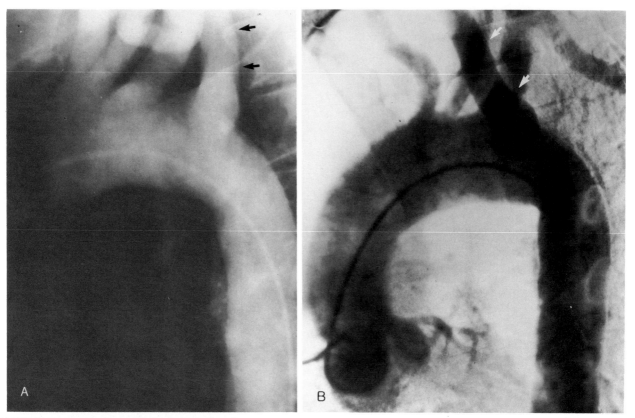

FIGURE 14–58. Aberrant Right Subclavian Artery

• • • •

A and *B*, An aberrant right subclavian artery arising as the fourth branch of the aortic arch *(arrows)* is demonstrated in two different patients (right posterior oblique view).

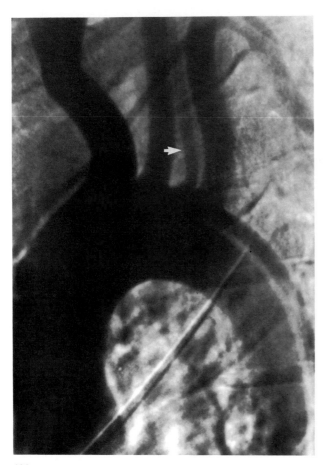

FIGURE 14–59. Origin of the Left Vertebral Artery Directly from the Aortic Arch

• • • •

This feature is a common anomaly seen in about 5% of patients *(arrows)*.

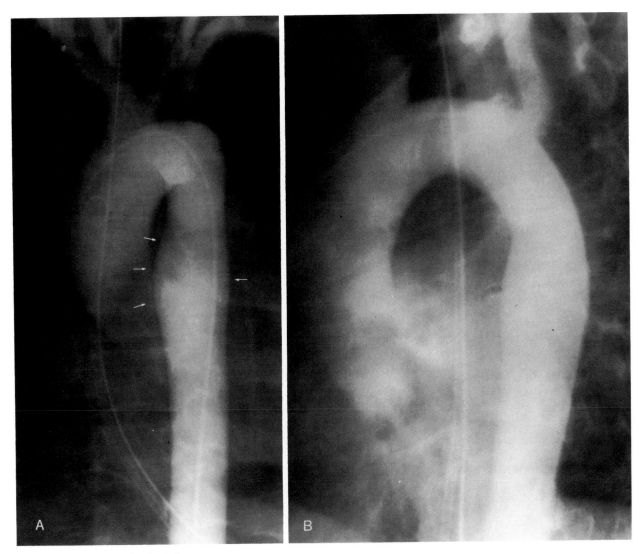

FIGURE 14–60. Postisthmic Bulge

• • • •

A and *B*, Anteroposterior and right posterior oblique views of a prominent postisthmic bulge *(arrows)*. This is a normal variant.

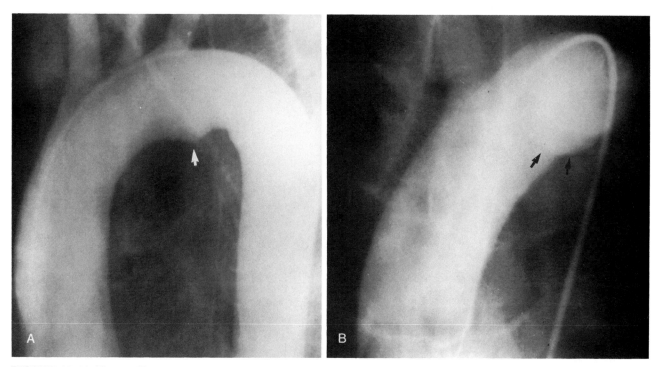

FIGURE 14–61. Ductus Bump

• • • •

A and *B,* The ductus bump is more proximal than usual *(arrow, A),* causing an abnormal edge on the anteroposterior aortogram *(arrows, B).*

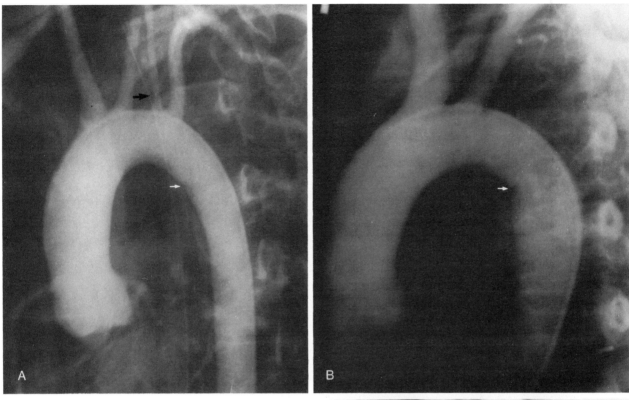

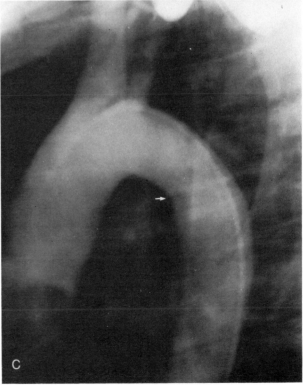

FIGURE 14–62. Angular Defects

• • • •

A–C, Angular defects in or near the ductus *(white arrows,
A–C)* may be difficult or impossible to distinguish from
intimal injuries. Computed tomography or magnetic resonance imaging may be reassuring if mediastinal hematoma
is not present. Note the aberrant origin of the left vertebral
artery from the aorta *(black arrow, A)*.

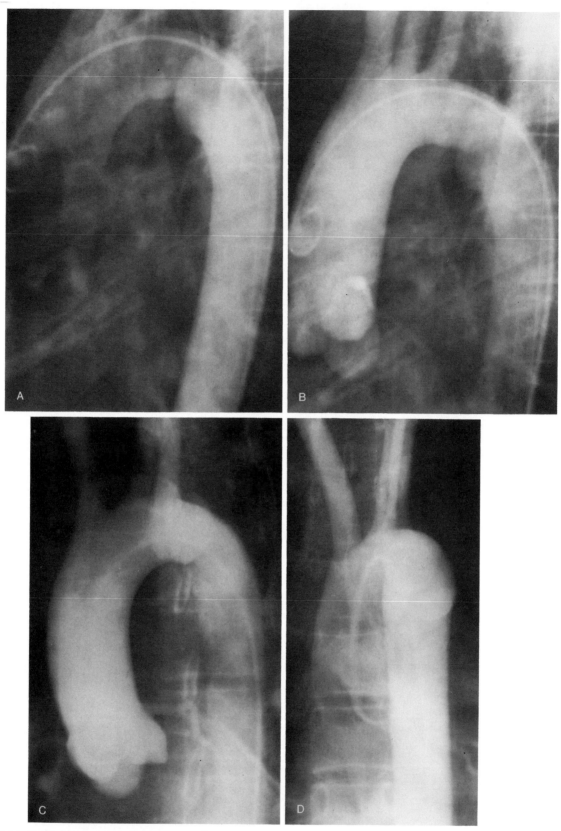

FIGURE 14–63. Prominent Lobulated Ductus Bump

• • • •

A–D, Multiple views of a very prominent lobulated ductus bump are shown in a patient with minimal deceleration trauma. This was considered very suspicious for injury, but because of the patient's poor clinical history and the lack of other injuries a computed tomography (CT) scan was performed; it showed no mediastinal hematoma. The patient subsequently underwent serial CT and repeat arteriography; these were unchanged. She has remained asymptomatic on follow-up.

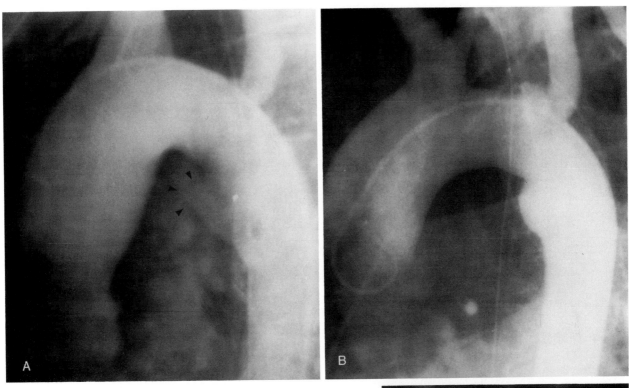

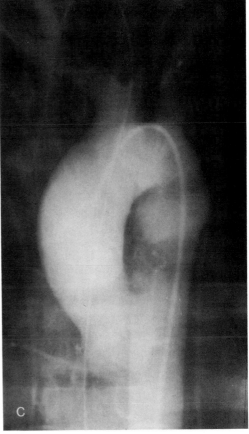

FIGURE 14–64. Ductus Bump with an Angular Superior Margin

• • • •

A–C, These views demonstrate a very prominent ductus bump with an angular superior margin *(arrowheads, A)*. They are considered very suspicious for injury, but the absence of significant associated trauma led to conservative treatment rather than to surgery. A computed tomography scan showed no mediastinal hematoma, and a follow-up arteriogram showed no change. The patient has remained well on clinical follow-up.

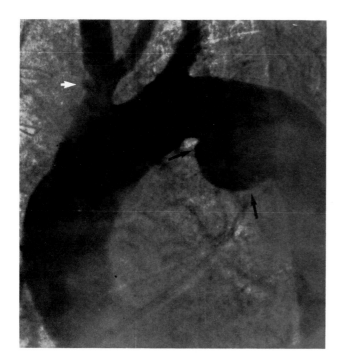

FIGURE 14–65. Atherosclerosis of the Ductus Bump

• • • •

Atherosclerosis with an ulcerated plaque in the anterior surface of the brachiocephalic trunk is visible *(white arrow)*, as is an aneurysm of the ductus bump *(black arrows)*. This patient had no history of trauma and was being studied for transient ischemic attacks.

from the aorta in the region of the aortic isthmus and particularly when they have an infundibular type origin may simulate partial aortic injuries or small pseudoaneurysms (Fig. 14–66). Anomalies of the aortic root may also simulate partial tears (Fig. 14–67). The angiogram itself may cause injury or be misinterpreted (Figs. 14–68 and 14–69).

Autopsy studies of victims of high-speed deceleration injuries demonstrate a very high incidence of nonisthmic aortic injuries. Ascending aortic injuries are more common than isthmic injuries in autopsy series, but nonisthmic injuries are relatively rare in patients who survive their accident long enough to be studied angiographically (see Fig. 14–53). Thoracic aortic transection may also occur at the diaphragmatic hiatus or at any point along the descending aorta (see Fig. 14–55).

The brachiocephalic arteries may be injured by deceleration forces alone or in combination with aortic injuries (Figs. 14–70 to 14–73).

Injuries of the brachiocephalic arteries and veins may cause displacement of mediastinal structures by pseudoaneurysms or hematomas, or they may be evidenced by nonspecific mediastinal hematoma or more specific pulse deficits.

Deceleration injuries of the abdominal aorta and its branches are rare but do occur. Transection of the abdominal aorta has usually been reported in association with injuries of the lumbar spine. The distractive torsional forces that displace the lumbar spine also tear the abdominal aorta, usually in proximity to the spinal injury. Deceleration injuries of the mesenteric vessels and renal arteries also occur, either as isolated phenomena or in association with other abdominal injuries (Figs. 14–74 to 14–77). Mesenteric vascular injuries are seldom diagnosed clinically and are most often found at exploratory laparotomy. Nontransmural injuries of the abdominal vessels may result in compromise or interruption of flow to the bowel or the kidney without associated hemoperitoneum or retroperitoneal hematoma. These lesions are extremely difficult to detect prior to organ damage from ischemia. Flow-limiting renal artery injuries may be detected on a postangiography kidney-ureter-bladder view or a "trauma series" intravenous pyelogram. If there is any asymmetry of the nephrograms, then lumbar aortography can be performed following evaluation of the thoracic aorta. CT is more sensitive than plain film radiography for detection of renal parenchymal and collecting system injuries (see Figs. 14–76 and 14–77). If a renovascular injury is suspected from the CT scan prior to arch aortography, then abdominal aortography may be indicated for further delineation.

Text continued on page 513

FIGURE 14–66. Intercostal Artery with an Infundibular Origin

• • • •

A–E, Several examples of an infundibular origin of the first intercostal artery *(arrows)* that arises near the ductus. This is a common anomaly that can be confused with traumatic rupture of the aorta.

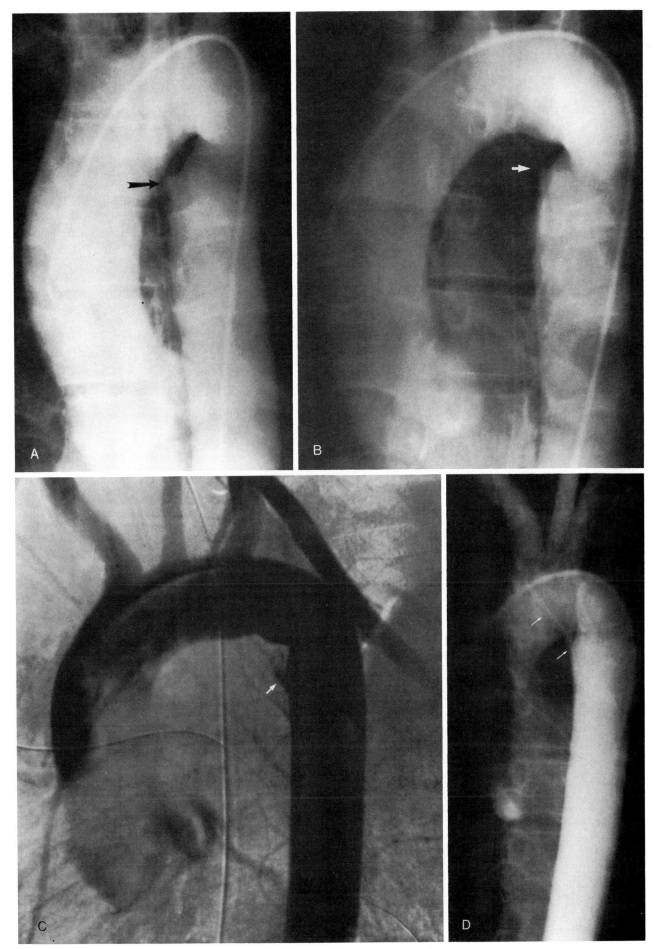

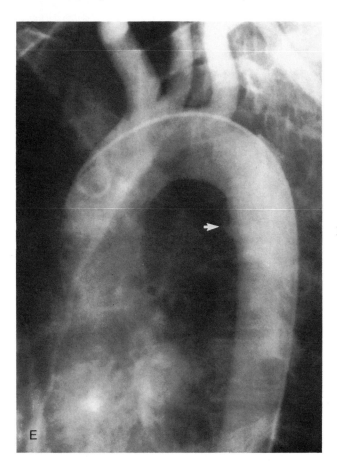

FIGURE 14–66 *Continued*

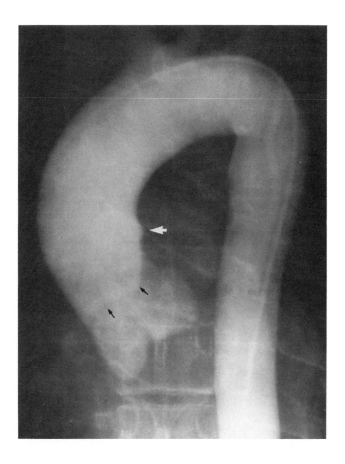

FIGURE 14–67. Coronary Artery Anomaly Simulating an Aortic Injury

• • • •

An aberrant origin *(white arrow)* of the right coronary artery *(black arrows)* is shown. This is a very uncommon anomaly that might be confused with an ascending aortic injury.

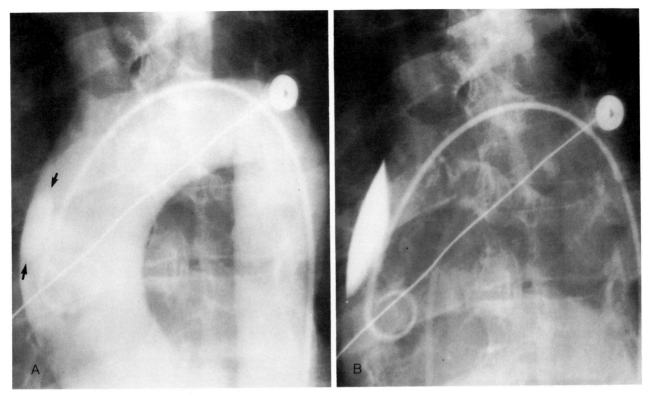

FIGURE 14–68. Subintimal Injection

• • • •

A, This view demonstrates subintimal injection *(black arrows, A)* through a side hole in a multihole pigtail catheter. B, The subintimal contrast material persists after the intravascular contrast has flowed away.

FIGURE 14–69. Simulated Pseudoaneurysm or Extravasation

• • • •

A, Contrast material trapped behind the aortic valve cusp during systole *(black arrowhead)* can simulate pseudoaneurysm or extravasation from the descending aorta. B, The key to avoiding confusion is to notice the presence of the filled valve cusp in the same position earlier or later in the filming sequence *(black arrow)*.

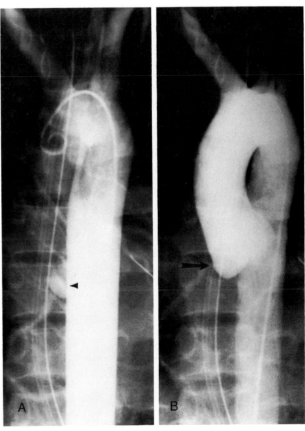

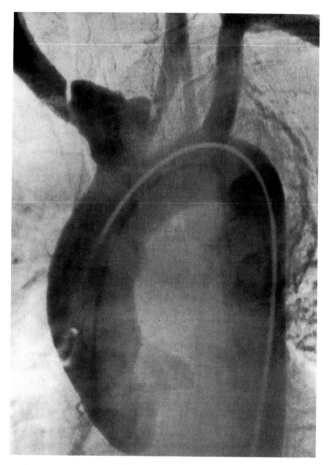

FIGURE 14–70. Deceleration Injury Resulting in the Avulsion of the Innominate Artery

• • • •

This patient has a common origin of the brachiocephalic and the left carotid arteries (so-called "bovine configuration") and an origin of the left vertebral artery from the aortic arch. There is a pseudoaneurysm between the brachiocephalic artery and the left common carotid artery caused by avulsion of the common trunk.

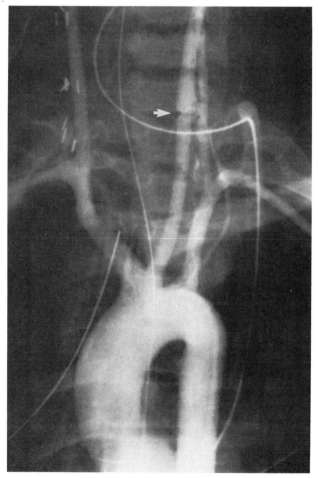

FIGURE 14–71. Deceleration Injury with Traction Injury of the Left Common Carotid Artery

• • • •

This type of injury (arrow) probably results from traction on the artery, which causes circumferential tearing of the intima or the media, or both. If more force were exerted on the artery, a complete avulsion would occur.

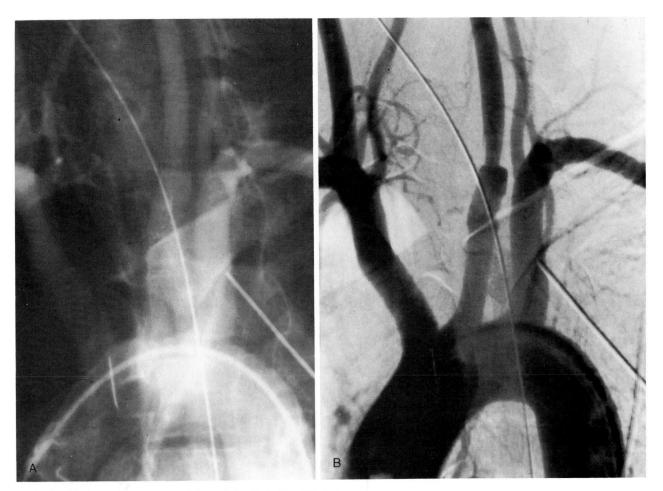

FIGURE 14–72. Incomplete Avulsion of the Left Carotid Artery

• • • •

A and *B,* An incomplete avulsion injury of the left common carotid artery appears similar to that in Figure 14–61. The image in *B* is a film subtraction made from the original film in *A.*

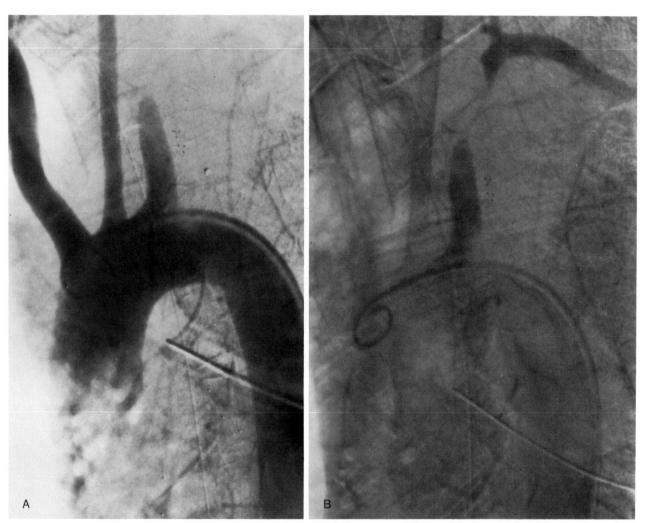

FIGURE 14–73. Occlusion and Reconstitution of the Left Subclavian Artery–Traumatic "Subclavian Steal"

• • • •

A, This view demonstrates occlusion of the left subclavian artery in a patient with a deceleration injury incurred in a motor vehicle accident. *B,* Reconstitution of the subclavian artery distal to the occlusion is accomplished by reversed flow in the left vertebral artery. This is a traumatic subclavian steal syndrome.

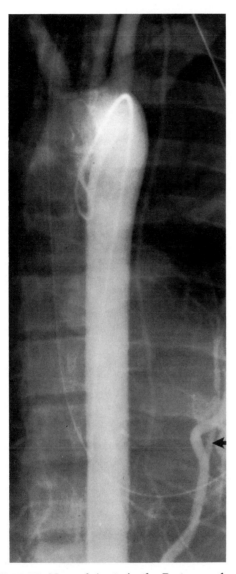

FIGURE 14–74. Normal Aorta in the Presence of Diaphragmatic Rupture

• • • •

This anteroposterior view from an arch aortogram shows a normal aorta. The splenic artery is seen in an abnormal position running vertically in the left thorax *(arrow)*. The patient had a ruptured diaphragm with herniation of the spleen into the left side of the chest.

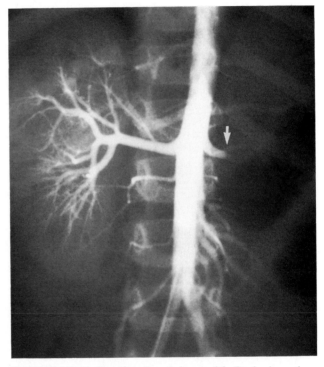

FIGURE 14–75. Deceleration Injury with Occlusion of the Left Renal Artery

• • • •

The occluded left renal artery *(arrow)* was completely avulsed.

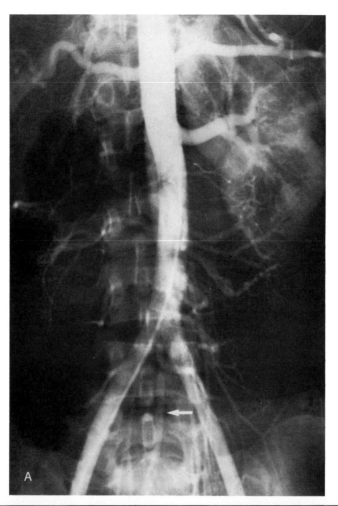

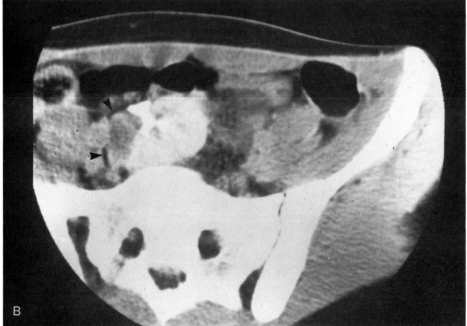

FIGURE 14–76. Pelvic Kidney

• • • •

A, This lumbar aortogram was performed owing to an absent right nephrogram on a trauma series intravenous pyelogram in a patient with a deceleration injury. The right renal artery is not in the expected position. Note the unusually large vessel running vertically between the common iliac arteries *(arrow).* This is the right renal artery supplying a pelvic kidney. *B,* This computed tomography scan shows the pelvic kidney with a segment of nonfunctioning parenchyma *(arrowheads).* This may have been caused by renal contusion or by a segmental artery occlusion/avulsion.

512

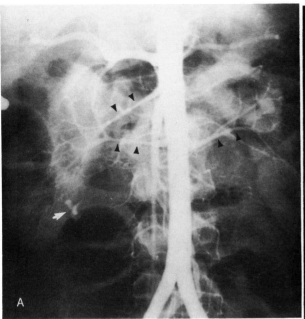
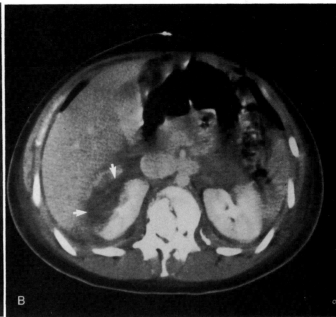

FIGURE 14–77. Segmental Renal Parenchymal Defect

• • • •

A, A lumbar aortogram in a patient with a deceleration injury is shown. There are two right renal arteries and a single left renal artery. All three main renal arteries show circumferential smooth narrowing compatible with vasospasm *(arrowheads).* A focal area of extravasation is seen near the lower pole of the right kidney *(arrow). B,* A computed tomography scan demonstrating a segmental parenchymal defect *(arrows).*

Bibliography

Peripheral Arterial and Venous Trauma

Hartling RP, McGahan JP, Lindfors KK, Blaisdell FW. Stab wounds to the neck: Role of angiography. Radiology 1989; 172:79–82.

McDonald EJ, Goodman PC, Winestock DP. The clinical indications for arteriography in trauma to the extremity. Radiology 1975; 116:45–47.

Perry MO, Thal ER, Shires GT. Management of arterial injuries. Ann Surg 1971; 173:403–408.

Reid JDS, Redman HC, Weigelt JA, et al. Wounds of the extremities in proximity to major arteries: Value of angiography in the detection of arterial injury. AJR 1988; 151:1035–1039.

Rose SC, Moore EE. Angiography in patients with arterial trauma: Correlation between angiographic abnormalities, operative findings and clinical outcome. AJR 1987; 149:613–619.

Sclafani SJA, Cooper R, Shaftan GW, et al. Arterial trauma: Diagnostic and therapeutic angiography. Radiology 1986; 161:165–172.

Transcatheter Therapy for Peripheral Arterial Injuries

Clark RA, Gallant TE, Alexander ES. Angiographic management of traumatic arteriovenous fistulas: Clinical results. Radiology 1983; 147:9–13.

Fisher RG, Ben-Menachem Y, Whigham C. Stab wounds of the renal artery branches: Angiographic diagnosis and treatment by embolization. AJR 1989; 152:1231–1235.

Hemingway AP, Allison DJ. Complications of embolization: Analysis of 410 procedures. Radiology 1988; 166:669–672.

Lawdahl RB, Routh WD, Vitek JJ, et al. Chronic arteriovenous fistulas masquerading as arteriovenous malformations: Diagnos-

tic considerations and therapeutic implications. Radiology 1989; 170:1011–1015.

Neal MP, Tisnado J, Cho S-R (eds). Emergency Interventional Radiology. Boston: Little, Brown & Co. Inc., 1989.

Sclafani SJA, Becker JA. Traumatic presacral hemorrhage: Angiographic diagnosis and therapy. AJR 1982; 138:123–126.

Sclafani SJA, Shaftan GW. Transcatheter treatment of injuries to the profunda femoris artery. AJR 1982; 138:463–466.

Deceleration Injuries of the Aorta

Akins CW, Buckley MJ, Daggett W, et al. Acute traumatic disruption of the aorta: A ten-year experience. Ann Thorac Surg 1981; 31:305–309.

Ayella RJ, Hankins JR, Turney SZ, Cowley RA. Ruptured thoracic aorta due to blunt trauma. J Trauma 1977; 17:199–205.

Bennett DE, Cherry JK. The natural history of traumatic aneurysms of the aorta. Surgery 1967; 61:516–523.

Finkelmeier BA, Mentzer RM, Kaiser DL, et al. Chronic traumatic thoracic aneurysm. J Thorac Cardiovasc Surg 1982; 84:257–266.

Flaherty TT, Wegner GP, Crummy AB, et al. Nonpenetrating injuries to the thoracic aorta. Radiology 1969; 92:541–546.

Parmley LF, Mattingly TW, Manion WC, Jahnke EJ. Nonpenetrating traumatic injury of the aorta. Circulation 1958; 17:1086–1101.

Sevitt S. Traumatic ruptures of the aorta: A clinicopathological study. Injury 1977; 8:159–173.

Stark P. Traumatic rupture of the thoracic aorta: A review. CRC Crit Rev Diagn Imaging 1985; 21:229–255.

Plain Film Findings in Traumatic Rupture of the Aorta

Cole DC, Knopp R, Wales LR, Morishima MS. Nasogastric tube displacement to the right as a sign of acute traumatic rupture of the thoracic aorta. Ann Emerg Med 1981; 10:623–626.

Fisher RG, Ward RE, Ben-Menachem Y, et al. Arteriography and the fractured first rib: Too much for too little? AJR 1982; 138:1059–1062.

Gerlock AJ, Muhletaler CA, Coulam CM, Hayes PT. Traumatic aortic aneurysm: Validity of esophageal tube displacement sign. AJR 1980; 135:713–718.

Gundry SR, Burney RE, Mackenzie JR, et al. Assessment of mediastinal widening associated with traumatic rupture of the aorta. J Trauma 1983; 23:293–299.

Kirshner R, Seltzer S, D'Orsi C, DeWeese JA. Upper rib fractures and mediastinal widening: Indications for aortography. Ann Thorac Surg 1983; 35:450–454.

Livoni JP, Barcia TC. Fracture of the first and second rib: Incidence of vascular injury relative to type of fracture. Radiology 1982; 145:31–33.

Poole GV. Fracture of the upper ribs and injury to the great vessels. Surg Gynecol Obstet 1989; 169:275–281.

Simeone JF, Deren MM, Cagle F. The value of the left apical cap in the diagnosis of aortic rupture. Radiology 1981; 139:35–37.

Simeone JF, Minagi H, Putman CE. Traumatic disruption of the thoracic aorta: Significance of the left apical extrapleural cap. Radiology 1975; 117:265–268.

Wilson RF, Arbulu A, Basset JS, Walt AJ. Acute mediastinal widening following blunt chest trauma. Arch Surg 1972; 104:551–558.

Woodring JH, Dillon ML. Radiographic manifestations of mediastinal hemorrhage from blunt chest trauma. Ann Thorac Surg 1984; 37:171–178.

Woodring JH, Fried AM, Hatfield DR, et al. Fractures of first and second ribs: Predictive value for arterial and bronchial injury. AJR 1982; 138:211–215.

Woodring JH, Pulmano CM, Stevens RK. The right paratracheal stripe in blunt chest trauma. Radiology 1982; 143:605–608.

Imaging Evaluation of Suspected Traumatic Rupture of the Aorta

Applebaum A, Karp RB, Kirklin JW. Surgical treatment for closed thoracic aortic injuries. J Thorac Cardiovasc Surg 1976; 71:458–460.

Barcia JC, Livonia JP. Indications for angiography in blunt thoracic trauma. Radiology 1983; 147:15–19.

Borman KR, Aurbakken CM, Weigelt JA. Treatment priorities in combined blunt abdominal and aortic trauma. Am J Surg 1982; 144:728–732.

Burney RE, Gundry SR, Mackenzie JR, et al. Chest roentgenograms in diagnosis of traumatic rupture of the aorta: Observer variation in interpretation. Chest 1984; 85:605–609.

Fishbone G, Robbins DI, Osborne DJ, Grnja V. Trauma to the thoracic aorta and great vessels. Radiol Clin North Am 1973; 11:543–554.

Gundry SR, Williams S, Burney RE, et al. Indications for aortography in blunt thoracic trauma: A reassessment. J Trauma 1982; 22:664–671.

Heiberg E, Wolverson MK, Sundarum M, Shields JB. CT in aortic trauma. AJR 1983; 140:1119–1124.

Kashuk JL, Moore EE, Millikan JS, Moore JB. Major abdominal vascular trauma: A unified approach. J Trauma 1982; 22:672–679.

Kirsh MM, Crane JD, Kahn DR, et al. Roentgenographic evaluation of traumatic rupture of the aorta. Surg Gynecol Obstet 1970; 131:900–904.

Kubota RT, Trip MD, Tisnado J, Cho S-R. Evaluation of traumatic rupture of descending aorta by aortography and computed tomography: Case report with follow-up. J Comput Tomogr 1985; 9:237–240.

Marnocha KE, Maglinte DDT. Plain-film criteria for excluding aortic rupture in blunt chest trauma. AJR 1985; 144:19–21.

Marsh DG, Sturm JT. Traumatic aortic rupture: Roentgenographic indications for angiography. Ann Thorac Surg 1976; 21:337–340.

Merine D, Brody WR. Critical review of Mirvis, Kostrubiak, et al. Role of CT in excluding major arterial injury after blunt thoracic trauma. AJR 1987; 149:601–605. Invest Radiol 1989; 24:733–734.

Mirvis SE, Bidwell JK, Buddemeyer EU, et al. Imaging diagnosis of traumatic aortic rupture: A review and experience at a major trauma center. Invest Radiol 1987; 22:187–196.

Mirvis SE, Kostrubiak I, Whitley NO, et al. Role of CT in excluding major arterial injury after blunt thoracic trauma. AJR 1987; 149:601–605.

Mirvis SE, Pais SO, Gens DR. Thoracic aortic rupture: Advantages of intra-arterial digital subtraction angiography. AJR 1986; 146:987–991.

Morgan PW, Goodman LR, Aprahamian C, et al. Evaluation of traumatic aortic injury: Does dynamic contrast-enhanced CT play a role? Radiology 1992; 182:661–666.

Raptopoulos V, Sheiman RG, Phillips DA, et al. Traumatic aortic tear: Screening with chest CT. Radiology 1992; 182:667–673.

Sefczek DM, Sefczek RJ, Deeb ZL. Radiographic signs of acute traumatic rupture of the thoracic aorta. AJR 1983; 141:1259–1262.

Seltzer SE, D'Orsi C, Kirshner R, DeWeese JA. Traumatic aortic rupture: Plain radiographic findings. AJR 1981; 137:1011–1014.

Sturm JT, Marsh DG, Bodily KC. Ruptured thoracic aorta: Evolving radiological concepts. Surgery 1979; 85:363–367.

White RD, Lipton MJ, Higgins CB, et al. Noninvasive evaluation of suspected thoracic aortic disease by contrast-enhanced computed tomography. Am J Cardiol 1986; 57:282–290.

Brachiocephalic Vessel Injuries

Ben-Menachem Y. Avulsion of the innominate artery associated with fracture of the sternum. AJR 1988; 150:621–622.

Bowers VD, Watkins GM. Blunt trauma to the thoracic outlet and angiography. Am Surgeon 1983; 49:655–659.

Castagna J, Nelson RJ. Blunt injuries to branches of the aortic arch. J Thorac Cardiovasc Surg 1975; 69:521–532.

Dula DD, Hughes HG, Majernick T. Traumatic disruption of the brachiocephalic artery. Ann Emerg Med 1983; 12:639–641.

Fisher RG, Hadlock F, Ben-Menachem Y. Laceration of the thoracic aorta and brachiocephalic arteries by blunt trauma. Radiol Clin North Am 1981; 19:91–110.

Atypical Traumatic Rupture of the Aorta

Asfaw I, Ramadan H, Talbert JG, Arbulu A. Double traumatic rupture of the thoracic aorta. J Trauma 1985; 25:1102–1104.

Di Summa M, Ottino GM, Trucano G, et al. Traumatic rupture of the thoracic aorta: Report of two unusual cases. J Cardiovasc Surg 1981; 22:181–186.

Fleckenstein JL, Schultz SM, Miller RH. Serial aortography assesses stability of "atypical" aortic arch ruptures. Cardiovasc Intervent Radiol 1987; 10:194–197.

Kirsh MM, Orringer MB, Behrendt DM, et al. Management of unusual traumatic ruptures of the aorta. Surg Gynecol Obstet 1978; 146:365–370.

SECTION

SIX

Pediatric Trauma

CHAPTER 15

Imaging of the Injured Child

NANCY K. ROLLINS, M.D.

Trauma is a leading cause of death and disability in infants and children.[1, 2] Blunt trauma is far more common than penetrating injury in preadolescents. A large proportion of blunt injuries are caused by motor vehicles in which the child is either a passenger or a pedestrian. Infants and young children tend to sustain multiple system injury with blunt trauma. The head and the extremities are injured most often, and about 25% of children with closed head injuries also have significant abdominal injury. Mortality increases from around 7% in children with injury to two body parts to virtually 100% when five body regions are injured.[3] Central nervous system (CNS) injuries in young children have the highest mortality rates when associated spinal injuries are present.[4, 5] Chest and abdominal injuries are associated with a higher mortality rate than are CNS injuries alone. As in adults, computed tomography (CT) is the initial and frequently the only imaging modality required in the evaluation of closed head injury in children.

Young children are generally uncooperative and require sedation to obtain CT images of diagnostic quality. However, sedation should be kept to a minimum in order to allow ongoing evaluation of a child's neurologic status. Furthermore, the child should be evaluated on an individual basis; sedation should not be prescribed for all patients routinely. Very young infants usually do not require any sedation and sleep if swaddled and given a pacifier. At the University of Texas Southwestern Medical Center at Dallas, those children who do require sedation receive oral choral hydrate in a dose of 50–80 mg/kg. Occasionally we use intravenous midazolam (Versed) in a dose of 0.07–0.08 mg/kg in an older child. We do not use intravenous midazolam in infants because of respiratory depression.

NEUROLOGIC TRAUMA

The diagnostic criteria established for the radiologic identification of intracranial sequelae of blunt trauma in adults also apply to children. However, the response of the pediatric brain to blunt trauma differs significantly from that of adults.[6, 7] Focal intracerebral hematomas due to shearing injury (Fig. 15–1) are relatively uncommon in children as compared with adults. Extra-axial hematomas are common in children. In our experience, traumatic subdural hematomas are more common than epidural hematomas,

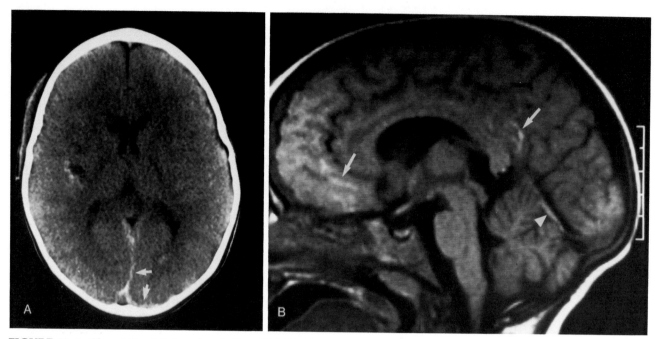

FIGURE 15–1. Closed Head Injury in a 3-Year-Old Child Involved in a Motor Vehicle Accident

• • • •

A, A nonenhanced axial computed tomography scan shows a partially hemorrhagic contusion deep in the right cerebral hemisphere with posterior interhemispheric and left occipital subarachnoid hemorrhage *(arrows)*. *B,* A sagittal T_1-weighted magnetic resonance image obtained 6 days after injury shows anterior and posterior interhemispheric subarachnoid hemorrhage *(arrows)* and a small posterior subdural hematoma *(arrowhead)*.

especially in younger children. Subdural hematomas are most frequently located over the convexity or in the posterior interhemispheric fissure. Acute subdural hematomas are frequently associated with cortical lacerations or contusions, and the degree of mass effect on the underlying brain may be greater than that predicted from the size of the extra-axial collection of blood. The pronounced mass effect that may be seen with small convexity subdural hematomas is therefore presumably related to underlying parenchymal injury that may not be detectable by CT. Subdural hematomas are usually venous in origin, whereas epidural hematomas in older children, as in adults, result from tearing of the meningeal artery. In young children, epidural hematomas may be venous in origin, and small nonexpanding epidural hematomas do not necessarily require surgical intervention. Children are also more prone to develop epidural hematomas of the posterior fossa than are adults.[8] Posterior fossa epidural hematomas usually result from venous bleeding from a torn dural sinus and may occur after only minor head trauma and without a skull fracture. Asymptomatic patients with small posterior fossa epidural hematomas do not require surgical drainage.

Ten to forty-four per cent of children with severe closed head injury, as defined by the Glasgow Coma Scale, have a normal head CT scan.[9, 10] Approximately one third of these patients subsequently develop CT evidence of brain contusion, cerebral edema, extra-axial hematomas, or cerebral atrophy. Subsequent outcome in patients with persistently negative head CT examinations appears to be related to the initial Glasgow Coma Score and the duration of time that the child is comatose, with about 75% of children leaving the hospital with a good recovery or only a moderate functional disability.[9]

Subarachnoid hemorrhage and cerebral edema are very common responses to closed head injury in children. The CT criteria of diffuse cerebral edema are small to absent ventricles and effacement of the basal cisterns. However, there is considerable variation in the size of the ventricles and cisterns in children, and a more sensitive criterion for cerebral edema is the loss of differentiation between the gray and the white matter (Figs. 15–2 and 15–3). Subarachnoid hemorrhage may coalesce to form clots and may be indistinguishable from subdural hemorrhage. Diffuse cerebral edema with or without frank areas of infarction is the most common CT finding in pediatric victims of head trauma and may be related to loss of the autoregulation of cerebral vasculature, which results in hyperemia and intracranial hypertension. The child may show flaccid or decerebrate posturing mimicking brain stem injury as a result of reversible cerebral edema. The outcome of closed head injury

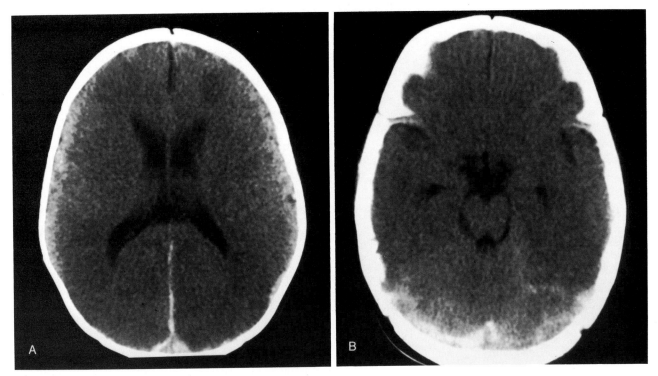

FIGURE 15–2. Cerebral Edema and Extra-axial Hemorrhage

• • • •

A, A nonenhanced axial computed tomography (CT) scan shows subarachnoid hemorrhage as well as a loss of gray-white differentiation and effacement of the sulci, indicating cerebral edema. *B*, An axial CT scan through the suprasellar cistern shows blood along the tentorium. Note the preservation of the basal cisterns despite diffuse severe cerebral edema.

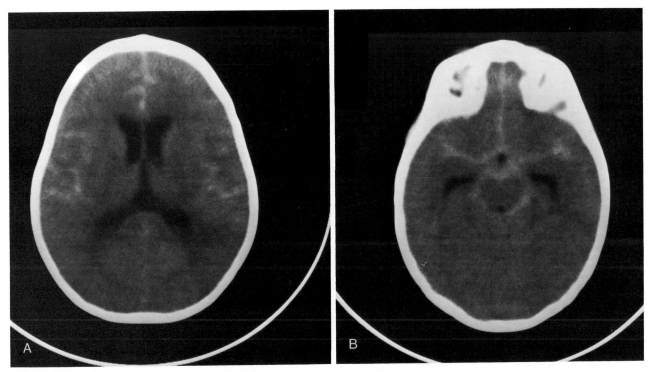

FIGURE 15–3. Subarachnoid Hemorrhage and Cerebral Edema in an Infant

• • • •

A, A nonenhanced axial cranial computed tomography scan of an abused infant shows subarachnoid hemorrhage, diffuse cerebral edema, and early hydrocephalus. Given the rarity of cerebral aneurysms and arteriovenous malformations in young children, this constellation of findings in an infant is the result of either accidental or abusive injury. *B*, Note the subarachnoid blood in the basal cisterns, the sylvian fissures, and the anterior interhemispheric fissure.

is better for children than that for adults. In one series,[6] children younger than 14 years of age had a 9% mortality rate as opposed to the nearly 50% mortality rate in the adult population when similar injuries and level of care were compared. Children 14–18 years of age have mortality rates similar to those of adults.[1, 6] A good to excellent recovery is expected in 88% of children younger than 14 years of age who have sustained primary head injury if these children are given aggressive care aimed at optimizing cerebral perfusion and controlling intracranial hypertension. The primary head injury itself is frequently not fatal; it is the hypotension, hypercarbia, and increased intracranial pressure that cause secondary, often fatal, damage.

Child Abuse

Child abuse is a relatively common cause of CNS mortality and morbidity in infants and young children,[11] and distinctive types of injury have been described,[12-15] some of which are virtually diagnostic of nonaccidental trauma. The most common findings are acute subdural hematomas, cerebral edema, and parenchymal contusions and hemorrhage (Fig. 15–4). The subdural hematomas are caused by tearing of the emissary veins during shaking of the young child. The head of an infant is relatively large and the neck muscles are weak, permitting tremendous acceleration and deceleration forces to be applied to the brain. Hemispheric infarcts and large infarcts confined to vascular distributions associated with subdural hematomas suggest direct compression of the common carotid artery in the neck by strangulation (Figs. 15–5 and 15–6). Bilateral cerebral infarcts result from diffuse hypoxic-ischemic injury and are manifest at CT by the "reversal sign."[16, 17] The CT scan demonstrates loss or reversal of the usual differentiation between the cerebral cortex and the white matter with preservation of the thalami, the brain stem, and the cerebellum. Other causes of the reversal sign on CT scans are accidental injury or asphyxia, infection, and degenerative brain disease.

The infant or the young child who has been abused may lack visible evidence of trauma and may be seen for the new onset of seizures, lethargy, or loss of consciousness or may be brain dead. The chronically abused child often has a large head as a result of subdural hematomas with both acute and chronic components (Figs. 15–7 and 15–8). Subdural hematomas are more common after abusive injury than are epidural hematomas. The findings of diffuse cerebral atrophy with subdural hematomas of variable ages are highly suggestive of repeated child abuse. The radiologist should not hesitate to raise the possibility of child abuse with the referring physician on the basis of these CT observations. A skeletal survey for fractures is suggested in all suspicious cases, especially when the severity of the injury is not explained by the proposed mechanism of trauma or when the caretaker of the child has delayed seeking medical attention. Magnetic resonance (MR) imaging may be useful when the CT scan is normal and the child has unexplained neurologic findings, when child abuse is strongly suspected on clinical grounds and the CT scan is normal, and when the child has split cranial sutures for no apparent reason (Fig. 15–9). MR imaging is more sensitive to small-convexity subdural subacute and chronic hematomas than is CT, and even small subdural hematomas may cause splitting of the cranial sutures. MR imaging is also more sensitive than CT to parenchymal contusions and subacute and chronic hemorrhages and to shear injuries.[18-21] However, MR imaging is not sensitive to acute parenchymal and subarachnoid hemorrhage, thus the acutely injured child should initially be evaluated with CT. MR imaging of the young child is time-consuming and usually requires a deep level of sedation that does not allow intensive monitoring.

The presence of a skull fracture is not diagnostic of child abuse. The characteristics of skull fractures that are more frequent with abuse are multiple fractures, bilateral fractures, and fractures that cross suture lines.[22] However, even these characteristics are not diagnostic of abuse. Skull fractures occurring from abuse cannot be differentiated from those resulting from accidental trauma on the basis of the fracture location, the depression of fracture fragments, the diastasis of the fracture, or the complexity of the fracture.[22]

Cervical spine injuries are uncommon in children. Injuries of the upper cervical spine are more common than those of the lower cervical spine, although Jefferson or burst fractures at the C1 level are rare. Lower cervical spine injuries tend to be associated with more severe trauma and a higher mortality rate. Unlike in adults, in whom compression or comminution fractures are common, cervical spine fractures in children younger than 8 years of age are associated with distraction of the osseous ring at the synchondroses. Although burst fractures, facet fractures, and facet dislocations are seen in teenagers, they are rare in young children.[23]

• • • •

THORACIC TRAUMA

Thoracic injuries in younger children tend to be a result of blunt trauma; teenagers, however, have a

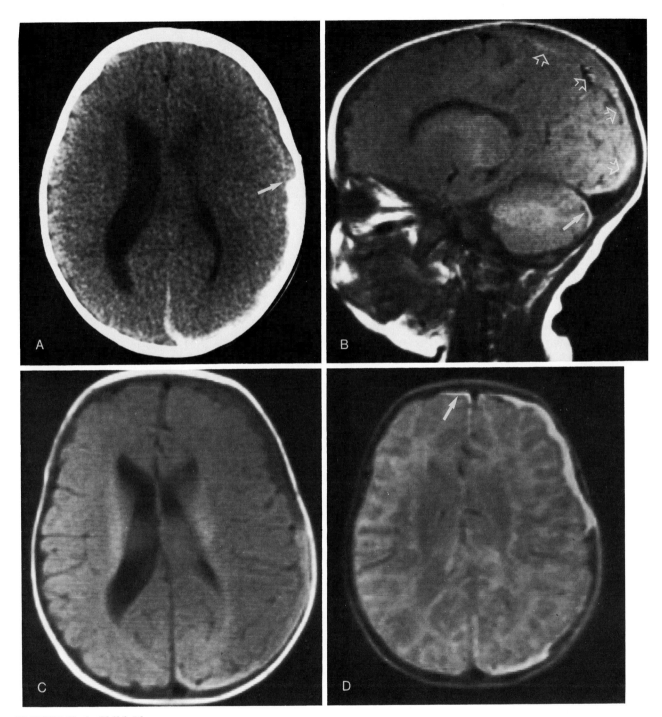

FIGURE 15–4. Child Abuse

• • • •

A, A 3-month-old infant presented with seizures. A nonenhanced computed tomography scan shows mild ventriculo-megaly and an acute left subdural hematoma having a blood-fluid level *(arrow).* Note the effacement of the ipsilateral lateral ventricle. *B,* A sagittal T_1-weighted image shows a small amount of infratentorial blood *(arrow)* and an isointense parietal hematoma *(open arrows).* Small infratentorial subdural hematomas are frequently missed at computed tomography. *C,* An axial T_1-weighted image shows a mild left-to-right shift and the left convexity subdural hematoma. *D,* On the axial T_2-weighted image a small right frontal subdural hematoma is also present *(arrow)* as is the subacute left subdural hematoma. There is no obvious cerebral edema, but the normal high brain water content of the infant may mask coexistent cerebral edema.

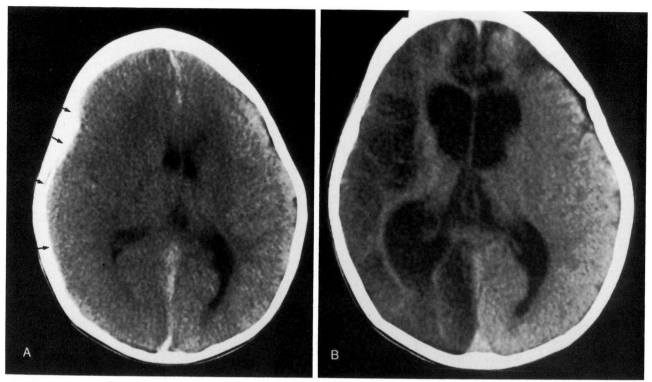

FIGURE 15–5. Strangulation Injury in an 8-Month-Old Comatose Infant with Seizures

• • • •

A, This nonenhanced computed tomography scan (CT) shows severe edema of the right cerebral hemisphere and the left frontal lobe with a convexity subdural hematoma *(arrows)* and blood along the falx. The radiographic appearance is virtually diagnostic of a strangulation injury. *B,* A CT scan obtained 7 months later shows extensive cystic encephalomalacia of the right cerebral hemisphere and a contralateral watershed infarct at the junction of the left anterior cerebral artery and the middle cerebral artery vascular distribution.

higher incidence of penetrating trauma.[24] The most common chest injuries are rib fractures, followed by pneumothorax, hemothorax, or both.[25] Flail chests are uncommon in children. Posterior rib fractures are highly specific for child abuse, whereas rib fractures resulting from accidental trauma are anterior or anterolateral. The posterior rib fractures of child abuse are believed to occur as a result of compression of the thorax by the abusing adult as the child is violently shaken. Child abuse, however, is an infrequent cause of intrathoracic injury. Following major trauma, lung lacerations and contusions occur without rib fractures more commonly in children than in adults, presumably owing to the greater compressibility of the child's chest wall. The flexibility of the thoracic cage and the elasticity of the child's tissues probably explain the low incidence of traumatic tears of the aorta in young children. Injury to the aorta following deceleration occurs most frequently at the level of the ligamentum arteriosus as in adults and is suggested by mediastinal widening on the chest radiograph. There may be no rib fractures. Mediastinal widening on a chest film may be due to venous bleeding rather than to an aortic injury. Mediastinal widening may also be secondary to injury to the upper thoracic spine. Given the low incidence of traumatic tears of the aorta in young children and the need for deep sedation or general anesthesia, thoracic aortography should not be done for mechanism of injury alone but should be reserved for children with an abnormal chest film demonstrating a widened mediastinum with rib fractures, displacement of the esophagus, indistinctness of the aortic knob, or other abnormalities. Injuries to the great vessels of the mediastinum are more common following penetrating injury than blunt trauma, and angiography is indicated in these cases.[24, 26]

• • • •

ORTHOPEDIC TRAUMA

The bones and joints of the extremities are injured frequently in children who have sustained major trauma. In older children, the injuries that result from accidental trauma cannot be differentiated reli-

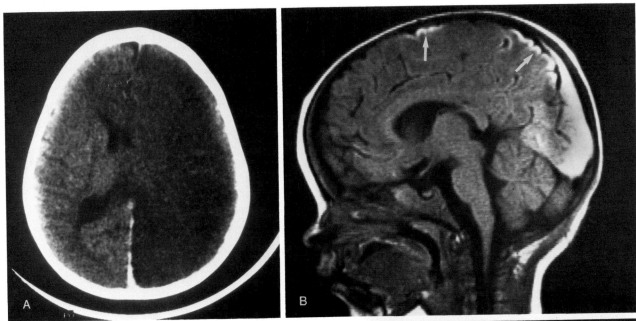

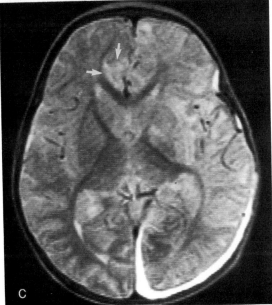

FIGURE 15–6. Strangulation Injury

• • • •

A, A 1-year-old boy presented comatose with seizure activity. The nonenhanced computed tomography scan shows extensive edema of the left cerebral hemisphere with posterior interhemispheric blood. The combination of cerebral infarction within a vascular territory and the presence of extra-axial blood in a young child in whom injury cannot be explained is virtually diagnostic of strangulation injury. The cerebral infarction results from the temporary occlusion of the cervical carotid artery by the abusive adult. Carotid angiography is not indicated in this setting as the carotid artery is only temporarily occluded. *B,* This sagittal T$_1$-weighted scan taken 9 days later shows hemorrhage or laminar necrosis within the cerebral cortex *(arrows)* as well as an occipital subdural hematoma. *C,* An axial T$_2$-weighted image reveals subtle edema throughout the left cerebral hemisphere and within the right frontal lobe *(arrows).*

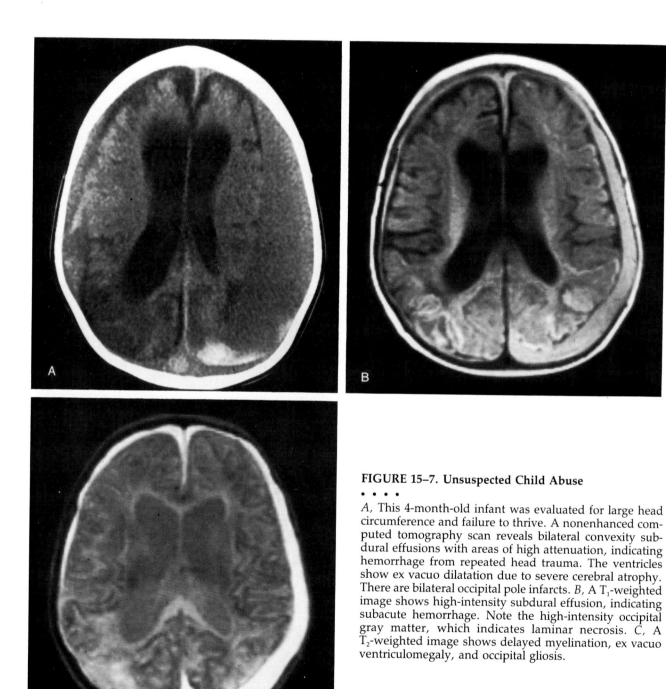

FIGURE 15–7. Unsuspected Child Abuse
• • • •

A, This 4-month-old infant was evaluated for large head circumference and failure to thrive. A nonenhanced computed tomography scan reveals bilateral convexity subdural effusions with areas of high attenuation, indicating hemorrhage from repeated head trauma. The ventricles show ex vacuo dilatation due to severe cerebral atrophy. There are bilateral occipital pole infarcts. *B*, A T_1-weighted image shows high-intensity subdural effusion, indicating subacute hemorrhage. Note the high-intensity occipital gray matter, which indicates laminar necrosis. *C*, A T_2-weighted image shows delayed myelination, ex vacuo ventriculomegaly, and occipital gliosis.

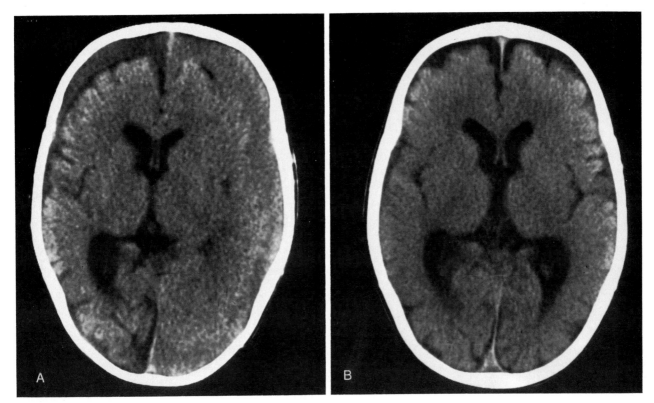

FIGURE 15–8. Unsuspected Child Abuse

• • • •

A, This nonenhanced computed tomography (CT) scan shows a chronic right convexity subdural hematoma and a left convexity subdural hematoma that is isodense with the regional brain. The child presented with a large head. *B,* The subdural hematomas resolved following repeated aspirations. A follow-up CT scan obtained 6 months later reveals mild ventriculomegaly. The child remains developmentally delayed, with chronic seizures as the sequelae of repeated closed head injury.

ably from those that result from an abusive injury. In children younger than 2–3 years of age, the metaphyseal bucket-handle and corner fractures of the extremities, scapular fractures, spinal process fractures, and posterior rib fractures are reliable indicators of child abuse and do not result from accidental trauma.

• • • •

ABDOMINAL TRAUMA

The management of children who have sustained blunt abdominal trauma differs considerably from that of adults.[27] Radical changes in the management of the traumatized child occurred in the 1980s, owing in part to the recognition of the high incidence of postsplenectomy sepsis especially in children younger than 5 years of age.[28–32] The spleen and the liver are the most commonly injured abdominal organs in children. Conservative management has shown that most splenic injuries heal without the need for surgical intervention because of the ability

of the pediatric spleen to spontaneously cease bleeding (Fig. 15–10). Even the most serious splenic lacerations can be treated with splenorrhaphy, and splenectomies are rarely performed in children today. The principles of conservative management in blunt abdominal trauma in children have been extended to hepatic (Fig. 15–11) and renal injuries[33] and have reduced the number of unnecessary laparotomies.

Although technetium nuclear scanning and ultrasound are used in some centers to screen for solid organ injury, CT has the ability to examine the solid organs, the bowel, and the mesentery more accurately,[34] relatively quickly, and without the need to move the traumatized child to different areas within the radiology department. The controversy over the use and the value of diagnostic peritoneal lavage (DPL) versus CT as the screening test of choice in the setting of blunt abdominal trauma continues in level one pediatric trauma centers much as in adult emergency rooms, with some centers advocating the routine use of DPL, some advocating CT, and others defining the roles of DPL and CT as complementary rather than mutually exclusive.[35–40] In children as in adults, DPL is sensitive to intra-abdominal injury,

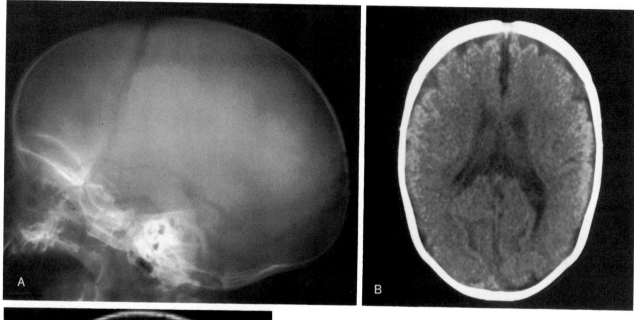

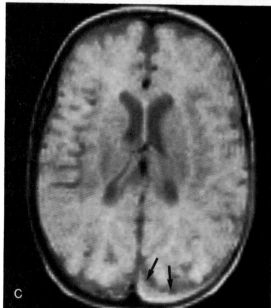

FIGURE 15–9. Split Cranial Sutures Demonstrated with Normal Computed Tomography and Abnormal Magnetic Resonance Scanning
• • • •
A, A lateral radiograph of the skull shows separation of the cranial sutures in a 5-month-old infant presenting with seizures and facial bruises. *B,* The nonenhanced cranial computed tomography scan is normal. *C,* An axial spin-density magnetic resonance image shows a high-density left occipital subdural hematoma *(arrows).*

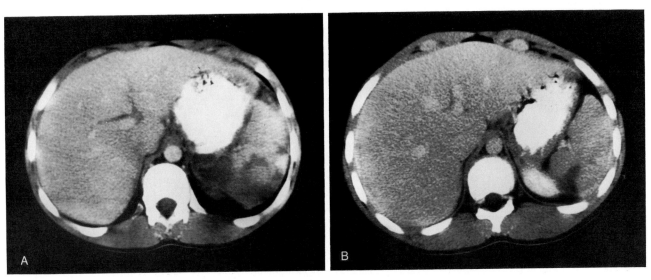

FIGURE 15–10. Nonsurgical Management of a Splenic Laceration

• • • •

A, This contrast-enhanced computed tomography (CT) scan through the upper abdomen of an 8-year-old boy shows a complex splenic laceration that abuts the capsule. *B,* The follow-up CT scan taken 6 weeks later shows a residual wedge-shaped infarct that healed completely 3 months later.

but it cannot reliably quantitate or identify the site of solid organ injury nor distinguish those children with self-limited hepatosplenic injury from those who require surgical intervention. DPL is probably more sensitive to bowel injury than is CT.[41] The technique is easily performed in the obtunded child, but the conscious young child requires fairly heavy sedation for the procedure to be performed safely. The statistics that support the superiority of CT over DPL in children come from dedicated pediatric trauma centers. Trauma centers that rely heavily on DPL cite the poor quality of trauma CT scans at their institutions as well as of preliminary interpretations given by residents or staff inexperienced in the performance and the interpretation of pediatric body imaging, which may lead to an unacceptable false-positive or false-negative rate.

Before the child undergoes a CT scan of the abdomen, a frontal chest radiograph should be taken as well as a supine view of the abdomen. If possible, the mechanism by which the child sustained the injury should be known. A lateral view of the lumbar spine should be added to screen for lap-belt injuries of the spine if the child was wearing a lap-belt at the time a motor vehicle accident occurred because abdominal CT is not sensitive to lumbar spine injuries.[42] Optimal CT imaging of the child requires careful attention to detail. The paucity of intra-abdominal and retroperitoneal fat in the child compared with that in the adult diminishes inherent tissue contrast and necessitates good opacification of the bowel and of blood vessels. Rapid respiratory rates in young children who do not understand the concept of breath holding, movement by the frightened and uncooperative child, and bowel motion may result in serious image degradation and a nondiagnostic study. The newer-generation conventional CT scanners have image acquisition times of less than 2 seconds, and the new ultrafast CT scanners permit subsecond scanning without a significant loss in resolution.[43] Shorter scan times reduce motion artifact and require less patient cooperation and, therefore, less sedation. Parenterally administered sedation should be kept to a minimum to permit ongoing clinical evaluation of the patient's mental status.

Criteria and indications for abdominal CT scan are stable vital signs, suspected intra-abdominal injury as evidenced by abdominal distention or tenderness, bruises on the anterior abdominal wall or known direct trauma to the abdomen, slowly declining hematocrit, concomitant neurologic injury that precludes accurate clinical assessment of the abdomen, the multiply injured patient, or significant hematuria (greater than 20–30 red blood cells per high-power field [RBC/hpf]). A nasogastric tube and a Foley catheter should be in place. Dilute water-soluble oral contrast medium should be given 10–15 minutes before the CT study. The dose of oral contrast agent is determined by approximate body weight and is 50–75% of the usual volume given,[44] although some centers do not routinely administer an oral contrast agent. There is some question in the literature as to whether children who have been resuscitated from hypovolemic shock should be given intravenous con-

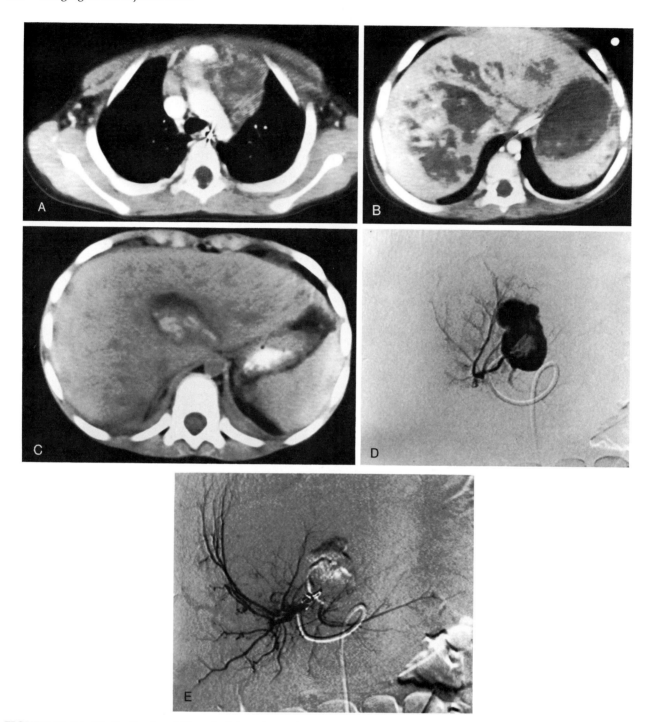

FIGURE 15–11. Mediastinal and Hepatic Injury in a 5-Year-Old Child Following a Crush Injury

• • • •

A, This axial contrast-enhanced computed tomography (CT) scan through the upper mediastinum shows an inhomogeneous thymus due to venous bleeding. *B,* An axial CT scan through the upper abdomen shows complex liver lacerations and numerous small splenic contusions. The child was managed conservatively. *C,* A falling hematocrit 4 weeks later prompted nonenhanced CT scanning that revealed near total healing of the hepatic and the splenic injuries, but an area of acute hemorrhage in the medial segment of the left lobe of the liver was found. Doppler ultrasound revealed pulsatile turbulent flow, suggesting a traumatic pseudoaneurysm. *D,* The selective injection of the artery supplying the medial segment of the left lobe of the liver confirms the presence of a large pseudoaneurysm. *E,* Thrombosis was achieved using a single Gianturco coil. Note the mass effect of the regional hematoma on the right hepatic arterial branches.

trast agents, since the return of normal blood pressure does not guarantee normal renal blood flow and the toxicity of contrast agents appears to be increased in the setting of renal ischemia.[45]

Many pediatric centers across the United States are now using nonionic intravenous contrast agents routinely, a practice that is recommended in all pediatric trauma patients. The intravenous contrast agent is administered by bolus in a dose of 2 ml/kg, and the Foley catheter is clamped. Contiguous 1-cm sections are taken through the abdomen and the pelvis immediately following administration of the contrast medium.

The CT images should be evaluated initially by the radiologist for their quality. The margins of the solid organs should be well defined, bowel should be opacified either with air or contrast, and bowel, fluid, and solid organs should be visually separate. The radiologist should make liberal use of different window and level settings to distinguish extraluminal air from fat and to detect subtle injuries of hepatic, splenic, and renal parenchyma. As suggested by Federle and Jeffrey,[46] the perisplenic space, the perihepatic space, the Morison pouch, the left paracolic gutter, and the pelvic cul-de-sac should be examined for fluid. Fluid found in only one of these spaces indicates a small-volume hemoperitoneum, fluid in two or more of these spaces indicates a moderate hemoperitoneum, and fluid filling all of these spaces indicates a large amount of intra-abdominal free blood. Even a large amount of free fluid does not necessarily mean the patient is still bleeding, and large volumes of intraperitoneal fluid do not correlate with a need for laparotomy,[47] although larger volumes of free fluid appear to correlate with a higher incidence of subsequent surgical intervention. A more accurate indication of ongoing bleeding is a falling hematocrit, which requires repeated transfusions of more than 40% of the total estimated circulating blood volume.[48]

An absolute indication for surgery is the presence of free intraperitoneal air, retroperitoneal air, or extraluminal contrast on the CT scan, which indicates bowel injury. There is no correlation between the severity of hepatic or splenic injury and the need for surgery.[47] Hepatosplenic injuries may be classified as parenchymal or subcapsular hematomas, single or multiple linear fractures, complex fractures, or vascular injuries.[48] Bowel, mesenteric, and pancreatic injuries are less common than hepatic and splenic injuries. Moderate to large amounts of intraperitoneal fluid without an obvious source may be an indication of intestinal injury,[41] and free intraperitoneal air may be lacking when bowel injury has occurred.[36] The presence of intraspinal air is suggestive of perforated small bowel trapped in a lumbar spine fracture.[44]

Several investigators[49, 50] have described a "hypoperfusion complex" seen on abdominal CT scans in young children who had suffered severe CNS injury, abdominal injury, or both, resulting in hypotension and metabolic acidosis and the need for massive fluid and respiratory support. Although the children were hemodynamically stable at the time of the CT study, all of the children who were described ultimately died of their injuries. The CT findings include a diffuse ileus with bowel wall thickening, abnormally intense enhancement of bowel wall, mesentery, and the kidneys, hypoperfusion or hyperperfusion of the pancreas, and decreased luminal diameter of the aorta, the inferior vena cava, the superior mesenteric artery and vein or a combination of these (Fig. 15–12). The dense enhancement of bowel wall and mesentery as well as the ileus are attributed to mesenteric vascular constriction, which results in slow flow. The prognosis with these CT findings is poor.

Hematuria is found frequently in the traumatized child.[51] The integrity of the ureters is best evaluated by intravenous pyelography, and that of the bladder is best evaluated by cystography. CT is more sensitive to subtle renal contusion and to small areas of extravasation than is intravenous pyelography. Karp and colleagues[52] have suggested a system for the grading of renal injuries in children by CT. A small parenchymal injury or contusion as evidenced by a focal area of decreased or increased opacification is a grade I injury. Contusions are not associated with extrarenal fluid collections. The presence of a small amount of subcapsular or perinephric fluid with a renal laceration indicates a grade II injury. Extensive laceration of the kidney with a large perinephric collection is a grade III lesion, and a grade IV injury is a kidney shattered into multiple fragments. Tears limited to the cortex are referred to as *lacerations*, and tears that extend into the collecting system are considered *renal fractures*. Perinephric fluid collections, which represent a mixture of urine and blood and which may be absent in renal arterial injury, may dissect around the ureter, within the interconal fascia, into the anterior pararenal space, and into the psoas muscle.[53] Unlike adults with ureteropelvic junction disruption in whom extravasated contrast material remains localized to the medial perinephric space, fluid tends to fill the perirenal, the perinephric, and the anterior pararenal spaces more readily in children. There appears to be a direct correlation between the amount of hematuria and the severity of renal injury with the mean number of RBC/hpf increasing with increasing grade of injury, although children with injury to the renal pedicle, like adults, may not have hematuria. Children with avulsed renal pedicles are frequently in shock, have expanding

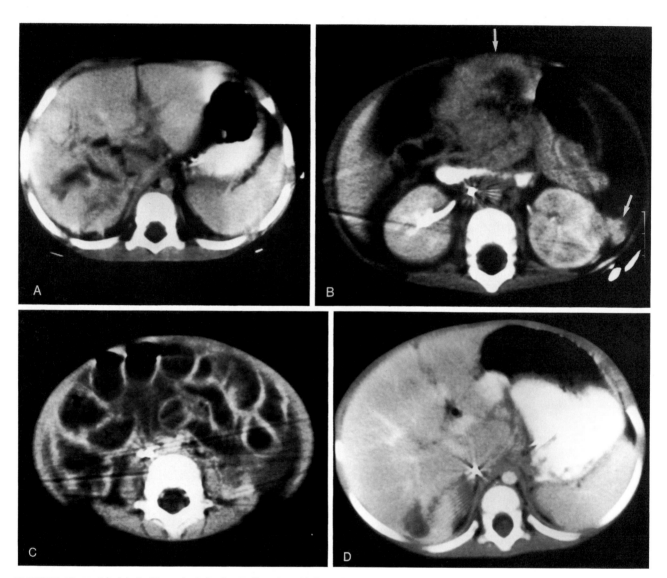

FIGURE 15–12. Multiple Hepatic Injuries Following Child Abuse

• • • •

This 18-month-old infant sustained multiple liver lacerations following direct blows to the abdomen during abusive injury. The child presented to the emergency room in shock 36 hours later and was resuscitated. *A,* A computed tomography (CT) scan reveals multiple lacerations in the caudate and the right lobe of the liver. *B,* An axial image through the midabdomen reveals hemorrhagic ascites *(arrows).* The left kidney is contused with delayed function. *C,* This axial image through the lower abdomen shows an adynamic ileus with abnormal enhancement of the bowel wall. Although this enhancement of the bowel wall is reported to be a poor prognostic indicator, the patient survived with intensive medical care. *D,* A follow-up CT scan obtained 2 weeks later reveals significant healing of the liver injury.

flank masses and bruises, or both.[54] In the normotensive asymptomatic child it appears that hematuria less than 30 RBC/hpf is unlikely to indicate significant renal injury, and CT performed solely on the basis of microscopic hematuria is not indicated. Intravenous pyelography also is of limited value in asymptomatic children with minimal hematuria and should be reserved for children with more than 20–30 RBC/hpf or with clinical findings suggestive of renal injury.[55-58]

Visceral abdominal injury occurs in about 20% of children known or suspected of being abused, and CT is the best screening tool in this setting.[59] However, abdominal CT should be reserved for those abused children with neurologic injury that precludes clinical assessment of the abdomen or for children with clinical signs and symptoms that are suggestive of abdominal injury.

References

1. Eichelberger MR, Randolph JG. Progress in pediatric trauma. World J Surg 1985; 9:222–235.
2. Beaver BC, Colombani PM, Fal H, et al. Efficacy of computed tomography in evaluating abdominal injuries in children with major head trauma. J Pediatr Surg 1987; 22:1117–1122.
3. Ramenofsky ML. Pediatric abdominal trauma. Pediatr Ann 1987; 16:318–326.
4. Eichelberger MR, Mangubat A, Sacco WJ, et al. Outcome analysis of blunt injury in children. J Trauma 1988; 28:1109–1117.
5. Snyder CL, Jain VN, Saltzman DA, et al. Blunt trauma in adults and children: A comparative analysis. J Trauma 1990; 30:1239–1245.
6. Bruce DA, Shut L, Bruno LA, et al. Outcome following severe head injury in children. J Neurosurg 1978; 48:679.
7. Bruce DA, Generalli MD, Longfitt TW. Resuscitation from coma due to head injury. Crit Care Med 1975; 6:254.
8. Koreaki M, Handa H, Munemitsu H, et al. Epidural hematomas of the posterior fossa in children. Childs Brain 1983; 10:130–140.
9. Lobato RD, Sarabia R, Rivas LL, et al. Normal computerized tomography scans in severe head trauma. J Neurosurg 1986; 65:784–789.
10. Kishore PRS, Lipper MH, Becker DP, et al. Significance of CT in head injury. AJNR 1981; 2:307–311.
11. McClelland CQ, Rekate H, Kaufman B, Persse L. Cerebral injury in child abuse: A changing profile. Childs Brain 1980; 7:225–235.
12. Merten DF, Osborne DRS, Radkowski MA, Leonidas JC. Craniocerebral trauma in the child abuse syndrome: Radiological observations. Pediatr Radiol 1984; 14:272–277.
13. Cohen RA, Kaufman RA, Myers PA, Towbin RB. Cranial computed tomography in the abused child with head injury. AJNR 1985; 6:883–888.
14. Sato Y, Yuh WTC, Smith WL, et al. Head injury in child abuse: Evaluation with MR imaging. Radiology 1989; 173:653–657.
15. Bird CR, McMahan JR, Gilles FH, et al. Strangulation in child abuse: CT diagnosis. Radiology 1987; 163:373–375.
16. Han KB, Towbin RB, DeCourten-Meyers G, et al. Reversal sign on CT. AJNR 1989; 10:1191–1198.
17. Bird CR, Drayer BP, Gilles FH. Pathophysiology of "reverse" edema in global cerebral ischemia. AJNR 1989; 10:95–98.
18. Kelly AB, Zimmerman RD, Snow RB, et al. Head trauma: Comparison of MR and CT: experience in 100 patients. AJNR 1988; 9:699–708.
19. Gentry LR, Godersky JC, Thompson B. MR imaging of head trauma: Review of the distribution and radiopathologic features of traumatic lesions. AJNR 1988; 9;101–110.
20. Sato Y, Yuh WTC, Smith WL, et al. Head injury in child abuse: Evaluation with MR imaging. Radiology 1989; 173:653–657.
21. Gaylon DD, Winfield JA. An unusual syndrome of brainstem trauma. Pediatr Neurosci 1988; 14:272–276.
22. Meserv CJ, Towbin R, McLaurin RL, et al. Radiographic characteristics of skull fractures resulting from child abuse. AJR 1987; 149:173–175.
23. Ehara S, El-Khoury GY, Sato Y. Cervical spine injury in children: Radiologic manifestations. AJR 1988; 151:1175–1178.
24. Meller JL, Little AG, Shermeta DW. Thoracic trauma in children. Pediatrics 1984; 74:813–819.
25. Levy JL. Management of crushing chest injuries in children. South Med J 1972; 65:1040–1044.
26. Bergman K, Dykes E, Spence L, Wesson D. Fatal thoracic vascular injuries in children (abstract). Pediatr Emerg Care 1990; 6:159.
27. Delius RE, Frankel W, Coran AG. A comparison between operative and nonoperative management of blunt injuries to the liver and spleen in adult and pediatric patients. Surgery 1989; 106:788–793.
28. Eichelberger MR, Randolph JG. Progress in pediatric trauma. World J Surg 1985; 9:222–235.
29. Karp MP, Cooney DR, Pros GA, et al. Nonoperative management of pediatric hepatic trauma. J Pediatr Surg 1983; 18:512–518.
30. Cywes S, Rode H, Millar AJW. Blunt liver trauma in children: Nonoperative management. J Pediatr Surg 1985; 20:14–18.
31. Oldham KT, Guile KS, Ryckman F, et al. Blunt liver injury in childhood: Evolution of therapy and current perspective. Surgery 1986; 100:542–549.
32. Buntain WL, Gould HR. Splenic trauma in children and techniques of splenic salvage. World J Surg 1985; 9:398–409.
33. Yale-Loehr AJ, Kramer SS, Quinlan DM, et al. CT of severe renal trauma in children: Evaluation and course of healing with conservative therapy. AJR 1989; 152:109–113.
34. Kaufman RA, Towbin R, Babcock DS, et al. Upper abdominal trauma in children: Imaging evaluation. AJR 1984; 142:449–460.
35. Fabian TC, Mangiante EC, White TJ, et al. A prospective study of 91 patients undergoing both computed tomography and peritoneal lavage following blunt abdominal trauma. J Trauma 1986; 26:602–608.
36. Marx JA, Moore EE, Jorden RC, Eule J. Limitations of computed tomography in the evaluation of acute abdominal trauma: A prospective comparison with diagnostic peritoneal lavage. J Trauma 1985; 25:933–937.
37. Goldstein AS, Salvatore JAS, Kupperstein NH, et al. The diagnostic superiority of computerized tomography. J Trauma 1985; 25:938–946.
38. Kearney PA, Vahey T, Burney RE, Glazer G. Computed tomography and diagnostic peritoneal lavage in blunt abdominal trauma. Arch Surg 1989; 124:344–347.
39. Sorkey AJ, Farnell MB, Williams HG Jr, et al. The complementary roles of diagnostic peritoneal lavage and computed tomography in the evaluation of blunt abdominal trauma. Surgery 1989; 106:794–801.
40. Rothenberg S, Moore EE, Marx JA, et al. Selective management of blunt abdominal trauma in children: The triage role of peritoneal lavage. J Trauma 1987; 27:1101–1106.
41. Sherck JP, Oakes DD. Intestinal injuries missed by computed tomography. J Trauma 1990; 30:1–7.
42. Taylor GA, Eggli KD. Lap-belt injuries of the lumbar spine in children: A pitfall in CT diagnosis. AJR 1988; 150:1355–1358.
43. Brody AS, Seidel FG, Kuhn JP. CT evaluation of blunt abdominal trauma in children: Comparison of ultrafast and conventional CT. AJR 1989; 153:803–806.
44. Kaufman RA. Technical aspects of abdominal CT in infants and children. AJR 1989; 153:549–554.

45. Schiffer MS. Use of contrast media in patients with hypovolemic shock (letter to editor). Radiology 1987; 166:579.

46. Federle M, Jeffrey B. Hemoperitoneum studied by computed tomography. Radiology 1983; 148;187–192.

47. Brick SH, Taylor GA, Potter BM, Eichelberger MR. Hepatic and splenic injury in children: Role of CT in the decision for laparotomy. Radiology 1987; 165:643–646.

48. Federle MP, Crass RA, Jeffrey B, Trunkey DD. Computed tomography in blunt abdominal trauma. Arch Surg 1982; 117:645–650.

49. Taylor GA, Fallat ME, Eichelberger MR. Hypovolemic shock in children: Abdominal CT manifestations. Radiology 1987; 164:479–481.

50. Kaufman RA, Stalker HP. Hypovolemic shock in children. Radiology 1988; 166:579–580.

51. Kuzmarov IW, Morehouse DD, Gibson S. Blunt renal trauma in the pediatric population: A retrospective study. J Urol 1981; 126:648–649.

52. Karp MP, Jewett TC, Kuhn JP, et al. The impact of computed tomography scanning on the child with renal trauma. J Pediatr Surg 1986; 21:617–623.

53. Siegel MJ, Balfe DM. Blunt renal and ureteral trauma in childhood: CT patterns of fluid collections. AJR 1989; 152:1043–1047.

54. Letsou GV, Gusberg R. Isolated bilateral renal artery thrombosis: An unusual consequence of blunt abdominal trauma: Case report. J Trauma 1990; 30:509–511.

55. Lieu TA, Fleisher GR, Mahboubi S, Schwartz JS. Hematuria and clinical findings as indications for intravenous pyelography in pediatric blunt renal trauma. Pediatrics 1988; 82:216–222.

56. Guice K, Oldham K, Eide B, Johansen K. Hematuria after blunt trauma: When is pyelography useful. J Trauma 1983; 23:305–311.

57. Taylor GA, Eichelberger MR, Potter BM. Hematuria: A marker of abdominal injury in children after blunt trauma. Ann Surg 1988; 208:688–693.

58. Stalker HP, Kaufman RA, Stedje K. The significance of hematuria in children after blunt abdominal trauma. AJR 1990; 154:569–571.

59. Sivit CJ, Taylor GA, Eichelberger MR. Visceral injury in battered children: A changing perspective. Radiology 1989; 173:659–661.

INDEX

· ·

Page numbers in *italics* refer to illustrations;
numbers followed by t indicate tables.

Abdomen. See also *Abdominal trauma*;
  specific organs.
  free air in, 379, *380*, 399, *399, 400*
    demonstration of, 377
    on computed tomography, 382–384,
      387, 400
Abdominal trauma, 375–447. See also
  Renal trauma; specific organs.
  angiography in, 378, 379
  appropriate radiographic studies for,
    378
  computed tomography in, 378, 379,
    382–384, *382–387*
  contrast studies in, 378, 379, 382
  in child, 525–531, *527, 528, 530*
  magnetic resonance imaging in, 378
  plain film radiography in, 377, 378,
    379–382, *380–381*
  radiographic findings in, 379–384
  scintigraphy in, 378
  ultrasound in, 378, 379, 382
  vascular, 504, *511–513*
  with thoracolumbar spine fracture, 267,
    277, 384
Abdominal wall trauma, 402, *402, 403*
Abducens nerve (VI), 4–7
  in skull base, 78–80, *81*
Abscess, retropharyngeal, with
  esophageal perforation, *357*
Acceleration injury, to brain, 21
  to cervical spine, 258
Adamkiewicz, artery of, 171
ADI (atlas-dens interval), 189–190
Adrenal gland trauma, 402
Alar ligament(s), 187
Amygdala, 16
Aneurysm, intracranial, rupture of,
  traumatic subarachnoid hemorrhage
  vs., 20
Angiography. See also *Aortography*;
  Venography.
  high-resolution selective arterial digital
    (IADSA), in peripheral arterial in-
    jury, 473
  in abdominal trauma, 378, 379
  in head trauma, 18–20, *20–23*, 27, 42
  in liver trauma, 389–391, *390*
    therapeutic applications of, 391, *391*
  in pancreatic injury, 398

Angiography *(Continued)*
  in penetrating injury of orbit, 154, *154*
  in peripheral arterial injury, 452–470,
    452t
    technique for, 470–473
    therapeutic applications of, 473–474,
      474–479
  in renal trauma, 408, 419–420
    findings on, 420, *421–428*
    therapeutic applications of, 420–428,
      425–426, 474, 479
  in skull base trauma, 78, 87, *88–91*
  in splenic trauma, 396–397
  of extra-axial fluid collections, 49, *49–53*
  subtraction techniques with, *90–91*
Annuloaortic ectasia, in Marfan's
  syndrome, *493*
Annulus of intervertebral disc, 169–170
  injury to, 171
Anterior atlantoaxial ligament, 170
Anterior atlanto-occipital membrane, 170
Anterior cerebral artery, normal magnetic
  resonance appearance of, *9*
Anterior cord syndrome, 259
Anterior cranial fossa, base of, 77
Anterior longitudinal ligament, 170
Anterior spinal artery(ies), 171
Anterolisthesis, of lower cervical spine,
  significance of, 232
  with hyperextension injury, 253
Anteroposterior view, in cervical spine
  evaluation, 180, 183, *184*
  in lower cervical spine trauma, 217
  open-mouth, in upper cervical spine
    trauma, 183, *184*, 190–191
Aorta, deceleration injuries of, 478–504
  abdominal, 504, *511–513*
  appropriate radiographic studies for,
    452
  in child, 522
  plain film radiography of, 452, 480–
    482, 482t, *483–487*
  screening for, 480
  developmental variants of, aortic tear
    vs., 483–504, *498–506*
  rupture of, in Marfan's syndrome, *493*
  traumatic rupture of (TRA), 478–480
    evaluation technique for, 482–483

Aorta *(Continued)*
  radiographic findings with, 483, *483–
    497*
Aortoesophageal fistula, due to
  esophageal foreign body, 364
Aortography, in deceleration injuries of
  aorta, 452
  interpretation of, 483–504
  technique for, 482–483
  injuries or artifacts due to, *507*
Aphasia, lesions associated with, 16
Aqueduct of Sylvius, normal magnetic
  resonance appearance of, *9, 14*
Arcuate fasciculus, 16
Arterial injury(ies), 451–474
  angiographic signs of, 452–470, 452t
  angiographic technique for, 470–473
  appropriate radiographic studies for,
    452
  atherosclerosis mimicking, 470, *473*
  blunt, 451
  deceleration. See also under *Aorta*.
    to abdominal vessels, 504, *511–513*
    to brachiocephalic arteries, 504, *508–
      510*
  penetrating, 451
  transcatheter interventions in, 473–474,
    474–479
  vasospasm and, 459–470, *470–472*, 471t
Arterial occlusion, on angiography, with
  peripheral arterial injury, 459, *466–
  469*
  therapeutic. See *Embolization, transcath-
    eter*.
Arteriography. See *Angiography*;
  Aortography.
Arteriovenous fistula(s), hepatic,
  angiographic treatment of, 391
  renal, angiographic imaging of, 420,
    424, 426, 427
    management of, 420–428
  with peripheral arterial injury, 452–454,
    453–455, 458
Artery of Adamkiewicz, 171
Artery of the cervical enlargement, 171
Arytenoid cartilage(s), *295, 296–297*
  dislocation of, with endotracheal intu-
    bation, 311, *312*

533

Atherosclerosis, arterial injury vs., 470, 473
of ductus bump, aortic tear vs., 483, 504
Atlantoaxial joint, 188
injury to, 203–204
Atlantoaxial ligament, anterior, 170
Atlanto-occipital joint, 187
injuries to, 191–193, 191–194
Atlanto-occipital membrane, anterior, 170
Atlas (C1), 187–188
bipartite, 188
congenital variations in, 188, 198–200
fractures of, 193–203
anterior arch, 191, 193–196, 194–197
Jefferson, 198–203, 200, 201
lateral mass, 202, 203
posterior arch, 194–195, 196–198, 198–200
transverse process, 203
occipitalization of, 188
Atlas spread index, 201
Atlas-dens interval (ADI), 189–190
Auditory cortex, 16
Axis (C2), 188–189. See also Dens.
fractures of, 204–213
body, 207–213, 210–213
transverse process, 210–211, 213
variations of, 189, 189
Axonal shearing, 22, 25

Barium studies. See Contrast studies.
Basal ganglia, 11
Basilar artery, normal appearance of, on computed tomography, 5, 6
on magnetic resonance imaging, 8, 12
Battery(ies), ingestion of, 362–363
Beam hardening, 5
BFD (bilateral facet dislocation), 234, 235–237, 238–239, 238
Bile, on computed tomography, 388
Bladder trauma. See Urinary bladder trauma.
Blood, on magnetic resonance imaging, 30
Blow-in fracture(s), 141
Blown pupil, 31
Blow-out fracture(s). See under Orbital fracture(s).
Body bagger syndrome, 363–364
Boerhaave's syndrome, 360–361, 361
Bone algorithm for computed tomography, in skull base trauma, 86
in spinal trauma, 174
Bougienage procedure(s), esophageal injury due to, 367
Bowel, herniation of, with diaphragmatic rupture, 338, 340, 343, 344
injury to, 382, 387, 399–400, 399–401
in child, 529
Brachiocephalic artery(ies), deceleration injury to, 504, 508–510
Brain. See also Brain trauma.
anatomy of, 3–17
on computed tomography, 5–7
on magnetic resonance imaging, 8–10
Brain stem, 3–7
Brain swelling, diffuse, increased intracranial pressure due to, 37
imaging of, 31–34, 34–36
in child, 518, 519
Brain trauma, 3–37
angiography in, 18–20, 20–23, 27, 42
appropriate radiographic studies for, 4

Brain trauma (Continued)
blunt, 21
brain's response to, 20–37
classification of, 23
computed tomography in, 4, 18, 19, 22–23, 25, 42
iatrogenic, 31, 33
imaging of, 17–37, 25–36
strategies for, 17–20, 19
in child, 517–520, 518, 519
due to child abuse, 520, 521–526
prognosis with, 518–519
ischemia secondary to, 23–30, 30, 34–37, 36
magnetic resonance imaging in, 4, 18, 19, 22–23, 25–27, 42
penetrating, 21, 24
types of, 20–22
Broca's area, 16
Bronchial injury. See Tracheobronchial injury.
Brown-Séquard syndrome, 259
Buckling force theory of orbital floor fracture, 123
Buckling of white matter, with isodense subdural hematoma, 67, 72
Burst fracture, 182, 218, 219, 219–220
defined, 217–218
stable, 275, 276
unstable, 275, 277

Caldwell projection, for facial trauma evaluation, 95, 96, 97, 99
Calvarium. See Skull fracture(s).
Carcinoma, squamous cell, of esophagus, after caustic ingestion, 366, 367
Cardiac trauma, 371, 372, 373
Carotid artery(ies). See also Internal carotid artery.
common, deceleration injury to, 508, 509
Carotid-cavernous sinus fistula, angiography of, 87, 88–89
balloon occlusion for, 87, 89–91
Cataract, traumatic, 153, 163–164, 164
Cauda equina, 170
Caudate nucleus, 11, 13
normal computed tomographic appearance of, 6
Caustic ingestion, esophageal injury due to, 365–366, 366, 367
Cavernous sinus, 80, 81
Cavitary pulmonary lesion(s), 324
Central cord syndrome, 259
Centrum, 169
Centrum semiovale, normal appearance of, on computed tomography, 7
on magnetic resonance imaging, 10
Cerebellar peduncle(s), inferior, 7
middle, 7
normal magnetic resonance appearance of, 8
superior, 7
Cerebellar tonsil(s), normal magnetic resonance appearance of, 8
Cerebellum, 7, 13
normal computed tomographic appearance of, 5
Cerebral artery, anterior, normal magnetic resonance appearance of, 9
middle, normal magnetic resonance appearance of, 9

Cerebral edema. See Brain swelling.
Cerebral embolism, with foreign body in chest or neck, 20, 20
Cerebral fissure, longitudinal, 13
transverse, 13
Cerebral herniation, due to epidural hematoma, 56, 57–58
transtentorial, due to trauma, 31–34, 35–36
Cerebral infarction, 23–30, 30, 34–37, 36
in child, 520, 522–524
Cerebral lobe(s), normal anatomy of, 11–17, 14–15
Cerebral peduncle(s), normal appearance of, on computed tomography, 6
on magnetic resonance imaging, 9
Cerebral vein(s), internal, normal magnetic resonance appearance of, 12
Cerebrospinal fluid, normal magnetic resonance appearance of, 12
Cerebrospinal fluid leak, cisternography for localization of, 87
with petrous bone fracture, 91
Cervical spine, 179–261. See also Atlas (C1); Axis (C2); Cervical spine trauma; Dens.
clearance of, 180–183
fractures of, lower, 239–258. See also Vertebral body fracture(s).
upper, 191–192, 191. See also under Atlas (C1); Axis (C2); Dens.
indications for imaging of, 173
lower, anatomy of, 213–214
vertical alignments in lateral view of, 181, 216
upper, anatomy of, 187–189
Cervical spine trauma, 179–261. See also Atlas (C1); Axis (C2); Dens.
appropriate radiographic studies for, 180
computed tomography in, 180, 214
geometric tomography in, 180
in child, 520
lower, 217–258
analysis of films in, 214–217
magnetic resonance imaging in, 180, 187
myelography in, 180
neurologic, 259–261
plain film radiography in, 180
projections for, 179–183, 181, 182, 184
upper, 191–213
analysis of films in, 189–191
with midface trauma, 113
Chance fracture, 277
Chest tube(s), computed tomography in localization of, 332, 333, 334
Chest wall trauma, 342–351
appropriate radiographic studies for, 316
Child(ren), 517–531. See also Infant(s).
abdominal trauma in, 526–531, 527, 528, 530
laryngeal trauma in, 286–287
neurologic trauma in, 517–520, 518, 519
due to abuse, 520, 521–526
prognosis with, 518–519
orthopedic trauma in, 522–525
sedation for imaging of, 517
thoracic trauma in, 520–522
Child abuse, abdominal injury in, 530, 531
neurologic injury in, 520, 521–526
orthopedic trauma in, 525
rib fractures in, 522

Child abuse (Continued)
skull fractures in, 520
suspected, imaging of head injuries in, 17
Chloral hydrate, for sedation of child, 517
Cholesteatoma, after petrous bone fracture, 90–91
Choroidal detachment, 164–165, 164
appropriate radiographic studies of, 127
Cingulate gyrus, 13, 16
Cisternography, 87
Claustrum, 11, 13
Clavicular dislocation, 351, 351
Clay-shoveler's fracture, 253, 255–257
Cocaine, ingestion of sealed packets of, 363–364
Coin(s), ingestion of, 362
Compression fracture. See also Wedge fracture.
defined, 217–218
Computed tomography (CT), cisternography using, 87
in abdominal trauma, 378, 379
findings on, 382–384, 382–387
in child, 525–531, 527, 528, 530
in blow-out fracture of orbit, 124, 125, 128–131, 131–133
in bowel injury, 400, 400, 401
in chest trauma, 331–332, 332–335
in deceleration injuries of the aorta, 452
in epidural hematoma, 54, 55–59, 55, 58
in esophageal trauma, 356, 369, 370
in facial trauma, 96, 97, 113
in head injury, 4, 18, 19, 22–23, 25, 42
in laryngeal trauma, 286, 289, 291, 292
in liver trauma, 384–389, 388, 389
in orbital fracture, 124, 125
in pancreatic injury, 397–398, 398
in penetrating injury of orbit, 151–154, 151–153
in renal trauma, 408, 415–417
findings on, 414, 417, 417–419
technique for, 415–417
in skull base trauma, 78, 84–87, 86
reconstruction algorithms for, 86
in soft tissue injury of orbit, 126, 127
in spinal trauma, 174–175
identification of vertebral level in, 214
in cervical region, 180, 214
in thoracolumbar region, 266, 267–268, 268, 269, 271–273
in splenic trauma, 392–396, 393–396
artifacts in, 392, 393
in ureteric injury, 408, 429, 430–431
in urinary bladder trauma, 409, 434, 436
of brain, normal anatomy on, 5–7
reversal sign on, 520
three-dimensional, in complex facial fractures, 119, 119–120
Concussion, spinal cord, defined, 260
Consciousness, brain stem in maintenance of, 4
Continuous diaphragm sign, 336, 336
Contrast agent(s), extravasation of. See Extravasation of contrast material.
for computed tomography, in child, 527–529
Contrast studies, in abdominal trauma, 378, 379
findings on, 382
in bowel injury, 399–400
in detection of diaphragmatic laceration, 342, 344–346
in esophageal trauma, 356, 358, 368–369

Contrast venography, 478, 480
Contrecoup injury, to brain, 22
to larynx, 297, 302–304
Contusion(s), brain, imaging of, 30–31
hepatic, 388, 388
parenchymal, in abdominal trauma, 382, 382
pulmonary, 316–318, 317–322
spinal cord, 260
splenic, 382, 394, 395
Conus medullaris, level of, 170
Coronary artery, anomalous origin of, aortic tear vs., 506
Corpus callosum, 13, 13
normal magnetic resonance appearance of, 14
Corpus striatum, 11
Cranial nerve(s), 4–7. See also Optic nerve(s) (II).
in middle cranial fossa, 78–80, 79, 81
in posterior cranial fossa, 81
Cranial suture(s), split, in child, imaging of, 520, 526
Craniofacial dissociation, 117, 119
Cricoid cartilage, 295, 296
fracture of, 297, 297–299
Cricothyroid membrane, 296
Cricothyroid muscle, 295, 296
CT. See Computed tomography (CT).
Cyst(s), spinal cord, imaging of, 268, 274
traumatic lung, 324
Cystography, in urinary bladder trauma, 409, 432–436
findings on, 432–436, 433–434
technique for, 433

Deceleration injury(ies), to abdominal vessels, 504, 511–513
to aorta. See under Aorta.
to brachiocephalic arteries, 504, 508–510
to brain, 21
Degenerative change, in spine, 214, 215
apparent, 172
Dens, 181, 188
fractures of, 204–206, 204–207
with atlas fracture, 194–197, 198
lordotic, 182, 190
normal computed tomographic appearance of, 5
Denticulate ligament(s), 170
Denture(s), computed tomography artifact due to, 5
Diaphragm, rupture of, 336–342, 339–348
arch aortogram in, 511
injuries associated with, 338
trauma to, appropriate radiographic studies for, 316
Diencephalon, 11
Diplopia, with blow-out fracture, of medial wall, 137
of orbital floor, 131, 135
Disc. See Intervertebral disc.
Dislocation(s). See also Fracture-dislocation; Subluxation.
arytenoid cartilage, with endotracheal intubation, 311, 312
atlanto-occipital, 192–193, 192–194
rotary, 193
clavicular, 351, 351
facet, 232–239
bilateral (BFD), 234, 235–237, 238–239, 238

Dislocation(s) (Continued)
unilateral (UFD), 223–225, 234–239, 234, 235
hyperextension (HED), of lower cervical spine, 230
thoracic spine, with thoracic injury, 346, 350
Dog's ears sign, 384
Double diaphragm sign, 327
DPL (diagnostic peritoneal lavage), in pediatric abdominal trauma, 525–527
Drug(s), esophageal trauma due to, 367
illegal, ingestion of sealed packets of, 363–364
Ductus bump, aortic tear vs., 483, 499–504
Dural tear(s), 268, 270

Edema, cerebral. See Brain swelling.
laryngeal, 297–307, 304–307
prevertebral, evaluation of, 183–187, 185t, 186t
Elderly patient(s), spine in, 172
Embolization, of foreign body, to brain, 20, 20
to heart, 371, 372, 373
transcatheter, for carotid-cavernous sinus fistula, 87, 89–91
for hepatic bleeding, 391, 391
for peripheral arterial injuries, 473–474, 474–479
for renal hemorrhage, 420–428, 425–426, 474, 479
for splenic hemorrhage, 397
Empyema, 335
Endoscopy, esophageal injury due to, 367
Endotracheal intubation, laryngeal trauma due to, 311, 312
Enophthalmos, 162
appropriate radiographic studies for, 127
Epidural hematoma, 52–59
angiography of, 49, 49, 52–53
clinicopathology of, 52–55, 54–58
computed tomography of, 54, 55–59, 55, 58
conservative treatment of, 56, 59
delayed, 56–59
in child, 518
of posterior fossa, 73–75, 75
parenchymal injury with, 55, 56
radiographic studies of, 48–49
spinal, 171
venous, 53–55
of posterior fossa, 73
Epiglottis, 295, 296
Esophageal stricture, due to caustic ingestion, 366, 366
Esophageal trauma, 355–370
appropriate radiographic studies for, 356, 368–369
classification of, 355
drug-induced, 367
due to caustic ingestion, 365–366, 366, 367
due to foreign body ingestion, 362–365, 363, 364
management of, 365
extrinsic, 355–360
iatrogenic, 367–368, 368
intrinsic, 360–361
laryngeal trauma with, 293

Esophageal trauma *(Continued)*
  recurrent leak after repair of, 360, *360*
  thermal, 366
  tracheobronchial injury with, 359–360
  vertebral artery injury with, 23
Esophagography, double-contrast,
  esophageal injury due to, 368
Esophagus. See also *Esophageal trauma.*
  perforation of, 355–358, *357, 358*
  rupture of, 358–359, *358, 359*
    due to double-contrast esophagogra-
     phy, 368
    in Boerhaave's syndrome, 360–361,
     361
    pneumomediastinum due to, 336
    squamous cell carcinoma of, after caus-
     tic ingestion, 366, *367*
ETF (extension teardrop fracture), 213,
  230, *230*
Ethmoid air cell injury, 101–105, *104*
  appropriate radiographic studies for, 96
Extension lateral view, in cervical spine
  evaluation, 183
Extension teardrop fracture (ETF), 213,
  230, *230*
External capsule, 13
Extra-axial space(s), appropriate
  radiographic studies for, 42, 49
  traumatic hemorrhage in, 48–75. See
    also *Epidural hematoma; Subdural he-
    matoma.*
  in child, 517–518, *518, 519*
Extravasation of contrast material, on
  angiography, in renal trauma, 420,
  422–423
  with peripheral arterial injury, 454–
    459, *456, 457*
  on urography in renal trauma, 411–412,
    413
Extreme capsule, 13
Eye(s), 147–165. See also *Globe(s).*
  appropriate radiographic studies for,
    126–127
  foreign body in, 147–154, *147–152*
  penetrating injury of, 147–154, *147–153*
  orbital fracture with, *146,* 147
Eye movement(s), control of, 7, 13, 16

Facet(s), vertebral, normal radiographic
  appearance of, 267
Facet dislocation(s), 232–239
  bilateral (BFD), 234, *235–237,* 238–239,
    238
  unilateral (UFD), *223–225,* 234–239, *234,*
    235
Facet fracture(s), *224, 233, 239,* 239–244
  facet dislocation vs., 234
Facet joint(s), 170
  alignment of, on lateral view of lower
    cervical spine, 216
Facet-pillar-pedicle complex injury(ies),
  232–253
Facial nerve (VII), 4
  in skull base, 81
  traumatic palsy of, 91
Facial smash, *104, 119,* 120–121
  appropriate radiographic studies for, 97
Facial trauma, 95–121
  appropriate radiographic studies for,
    95–97, *98–100*
  computed tomography in, 96, 97, 113

Falx, normal appearance of, on computed
  tomography, 7
  on magnetic resonance imaging, *9*
Fetal lobulation(s) of spleen, 394–396, *396*
Fetus, exposure of, to radiation, with
  maternal pelvic injury, 404
Flail chest, 346
Flaval ligament(s), 170
Flexion distraction injury, *267–268,* 277
Flexion lateral view, in cervical spine
  evaluation, 183
Flexion-teardrop fracture, 221–228, *221–
  227*
  defined, 217–218
Football sign, 399
Foramen of Monro, 17, *18*
Foreign body(ies), esophageal injury due
  to, 362–365, *363, 364*
  management of, 365
  in bladder, 436, *437*
  in orbit, 147–154, *147–152*
    appropriate radiographic studies for,
     126
  laryngeal, 309, *309, 310*
  urethral, *441*
Fornix, 13
Fourth ventricle, 17, *18*
  normal appearance of, on computed to-
    mography, *5*
  on magnetic resonance imaging, *8, 14*
Fracture(s), atlas. See under *Atlas (C1).*
  axis. See under *Axis (C2); Dens.*
  blow-in, 141
  blow-out. See under *Orbital fracture(s).*
  burst. See *Burst fracture.*
  cervical spine, lower, 239–258. See also
    Vertebral body fracture(s).
    upper, 191–192, *191.* See also under
     Atlas (C1); Axis (C2); Dens.
  Chance, 277
  clay-shoveler's, 253, *255–257*
  compression. See also *Wedge fracture.*
    defined, 217–218
  cricoid cartilage, 297, *297–299*
  facet, *224, 233, 239,* 239–244
    facet dislocation vs., 234
  facial, signs suggestive of, 95–101
  hangman's, 206–207, *208, 209*
    simulated, 189, *189*
  horizontal fissure, 277
  hyoid, *296*
  Jefferson, 198–203, *200, 201*
  lamina, of lower cervical spine, 253–
    258, *258*
  Le Fort, 117–119, *117–120*
    appropriate radiographic studies for,
     97
  mandibular, 105–110, *108–111*
    treatment of, 110–113, *112*
  nasal, 101–105, *102–104*
    appropriate radiographic studies for,
     96
  occipital condyle, 191–192, *191*
  odontoid, 204–206, *204–207*
    with atlas fracture, *194–197,* 198
  pedicle, of lower cervical spine, *225,
    227,* 253, *254–255*
  pelvic, bladder trauma and, *432, 432,*
    434
    transcatheter intervention for hemor-
     rhage with, *456, 457,* 473–474,
     474
  petrous bone, *86,* 90–91, *92–93*
  pillar, *205, 239,* 245–252

Fracture(s) *(Continued)*
  posterior distraction, 275–277, *278*
  pyramidal, 117–119, *117–120*
  renal, defined, 529
  rib. See *Rib fracture(s).*
  sacral, 277, *280*
  sagittal, *220–227, 228, 229*
    defined, 217–218
  skull. See *Skull fracture(s).*
  skull base. See under *Skull base.*
  Smith, 275–277, *278*
  spinous process, of lower cervical
    spine, 253, *255–257*
  sternal, 346–351
  teardrop, extension (ETF), 213, 230, *230*
    flexion, 217–218, 221–228, *221–227*
  thoracolumbar spine. See *Thoracolumbar
    spine fracture(s).*
  thyroid cartilage, 297, *297–302*
  transverse process. See under *Transverse
    process(es).*
  tripod, 113–117, *115–116, 141, 142*
    appropriate radiographic studies for,
     125
  uncinate process, 231
  vertebral body. See *Vertebral body frac-
    ture(s).*
  wedge. See *Wedge fracture.*
  zygomatic, 113–117, *114–116*
    appropriate radiographic studies for,
     97
Fracture-dislocation, of lower cervical
  spine, flexion, 221–228, *221–227*
  hyperextension, 253
  hyperflexion, 232, *232, 233*
Frontal horn(s), 17, *18*
Frontal lobe(s), 13–15, *15*
  inferior, normal computed tomographic
    appearance of, *6*
Frontal sinus injury, 101
  appropriate radiographic studies for, 96

Gastrointestinal system, 377–404. See also
  Abdominal trauma.
Geniculate body, lateral, 11
  medial, 11
Genitourinary system, 407–447. See also
  Renal trauma; specific structures.
  appropriate radiographic studies for,
    408–409
Genu of corpus callosum, normal
  magnetic resonance appearance of, *10*
Geometric tomography, in spinal trauma,
  174, 180
Glasgow Coma Scale, prognosis for child
  with head injury and, 518
Globe(s). See also *Eye(s).*
  normal magnetic resonance appearance
    of, *8*
  rupture of, 154–155, *155–158*
    appropriate radiographic studies for,
     126
Globus pallidus, 11, 13
Glossopharyngeal nerve (IX), 4
  in skull base, 81
Gott, tetrad of, 360–361
Gray matter, normal appearance of, on
  computed tomography, 7
  on magnetic resonance imaging, 10,
    12
Gunshot wound, cardiac embolism with,
  371, *372, 373*

Gunshot wound *(Continued)*
  cerebral embolism with, 20, *20*
  to brain, tracking path of, 31, *31, 32*

Hangman's fracture, 206–207, *208, 209*
  simulated, 189, *189*
Head trauma, 1–165. See also *Brain trauma.*
  plain film radiography in, 4, 22, 41, 42, 49
  ultrasound in, 49
Hearing loss, with petrous bone fracture, 90, 91
Heart trauma, 371, *372, 373*
HED (hyperextension dislocation), of lower cervical spine, 230
Hematocele, with testicular injury, 445
Hematocrit effect, in subdural hematoma, 67
Hematoma(s), body wall, 402, *402, 403*
  epidural. See *Epidural hematoma.*
  hepatic subcapsular, 388, *388, 391*
  mediastinal, 482
  optic nerve, 155–159, *159, 160*
  paraspinal, 171
  pelvic, bladder imaging in presence of, 434–436, *435, 436*
  prevertebral, 171
  pulmonary, 319–325, *321–325*
  renal, 412, *414, 419*
  retrobulbar, 159
  splenic subcapsular, 394, *395*
  subdural. See *Subdural hematoma.*
  subperiosteal, of orbit, 159–160, *161*
    appropriate radiographic studies for, 127
  testicular, 445, *445*
Hematomyelia, defined, 260
Hematuria, in child, 529–531
  injuries causing. See site-specific entries, e.g., *Renal trauma; Urinary bladder trauma.*
Hemoperitoneum, *385, 386*
  with splenic trauma, 392, *393*
Hemorrhage, extra-axial, 48–75. See also *Epidural hematoma; Subdural hematoma.*
  in child, 517–518, *518, 519*
  hepatic, angiographic embolization of, 391
  in abdominal trauma, 382, *384–386*
  internal iliac artery, 457, 473–474, *474*
  renal, angiographic embolization for, 420–428, *425–426, 474, 479*
  splenic, angiographic embolization for, 397
  subarachnoid. See *Subarachnoid hemorrhage.*
  subchoroidal, 152, *153*
  subconjunctival, 160–162, *163*
    appropriate radiographic studies for, 127
  vitreous, *153,* 160, *162*
    appropriate radiographic studies for, 127
Hemothorax, 330–331
Hernia(s), traumatic diaphragmatic, 338–342, *339–348*
  arch aortogram in, *511*
Herniation, cerebral, due to epidural hematoma, 56, *57–58*
  transtentorial, 31–34, *35–36*
  intervertebral disc, 171

Herniation *(Continued)*
  acute traumatic, 231
Hippocampal formation, *13, 16*
Hydraulic theory of orbital floor fracture, 123
Hydrocephalus, due to brain trauma, 34
Hygroma, subdural, subdural hematoma vs., 59–62
Hyoepiglottic ligament, 296
Hyoid bone, *291, 292, 295,* 296
  fracture of, *296*
Hyperextension dislocation (HED), of lower cervical spine, 230
Hyperextension fracture-dislocation, of lower cervical spine, 253
Hyperextension sprain, of lower cervical spine, 231
Hyperflexion sprain, of lower cervical spine, 232, *232, 233*
Hyphema, 165, *165*
Hypocycloidal polytomography, in spinal trauma, 174
Hypoglossal nerve (XII), 4
  in skull base, 81
Hypoperfusion complex, on abdominal computed tomography in young child, 529, *530*
Hypothalamus, 11

IADSA (high-resolution selective arterial digital angiography), in peripheral arterial injury, 473
Iliac artery(ies), internal, hemorrhage from, 457, 473–474, *474*
Incontinence, frontal lobe lesions associated with, 13
Infant(s). See also *Child(ren).*
  spine in, 172
Infarction, cerebral, 23–30, *30,* 34–37, *36*
  in child, 520, *522–524*
Inferior cerebellar peduncle, 7
Inferior rectus muscle of eye, entrapment of, with blow-out fracture, 131, *133,* 135, *135–137*
Ingestion injury, 361–367
Inhalation injury, 307, *307*
Inner laminar line, 187, *190*
Innominate artery, deceleration injury to, *508*
Insula, *13, 17*
  normal appearance of, on computed tomography, *6*
  on magnetic resonance imaging, *9, 15*
Intercostal artery, anomalous origin of, aortic tear vs., *504–506*
Intermaxillary fixation, for mandibular fracture, 110, *112*
Internal capsule, 13
  normal computed tomographic appearance of, *6*
Internal carotid artery, in skull base, 79, 80, *81*
  injury to, with skull base trauma, 87, *88–91*
  stretch injury to, 20, *21*
Internal cerebral vein(s), normal magnetic resonance appearance of, *12*
Internal iliac artery(ies), hemorrhage from, 457, 473–474, *474*
Internuclear ophthalmoplegia, 7
Interspinous ligament(s), 170
Intertransverse ligament(s), 170

Interventricular foramen of Monro, 17, *18*
Intervertebral disc, 169–170
  acute injury to, 231
  distractive injury to, 231
  protrusion of, causes of, 171
Intervertebral foramen(ina), 169
Intimal flap(s), on angiography, with peripheral arterial injury, 459, *465*
Intracranial aneurysm, rupture of, traumatic subarachnoid hemorrhage vs., 20
Intracranial pressure, increased, due to diffuse brain swelling, 37
Intubation, endotracheal, laryngeal trauma due to, 311, *312*
  nasogastric, esophageal injury due to, 367
    in identification of diaphragmatic laceration, 338–342, *339, 341–343*

Jefferson fracture(s), 198–203, *200, 201*
Jugular foramen, 81

Kidney(s). See also *Renal trauma.*
  hematoma of, 412, *414, 419*
  laceration of. See *Laceration(s), renal.*
  pseudoaneurysm in, 420, *424–426*

Labyrinth, evaluation of, 91
Laceration(s), diaphragmatic. See *Diaphragm, rupture of.*
  hepatic, *383, 384,* 388, *389*
  of brain, imaging of, 31, *31, 32*
  parenchymal, in abdominal trauma, 382, *383*
  pulmonary, 318–325, *319–321, 324–325*
  renal, computed tomography findings with, *417–419*
    defined, 529
    intravenous urography findings with, 409, *410,* 415, *415, 416*
  spinal cord, defined, 260
  splenic, *383, 384,* 392–394, *394*
    in child, 527
  testicular, *445*
Lamina fracture(s), of lower cervical spine, 253–258, *258*
Language, cerebral areas for, 16
Laryngeal edema, 297–307, *304–307*
Laryngeal nerve(s), 296
Laryngeal stenosis, 311–313
Laryngeal trauma, 285–313
  appropriate radiographic studies for, 286, *287–293*
  blunt, 297–307, *297*
    changing incidence of, 287
  classification of, 287
  clinical signs of, 285
  due to foreign bodies, 309, *309, 310*
  examinations for associated injuries with, 293, *293–294*
  extrinsic, 287
  iatrogenic, 311, *312*
  in child, 286–287
  inhalation, 307, *307*
  intrinsic, 287
  management of, 311–313
  penetrating, 308–309, *308*
    changing incidence of, 287

Laryngography, in laryngeal trauma, 286, 287–289, 290
Larynx. See also Laryngeal trauma.
  anatomy of, 293–297, 295
Lateral geniculate body, 11
Lateral sulcus, 13
Lateral ventricle(s), 13, 17, 18
  normal computed tomographic appearance of, 6
Lateral view, flexion and extension, in cervical spine evaluation, 183
  in cervical spine evaluation, 179, 180, 181, 182
  in facial trauma evaluation, 95, 96, 97, 99
  in lower cervical spine trauma, 214–217
  in upper cervical spine trauma, 181, 182, 189–190
Le Fort fracture(s), 117–119, 117–120
  appropriate radiographic studies for, 97
Lee's X, 192–194
Left-to-right shunt, with cardiac trauma, 371, 372
Lens injury, 153, 162–164, 163, 164
  appropriate radiographic studies for, 127
Ligamentum(a) flavum(a), 170
Limbic lobe, 16
Liver. See also Liver trauma.
  contusions of, 388, 388
  herniation of, with diaphragmatic rupture, 342, 347, 348
  laceration of, 383, 384, 388, 389
  subcapsular hematoma of, 388, 388, 391
Liver trauma, 384–392
  angiography in, 389–391, 390
    therapeutic applications of, 391, 391
  computed tomography in, 384–389, 388, 389
  in child, 528, 529, 530
  plain film radiography in, 384
  scintigraphy in, 391–392
  ultrasound in, 392
Longitudinal cerebral fissure, 13
Longitudinal fasciculus, medial, 7
Longitudinal ligament(s), anterior, 170
  posterior, 170
Lordotic dens, 182, 190
Lumbar spine trauma. See Thoracolumbar spine trauma.
Lung(s), cavitary lesion of, 324
  contusion of, 316–318, 317–322
  hematoma of, 319–325, 321–325
  laceration of, 318–325, 319–321, 324–325
  trauma to, 316–325
    appropriate radiographic studies for, 316
Lung cyst, traumatic, 324
Lung torsion, 325
Luschka, uncovertebral joint of, 213

Mach line(s), from oropharyngeal space, 105, 110
Magnetic resonance imaging (MRI), in abdominal trauma, 378
  in blow-out fracture of orbital floor, 124, 131–135, 133, 134
  in cervical spine trauma, 180
    for soft tissue evaluation, 187
  in deceleration injuries of the aorta, 452
  in esophageal trauma, 356, 369

Magnetic resonance imaging (MRI) (Continued)
  in head injury, 4, 18, 19, 22–23, 25–27, 42
  in laryngeal trauma, 286, 289–293
  in orbital fracture, 124
  in soft tissue injury of orbit, 126, 127
  in spinal cord injury, 252, 260–261
  in spinal trauma, 175–176
    contraindications to, 175
  in suspected child abuse, 520, 526
  in thoracolumbar spine trauma, 266, 267–268, 269, 271–274
    contraindications to, 268t
  of brain, midline and lateral sagittal, 14–15
    T₁-weighted, 8–10
    T₂-weighted, 12
Mallory-Weiss tear(s), 360
Mandible, 105, 105
  injury to, 105–113
    appropriate radiographic studies for, 96–97
    panoramic film of, 105, 107
    plain film evaluation of, 105–110, 106, 107, 109–112
Marfan's syndrome, spontaneous aortic rupture in, 493
Medial geniculate body, 11
Medial longitudinal fasciculus, 7
Medial rectus muscle of eye, entrapment of, with blow-out fracture, 137, 140
Mediastinal hematoma, 482
Medulla, normal magnetic resonance appearance of, 8
Memory, recent, cerebral area for, 16
Meningeal artery, middle, injury to, with skull fracture, 42, 49, 49, 53
Mesenteric vessel(s), deceleration injury to, 504
Mesentery, injury to, 382, 387, 399–400, 400
Midazolam (Versed), for sedation of child, 517
Midbrain, normal appearance of, on computed tomography, 6
  on magnetic resonance imaging, 8, 9, 12
Middle cerebellar peduncle(s), 7
  normal magnetic resonance appearance of, 8
Middle cerebral artery, normal magnetic resonance appearance of, 9
Middle cranial fossa, base of, 77–80
  complex fracture of floor of, 92–93
Middle meningeal artery, injury to, with skull fracture, 42, 49, 49, 53
Midface separation, 117, 119
Midface trauma, 113
  appropriate radiographic studies for, 97
Monro, foramen of, 17, 18
Motor cortex, 13
Motor pathway, 13–15
MRI. See Magnetic resonance imaging (MRI).
Myelography, in spinal cord injury, 260
  in spinal trauma, 176–177
    cervical, 180
    thoracolumbar, 266, 267–268, 270
Myocardial rupture, 371

Naked facet sign, 267, 268
Nasal fracture(s), 101–105, 102–104

Nasal fracture(s) (Continued)
  appropriate radiographic studies for, 96
Nasofrontal duct, fractures involving, 101
Nasogastric tube, esophageal injury due to, 367
  in identification of diaphragmatic laceration, 338–342, 339, 341–343
Nasolacrimal duct, fractures involving, 101
Neck. See also Cervical spine.
  soft tissue trauma in, 285–313
Neural arch of vertebra, 169
  injury to, 232–258
Neurapraxia of the cervical spinal cord, 259
Neurologic trauma. See Brain trauma; Spinal cord, injury to.
Niclerio's sign, 361, 368
Nuchal ligament, 170
Nuclear medicine technique(s). See also Scintigraphy.
  for cerebrospinal fluid leak detection, 87
Nucleus pulposus, 170

Occipital condyle fracture(s), 191–192, 191
Occipital horn, 17
Occipital lobe, 15, 16–17
  normal magnetic resonance appearance of, 9
Occipital vertebra, 188
Occipitoaxial joint, 187
Oculomotor nerve (III), 4–7
  in skull base, 78–80, 81
Odontoid process. See Dens.
Olfactory nerve (I), in skull base, 79, 81
Open-mouth view, in cervical spine evaluation, 183, 184, 190–191
Ophthalmoplegia, internuclear, 7
Optic nerve(s) (II), avulsion or hematoma of, 155–159, 159, 160
  in skull base, 78, 79, 81
  injury to, appropriate radiographic studies for, 126
  normal magnetic resonance appearance of, 8
Orbit, 123–165
  appropriate radiographic studies for, 124–127
  foreign bodies in, 147–154, 147–152
  fractures of. See Orbital fracture(s).
  normal computed tomographic appearance of, 145
  penetrating injury of, 147–154, 147–153
    angiography in, 154, 154
    computed tomography in, 151–154, 151–153
    orbital fracture with, 146, 147
  soft tissue of. See Eye(s); Globe(s).
  subperiosteal hematoma of, 159–160, 161
    appropriate radiographic studies for, 127
Orbital fracture(s), 123–147
  apex, 143, 143, 144
    appropriate radiographic studies for, 125
  appropriate radiographic studies for, 124–125
  blow-in, 141
  blow-out, appropriate radiographic studies for, 124–125

Orbital fracture(s) (Continued)
computed tomography in, 124, 125, 128–131, 131–133
indications for surgery with, 135
magnetic resonance imaging in, 124, 131–135, 133, 134
of medial wall, 134, 137, 138–140
of orbital floor, 123–135, 128–137
of orbital roof, 137–141, 141, 142
plain film radiography in, 124, 125, 128, 128–130
with penetrating injury, 146, 147
Orthopedic trauma, in child, 522–525
Os odontoideum, 189
Ossicle(s), traumatic disruption of, 90
Ossification, degenerative, in spine, 214, 215
Osteophyte(s), 214, 215

Pancreatic injury, 397–399, 398
Panorex view, for mandibular injury, 105, 107
Papain, for meat impacted in esophagus, 365
Parahippocampal gyrus, 16
Paranasal sinus(es), injury to, 101–105, 104
appropriate radiographic studies for, 96
opacification of, with skull base fracture, 83–84
Paraspinal hematoma, 171
Parietal lobe, 15–16, 15
Parieto-occipital center, 16
Pars interarticularis of vertebra, 169
Pedicle fracture, of lower cervical spine, 225, 227, 253, 254–255
Pelvic fracture(s), bladder trauma and, 432, 432, 434
transcatheter intervention for hemorrhage with, 456, 457, 473–474, 474
Pelvic hematoma, bladder imaging in presence of, 434–436, 435, 436
Penile clamp(s), in retrograde urethrography, 437
Penile injury, 438–445, 444
appropriate radiographic studies for, 409
Peritoneal lavage, diagnostic (DPL), in pediatric abdominal trauma, 525–527
Petrous bone fracture, 86, 90–91, 92–93
Pillar fracture(s), 205, 239, 245–252
Pineal gland, 11
normal computed tomographic appearance of, 6
Piston fragment, with burst fracture of vertebra, 218, 219, 219–220
Piston stenosis, 217
Pituitary gland, normal magnetic resonance appearance of, 8, 14
Pituitary stalk, normal magnetic resonance appearance of, 9
Plain film radiography, in abdominal trauma, 377, 378
findings on, 379–382, 380–381
in blow-out fracture, 124, 125, 128, 128–130
in bowel injury, 399, 399, 400
in deceleration injuries of the aorta, 452, 480–482, 482t, 483–487
in esophageal trauma, 356, 368
in facial trauma, 96–97

Plain film radiography (Continued)
in head injury, 4, 22, 41, 42, 49
in laryngeal trauma, 286, 287, 288, 289
in liver trauma, 384
in orbital fracture, 124, 125
in pancreatic injury, 397
in pulmonary trauma, 316
in skull base trauma, 78, 83–84, 84–85
in soft tissue injury of orbit, 126
in spinal trauma, 173–174
cervical, projections for, 179–183, 181, 182, 184
thoracolumbar, 265–267, 267, 267t
in splenic trauma, 392
in tripod fracture, 125
with portable equipment, in laryngeal trauma, 288
in thoracic trauma, 315–316, 325
Pleura, trauma to, 325–332
appropriate radiographic studies for, 316
computed tomography in, 331–332, 332–335
Pleural effusion, 331, 331
computed tomography in detection of, 331–332, 333
Plummer-Vinson syndrome, drug-induced esophageal injury and, 367
Pneumatocele(s), 324
Pneumocephalus, with skull base fracture, 82, 84
Pneumomediastinum, 335–336, 336, 337
Pneumoperitoneum, 380, 382–384, 387
Pneumothorax, 323, 325–330, 326
anteromedial, 325–327, 327, 328, 330
computed tomography in detection of, 331, 332
subpulmonic, 327, 329, 330
tension, 328, 330
with tracheobronchial injury, 336, 337, 338
Polytomography, hypocycloidal, in spinal trauma, 174
in blow-out fracture of orbital floor, 124, 128
in facial trauma, 97
in orbital fractures, 124, 125
Pons, normal computed tomographic appearance of, 5
Ponticulus posticus, 188, 198, 200
Postcentral gyrus, 15, 16
Posterior cranial fossa, base of, 81
epidural hematoma in, in child, 518
extra-axial hematoma in, 73–75, 75
Posterior ligament avulsion, without fracture, due to seat belt injury, 275
Posterior longitudinal ligament, 170
Posterior spinal artery(ies), 171
Posterolateral spinal artery(ies), 171
Postural disimpaction, for esophageal foreign body, 365
Precentral gyrus, 13, 15
Precentral motor area, 13
Pregnant uterus, 402–404
Prevertebral fat stripe, 187
Prevertebral hematoma, 171
Prevertebral soft tissue swelling, evaluation of, 183–187, 185t, 186t
Proptosis, 162
appropriate radiographic studies for, 127
Pseudoaneurysm(s), chronic, with traumatic rupture of the aorta, 478, 480–481

Pseudoaneurysm(s) (Continued)
hepatic, 390
angiographic treatment of, 391
renal, 420, 424–426
with peripheral arterial injury, 454–459, 454, 455, 458–464, 475
transcatheter intervention for, 476–479
with traumatic rupture of the aorta, aortographic findings with, 483, 483, 484, 486–491, 494, 495, 497
plain film radiographic findings with, 482, 483–487
Pseudocyst(s), pancreatic, after injury, 397
traumatic lung, 324
Pseudomeningocele, cervical, 261
thoracolumbar, 269, 270
Pulmonary interstitial emphysema, pneumomediastinum due to, 336
Putamen, 11, 13
normal computed tomographic appearance of, 6
Pyelography, antegrade, in ureteric injury, 429, 430
intravenous, indications for, in child, 531
retrograde, in ureteric injury, 408, 429–430, 431
Pyramidal fracture, 117–119, 117–120
Pyramidal tract(s), 7
Pyriform sinus(es), 296

Quadrigeminal plate, normal appearance of, on computed tomography, 6
on magnetic resonance imaging, 14

Radiation, esophageal injury due to, 367–368
fetal exposure to, with maternal pelvic injury, 404
Radiography, plain film. See Plain film radiography.
Radionuclide imaging. See Scintigraphy.
Rectus muscle of eye, inferior, entrapment of, with blow-out fracture, 131, 133, 135, 135–137
medial, entrapment of, with blow-out fracture, 137, 140
Recurrent laryngeal nerve, 296
Renal artery(ies), deceleration injury to, 504, 511
intimal injury to, 420, 427–428
occlusion of, angiographic findings with, 420, 421–423
intravenous urography findings with, 411, 411
Renal fracture(s), defined, 529
Renal trauma, 407–432
appropriate radiographic studies for, 408
computed tomography in, 408, 414, 415–417, 417–419
in child, 529–531
intravenous urography in, 407–415, 410–416
renal angiography in, 408, 419–420, 421–428
therapeutic applications of, 420–428, 425–426, 474, 479
ultrasound in, 428

Renal trauma (*Continued*)
    vascular, with deceleration injury, 504, *511–513*
Retinal detachment, 165
Retrobulbar hematoma, 159
Retropharyngeal abscess, with esophageal perforation, *357*
Retropharyngeal soft tissue thickness, measurement of, 183–187
    normal values for, in adult, 185t
        in child, 186t
Retrotracheal soft tissue thickness, measurement of, 183–187
    normal values for, in child, 186t
Reversal sign, 520
Rib fracture(s), *326*, 342–346
    hepatic trauma with, 384
    in child, 522
    tracheobronchial injury and, 336
Ring apophysis(es), *181*, 214
Rotary fixation, atlantoaxial, 203–204
Rotation, of upper cervical spine, assessment of, 190–191

Sacral fracture(s), 277, *280*
Sagittal fracture, 220–227, *228, 229*
    defined, 217–218
Sagittal sinus thrombosis, *28–29*
Scintigraphy, in abdominal trauma, 378
    in esophageal trauma, 356
    in extra-axial fluid collections, 49
    in hepatic trauma, 391–392
    in renal trauma, 428
    in splenic trauma, 397
    in testicular injury, 445
Scrotal injury, 445–447
    appropriate radiographic studies for, 409
Seat belt injury(ies), to thoracolumbar spine, 275–277, *278*
Sedation, for imaging child, 517
Sensory cortex, 16
Septum pellucidum, *13*
Shearing, axonal, 22, *25*
Shearing stenosis, 217
Short tau inversion recovery (STIR) sequences, in orbital evaluation, 131
    in spinal trauma, 176
Skin fold(s), mistaken for pneumothorax, 327–330, *331*
Skull base. See also *Skull base trauma.*
    anatomy of, 77–81, *79, 81*
    fractures of, computed tomography of, *80,* 84–87, *86*
        involving clivus, *82–83, 86*
        plain film radiography of, 83–84, *84–85*
        radiologic management of, 81–83
Skull base trauma, 77–93
    angiography in, 78, 87, *88–91*
    appropriate radiographic studies for, 78
    computed tomography in, 78, 84–87, *86*
    plain film radiography in, 78, 83–84, *84–85*
    radiologic management of, 81–87
Skull fracture(s), 41–48
    appropriate radiographic studies for, 42
    depressed, 42–48, *46–48*
    in child abuse, 520
    linear, 41–42, *43–45*
Skull series, in head injury assessment, 4, 22, 41, 42, 49

Smith fracture, 275–277, *278*
Spinal accessory nerve (XI), 4
    in skull base, 81
Spinal artery(ies), 171
Spinal canal, contents of, 170–171
    normal diameter of, 214
Spinal cord, arterial supply to, 171
    avulsion of, 281, *281*
    cervical, neurapraxia of, 259
    compression of, 272
    imaging of, 260–261
    injury to, 259–261
        causes of, 171–172
        clinical syndromes of, 259–260
        pathology of, 260
    level of, 170–171
    organization of, 170
    transverse attachments of, 170
Spinal cord cyst(s), post-traumatic, 268, *274*
Spinal nerve root(s), cervical, injury to, 261
    numbering of, 171
    post-traumatic avulsion of, *270*
Spinal stenosis, 214–216
    piston, 217
    shearing, 217
Spinal trauma. See also *Cervical spine trauma; Thoracolumbar spine trauma.*
    characterization of, 171–173
    computed tomography in, 174–175
    designation of level of, 171
    geometric tomography in, 174
    magnetic resonance imaging in, 175–176
    myelography in, 176–177
    plain film radiography in, 173–174
    principles of imaging of, 173–177
    radiographic signs of, 173
    types of, 171–172
    vascular imaging in, 177
Spine, 167–281. See also *Cervical spine; Spinal trauma.*
    anatomy of, 169–171
    arterial supply to, 171
    clinical stability of, defined, 172
    indications for imaging of, 173
    motion segments of, 170
    normal motions of, 172
Spinolaminar line(s), *181,* 216–217
    of axis, 190
Spinous process, 169
    fracture of, in lower cervical spine, 253, *255–257*
Spleen, contusion of, *382, 394, 395*
    developmental variations of, 394–396, *396*
    herniation of, with diaphragmatic rupture, *511*
    laceration of, *383, 384,* 392–394, *394*
        in child, 527
    subcapsular hematoma of, 394, *395*
    trauma to, 392–397, *393–396*
        angiography in, 396–397
        in child, 525, *527*
        treatment of, 396, 397
Splenium of corpus callosum, normal magnetic resonance appearance of, *10*
Spondylolisthesis, 189
Sprain, of lower cervical spine, hyperextension, 231
    hyperflexion, 232, *232, 233*
Squamous cell carcinoma, esophageal, after caustic ingestion, 366, *367*
Stability, spinal, defined, 172

Sternal fracture(s), 346–351
STIR sequences, in orbital evaluation, 131
    in spinal trauma, 176
Stomach, herniation of, with diaphragmatic rupture, 338–342, *339–343, 345–346*
Strangulation injury, in child, 520, *522, 523*
Streak artifact(s), on computed tomography, due to bullet fragment, *151*
    due to radiodense objects, 415, *417*
    vitreous hemorrhage vs., 160, *162*
Stretch injury, to carotid artery, 20, *21*
    to optic nerve, 159
Subarachnoid hemorrhage, in child, 518, *518, 519*
    subdural hematoma vs., 64, 67
    traumatic, aneurysmal hemorrhage vs., 20
    vasospasm due to, 37
Subchoroidal hemorrhage, 152, *153*
Subclavian artery(ies), aberrant, aortic tear vs., *498*
    deceleration injury to, *510*
Subclavian steal, traumatic, 510
Subconjunctival hemorrhage, 160–162, *163*
    appropriate radiographic studies of, 127
Subdural effusion(s), subdural hematoma vs., 59
Subdural hematoma, 59–73
    acute, 62–72
        bilateral, 64, *66*
        conservative treatment of, 62–64, *65*
        epidemiology of, 59
        mortality due to, 59, 62
        parenchymal injury with, 62, *63–64*
    angiography of, 49, *50–51*
    chronic, 69, 72–73
        epidemiology of, 59
    clinicopathology of, 59–62, *60–62*
    hypodense, 67, *69*
    imaging of, 25–27
    in child, 517–518, *518*
        due to abuse, 520, *521–525*
    interhemispheric fissure, *61–62,* 64–67
    isodense, 67–72, *68, 71–73*
    layering in, *66,* 67, *70,* 73
    magnetic resonance imaging of, 72, *74*
    of posterior fossa, 75
    radiographic studies of, 48–49
Subdural hygroma, subdural hematoma vs., 59–62
Subluxation. See also *Dislocation(s).*
    anterior, of lower cervical spine, 232, *232, 233*
    atlantoaxial, 203
Submentovertex view, for facial trauma evaluation, 95, 96, 97, *100*
Subperiosteal hematoma of orbit, 159–160, *161*
    appropriate radiographic studies for, 127
Substantia nigra, 11
Superior cerebellar peduncle, 7
Superior laryngeal nerve, 296
Superior temporal gyrus, 16
Supplementary motor area, 13
Supraspinous ligament, 170
Swimmer's view, in cervical spine evaluation, 179–180, *182*
Sylvian aqueduct, normal magnetic resonance appearance of, *9, 14*

Sylvian fissure, normal appearance of, on computed tomography, 6
  on magnetic resonance imaging, 9
Sylvian triangle, 17

TAR (titratable acid/alkaline reserve), potential for esophageal injury and, 366
Targeting, in computed tomography, 86
Teardrop fracture, extension (ETF), 213, 230, 230
  flexion, 221–228, 221–227
  defined, 217–218
Temporal gyrus, superior, 16
Temporal horn, 17
Temporal lobe, 15, 16
  normal appearance of, on computed tomography, 5
  on magnetic resonance imaging, 9
Temporomandibular joint(s), injury to, with mandibular injury, 105, 108, 110, 112
  radiographic evaluation of, 105
Tentorium, normal computed tomographic appearance of, 6
Testicular injury, 444, 445–447, 445, 446
  appropriate radiographic studies for, 409
Tetrad of Gott, 360–361
Thalamus, 11
  normal appearance of, on computed tomography, 6
  on magnetic resonance imaging, 9, 14
Thermal injury, esophageal, 366
Third ventricle, 17, 18
  normal appearance of, on computed tomography, 6
  on magnetic resonance imaging, 9
Thoracolumbar spine fracture(s), 265, 267–268, 271–273
  classification of, 274, 275
  hepatic trauma with, 267, 277, 384
  thoracic injury with, 346, 349, 350
Thoracolumbar spine trauma, 265–281. See also Thoracolumbar spine fracture(s).
  appropriate radiographic studies for, 266
  clinical findings with, 277–281
  mechanisms of, 275–277
  myelography in, 266, 267–268, 270
  penetrating, 281
  radiologic evaluation of, 265–268, 267t
Thorax, trauma to, 315–351
  appropriate radiographic studies for, 316
  causes of, 315
  computed tomography in, 331–332, 332–335
  in child, 520–522
  portable chest film in detection of, 315–316, 325
Three column classification of spinal fractures, 274, 275
Thrombosis, venous sinus, 23, 28–29
Thyroarytenoid ligament(s). See Vocal cord(s).
Thyrohyoid membrane, 293, 295
Thyroid cartilage, 293, 295
  fracture of, 297, 297–302
Titratable acid/alkaline reserve (TAR), potential for esophageal injury and, 366

Tomography. See also Polytomography.
  geometric, in spinal trauma, 174, 180
  in laryngeal trauma, 286
  in thoracolumbar spine trauma, 266
TRA. See Aorta, traumatic rupture of (TRA).
Tracheobronchial injury, 332–336, 336–338
  appropriate radiographic studies for, 316
  esophageal injury with, 359–360
Transcatheter embolization. See under Embolization.
Translational injury, 277, 279
Transoral odontoid view, 183, 184, 190–191
Transtentorial herniation, 31–34, 35–36
Transverse cerebral fissure, 13
Transverse foramen(ina) of vertebra(e), 169
Transverse process(es), 169
  fracture of, of atlas, 203
    of axis, 210–211, 213
    of lower cervical spine, 214, 225, 227, 258
Trigeminal nerve (V), 4
  in skull base, 78–80, 81
Tripod fracture, 113–117, 115–116, 141, 142
  appropriate radiographic studies for, 125
Trochlear nerve (IV), 4–7
  in skull base, 78–80, 81

UFD (unilateral facet dislocation), 223–225, 234–239, 234, 235
Ultrasound, for foreign body localization in orbit, 149–151
  in abdominal trauma, 378, 379
    findings on, 382
  in evaluation of pregnant uterus, 404
  in liver trauma, 392
  in pancreatic injury, 397
  in renal trauma, 428
  in splenic trauma, 396
  in testicular injury, 445, 445, 446
    normal findings on, 444, 445
  midline, in head injury assessment, 49
Uncinate process fracture, 231
Uncovertebral joint of Luschka, 213
Ureteric injury, 428–432
  appropriate radiographic studies for, 408
  blunt, 429, 429
  management of, 430–432
  penetrating, 429, 430
Urethral injury, 436–438, 438–443
  appropriate radiographic studies for, 409
Urethrography, retrograde, in urethal injury, 437–438, 439–443
  technique for, 437, 438
Urinary bladder trauma, 432–436
  appropriate radiographic studies for, 408–409
  computed tomography in, 409, 434, 436
  cystography in, 408, 432–434, 432–436
  due to foreign body, 436, 437
Urography, intravenous, in renal trauma, 407–415, 410–416
  in ureteric injury, 408, 429–430, 429, 430
  in urinary bladder trauma, 409
  normal findings on, 410

Uterus, pregnant, 402–404

Vagus nerve (X), 4
  in skull base, 81
Vascular imaging. See also Angiography; Aortography; Venography.
  in spinal trauma, 177
Vascular injury(ies), 451–513. See also Aorta; Arterial injury(ies); Venous injury(ies).
  appropriate radiographic studies for, 452
  types of, 451
Vasodilator(s), response to, in distinction of vasospasm from arterial injury, 470, 472
Vasospasm, arterial injury and, 459–470, 470–472, 471t
  due to subarachnoid hemorrhage, 37
Venography, contrast, 478, 480
Venous injury(ies), 462, 474–478, 480
  appropriate radiographic studies for, 452
Venous sinus thrombosis, 23, 28–29
Ventricular system, 17, 18. See also Fourth ventricle; Lateral ventricle(s); Third ventricle.
Ventricular trigone, normal magnetic resonance appearance of, 9
Versed (midazolam), for sedation of child, 517
Vertebra(e). See also Atlas (C1); Axis (C2); Vertebra prominens (C7).
  anatomy of, 169
  linkages between, 169–170
  occipital, 188
Vertebra prominens (C7), 181, 213, 214
Vertebral artery(ies), 171
  anomalous origin of, aortic tear vs., 498, 501
  assessment of, in cervical spine trauma, 187
  injury to, with cervical spine trauma, 187
    with esophageal injury, 23
    with penetrating neck injury, 22
Vertebral body(ies), 169. See also Vertebral body fracture(s).
Vertebral body fracture(s), 217–231
  burst. See Burst fracture.
  flexion-teardrop, 221–228, 221–227
    defined, 217–218
  margin, 228–231, 249
  sagittal, 220–227, 228, 229
    defined, 217–218
  types of, 217–218
  wedge. See Wedge fracture.
Vertebral column. See Spine.
Vertebral foramen(ina), 169
Vertigo, with petrous bone fracture, 91
Vestibulocochlear nerve (VIII), 4
  in skull base, 81
Visual cortex, 17
Vitreous hemorrhage, 153, 160, 162
  appropriate radiographic studies for, 127
Vocal cord(s), 295, 297
  paralysis of, prognosis with, 313

Waters' view, for facial trauma evaluation, 95, 96, 97, 98

Waters' view *(Continued)*
  stereo, for facial trauma, 113
Watershed area, 24
Wedge fracture, defined, 217–218
  of cervical spine, 218–219, *218*
  of thoracolumbar spine, 275, *275*
Wernicke's area, 16
Whiplash, 258

White matter, buckling of, with isodense
    subdural hematoma, 67, *72*
  normal appearance of, on computed to-
    mography, *7*
  on magnetic resonance imaging, *10,
    12*
  shearing injury to, imaging of, *19*

Zygapophyseal joint(s). See *Facet joint(s).*
Zygoma, 113
  fracture of, 113–117, *114–116*
    appropriate radiographic studies for,
    97